NMS Pediatrics

5th ... N

H. Dworkin, MD
...ssor and Chairman
...artment of Pediatrics
...versity of Connecticut School of Medicine
...mington, Connecticut
...ysician-in-Chief
...necticut Children's Medical Center
...tford, Connecticut

Paula S. Algranati, MD
Professor of Pediatrics
Director of Medical Student Education
Department of Pediatrics
University of Connecticut School of Medicine
Farmington, Connecticut

Wolters Kluwer | Lippincott Williams & Wilkins
Health
Philadelphia • Baltimore • New York • London
Buenos Aires • Hong Kong • Sydney • Tokyo

Senior Managing Editor: Stacey Sebring
Marketing Manager: Jennifer Kuklinski
Managing Editor, Production: Eve Malakoff-Klein
Designer: Holly Reid McLaughlin
Compositor: Aptara
Printer: R.R. Donnelley Shenzhen

Fifth Edition

351 West Camden Street
Baltimore, MD 21201

530 Walnut Street
Philadelphia, PA 19106

Printed in China

9 8 7 6 5 4 3 2 1

Library of Congress Cataloging-in-Publication Data

NMS pediatrics / editors, Paul H. Dworkin, Paula S. Algranati. — 5th ed.
p. ; cm. — (National medical series for independent study)
Rev. ed. of: Pediatrics / editor, Paul H. Dworkin. 4th ed. c2000.
Includes index.
ISBN 978-0-7817-7075-0 (alk. paper)
1. Pediatrics—Outlines, syllabi, etc. 2. Pediatrics—Examinations, questions, etc. I. Dworkin, Paul H. II. Algranati, Paula S. III. Pediatrics. IV. Title: Pediatrics. V. Series.
[DNLM: 1. Pediatrics—Examination Questions. 2. Pediatrics—Outlines. WS 18.2 N738 2009]
RJ48.3.P44 2009
618.920076—dc22

2008024068

DISCLAIMER

Care has been taken to confirm the accuracy of the information present and to describe generally accepted practices. However, the authors, editors, and publisher are not responsible for errors or omissions or for any consequences from application of the information in this book and make no warranty, expressed or implied, with respect to the currency, completeness, or accuracy of the contents of the publication. Application of this information in a particular situation remains the professional responsibility of the practitioner; the clinical treatments described and recommended may not be considered absolute and universal recommendations.

The authors, editors, and publisher have exerted every effort to ensure that drug selection and dosage set forth in this text are in accordance with the current recommendations and practice at the time of publication. However, in view of ongoing research, changes in government regulations, and the constant flow of information relating to drug therapy and drug reactions, the reader is urged to check the package insert for each drug for any change in indications and dosage and for added warnings and precautions. This is particularly important when the recommended agent is a new or infrequently employed drug.

Some drugs and medical devices presented in this publication have Food and Drug Administration (FDA) clearance for limited use in restricted research settings. It is the responsibility of the health care provider to ascertain the FDA status of each drug or device planned for use in their clinical practice.

To purchase additional copies of this book, call our customer service department at **(800) 638-3030** or fax orders to **(301) 223-2320**. International customers should call **(301) 223-2300**.

Visit Lippincott Williams & Wilkins on the Internet: http://www.lww.com. Lippincott Williams & Wilkins customer service representatives are available from 8:30 am to 6:00 pm, EST.

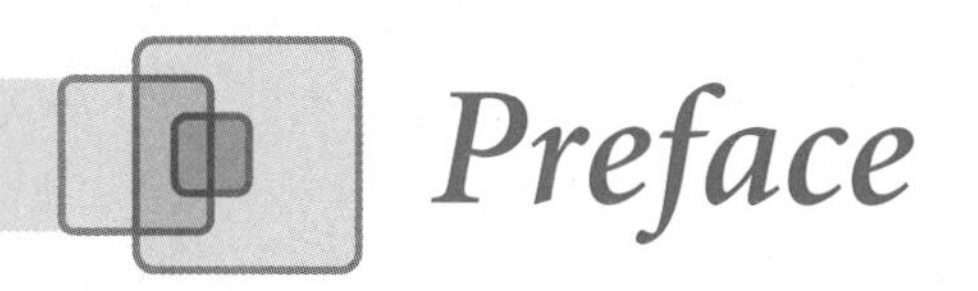

Preface

Casual review of the fifth edition of *NMS Pediatrics* suggests many similarities to prior editions. As with the earlier editions, our goal is to ensure that the text remains useful as an in-depth review of pediatrics for students preparing for the United States Medical Licensing Examination (USMLE)—Step 2, as well as a helpful supplement during pediatric clerkships. We have retained the signature outline format of the NMS series, as well as the characteristic features, including study questions, case studies in clinical decision making, and a comprehensive examination. Chapter content has been updated to include new and current information.

The fifth edition is notable for several important changes. Medical student feedback on both the NMS series and our specific text encouraged us to "streamline" the content to "just tell readers what they need to know." Students encouraged us to shorten the printed text and use online capacity for supplemental materials. They also urged us to commit to a more frequent revision cycle, to ensure that content remains timely and accurate.

The fifth edition of *NMS Pediatrics* benefits from adherence to these recommendations. As with prior editions, all chapters in the text have been thoroughly revised and updated to include new and current information. In response to feedback, however, authors were directed to align their chapters to better reflect medical student knowledge competencies as captured in the 2005 revision of the *General Pediatric Clerkship Curriculum* by the Curriculum and Evaluation Task Forces of the Council on Medical Student Education in Pediatrics (COMSEP), in collaboration with the Medical Student Education Special Interest Group of the Ambulatory Pediatric Association (APA). As a result, the chapters are less dense, less comprehensive, and more focused on the core knowledge expected of medical students by the completion of their pediatric training. In keeping with the electronic format of the USMLE and to shorten the length of the printed text, this new edition places online its supplemental learning materials, including case studies and comprehensive exam questions and annotated answers.

As with prior editions, I am very pleased that current and former faculty members of the Department of Pediatrics of the University of Connecticut School of Medicine serve as the contributing authors to this text. The willingness of our busy faculty to prepare and revise chapters reflects their ongoing commitment to medical education. Selection of new authors for this edition was based on their involvement with and contributions to medical student education in our clerkships.

I am particularly pleased to welcome my friend and colleague, Paula S. Algranati, MD, as coeditor of this text. Dr. Algranati is Professor and Director of Medical Student Education in our Department of Pediatrics of the University of Connecticut School of Medicine. In addition to her leadership of our medical student curriculum and clerkship experiences, Dr. Algranati's extensive involvement with COMSEP, the APA, and the National Board of Medical Examiners (NBME) has proven invaluable to the revision of this text. Her expertise in evaluation informed her meticulous editing of the text's study questions, comprehensive exam, and case studies.

As always, we hope that this text remains useful and relevant for pediatric trainees. We are particularly hopeful that the major revisions of this fifth edition enhance the usefulness of the text for medical students.

Paul H. Dworkin, MD

Contributors

Mary-Alice Abbott, MD, PhD
Assistant Professor of Pediatrics
Tufts University School of Medicine
Boston, Massachusetts
Pediatric Geneticist
Baystate Medical Center
Springfield, Massachusetts

Paula S. Algranati, MD
Professor of Pediatrics
Director of Medical Student Education
Department of Pediatrics
University of Connecticut School of Medicine
Farmington, Connecticut

Frederick J. Bogin, MD
Assistant Professor of Pediatrics
University of Connecticut School of Medicine
Farmington, Connecticut
Director of Pediatric Primary Care Center
Saint Francis Hospital and Medical Center
Hartford, Connecticut

Christopher L. Carroll, MD
Assistant Professor of Pediatrics
University of Connecticut School of Medicine
Farmington, Connecticut
Division of Pediatric Critical Care
Connecticut Children's Medical Center
Hartford, Connecticut

John Casey, MD, CM
Clinical Assistant Professor of Pediatrics
New York University School of Medicine
Division of Neonatology
NYU Langone Medical Center
New York, New York

Zoe Casey, MBBS
Assistant Professor of Pediatrics and Traumatology/Emergency Medicine
University of Connecticut School of Medicine
Farmington, Connecticut
Division of Emergency Medicine
Connecticut Children's Medical Center
Hartford, Connecticut

Leon Chameides, MD
Emeritus Clinical Professor of Pediatrics
University of Connecticut School of Medicine
Farmington, Connecticut
Former Director, Division of Cardiology
Connecticut Children's Medical Center
Hartford, Connecticut

Karen L. Daigle, MD
Department of Pediatrics
The Warren Alpert Medical School of Brown University
Division of Pulmonary Medicine
Hasbro Children's Hospital/Rhode Island Hospital
Providence, Rhode Island

Daniel J. Diana, MD
Clinical Professor of Pediatrics
University of Connecticut School of Medicine
Farmington, Connecticut
Former Director, Division of Cardiology
Connecticut Children's Medical Center
Hartford, Connecticut

Barbara S. Edelheit, MD
Assistant Professor of Pediatrics
University of Connecticut School of Medicine
Farmington, Connecticut
Division of Rheumatology
Connecticut Children's Medical Center
Hartford, Connecticut

Karan Emerick, MD
Associate Professor of Pediatrics
University of Connecticut School of Medicine
Farmington, Connecticut
Division of Digestive Diseases, Hepatology and Nutrition
Connecticut Children's Medical Center
Hartford, Connecticut

Elizabeth D. Estrada, MD
Associate Professor of Pediatrics
University of Connecticut School of Medicine
Farmington, Connecticut
Division of Endocrinology and Diabetes
Connecticut Children's Medical Center
Hartford, Connecticut

Marshall P. Grodofsky, MD
Assistant Clinical Professor of Pediatrics
University of Connecticut School of Medicine
Farmington, Connecticut
Connecticut Allergy and Asthma Center
West Hartford, Connecticut

J. Nathan Hagstrom, MD
Associate Professor of Pediatrics
Head, Division of Hematology/Oncology
University of Connecticut School of Medicine
Farmington, Connecticut
Director, Division of Hematology/Oncology

Connecticut Children's Medical Center
Hartford, Connecticut

Melissa Held, MD
Assistant Professor of Pediatrics
University of Connecticut School of Medicine
Farmington, Connecticut
Divisions of Hospitalist Care and Infectious Diseases
Connecticut Children's Medical Center
Hartford, Connecticut

Felice A. Heller, MD
Assistant Clinical Professor of Pediatrics
University of Connecticut School of Medicine
Farmington, Connecticut
Division of Cardiology
Connecticut Children's Medical Center
Hartford, Connecticut

Hillary Hernandez-Trujillo, MD
Pediatric Residency Training Program
University of Connecticut School of Medicine
Farmington, Connecticut

Michael S. Isakoff, MD
Assistant Professor of Pediatrics
University of Connecticut School of Medicine
Farmington, Connecticut
Division of Hematology/Oncology
Connecticut Children's Medical Center
Hartford, Connecticut

Patricia Joyce, MD
Associate Professor of Pediatrics
University of Connecticut School of Medicine
Farmington, Connecticut
Director, Pediatric Clinic
Burgdorf/Bank of America Health Center
Hartford, Connecticut

Thomas L Kennedy III, MD
Clinical Professor of Pediatrics
Section of Pediatric Nephrology
Yale University School of Medicine
New Haven, Connecticut
Chairman
Department of Pediatrics
Bridgeport Hospital
Bridgeport, Connecticut

Peter J. Krause, MD
Professor of Pediatrics
Head, Division of Infectious Diseases
University of Connecticut School of Medicine
Farmington, Connecticut
Director, Division of Infectious Diseases
Connecticut Children's Medical Center
Hartford, Connecticut

Carol R. Leicher, MD
Associate Professor of Pediatrics and Neurology
University of Connecticut School of Medicine
Farmington, Connecticut
Medical Director of Neurology
Connecticut Children's Medical Center
Hartford, Connecticut

Harris B. Leopold, MD
Associate Clinical Professor of Pediatrics
Head, Division of Cardiology
University of Connecticut School of Medicine
Farmington, Connecticut
Director, Division of Cardiology
Connecticut Children's Medical Center
Hartford, Connecticut

Ted S. Rosenkrantz, MD
Professor of Pediatrics
University of Connecticut School of Medicine
Division of Neonatal and Perinatal Medicine
University of Connecticut Health Center
Farmington, Connecticut

Aric Schichor, MD
Associate Professor of Pediatrics
Head, Division of Adolescent Medicine
University of Connecticut School of Medicine
Farmington, Connecticut
Director, Section on Adolescent Medicine
Saint Francis Hospital and Medical Center
Hartford, Connecticut

Francisco Sylvester, MD
Associate Professor of Pediatrics
University of Connecticut School of Medicine
Farmington, Connecticut
Division of Digestive Diseases, Hepatology and Nutrition
Connecticut Children's Medical Center
Hartford, Connecticut

Catherine C. Wiley, MD
Associate Professor of Pediatrics
University of Connecticut School of Medicine
Farmington, Connecticut
Division of General Pediatrics
Connecticut Children's Medical Center
Hartford, Connecticut

James F. Wiley II, MD, MPH
Professor of Pediatrics and Traumatology/Emergency Medicine
University of Connecticut School of Medicine
Farmington, Connecticut
Division of Emergency Medicine
Connecticut Children's Medical Center
Hartford, Connecticut

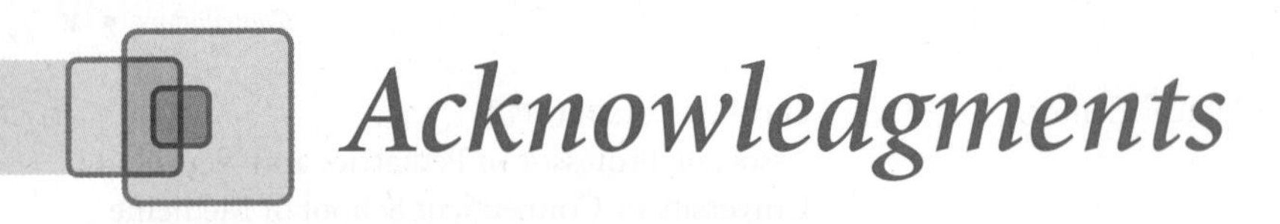

Acknowledgments

The editors and contributing authors thank Donna M. Balado, Senior Acquisitions Editor at Lippincott Williams & Wilkins, for sharing the findings from medical student focus group discussions on the NMS texts and for providing feedback from student reviews of the fourth edition of *NMS Pediatrics.* Stacey Sebring, Senior Managing Editor, and Oakley Julian, Editorial Assistant at Lippincott Williams & Wilkins, provided valuable oversight and support throughout the preparation of this text.

The most recent revision of the *General Pediatric Clerkship Curriculum* of the Council on Medical Student Education in Pediatrics (COMSEP) and the Ambulatory Pediatric Association (APA) greatly informed the content of this edition. We wish to acknowledge William Raszka, MD, chair of the COMSEP Curriculum Task Force; Paula Algranati, MD, and Lindsey Lane, MD, cochairs of the COMSEP Evaluation Task Force; Bill Raszka, MD, and Lindsey Lane, MD, cochairs of the APA Medical Student Education SIG; and the late Steve Miller, MD, past-president of COMSEP, for the their leadership in curriculum reform.

We are also grateful to Esperanza Lesmes for her impeccable administrative assistance in the preparation of this fifth edition.

Paul H. Dworkin, MD
Paula S. Algranati, MD

Contents

chapter **1**

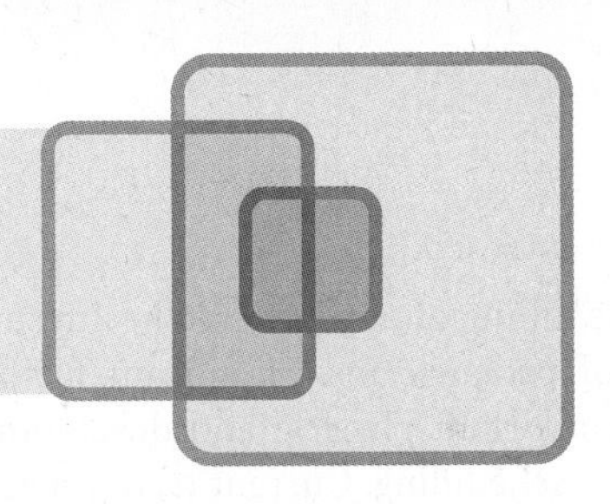

Child Health Supervision

CATHERINE WILEY • PAULA S. ALGRANATI

I GOAL AND SCOPE OF PEDIATRIC PRACTICE

The goal of child health supervision is promotion of optimal growth and development of children. A long-term partnership between the clinician and patient and family provides the vehicle for meeting this challenge. Ambulatory practice time is typically divided as follows:

A **Child health supervision** (i.e., well-child "check-ups") accounts for approximately 50% of practice time.

B **Infectious diseases** represent a major proportion of practice time devoted to "problem" visits, and the most common problems are upper respiratory tract illness, otitis media, and gastroenteritis.

C **Other disorders** that account for the remainder of practice time include injuries, skin disorders, asthma and allergies, and behavioral and developmental concerns.

D **Recent trends** As time spent caring for hospitalized children diminishes, areas that are receiving increased attention from pediatricians include asthma and allergies, obesity, effects of environmental pollutants such as lead, school functioning, child behavior, substance abuse, family functioning, and child health supervision.

E **Clinical disorders commonly encountered within the office setting** In this chapter, we will address some of the more common concerns that are raised within the context of child health supervision. Examples of such topics include:

1. **Newborn** (see Chapter 6): Jaundice, birthmarks, and developmental dysplasia of the hip *(see III C 7)*
2. **Early infancy:** Diaper rash (*see III F 4*) and colic (*see III F 5*)
3. **Late infancy:** Intoeing (*see IV C 5 a*), temper tantrums (*see IV F 1*), and night crying (*see IV F 2, V F 3*)
4. **Preschool age:** Innocent heart murmurs (*see V C 5*) and stuttering (*see V F 4*)
5. **School age:** Recurrent pains (*see VI F 3*; Chapter 4) and poor school performance (*see VI F 4*; Chapter 4)
6. **Adolescence:** Puberty (*see VII* and Chapter 5)

II HEALTH SUPERVISION VISITS

A **Goals** Priority is given to parents' agendas, and an emphasis is placed on longitudinal surveillance and screening at targeted ages.

1. Assess the child's current biopsychosocial functioning.
2. Address parents' concerns.
3. Identify, diagnose, and manage current problems.
4. Prevent or diminish future problems.
5. Provide support and encouragement to families and children.

B Schedule and content

1. Recommendations for the timing of routine child health supervision visits have evolved through consensus on the part of pediatricians. Significant factors include immunization schedules (Figure 1-1), timing of important physical and developmental issues, and pediatricians' own perceptions of appropriate scheduling. Current recommendations for routine visits include:
   a. **Newborn/early infancy:** By 5 days of age (within 48 hours for infants discharged < 48 hours after delivery); 2 to 4 weeks; 2, 4, and 6 months
   b. **Late infancy:** 9, 12, 15, 18, 24, and 30 months
   c. **Preschool:** 3, 4, and 5 years
   d. **School age:** 6, 8, 10, 11, and 12 years
   e. **Adolescent:** Yearly beginning at 13 years of age
2. Recommendations for the **content** of visits have also evolved through pediatrician consensus. Significant contributing factors include immunization schedules, evidence for the efficacy of certain procedures and screening tests, expectations of parents and patients, and pediatricians' own experience with delivering well-child care. Specific recommendations are discussed within each age-related section of this chapter (*see also II F*).

C History seeks to determine the child's current functioning in biopsychosocial spheres. Parents' overall assessment of their child's functioning is solicited, in addition to specific information. Parents and children are encouraged to ask questions, discuss concerns, and guide the agenda for the visit. Initial visits include a comprehensive review of medical history, family health history, and family psychosocial history. Interval visits require an update in each of these areas. Over time, the interview is directed increasingly toward the child, commensurate with communication and interpersonal abilities.

D Physical examination A complete physical examination is performed at each visit. Particular areas receive emphasis, depending on the age of the child. Priority is given to systems undergoing rapid change (e.g., head growth in the infant, pubertal manifestations in the adolescent), areas with a high incidence of pathology (e.g., tympanic membranes in the toddler), and areas most responsive to early intervention (e.g., hearing and vision deficits in the infant).

1. Examination **sequence** is determined by the child's age and developmental stage, state of health, previous experiences, and individual temperament.
2. Measurements should ideally be obtained and plotted on the appropriate growth charts at the onset of the visit, so that problems can be pursued via relevant history and physical examination (see Chapter 4). Current measurements are compared to age-related norms, as well as to the child's own previous values.

E Developmental monitoring is performed during each well-child visit through a combination of history, observation, and screening at targeted ages. Monitoring occurs within the context of longitudinal surveillance, including:

1. **History** that elicits parents' assessment of their child's developmental progress, explores concerns, and reviews specific, relevant developmental milestones. A reliable question is, "Do you have any concerns about your child's learning, behavior, or development?"
2. **Observations** during the history and physical examination to confirm developmental history and reveal actual levels of functioning. The pediatrician may encourage the child to demonstrate a specific skill (e.g., by holding out a small object to elicit a pincer grasp or by placing the toddler on his or her feet to observe gait).
3. **Screening.** The American Academy of Pediatrics (AAP) recommends developmental screening with a standardized instrument, minimally at ages 9, 18, and 30 months (24 months when 30-month visits are not routine), and more frequently for children at increased risk of developmental problems. A variety of tools may be used, including parent questionnaires and clinician-administered screening instruments (e.g., **Denver II**) (Figure 1-2).
   a. The well-recognized limitations of such tools must be considered when interpreting results. Whenever possible, efforts should be made to compare findings with the opinions of the child's parents, day care provider, preschool or school teacher, social worker, or public health

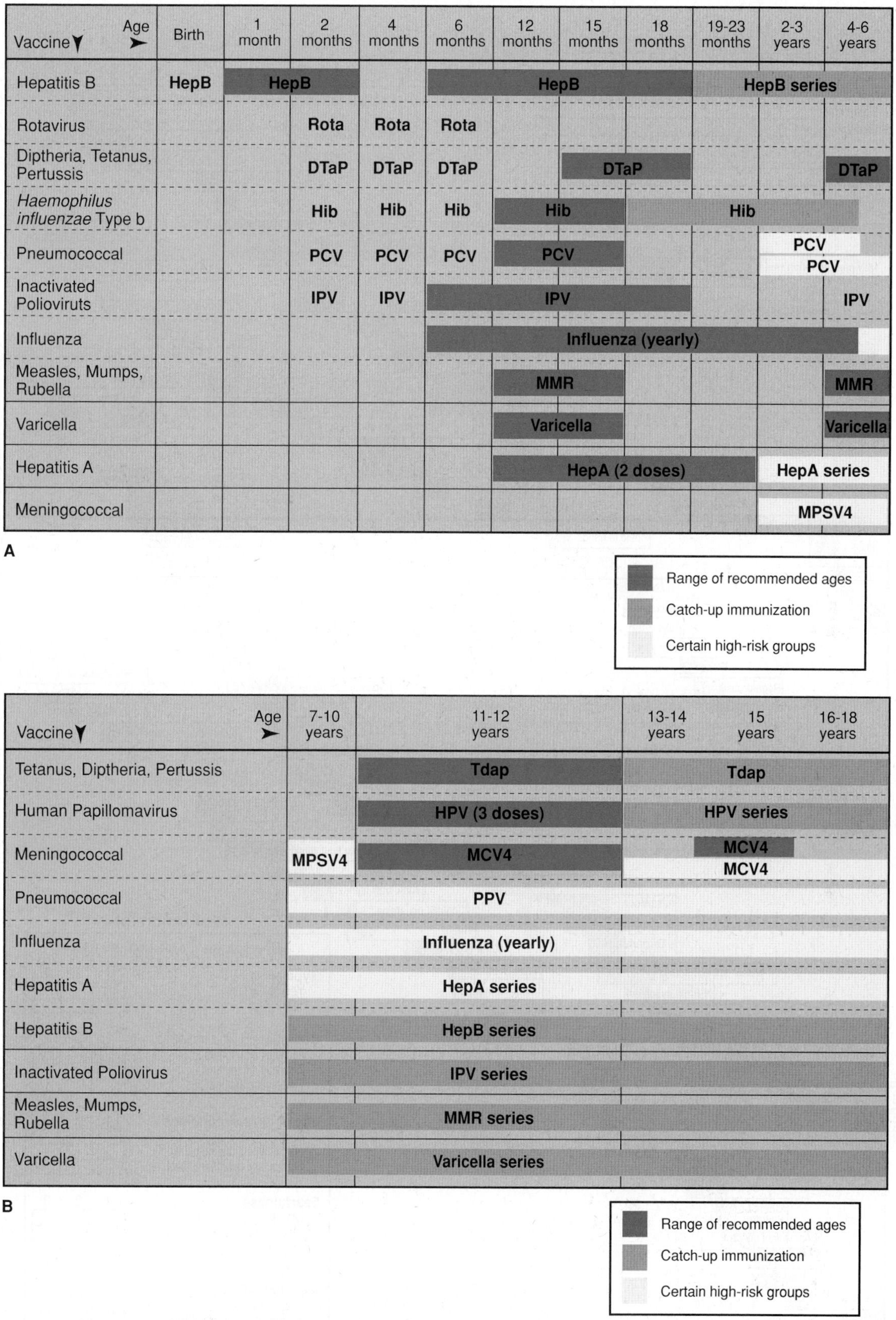

Vaccine ▼ / Age ►	Birth	1 month	2 months	4 months	6 months	12 months	15 months	18 months	19-23 months	2-3 years	4-6 years
Hepatitis B	HepB	HepB				HepB				HepB series	
Rotavirus			Rota	Rota	Rota						
Diptheria, Tetanus, Pertussis			DTaP	DTaP	DTaP		DTaP				DTaP
Haemophilus influenzae Type b			Hib	Hib	Hib	Hib			Hib		
Pneumococcal			PCV	PCV	PCV	PCV				PCV	PCV
Inactivated Poliovirus			IPV	IPV		IPV					IPV
Influenza								Influenza (yearly)			
Measles, Mumps, Rubella						MMR					MMR
Varicella						Varicella					Varicella
Hepatitis A							HepA (2 doses)			HepA series	
Meningococcal										MPSV4	

A

Range of recommended ages

Catch-up immunization

Certain high-risk groups

Vaccine ▼ / Age ►	7-10 years	11-12 years	13-14 years	15 years	16-18 years
Tetanus, Diptheria, Pertussis		Tdap		Tdap	
Human Papillomavirus		HPV (3 doses)		HPV series	
Meningococcal	MPSV4	MCV4		MCV4 MCV4	
Pneumococcal		PPV			
Influenza		Influenza (yearly)			
Hepatitis A		HepA series			
Hepatitis B		HepB series			
Inactivated Poliovirus		IPV series			
Measles, Mumps, Rubella		MMR series			
Varicella		Varicella series			

B

Range of recommended ages

Catch-up immunization

Certain high-risk groups

FIGURE 1-1 Vaccines are listed under routinely recommended ages. Bars indicate range of recommended ages for immunization. Any dose not given at the recommended age should be given as a "catch-up" immunization at any subsequent visit when indicated and feasible. DTaP, diphtheria-tetanus-acellular pertussis vaccine; Hep A, hepatitis A vaccine; Hep B, hepatitis B vaccine; Hib, *Haemophilus influenzae* type b vaccine; IPV, inactivated poliomyelitis vaccine; MCV4, meningococcal conjugate vaccine; MMR, measles, mumps, and rubella vaccine; MPSV, meningococcal polysacchiaride vaccine; PCV, pneumococcal conjugate vaccine; Rota, rotavirus vaccine. (Adapted from Recommended Immunization Schedules for Persons 0–18 years—United States, 2007. *MMWR* 55:Q1–Q4, 2007. Approved by the Advisory Committee on Immunization Practices [ACIP], the American Academy of Pediatrics [AAP], and the American Academy of Family Physicians [AAFP]. Consult full recommendations for updates and specific details.)

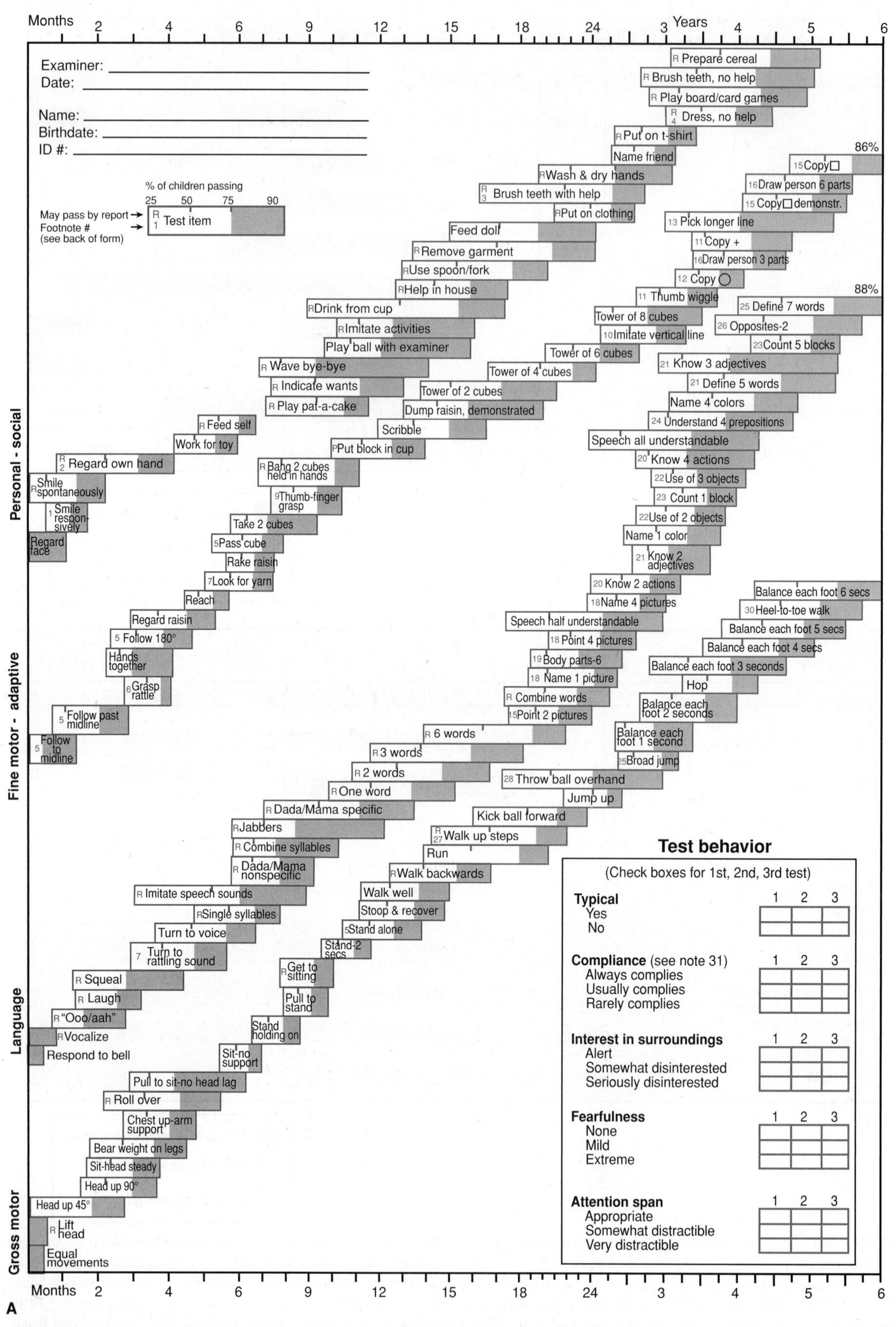

FIGURE 1-2 Denver II. (Reprinted with permission from Frankenburg WK, Dodds J, Archer P, et al.: The Denver II: a major revision and restandardization of the Denver Developmental Screening Test. *Pediatrics* 89:93, 1992.) (*continued*)

Directions for administration

1. Try to get child to smile by smiling, talking, or waving. Do not touch him/her.
2. Child must stare at hand several seconds.
3. Parent may help guide toothbrush and put toothpaste on brush.
4. Child does not have to be able to tie shoes or button/zip in the back.
5. Move yarn slowly in arc from one side to the other, about 8" above child's face.
6. Pass if child grasps rattle when it is touched to the backs or tips of fingers.
7. Pass if child tries to see where the yarn went. Yarn should be dropped quickly from sight from tester's hand without arm movement.
8. Child must transfer cube from hand to hand without help of body, mouth, or table.
9. Pass if child picks up raisin with any part of thumb or finger.
10. Line can vary only 30 degrees or less from tester's line.
11. Make a fist with thumb pointing upward and wiggle only the thumb. Pass if child imitates and does not move any fingers other than the thumb.

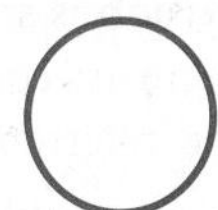

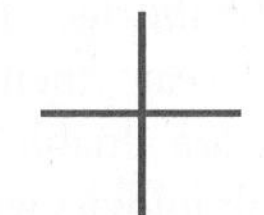

12. Pass any enclosed form. Fail continuous round motions.
13. Which line is longer? (Not bigger.) Turn paper upside down and repeat. (pass 3 of 3 or 5 of 6)
14. Pass any lines crossing near midpoint.
15. Have child copy first. If failed, demonstrate.
16. When scoring, each pair (2 arms, 2 legs, etc.) counts as one part.
17. Place one cube in cup and shake gently near child's ear, but out of sight. Repeat for other ear.
18. Point to picture and have child name it. (No credit given for sounds only.)

If less than 4 pictures are named correctly, have child point to picture as each is named by tester.

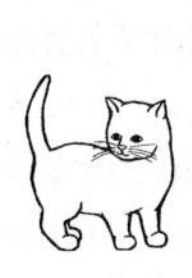
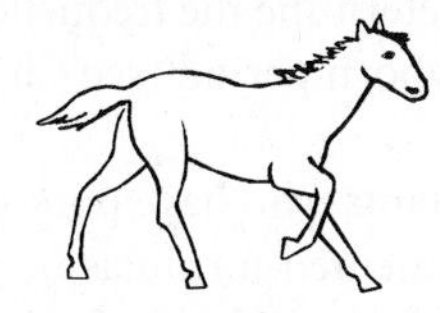
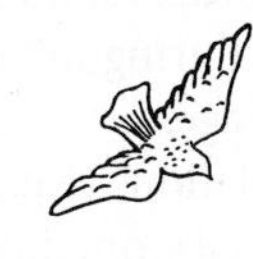
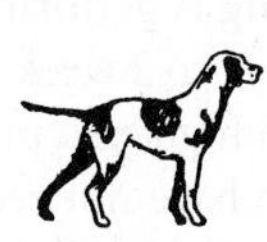
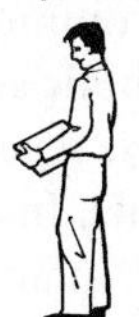

19. Using doll, tell child: Show me the nose, eyes, ears, mouth, hands, feet, tummy, hair. (Pass 6 of 8)
20. Using pictures, ask child: Which one flies?... says meow?... talks?... barks?... gallops? (Pass 2 of 5, 4 of 5)
21. Ask child: What do you do when you are cold?... tired?... hungry? (Pass 2 of 3, 3 of 3)
22. Ask child: What do you do with a cup?... What is a chair used for?... What is a pencil used for? Action words must be included in answers.
23. Pass if child correctly places and says how many blocks are on paper. (1, 5)
24. Tell child: Put block **on** table, **under** table, **in front of** me, **behind** me. (Pass 4 of 4) (Do not help child by pointing, moving head or eyes.)
25. Ask child: What is a boat?... lake?... desk?... house?... banana?... curtain?... fence?... ceiling? Pass if defined in terms of use, shape, what it is made of, or general category (such as banana is a fruit, not just yellow). (Pass 5 of 8, 7 of 8)
26. Ask child: If a horse is big, a mouse is ______? If fire is hot, ice is ______? If the sun shines during the day, the moon shines during the ______? (Pass 2 of 3)
27. Child must walk up steps. Child may use wall or rail only, not person. May not crawl.
28. Child must throw ball overhand 3 feet to within arm's reach of tester.
29. Child must perform standing broad jump over width of test sheet (8 1/2").
30. Tell child to walk forward, → heel to within 1 inch of toe. Tester may demonstrate. Child must walk 4 consecutive steps.
31. In the second year, half of normal children are noncompliant.

Observations:

B

FIGURE 1-2 *Continued.*

nurse and interpret findings in the context of knowledge of the child through longitudinal surveillance.

b. A developmental screening test must not be considered equivalent to intelligence quotient testing, nor a definite predictor of current or future abilities. Screening merely identifies children at risk for possible developmental problems and in need of further evaluation or closer monitoring.

F Procedures

1. **Sensory screening.** During infancy, sensory screening is accomplished via relevant history from parents and observations during physical examination.
   a. Objective **visual acuity screening** using pictures, the "Tumbling E" test, or other measures is recommended for all children beginning at age 3 years, with a repeat attempt 4 to 6 months later for children unable to cooperate. Visual acuity should be 20/40 or better by the age of 3 to 5 years and 20/30 by the age of 6 years. In otherwise healthy children, vision is screened annually through age 6 years, then at 8, 10, 12, and 15 years, or whenever there are concerns. Children who fail or are unable to complete vision screening should be referred to an optometrist or ophthalmologist with pediatric expertise.
   b. Universal newborn **hearing screening** is now routine (see Chapters 4 and 6). Hearing can be screened objectively using a pure tone stimulus beginning at approximately age 4 years. Failure of audiometric screening is defined as inability to hear in either ear sounds of 1000 Hz or 2000 Hz at 20 dB, or 4000 Hz at 25 dB. In otherwise healthy children, hearing is screened annually through age 6 years, then at 8, 10, 12, and 15 years, or whenever there are concerns. Formal audiologic testing should be requested when a child fails screening.
2. **Laboratory** screening tests should be performed selectively. The individual needs of the child and the community prevalence of disorders should determine the frequency of such tests.
   a. **Metabolic screening** is performed during the newborn period (see Chapter 6), and in some states is repeated at 1 to 2 weeks of age.
   b. **Anemia.** In certain high-risk populations (e.g., infants who have poor growth or nutritional status, infants who have not received iron-supplemented formulas or iron-fortified cereals, infants weaned to whole milk before 9 months of age), screening for iron deficiency anemia should be performed near the end of the first year when depletion of iron stores is maximum. Hemoglobin, hematocrit, red blood cell indices, or free erythrocyte protoporphyrin can be measured. Screening of economically disadvantaged children (presumed to be at higher risk) is performed annually to age 6 years, once between 7 and 11 years, and once in adolescence. Annual screening is advised for menstruating females. Some school districts require screening for anemia at specified ages (e.g., kindergarten, middle school, and high school entry).
   c. **Lead screening.** At 1 and 2 years of age, the AAP currently recommends universal blood lead screening for economically disadvantaged children and children living in areas lacking specific screening guidelines. Pediatricians must be aware of locale-specific screening recommendations. Often, such guidelines include targeted screening based on risk, such as residence in homes built before 1978 (see Chapter 2).
   d. **Cholesterol testing.** Currently, universal cholesterol screening is not recommended. Screening is indicated for those children at highest risk for the development of early atherosclerosis based on family history (e.g., parent or grandparent who has history of premature [$\leq$ 55 years of age] atherosclerotic heart disease, vascular disease, stroke, or sudden death from heart disease, or a parent who has hypercholesterolemia). Other children to consider as candidates for screening include those who do not have adequate data regarding family history or those who have other identified risk factors (see Chapter 17).
   e. **Although relatively inexpensive and easy to perform,** periodic routine **urinalysis** screening is probably not cost effective. Nevertheless, some school systems continue to require this test on school entry and periodically thereafter.
3. **Tuberculosis.** Children should be screened for risk factors for exposure to tuberculosis, including foreign travel (Table 1-1), and tuberculin skin testing performed only when risk is identified or when required by local regulations. Screening should use the **intradermal (Mantoux) test,** which contains purified protein derivative. All results should be read by qualified medical personnel.

TABLE 1-1 Tuberculin Skin Testing Recommendations for Children[a]

Validated Questions for Determining Need for Tuberculin Skin Testing
- Has a family member or contact had tuberculosis disease?
- Has a family member had a positive tuberculin skin test?
- Was your child born in a high-risk country (countries other than the United States, Canada, Australia, New Zealand, or Western Europe)?
- Has your child traveled (had contact with resident populations) to a high-risk country for more than 1 week?

Risk Factors that Indicate Need for Immediate Skin Testing
- Contact with persons who have confirmed or suspected infectious tuberculosis (contact investigation); this includes children identified as contacts of family members or associates who have been in prison the last 5 years
- Radiographic or clinical findings suggesting tuberculosis
- Immigration from endemic countries (e.g., Asia, Middle East, Africa, Latin America)
- Travel history to endemic countries and/or significant contact with indigenous persons from such countries
- Prior to initiation of immunosuppressive therapy

Risk Factors that Indicate Need for Periodic Testing (Variable Frequency of Testing According to Specific Risk Factors)
- HIV infection or exposure to HIV-infected individuals
- Incarceration (adolescents)
- Exposure to members of high-risk groups (e.g., homeless; adults or adolescents who reside in institutions, penal institutions, or nursing homes; migrant farm workers; illicit drug users)
- Association with parents or household contacts whose tuberculin skin test status is unknown and who immigrated from endemic country or who travel to endemic area
- Residence in a high-risk neighborhood or community

HIV, human immunodeficiency virus.
[a]Immunization with bacille Calmette-Guérin is not a contraindication to tuberculin skin testing.
Adapted with permission from American Academy of Pediatrics: *2006 Red Book: Report of the Committee on Infectious Diseases*, 24th ed. Edited by Pickering L. Elk Grove Village, IL, American Academy of Pediatrics, 2006, pp 683–684.

4. **Immunizations** (see Figure 1-1). At present, children are recommended to be routinely immunized against diphtheria, tetanus, pertussis, polio, rotavirus, measles, mumps, rubella, varicella, hepatitis A and B, influenza, human papilloma virus, and infections due to *Haemophilus influenzae* type b, *Streptococcus pneumoniae*, and *Neisseria meningitidis* (see Figure 1-1 and Tables 1-2 and 1-3). Key concepts include:
   a. **Counseling consent.** Past reactions to vaccines and contraindications and precautions are important considerations prior to administration of any vaccine (see Figure 1-2 and Tables 1-2 and 1-3). The Centers for Disease Control and Prevention (CDC) require that all parents be given the appropriate Vaccine Information Statement for each dose of each vaccine. Benefits and risks of immunization should be discussed, including common and unusual reactions, and the parents must have the opportunity to give their informed consent before immunization.
   b. **Timing.** Careful attention to requirements for minimum age and interval between doses and need for "catch-up" of missed vaccines is important. Children may receive all needed routine vaccines during a single visit. Deferring vaccines to avoid multiple injections or during minor illness is an important cause of incomplete immunizations. Immunization status should be a consideration at all visits, not solely at health supervision visits. Periods of increased vaccine activity include ages 2 to 18 months (primary immunizations), ages 4 to 6 years (booster doses), and 11 to 12 years (a single dose each of tetanus-diphtheria-acellular pertussis and meningococcal vaccines and, for females, a three-dose series against human papilloma virus). The intervening years provide opportunities for "catch-up" due to missed immunizations or changes in the immunization schedule.

G **Anticipatory guidance** is the process by which pediatricians offer counseling during health supervision (e.g., on such topics as nutrition, safety, child behavior and development, parent-child interaction, various medical issues). Experienced pediatricians capitalize on "teachable moments" to offer guidance that is meaningful in the context of the parent's current concerns and child's emerging

TABLE 1-2 Routine Immunizations

Immunization	Type	Usual Reactions	Route
Hepatitis B	Recombinant viral antigen	Soreness at injection site, and fever in 1%–6%	IM
DTaP, TdaP	Bacterial toxoid (diphtheria, tetanus, inactivated bacterial subunits [pertussis])	Transient local and minor systemic reactions in 25%–33%, more common after doses 4 and 5 of DTaP	IM
Hib	Polysaccharide-protein conjugate	Transient local reaction, mild fever in 25%	IM
IPV	Inactivated virus	Transient local reactions	IM
PCV7	Polysaccharide-protein conjugate	Transient local reactions (25%), fever (33%)	IM
Rotavirus	Live-attenuated virus	Diarrhea, vomiting (1%–3%)	PO
MMR	Live-attenuated virus	5–7 d after dose: 5%–15% fever lasting 1–2 d, transient rash, adenopathy 7–21 d after dose: transient arthralgia (0.5% of children, 25% of postpubertal females with or without arthritis)	SC
Varicella	Live-attenuated virus	Transient pain or redness at injection site, occurrence: 20%–35% Mild maculopapular or vesicular rash, occurrence: 7%–8%	SC
Hepatitis A	Inactivated viral antigen	Local reactions 20%–50%, mild systemic reactions < 10%	IM
MCV4	Polysaccharide-protein conjugate		IM
HPV		Pain at site (80%), local reaction (25%, usually minor)	IM
Influenza	Inactivated viral, or live-attenuated	Local reactions, fever, myalgia, rhinorrhea with intranasal vaccine	IM (inactivated) IN (live)

DTaP, diphtheria-tetanus-acellular pertussis; TdaP, tetanus-diphtheria-acellular pertussis (adolescents); Hib, *Haemophilus influenzae* type B; IPV, inactivated polio vaccine (types 1, 2, 3); PCV, pneumococcal conjugate vaccine; IM, intramuscular; PO, oral; MMR, measles-mumps-rubella; SC, subcutaneous; MCV4, meningococcal conjugate vaccine; HPV, human papilloma virus vaccine; IN, intranasal.

abilities (e.g., a parent's concern about picky eating offers the opportunity to discuss the toddler's reduced caloric needs and struggle for independence). Through such counseling, the pediatrician helps parents anticipate impending changes in the child's behavior, thereby easing parental concern and enhancing appropriate parental responses to each new phase of development.

III EARLY INFANCY HEALTH SUPERVISION (2–5 DAYS TO 6 MONTHS)

A Goals

1. Assess the infant's and mother's recovery from the birth process.
2. Assess the infant's progress during this period of rapid growth and intense developmental progress.
3. Assess the family's adjustment to the new infant and quality of initial parent-child interactions.
4. Administer the primary series of immunizations.
5. Foster new parents' sense of competency.

B Interval history

1. **Daily functioning.** Inquire about patterns and adequacy of breastfeeding or formula feeding, sleep location and schedule, bowel and bladder functioning, injury prevention, and toys

TABLE 1-3 Contraindications to Routine Immunizations

Contraindications for all routine vaccines: Anaphylactic reaction to a vaccine contraindicates further doses of that vaccine. Anaphylactic reaction to a vaccine constituent contraindicates the use of vaccines containing that substance.

Decisions regarding vaccines in the event of intercurrent illness and fever: Vaccines should not be used if an undesirable side effect or adverse reaction to the vaccine may seriously affect or be confused with an underlying illness. A common situation is the child needing immunization who has an acute illness. Minor illness, with or without fever (≤ 100.4°F [38°C]), does **not** contraindicate immunization. Deferring immunization in such situations constitutes a missed opportunity and frequently results in unimmunized children. For the child who has an acute, febrile illness, guidelines for immunization are based on the physician's assessment of the child's illness and the specific vaccines the child is scheduled to receive. If fever or other manifestations suggest a moderate or serious illness, the child should not be vaccinated until recovered.

Precautions: For individual vaccines, a variety of events or conditions may justify exercising precaution before immunization. Precautions are not absolute contraindications. Rather, a precaution mandates careful review of the risks vs. benefits, depending on the specific circumstances of the individual patient and the vaccine in question. For further elaboration on precautions for individual vaccines, the clinician is advised to consult the most recent edition of the American Academy of Pediatrics *Red Book: Report of the Committee on Infectious Diseases.*

True Contraindications for Individual Vaccines

Vaccine	Contraindications
DTaP, TdaP	Encephalopathy within 7 d of administration of previous dose of DTaP or pertussis-containing vaccine
IPV	Anaphylactic reaction to neomycin or streptomycin
PCV	Anaphylactic reaction to a previous dose of vaccine or vaccine component
Hib	None
Hepatitis B	Anaphylactic reaction to baker's yeast
Rotavirus	Altered immunocompetence, including HIV and infants under evaluation for perinatal HIV exposure, fever > 100.3°F, moderate to severe gastroenteritis, chronic gastrointestinal disease, intussusception
MMR	Anaphylactic reaction to neomycin or gelatin; pregnancy; known altered immunity, including HIV if severe immunocompromise
Varicella	Anaphylactic reaction to neomycin or gelatin; pregnancy; known altered immunity, including HIV
MCV4	Anaphylaxis to any component, including diphtheria toxoid or latex
HPV	Anaphylaxis to baker's yeast or previous dose of vaccine
Influenza, inactivated	Anaphylactic reaction to previous dose or to eggs
Influenza, live-attenuated	Any underlying chronic health condition in recipient, severe immunocompromise in household contact

DTaP, diphtheria-tetanus-acellular pertussis; TdaP, tetanus-diphtheria-acellular pertussis; IPV, inactivated poliovirus vaccine; PCV, pneumococcal conjugate vaccine; Hib, *Haemophilus influenzae* type B; HIV, human immunodeficiency virus; MMR, measles-mumps-rubella; MCV4, meningococcal conjugate vaccine

Adapted with permission from American Academy of Pediatrics: *2006 Red Book: Report of the Committee on Infectious Diseases,* 27th ed. Edited by Pickering L. Elk Grove Village, IL, American Academy of Pediatrics, 2006, pp 847–851.

provided. The first newborn visit is particularly focused on review of the prenatal and birth history, evidence of adequate hydration, successful adaptation to extrauterine existence (e.g., spontaneous waking to feed), and presence of jaundice.

2. **Health concerns.** Inquiry may focus on parents' assessment of the infant's growth rate and physical appearance. Consider specific inquiry about healing of umbilicus and circumcision sites, rashes, first illnesses such as colds or fevers, teething, use of medicines and vitamins, and assessment of infant's vision and hearing.

3. **Development**

   a. **Affective.** Parents are encouraged to discuss their assessment of the infant's temperament (e.g., easy vs. difficult, predictability of behaviors) and their response to typical behaviors (e.g., crying or fussing). Other topics include evidence for increasing mutual attachment between infant and caretakers and, after the first few weeks of life, evidence for increasing regularity of schedules.

b. **Milestones.** This begins with a general question such as, "What's he doing lately?" Topics may also include emerging motor skills ("What's he doing with his head or his body?"); social skills ("What does he do when he sees you?"); and language ("Does he make any sounds?"). (See Figure 1-2 for age-related milestones.)

4. **Family health** and **family psychosocial histories.** Topics may include the family's adjustment to the new baby, spouse involvement in child care, parent returning to work, day care arrangements, sibling rivalry, and tobacco and drug use.

C Physical examination Physical examination of the young infant should focus on recovery from birth trauma, continued surveillance for congenital anomalies, evidence of rapid progress in physical growth and motor development, confirmation of intact senses, and assessment of parent-child attachment and interactions. The following areas are emphasized:

1. **General appearance** and **measurements.** General appearance and state of hygiene are observed. Weight, length, and head circumference are measured and plotted on the appropriate charts. The first newborn office examination is particularly focused on evidence of adequate hydration, inspection for extent of jaundice, and evidence of successful adaptation to extrauterine life (e.g., absence of cyanosis, pallor, lethargy).

2. **Skin. Rashes** are particularly common in this age group. Their presence, appearance, and distribution are noted.
   a. **Infantile acne** resembles the adolescent form of acne vulgaris. It appears during the first few months of life and resolves spontaneously. It probably results from the hormonal stimulation of sebaceous glands that have not yet involuted to their childhood state of immaturity.
   b. **Miliaria rubra.** Also known as heat rash, these red papulovesicular lesions may be found anywhere on the body but typically predominate in clothed areas.
   c. **Infantile seborrheic dermatitis.** This condition appears during the first few months of life as a greasy, yellow-tinged, scaly rash on the face, eyebrows, skin folds, and scalp (cradle cap).
   d. **Atopic dermatitis.** The infantile form usually begins when the infant is 2 to 6 months of age and is characterized by erythema, scaling, papules, vesicles, crusting, and pruritus. The rash usually begins on the cheek, forehead, or scalp and extends to the trunk or extremities.
   e. If **jaundice** persists, its presence and distribution are noted, and measurement of serum bilirubin levels is considered.

3. **Head and neck**
   a. **Sutures** are usually palpable as ridges until the infant is approximately 6 months of age. The **posterior fontanelle** closes by the second month, but the anterior fontanelle is patent for 1 to 2 years.
   b. **Vision** may be assessed grossly by noting the infant's response to a light or bright object and by noting fixation on faces and inanimate objects. By the age of 2 months, infants follow an object past the midline and by age 4 months they follow an object to a full arc of 180 degrees. Screening for strabismus begins at 3 to 4 months of age and includes both querying parents for presence of crossed eyes or lazy eye and examination for symmetry of the corneal light reflex. Observation for conjugate movement of eyes begins once the infant is able to fix and follow an object.
   c. **Hearing** may be assessed grossly by noting the infant's response to sound and, at 2 months, observing for a turning of the head and eyes. Examination of the tympanic **membranes** in infants is facilitated by pulling the auricle down, because the canal is directed upward. Mobility of the eardrum should be evaluated by pneumatic otoscopy.
   d. White patches on the buccal mucosa and tongue that cannot be scraped off indicate **candidal infection (thrush).**
   e. **Congenital muscular torticollis** results from a unilateral shortening of the sternocleidomastoid muscle. Typical features include a head tilt toward and chin rotation away from the affected muscle. Abnormalities of the cervical spine and cranial nerves must be ruled out. This condition usually resolves during the first year and responds to physical therapy. Untreated, flattening of the skull may develop on the affected side (**positional plagiocephaly**).

4. **Chest.** Cardiac auscultation during the first 6 months of life may reveal **functional murmurs** (i.e., physiologic sounds of turbulence) or murmurs of such disorders as patent ductus arteriosus, atrial septal defect, and ventricular septal defect (Chapter 12).
5. **Abdomen.** The **umbilical site** heals by 1 month of age. Once the cord has separated and healed, fluid drainage suggests an abnormal connection between the surface of the abdomen and underlying structures, such as a patent urachus. **Umbilical hernias** are commonly noted in infants, often with **diastasis** of the rectus muscles. Most umbilical hernias resolve by school age.
6. **Genitalia.** A **hydrocele** is manifested by a swollen, nontender scrotum that easily transilluminates. The presence of an accompanying hernia may be difficult to ascertain. Many hydroceles spontaneously resolve by the end of the first year. The urinary stream is observed for forcefulness and straightness.
7. The **hips** of all infants must be carefully examined for **dislocation,** even if the newborn examination was reported to be normal. After the first few weeks of life, the principle screening maneuver for developmental hip dysplasia consists of testing for symmetric and full 90-degree abduction of hips while positioned in 90 degrees of flexion.
8. **Neurologic examination.** By approximately 2 months of age, the healthy infant should be alert and display interest in the examiner, often through eye contact and a social smile. Primitive reflexes elicited during the first months of life include Moro, grasping, and tonic neck reflexes (Chapter 18). By 4 to 6 months of age, these reflexes diminish.
   a. **Developmental monitoring.** History is confirmed by direct observation. Wide variations in normal development are the rule. The significance of an infant's failure to achieve a milestone must be interpreted with caution.
   b. Specific assessments should include **vision, hearing, vocalization,** and **gross and fine motor skills.** (For specific milestones, see Figure 1-2.)

D **Procedures: Metabolic screening** (*see II F 2*) and **immunizations** (*see II F 4*, Figure 1-1, and Tables 1-2 and 1-3).

E **Anticipatory guidance**

1. **Feeding.** As the optimal source of infant nutrition, breast milk offers numerous health advantages. Breast milk provides protection against a host of infectious diseases, decreases infant mortality, improves neurodevelopmental outcomes, and confers additional maternal health benefits. Observation of breastfeeding affords the opportunity to provide guidance about appropriate positioning, latching, suckling, and swallowing. Pacifier use should be deferred until after 1 month of age, to avoid interference with proper suckling and to establish sufficient milk supply. While new mothers frequently are concerned about milk supply, insufficient production of breast milk is an uncommon phenomenon. Infants who are successfully breastfeeding should have a minimum weight gain of 20 g/day and should void and stool at least four to six times daily by day 4 of life. Proper positioning and frequent, on-demand, rather than scheduled feedings at least every 2 to 3 hours in the first weeks of life help to empty the breast and establish milk supply. Commercially prepared formula is an acceptable alternative to breast milk. Whole cow's milk is inappropriate for use during the first 12 months of life. Parents should be cautioned to precisely follow directions for formula mixing. During the first 6 months of life, normal healthy infants require approximately **100 to 110 kcal/kg/day** of breast milk or formula for adequate growth. Solid food should not be introduced until the infant is at least 4 to 6 months of age. Because of the risk of infant botulism, infants under 1 year of age should never be fed **honey.**
   a. Healthy, full-term infants consuming at least 500 mL daily of commercially prepared formula fortified with iron generally require no vitamin or mineral supplementation.
   b. Breast-fed infants should receive a supplement containing at least 200 IU of **vitamin D** per day. Most liquid multiple vitamin preparations contain 400 IU/mL and are appropriate for this purpose. **Iron supplementation** is generally not required in this age group because of the increased bioavailability of iron in breast milk. However, infants who have low iron stores, those who have anemia, and those not consuming iron-fortified infant cereal by 6 months of age should receive iron supplementation.

TABLE 1-4 Recommended Fluoride Supplementation

	Local Water Fluoride Concentration Parts per Million (ppm)		
Age	<0.3	0.3–0.6	> 0.6
6–36 mo	0.25 mg	None	None
3–6 y	0.5 mg	0.25 mg	None
6–16 y	1 mg	0.5 mg	None

c. **Fluoride.** Beginning at 6 months of age, a daily supplement of 0.25 mg of fluoride is prescribed for exclusively breast-fed infants and those infants whose local water supply contains a fluoride concentration of < 0.3 parts per million (ppm) (Table 1-4).

2. **Safety and injury prevention: Crib safety.** The incidence of sudden infant death syndrome (SIDS) has dropped by over 50% since 1992 when the American Academy of Pediatrics advised that infants be positioned supine for sleep. This concept is reinforced by the nationwide safety campaign "Back to Sleep." Side sleeping is not recommended, as this position is associated with a higher risk of SIDS. The mattress should be firm, covered by a tight-fitting sheet, and there should be no soft objects or pillows underneath or around the infant. Crib bars should be no further than 2.38 inches apart. To further avoid suffocation, objects such as pacifiers and mobiles should not be hung within the crib. The use of a pacifier at bedtime (beginning after 1 month of age for breast-fed infants), avoidance of maternal smoking, and having mother and infant sleep in the same room but not the same bed are additional measures that have been associated with a reduced risk of SIDS.

3. **Elimination.** Breast-fed infants tend to have thin, yellow, seedy stools with almost every feeding, whereas formula-fed infants tend to have stools with more form but less frequency. There is, however, considerable variation in elimination patterns.

4. **Sleep habits.** Most infants sleep through the night by 4 months of age. Problematic night waking later in infancy may be avoided if parents routinely place the baby in bed sleepy but awake, thus encouraging a habit of self-soothing at bedtime. Nighttime bottles may cause milk-bottle caries and should be avoided.

5. **Developmental issues**

   a. **Affective**

   (1) **State organization.** The "predictable unpredictability" of the newborn gradually gives way to increasing regularity of demands. By approximately 2 months of age, feeding and sleep schedules may be established.

   (2) **Synchrony.** Parent-infant interaction is reciprocal in nature, and a sense of mutual awareness and expectations evolves during the first months of the infant's life.

   (3) **Attachment** becomes the main affective issue by 2 to 3 months of age. By this time, the infant both recognizes and uniquely responds to parents.

   (4) **Temperament.** The infant's behavioral style becomes increasingly evident during this time. The regular patterns, adaptability, and positive mood of the "easy" infant contrast with the irregularity, unpredictability, and intensely negative mood of the "difficult" infant. The wide range of normal behavior should be stressed.

   b. **Motor skills.** The infant's increasing mobility is usually evident by 4 to 6 months of age as the infant rolls over, sits with support, grasps a rattle, and places objects within the mouth.

F Common problems and concerns in young infants

1. **Breastfeeding concerns** (see also Chapter 6)

   a. **Ineffective breastfeeding** may present with reduced frequency of voiding and stooling, jaundice, dehydration, and inadequate weight gain. Direct observation of breastfeeding followed by management of identified problems is essential. Treatment may include more frequent feeding, treatment of engorgement or sore/cracked nipples, use of galactogogues (milk production enhancers), breast pumping, and breast milk (or, as a last resort, formula) supplementation. A lactation consultant may provide advice and support to optimize the chances of successful breastfeeding.

b. **Jaundice. Breastfeeding-associated jaundice** most often occurs in the first 2 to 5 days of life, due to insufficient breast milk transfer (see "ineffective breastfeeding" above), whereas **breast milk jaundice** occurs after day 3 to 5 and may persist for 2 to 4 weeks. While the mechanism of breast milk jaundice is unknown, the cause is likely to be genetically determined differences in the composition of breast milk. Discontinuation of breastfeeding for 24 to 48 hours will result in a decline in serum bilirubin, confirming the suspicion of breast milk jaundice; however, this strategy is reserved for management of newborns with severely elevated bilirubin levels.

2. **Eye drainage,** typically from one eye, may indicate a blocked tear duct, or **dacryostenosis.** Swelling, erythema, and induration around the lacrimal sac may indicate an acquired infection, or **dacryocystitis.**
3. **Conjunctivitis.** Ophthalmia neonatorum is conjunctivitis occurring within the first 4 weeks of life (see Chapter 6).
4. **Diaper rash.** Common varieties of diaper dermatitis include the following:
   a. **Irritant** diaper rash spares the skin folds and produces red, dry, wrinkled skin and shallow erosions over the buttocks.
   b. **Candidal** rash is characterized by beefy redness of the deep skin folds and satellite lesions.
   c. **Infantile seborrheic dermatitis** starts as erythematous, well-demarcated patches in the diaper area and typically spreads to involve the face, scalp, and flexural areas. Greasy or crusty scales are characteristic (*see III C 2 c*).
   d. **Staphylococcal** diaper rash is characterized by erythematous pustules and bullae with surrounding erythema.
   e. **Intertrigo** is a poorly understood dermatitis that is characterized by confluent erythema and white or yellow exudate involving the deep skin folds.
5. **Colic.** Healthy infants cry up to 3 hours per day. Colic is defined as intermittent, unexplained crying exceeding this amount (see Chapter 4). Excessive crying usually begins in the first month and typically occurs in the late afternoon and evening hours. During this time, the infant is difficult to console. Formula intolerance, constipation, teething, illness, and so forth usually do not explain episodes of colic. Spontaneous resolution usually occurs by the age of 3 months.
6. **Constipation.** Infants may commonly have a bowel movement only once every several days. Unless stools are hard and pellet-like and are accompanied by significant infant distress, parents should be reassured. The amount of iron found in formula does not cause constipation. True constipation in an otherwise healthy infant may be treated by offering apple or prune juice between feedings.
7. **Teething.** Infants may begin teething by 6 months of age. Excessive drooling, rhinorrhea, mild diarrhea, irritability, and decreased appetite may be associated with teething. High fevers should not be attributed to teething.

IV LATE INFANCY HEALTH SUPERVISION (6 MONTHS TO 2 YEARS)

A Goals

1. Assess the infant's progress during this period of changing nutritional requirements and frequently diminishing appetite.
2. Assess the infant's progress in becoming a mobile, verbal, and autonomously functioning individual.
3. Assess the "goodness of fit" between the family's expectations and the infant's increasingly visible behavioral style and emerging abilities.
4. Administer booster doses of important immunizations and primary measles-mumps-rubella (MMR), varicella, and hepatitis A vaccines.

B Interval history

1. **Daily functioning.** Feeding questions center around quantity and type of milk, juice, and solids consumed; weaning from breast or bottle; use of a cup and spoon; finger foods; and number of meals offered per day. Beginning at approximately 1 year of age, conflicts during mealtimes and diminishing appetite are topics of concern for parents. Other issues include sleep concerns,

bowel and bladder functioning (including attempts at toilet training), care of newly emerging teeth, age-appropriate toys, sharing books, and injury prevention measures.

2. **Health concerns.** Inquiry may include parents' assessment of the infant's overall health, with focus on common infections such as upper respiratory tract infections and otitis media. Other topics may include diminishing growth rate, appearance of extremities as gait emerges, hearing ability and speech development, presence of crossed or lazy eye, use of medicines, avoiding lead exposure, and iron deficiency.
3. **Development**
   a. **Affective.** The infant's emerging struggle to achieve autonomy and independence may manifest as resistance to passive feeding, bedtime struggles, or disturbing night awakening, and the appearance of temper tantrums. Goodness of fit between parents' expectations and the infant's abilities and behavioral style is assessed by exploring parents' management of problem behaviors and overall expressions of approval, flexibility, and satisfaction with respect to their child.
   b. **Milestones.** Topics include emergence and content of language; evidence of independent sitting, cruising, and walking; manipulation of small objects; ability to indicate needs without crying; and enjoyment of simple games such as peek-a-boo (see Denver II , Figure 1-2).
4. **Family health** and **family psychosocial histories.** Stage-related inquiry may include adjustment to day care, parental return to work, and the family's response to the infant's struggle between dependence and independence.

C Physical examination Physical examination of the older infant emphasizes evaluation of the sensory systems (hearing, vision, and language), motoric functioning, the appearance of the extremities, and dentition. The pediatrician may observe for the parents' management of the child's negative responses to the examination maneuvers. The following areas are emphasized:

1. **General appearance.** Attention to both physical and behavioral characteristics such as motoric activity and verbal expression, general hygiene, attachment between infant and caretaker, and overall mood are important. Weight, length, and head circumference are measured and plotted on the appropriate charts.
2. **Skin. Carotenemia** is a benign orange discoloration of the skin seen in infants who consume large quantities of orange and yellow vegetables and fruits. The absence of scleral discoloration and a supporting dietary history distinguish this spontaneously resolving phenomenon from jaundice.
3. **Head and neck**
   a. **Eyes. Strabismus** screening, with observation for conjugate movement of eyes and a symmetric corneal reflex, may be supplemented by the **alternate cover test.** Vision is subjectively evaluated as the child reaches out for and manipulates objects. In some young children, a flat nasal bridge or epicanthal folds may obscure the medial sclerae, giving the false impression of strabismus (i.e., pseudostrabismus). In these children, the corneal light reflex is symmetric.
   b. **Ears.** Given the high incidence of middle ear disease that occurs during this age period, careful inspection of the **tympanic membranes** includes color, landmarks, and mobility as assessed by pneumatic otoscopy. Distraction during insertion of the otoscope may enhance cooperation during this examination. The child's response to sound is observed. Tympanometry may be used to detect middle ear effusions (see Chapter 10).
   c. **Teeth.** The first teeth to erupt are usually the lower central incisors at approximately 6 to 8 months. By 2 to 2 1/2 years of age, most children have acquired the full set of 20 primary teeth. Decay, particularly involving the upper central and lateral incisors, suggests milk-bottle caries resulting from inappropriate bedtime practices. Mottled, pitted teeth may suggest excessive fluoride ingestion.
4. **Genitalia**
   a. **Boys.** Surgical referral at 1 year of age is indicated if either a hydrocele has not resolved or a testicle cannot be manipulated into the scrotum.
   b. **Girls.** Labial adhesions, which form postnatally, require no treatment unless there is obstruction to flow of urine. Most adhesions disappear spontaneously, either with repeated minor trauma of diaper changes or during puberty, under the influence of estrogen.

5. **Extremities**
   a. The novice walker demonstrates a wide-based gait for stability, and frequently the feet point outward secondary to external rotation of the hips. With increased confidence in walking, the legs come together. Intoeing, usually caused by torsional deformities, often appears in toddlers. The most common torsional deformities are femoral anteversion, internal tibial torsion, and metatarsus adductus. With the exception of rigid metatarsus varus, these deformities improve with age.
      (1) **Increased femoral anteversion** results when the femoral neck is internally rotated relative to the rest of the femur.
      (2) **Internal tibial torsion** produces intoeing, because the tibia is twisted inward on its longitudinal axis.
      (3) **Metatarsus adductus** may not be detected until later infancy. A rigid varus deformity of the forefoot may require casting.
   b. During late infancy and early toddler years, the feet appear to be **flat.** This impression is caused by normal fat pads present under the arch of the foot.
6. **Neurologic** assessment and **developmental monitoring.** Intact cranial nerve function is observed, with special attention to assessing vision and hearing. New skills are acquired in a cephalocaudal progression (e.g., head control before reaching, then sitting). Observation of milestones such as sitting, standing, walking, and manipulation of objects provides evidence of gross and fine motor functioning. In a nonambulatory child, the degree of head control when pulled from supine to sitting is also observed. Deep tendon reflexes can be assessed with either a reflex hammer or the examiner's fingers tapping directly on the tendon.
   a. Most **primitive reflexes** of early infancy disappear during the middle of the first year (e.g., Moro, sucking, rooting, tonic neck). Significant delay in timing of disappearance of early reflexes or failure to demonstrate full and symmetric reflexes that normally manifest later during the first year (e.g., lateral prop, parachute) is a nonspecific sign of neurologic abnormality (see Chapter 18).
   b. **Developmental assessment** is completed by observing for age-appropriate vocalization and language, gross and fine motor activities, and interactions between infant, parent, and examiner (see Denver II, Figure 1-2).

D Procedures

1. **Immunizations** (see Figure 1-1 and Tables 1-2 and 1-3). Consider **anemia screening** (*see II F 2 b*), **lead screening** (*see II F 2 c*), and **tuberculosis screening** (*see II F 3*).

E Anticipatory guidance

1. **Feeding**
   a. By the end of the first year, a schedule of three meals per day is feasible.
   b. **Table foods** are introduced slowly, adding one new food every 5 to 7 days while observing for any adverse reactions. With increasing fine motor control, finger foods should be encouraged. Foods should be prepared without added salt.
   c. Weaning from bottle to cup should commence by the end of the first year. Beginning use of a spoon is possible by the age of 15 months.
   d. Whole cow's milk may replace iron-fortified formula or breast milk beginning at 12 months of age. Low-fat or skimmed milk is not recommended until after 2 years of age.
   e. Juice is limited to 4 to 6 ounces per day, offered only in a cup. "Fast food" and soda should never be part of the infant diet.
   f. With physical growth slowing by the end of the first year of life, a normal decrease in appetite occurs.
2. **Safety and injury prevention**
   a. Potential dangers for the child include stairways, open windows, electric sockets, hanging tablecloths, and electric cords. Use of a playpen, high chair, expandable gates, and covers for wall sockets reduces dangers. Infant walkers are highly discouraged; parents must specifically be reminded that walkers should never be used in an area with stairs (see Chapter 2).
   b. When the infant reaches both 12 months and 20 pounds, use of a forward-facing toddler **car seat** is appropriate.

c. Due to the possible danger of **accidental ingestion** of poisonous substances, parents should have the telephone number of the poison control center on hand. Household plants and common remedies (e.g., acetaminophen) are potential toxins (see Chapter 2).

d. Participation in **infant "swim" programs** is discouraged. These programs are of no proven benefit and may expose infants to a variety of risks, including water intoxication (causing hyponatremic seizures) and infections (such as giardiasis). In addition, parents should be advised that it is extremely unlikely that infants can become "water safe."

e. Guns should not be kept in homes with children. Parents who own firearms should be advised to store ammunition separately from guns and keep all equipment locked and unavailable.

3. **Sleep habits.** If night awakening occurs, the child should not be brought into the parents' bed or offered a nighttime bottle. Rather, after the child's safety is ensured, he or she should be put back to bed in a loving but firm manner and allowed to fall back asleep without assistance (*see III E 4*).

4. **Toilet training** should be child oriented and deferred until at least 18 months of age. Signs of readiness include a desire to please, pleasure in imitating adults, desire to develop autonomy, and adequate motor development, including the ability to sit and walk.

5. **Dental care.** After eruption, teeth should be cleaned with gauze or a soft cloth. Beginning around 12 months of age, a soft brush and nonfluoride toothpaste may be used, and a first dental visit is advised. A daily supplement of 0.25 mg of fluoride should be prescribed for children residing in areas where the local water supply is severely fluoride deficient, beginning at 6 months of age (see Table 1-4).

6. **Developmental issues**

a. **Autonomy.** Negativism, refusal of passive spoon feedings, and the appearance of temper tantrums (beginning around 15–18 months) are examples of the toddler's struggle for independence. The toddler continually explores the limits of the environment.

b. **Temperament** remains highly discernible and may allow parents to predict the child's responses to certain circumstances.

c. **Attachment.** Behaviors reflecting the continued importance of attachment include clinging to parents, night awakening, and stranger and separation anxiety.

d. **Motor skills.** Evolving motor skills parallel the development of autonomy. However, increased mobility renders the environment a potentially greater threat to the child's safety.

e. **Cognitive development**

(1) **Object permanence** is reflected by the infant's ability to uncover a hidden toy, which develops at approximately 9 to 10 months of age.

(2) Also at approximately 9 to 10 months of age, the infant's interest in a wind-up toy relates to **an understanding of causality.**

(3) At approximately 18 months of age, the toddler is able to represent mentally an object or action that is not perceptually present (e.g., "pretend play"). Symbolic play is now possible because the child is capable of **thought.**

F Common problems and concerns

1. **Temper tantrums** are a normal manifestation of the toddler's struggle between autonomy and dependence. Distracting the child or ignoring behavior after ensuring the child's safety are reasonable approaches to a temper tantrum (see Chapter 4).

2. **Night crying.** Many infants 6 to 12 months of age cry at night, despite a previously good sleep pattern. Such awakening typically resolves within 1 to 4 weeks if parents provide brief reassurance and avoid reinforcing the crying by picking up or feeding the child.

3. **Stranger** and **separation anxiety** are typical manifestations of attachment during the latter half of the first year of life.

4. **Poor appetite is a common parental concern.** A decrease in appetite should be anticipated because the child's slower physical growth demands fewer calories (see Chapter 4). The child's daily needs are met by intake of a pint of milk, an ounce of fruit juice or a piece of fruit, 2 ounces of iron-containing protein, and possibly a multivitamin for the "picky" eater.

5. **Teething** (*see III F 7*)

6. The incidence of acute **otitis media** is highest in this age group. Recurrent infection and persistent middle ear effusion (serous otitis media) may be associated with poor growth, behavior problems, diminished hearing, and interference with normal language development. Avoiding recumbent milk feeding (e.g., bottle in bed) and exposure to cigarette smoke may diminish the risk of infection.

V PRESCHOOL YEARS HEALTH SUPERVISION (2–5 YEARS)

A Goals

1. Assess the younger preschool-age child's progress through this rough-and-tumble period of high motor activity and rapid emergence of speech and language abilities.
2. Assess the older preschool-age child's readiness for school.
3. Assess the goodness of fit between the child's personal style and the family.
4. Administer formal sensory screenings.
5. Administer booster immunizations.
6. Lay the foundation for future independent relationship between child and physician, by directing the interview to the child at 3 to 4 years of age.

B Interval history

1. **Daily functioning.** Feeding questions center around participation in family meals, typical diet, snacking patterns, food refusal, and management of conflicts. Other topics include sleep concerns, especially disturbing night awakening; progress and problems in toilet training; dental care; and injury prevention measures.
2. **Health concerns.** Inquiry may include parents' assessment of the preschooler's overall health, with particular focus on frequency of common infections, issues related to motor activity and gait, and occurrence of injuries and unintentional ingestions. Other important topics include hearing and vision concerns, use of medicines, and avoidance of lead exposure.
3. **Development**
   a. **Affective.** The preschooler's continuing struggles between autonomy and dependence gradually become less intense. Additional topics include peer interactions (particularly aggression and sharing), play preferences, and overall goodness of fit between preschooler and other family members.
   b. **Cognitive development.** A major focus of inquiry centers on the content, intelligibility, and complexity of language. Other topics include evidence for emerging curiosity and interest in objects or people not actually present (representation). Parents' and child's perceptions of school readiness become paramount concerns as the child prepares to begin formal schooling.
   c. **Milestones** (see Denver II, Figure 1-2)
4. **Family health** and **family psychosocial histories.** Stage-related inquiry may include adjustment to preschool, sibling rivalry, and anticipated changes in family life with school entry.

C

Physical examination of the preschool-age child emphasizes observations of overall motoric activity (active vs. quiet); appearance of teeth, tympanic membranes, and extremities; and speech. The older preschooler is also assessed for degree of cooperation and resistance to examination as well as ability to separate from parent and engage in independent interaction with the physician. The following areas are emphasized:

1. **General appearance** is assessed, with attention to both physical and behavioral characteristics such as general hygiene, interest and curiosity, and overall mood. Weight and length (supine measurement) and height (standing measurement) are obtained and plotted on the appropriate charts. Care should be taken to plot the 2- to 3-year-old child on the chart appropriate to the method used to obtain length (0–36 months) or height (2–18 years). The body mass index (BMI) is calculated (weight in kg/height in meters^2) and plotted. A BMI over the 95th percentile is defined as obese; BMI at the 85th to 95th percentile identifies overweight children (see Chapter 4).

2. **Ears** (*see IV C 3 b*)
3. **Teeth.** The number and condition of the primary teeth and the type of occlusion should be noted.
4. **Speech.** By 2 years of age, approximately 50% of the child's speech should be intelligible, and by 3 years of age, 75% should be intelligible. By 4 years of age, almost all of the child's speech should be intelligible. Articulation errors, such as substituting "w" for "r" in rabbit, or "d" for "th," are normal in the toddler age group.
5. **Chest. Innocent heart murmurs** are frequently discovered in this age group and reflect sounds of blood flowing through normal cardiac and great vessel architecture. The most common innocent heart murmur of childhood is the Still murmur. This systolic ejection murmur is low-pitched, musical, or vibratory in quality and is loudest at the lower left sternal border or midway between the lower left sternal border and cardiac apex. A cardinal feature of an innocent murmur is an increase in intensity in the supine position and in states of increased cardiac output such as fever or after exercise. By definition, there are no associated symptoms or signs of cardiac disease (see Chapter 12).
6. **Blood pressure** is measured annually beginning at 3 years of age.
7. **Back.** The combination of lumbar lordosis and relative laxity of the abdominal musculature explains the classic pot-bellied appearance of the toddler.
8. **Extremities.** With ambulation, torsional deformities of the legs as well as flat feet may be noted (*see IV C 5*).
   a. **Increased femoral anteversion** is a relatively common cause of intoeing in children 3 to 7 years of age (*see IV C 5*).
   b. **Flat feet.** Young children universally have flat feet as the medial longitudinal arch does not develop until about 4 to 5 years of age.
9. **Developmental assessment.** The 3-year-old child begins to share toys and play interactive games. By the time of school entry, the child should easily separate from the mother. (For milestones see Denver II , Figure 1-2.)

D **Procedures: Immunizations** (see Figure 1-1 and Tables 1-2 and 1-3) and **vision and hearing screening** (*see II F 1*). Consider **urinalysis** and screenings for **tuberculosis, anemia, lead poisoning,** and **cholesterol** (*see II F 2 and 3*).

E Anticipatory guidance

1. **Safety** and **injury prevention.** Topics for discussion include traffic and playground safety, animal bites, fire, and water safety. Because bicycle helmets have been proven to reduce head injuries, children should always wear an approved helmet while riding.
2. **Toilet training.** Maintaining a child-oriented approach is important (*see IV E 4*). Allowing the child to sit undressed on a potty-chair and dropping soiled diapers into the chair's bowl are helpful.
3. **Dental care.** The child should be instructed in the use of a toothbrush with a "pea-sized" amount of toothpaste. Daily fluoride supplements are continued for children residing in areas where the local water is fluoride deficient, taking into account all sources of dietary fluoride (see Table 1-4).
4. **Play.** The 2-year-old child is not capable of sharing and engages in solitary, parallel play. During successive years, the child's interest in and ability to engage in interactive play with peers emerge.
5. **Television.** Parents should be advised to limit television viewing to a maximum of 1 to 2 hours per day and to monitor the content of programs watched. Television viewing reduces time available for other activities (e.g., physical exercise) and promotes consumption of unhealthy foods. Violent program content is believed to promote aggression.
6. **School readiness.** Attitudes concerning separation and readiness for school should be discussed with the parents and child. Parent-child book sharing has been demonstrated to improve oral language skills and school readiness.
7. **Developmental issues**
   a. **Autonomy.** Continuing negativism may be encountered during such activities as eating, toilet training, and tooth care, as well as in play groups.

b. **Attachment.** As school entry approaches, the child's ability to separate from the parent becomes increasingly important.

c. **Temperament.** Sensitivity to the child's behavioral style allows parents to predict the child's responses to certain situations. For example, responses to school entry may differ greatly for the "slow-to-warm-up" child as opposed to the "difficult" child.

d. **Impulse control.** Wide variability in impulse control among children is apparent. Increasing demands are placed on the child as school entry approaches.

e. **Motor skills.** The "motor-minded" toddler enjoys rough-and-tumble play, whereas more passive activities are enjoyed by the calm child.

f. **Cognitive development.** This age period is the preoperational period of cognitive development, and mastery of language is the major cognitive issue. The 2-year-old's incessant asking of "What's this?" and "What's that?" is followed by "Why do I have to?" at the age of 4 years. Rational thinking is not yet possible.

g. **Gender identity.** The concept of gender as fixed and stable emerges at approximately 4 to 5 years of age and reflects the child's ability to establish a stable definition of physical concepts.

h. **Peer interactions.** At 3 to 4 years of age, sharing and interactive play emerge. Sibling rivalry is typical at this age. As school entry nears, values and attitudes of those outside the family, particularly a child's peers, become increasingly important.

F Common problems and concerns

1. **Separation anxiety** (*see IV F 3*)
2. **Sibling rivalry.** Parents should be encouraged to spend "special time" alone with each child and to avoid comparing siblings.
3. **Night awakening** (*see IV F 2*). Night feeding or allowing the child to sleep in the parent's bed will serve to reinforce night awakening.
4. **Stuttering.** Between 2 and 5 years of age, many children experience normal disfluency, which is characterized by repetitions of whole words and phrases and typically continues for less than a year. In contrast, stuttering is characterized by partial-word repetitions; multiple rather than single repetitions; irregular, rapid, or abrupt repetitions; and a high frequency of nonfluency. By late childhood, many children have recovered from stuttering. Parents should not correct the child or interrupt the child's efforts to speak, but may assist by modeling slower speech and allowing the child adequate time to respond.

VI SCHOOL-AGE YEARS HEALTH SUPERVISION (5–12 YEARS)

A Goals

1. Assess the school-age child's overall health status through this period of relatively slow, steady growth and diminishing frequency of intercurrent illness.
2. Assess the child's adjustment and progress in school.
3. Assess the child's social functioning, with particular attention to peer interactions and extracurricular activities.
4. Assess the older school-age child for signs of puberty and discuss upcoming changes with both child and family.
5. Administer immunizations.
6. Nurture an independent relationship between child and physician and foster the child's self-monitoring of healthy habits.

B Interval history

1. **Daily functioning.** Potential topics include typical diet, concerns about body image, sleep patterns, independence in toileting, dental care, sports and exercise participation, leisure activities, and safety habits.
2. **Health concerns.** Inquiry may include recent illnesses; recurrent pains and aches; sports injuries; speech, hearing, or vision problems; questions about upcoming puberty; and use of medicines.

3. **Development**
   a. **Affective.** For the younger school-age child, questions center around descriptions of behavioral style (e.g., outgoing, shy); adaptation to the rhythm of a formal school year; and peer interactions. For the older school-age child, attention focuses on extent of involvement with peers and peer values, conflicts with authority figures, and increasing evidence of self-reliance for personal needs and home and school responsibilities.
   b. **Cognitive development.** School performance, classroom behavior, relationship to peers, and athletic activities are important indicators of cognitive and social development. Areas to explore include the child's likes and dislikes about school, grades, absenteeism, and retention (i.e., needing to repeat a grade). Inquire about areas of difficulty and plans for remediation.
   c. **Milestones.** Inquiries about school performance, athletic ability, and hobbies constitute major areas of focus.
4. **Family health** and **family psychosocial histories.** Stage-related inquiry may include the family's adjustment to the child's school entrance, after-school supervision, activities shared by family members, and rules and conflicts at home.

C **Physical examination** Height, weight, and blood pressure should be recorded. BMI is calculated and plotted (*see V C 1*). Areas deserving special emphasis during the complete examination include the following:

1. **General appearance.** The overall mood, facial appearance, degree of eye contact with the examiner, and relationship to the parent are observed. For the older child, a "weather report" assessment may be requested (e.g., "In general, if you were to give me a weather report to describe your life, what would you say? For example, would you say things for you are generally sunny, cloudy, or stormy?").
2. **Skin.** With the onset of puberty, acne may develop (see Chapter 5).
3. **Teeth.** The secondary teeth begin to erupt when the child is approximately 7 to 8 years of age. The top teeth should overlap the bottom teeth all the way around the mouth, and the child should bite down on the back teeth.
4. **Pharynx.** Relative to adults, the tonsils in this age group frequently appear enlarged. This is the result of normal, age-related lymphoid hyperplasia that is often exacerbated by upper respiratory tract infections. If swallowing or breathing functions are not affected, no intervention is required.
5. **Genitalia** and **breast development.** Documenting pubertal changes is important (see Chapter 5).
6. **Back.** The usefulness of screening for scoliosis in otherwise healthy children and adolescents is controversial, but screening continues to be required by many school districts (see Chapter 5).

D **Procedures: Immunizations** (see Figure 1-1 and Tables 1-2 and 1-3) and **vision and hearing screenings** (*see II F 1*). Consider **urinalysis** (*see II F 2 e*), **cholesterol** testing (see *II F 2 d*), and screening for **tuberculosis** (see *II F 3*).

E Anticipatory guidance

1. **School progress.** Asking both parent and child about school performance is important.
2. **Safety** and **injury prevention.** Important topics include seat belt use, bicycle and pedestrian safety, protective equipment for sports, supervision outside of school hours, and water and firearm safety.
3. **Sex education.** Topics to be discussed with parents include their attitudes toward sex education and plans for discussing sexuality with their children.
4. **Health** and **dental habits.** With increasing autonomy and separation, the child is making decisions and developing his or her own health habits. The child should be encouraged to make wise decisions about diet, exercise, safety, and so forth. Children residing in communities with inadequate water fluoride concentrations should continue to receive supplements through 16 years of age (see Table 1-4).
5. **Developmental issues**
   a. **Autonomy.** The challenging of limits precedes the ability to make wise decisions and thus requires parental limit setting. By approximately 8 years of age, the child declares his or her

independence by transferring allegiance to a peer group. The development of a "best friend" is a milestone in interpersonal growth. Allowing the child to assume increasing responsibility may lessen family conflict. By early adolescence, the drive for autonomy culminates in the child's challenging of long-standing beliefs.

b. Cognitive development

(1) **Concrete operations.** At approximately 8 years of age, the child is able to focus on multiple aspects of a problem, establish hierarchies, use logic, and see the viewpoints of others.

(2) **Formal operations.** By 12 years of age, the ability to use hypothetical and abstract reasoning emerges.

c. Physical development. The onset or timing of pubertal changes may cause concern on the part of the parents or child.

F Common problems and concerns

1. **Acting-out behavior.** As the child strives for independence, some challenging of limits is likely. With increasing peer influence, confrontations with authority figures (i.e., teachers, parents) occur.
2. **Separation anxiety.** If the child is unsuccessful in securely achieving independence from home and family, school avoidance and school phobia may become problems (see Chapter 4).
3. **Recurrent pains.** During the middle childhood years, children may have recurrent somatic complaints such as headache, abdominal pain, and limb pain. Pains of this sort typically have no clear-cut organic cause. They are usually the consequence of environmental, temperamental, and constitutional factors (see Chapter 4).
4. **Poor school performance.** The role of the provider includes helping the parents understand special education programs and services as well as the law requiring that school systems evaluate children who experience difficulties in both learning and behavior. The pediatrician should also provide the names of local resources for help (see Chapter 4).
5. **Obesity**. Parents may raise concern about their child's weight, or the pediatrician may identify the problem, referring to growth and BMI charts for confirmation. Assessment must include attention to family history and secondary complications (e.g., obstructive sleep apnea, hypertension, type II diabetes). It is important to determine whether parent and child appear receptive to intervention. Counseling should include proper diet and exercise, and treatment must involve the entire family (see Chapter 4).

VII ADOLESCENCE (SEE CHAPTER 5)

Issues such as entry into puberty, confidentiality, reproductive health, at-risk behaviors, mental health, and transition to adulthood significantly impact the scope and focus of health supervision visits for adolescents. Central to these visits is the creation of an environment of mutual trust, where the adolescent is empowered to ask difficult questions and discuss sensitive issues.

BIBLIOGRAPHY

Algranati PS: Effect of developmental status on the approach to physical examination. *Pediatr Clin North Am* 45:1–23, 1998.

Algranati PS: Pediatric clinical encounter. In: *Introduction to Clinical Medicine.* Edited by Willms JL, Lewis J. Baltimore, MD, Williams & Wilkins, 1991, pp 121–153.

Algranati PS: *The Pediatric Patient: An Approach to History and Physical Examination.* Baltimore, MD, Williams & Wilkins, 1992.

American Academy of Pediatrics Committee on Environmental Health: Lead exposure in children: prevention, detection, and management. *Pediatrics* 116:1036–1046, 2005.

American Academy of Pediatrics Committee on Nutrition: Prevention of pediatric overweight and obesity. *Pediatrics* 112:424–430, 2003.

American Academy of Pediatrics Committee on Psychosocial Aspects of Child and Family Health: *Guidelines for Health Supervision III.* Elk Grove Village, IL, American Academy of Pediatrics, 2002.

American Academy of Pediatrics Committee on Psychosocial Aspects of Child and Family Health: The new morbidity revisited: a renewed commitment to the psychosocial aspects of pediatric care. *Pediatrics* 108:1227–1229, 2001.

American Academy of Pediatrics Council on Children With Disabilities: Identifying infants and young children with developmental disorders in the medical home: an algorithm for developmental surveillance and screening. *Pediatrics* 118:405–420, 2006.

American Academy of Pediatrics Section on Breast Feeding: Breast feeding and the use of human milk. *Pediatrics* 115:496–506, 2005.

American Academy of Pediatrics Subcommittee on Hyperbilirubinemia: Management of hyperbilirubinemia in the newborn infants 35 or more weeks of gestation. *Pediatrics* 114:297–316, 2004.

American Academy of Pediatrics Task Force on Sudden Infant Death Syndrome: The changing concept of sudden infant death syndrome: diagnostic coding shifts, controversies regarding the sleeping environment, and new variables to consider in reducing risk. *Pediatrics* 116:1245–1255, 2005.

Kleinman R: *Pediatric Nutrition Handbook,* 4th ed. Committee on Nutrition. Elk Grove Village, IL, American Academy of Pediatrics, 1998.

Willms JL, Schneiderman H, Algranati PS: *Physical Diagnosis: Bedside Evaluation of Diagnosis and Function.* Baltimore, MD, Williams & Wilkins, 1994.

Zuckerman B, Parker S: Teachable moments: assessment as intervention. *Contemp Pediatr* 14:103–118, 1997.

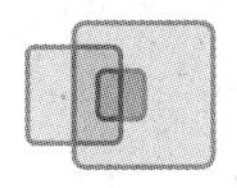

Study Questions

Directions: *Each of the numbered items or incomplete statements in this section is followed by answers or completions of the statement. Select the ONE lettered answer or completion that is BEST in each case.*

1. A 12-month-old girl has had a diaper rash for a week. She completed a 10-day course of cephalexin for treatment of impetigo several days ago. The rash is beefy red and most prominent in the skin folds, and superficial peeling is present at the margins. There are scattered erythematous "satellite" papules. Which of the following is the most likely diagnosis for this infant's diaper rash?

- A Atopic dermatitis
- B Candidal diaper rash
- C Staphylococcal diaper rash
- D Intertrigo
- E Irritant diaper dermatitis

2. A 5-year-old boy is scheduled for routine health supervision 2 months before starting kindergarten. In order to prepare him for the upcoming visit, his mother calls the nurse to inquire about the usual procedures. Which of the following screening procedures should be routinely included in all pre–kindergarten-age health supervision visits?

- A Blood lead level
- B Vision testing
- C Tuberculosis skin test
- D Serum cholesterol level
- E Dyslexia testing

3. A 16-month-old child has a diet that consists almost exclusively of breast milk. Which of the following physical findings is consistent with this dietary history?

- A Head circumference $>$ 95th percentile for age
- B Low weight for age
- C Yellow discoloration of the skin
- D Pallor
- E Erythematous scaling rash over the hands, feet, and diaper area

QUESTIONS 4 AND 5

During a health maintenance visit, the mother of a 12-year-old boy mentions that she and her husband are concerned about their son's reluctance to try out for the local swim team. Despite the boy's ability to compete effectively, he becomes upset whenever his parents raise the topic. The results of his physical examination are entirely normal, although he is prepubertal. A review of the boy's early health records reveals concerns about past behavior (his parents were initially reluctant to leave him with sitters because of his difficulties with separation; he adapts slowly to new situations such as school and camp).

4. In offering anticipatory guidance to this family, which of the following developmental issues is most important for the pediatrician to address?

- A Gender identity
- B Temperament
- C Impulse control
- D Synchrony
- E Acting-out behavior

5. On the basis of this information, which of the following is the most developmentally appropriate advice to offer the boy's parents?

- A Ask about the possibility of the boy competing with a younger group of children
- B Allow the boy to make up his own mind about trying out for the team

C Request that the boy's friends encourage him to try out for the team
D Urge the boy to attend the tryout sessions
E Arrange for mental health counseling for the boy

6. Which of the following etiologies is the most commonly accepted explanation for infantile colic?

A Formula intolerance
B Otitis media
C Constipation
D Teething
E Unexplained crying

7. A 4-month-old boy develops a temperature of 101°F (38.4°C) and is fussy for 2 hours after immunization with the diphtheria-tetanus-acellular pertussis (DTaP) vaccine. Which of the following is the correct approach to routine immunizations at this boy's 6-month health supervision visit?

A Defer immunization with the acellular pertussis vaccine, and instead administer diphtheria and tetanus toxoid vaccine (DT)
B Defer immunization with the acellular pertussis vaccine, and instead administer tetanus toxoid and reduced-dose diphtheria toxoid vaccine (Td)
C Administer half the usual dose (i.e., split dose) of the DTaP vaccine
D Defer all immunizations until the infant is 12 months old
E Administer the DTaP vaccine with instructions for fever control

8. During the health supervision visit of a healthy 6-month-old girl, history discloses that the infant's daily intake consists of breast milk and approximately 1/2 cup of infant cereal, mixed with breast milk. The infant has been growing steadily along the 25th percentile for height, weight, and head circumference. Past medical history is significant only for a single episode of otitis media. Which of the following recommendations regarding nutritional supplementation with vitamins and minerals is most appropriate for this infant?

A Begin a daily supplement of vitamin D and iron
B Begin a daily supplement containing vitamin D and fluoride
C Begin a daily supplement containing fluoride and iron
D Begin a daily supplement containing vitamin D, iron, and fluoride
E No supplement is needed at this time

Directions: *Each set of matching questions in this section consists of a list of 4 to 6 lettered options followed by several numbered items. For each numbered item, select the ONE lettered option that is most closely associated with it. Each lettered option may be selected once, more than once, or not at all.*

QUESTIONS 9–13

For each of the following behavior patterns described below, select the most relevant developmental issue.

A Synchrony
B Temperament
C Attachment
D Autonomy/independence
E State organization

9. A 3-week-old infant with markedly irregular sleeping and feeding schedules

10. An 8-month-old infant with night awakening and night crying

11. A 15-month-old toddler with temper tantrums who is not allowed to climb on a chair

12. A 2-year-old who is resistant to toilet training

13. A "slow-to-warm-up" child who displays quiet, subdued classroom behavior in early September

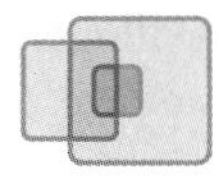

Answers and Explanations

1. The answer is B (*III F 4*). Involvement of the skin folds, beefy red skin, and satellite lesions are characteristic findings in candidal diaper rash. Recent antibiotic treatment is a common risk factor. Atopic dermatitis involves extensor surfaces in infants and typically spares the diaper area; flexural involvement usually develops after the first year of life. Pustules, bullae, and erosions (ruptured bullae) are signature features of staphylococcal diaper dermatitis. Intertrigo involves the skin folds, but whitish exudates are usually present and satellite lesions are not expected. Irritant diaper dermatitis spares the skin folds and produces dry, wrinkled skin.

2. The answer is B (*II F*). Objective sensory evaluation (which includes both formal vision and hearing screening) is an important component of the prekindergarten physical exam. Universal screening for lead intoxication and tuberculosis is no longer recommended; these screenings should be performed in children deemed at risk based upon criteria previously discussed. Measurement of serum cholesterol is indicated based on family history of increased risk, but is not routine for all children. Dyslexia testing is not a routine component of child health supervision at any age.

3. The answer is D (*III E 1 b, IV C 2*). Term infants have significantly depleted their prenatally acquired supply of iron by age 6 months. For this reason, the first solid food that is recommended for introduction at age 6 months is iron-fortified cereal. Thus, by age 9 to 12 months, exclusively breast-fed infants predictably develop iron deficiency and may exhibit signs of anemia such as pallor. Severe iron deficiency can cause frontal bossing, but it does not cause macrocephaly. Body weight depends upon both total calories per kilogram ingested and energy expended; thus, exclusively breast-fed infants can be underweight, overweight, or normal weight. Yellowish skin discoloration without scleral icterus (carotenemia) is a common finding in toddlers consuming large quantities of yellow and orange fruits and vegetables, but is not a feature of breast milk consumption. Exclusive breastfeeding is not associated with dermatitis.

4 and 5. The answers are: 4-B (*VI E 5, VI F 1, V E 7*). **5-B** (*VI E 5*). At 12 years of age, important developmental issues to consider during anticipatory guidance include autonomy/independence, temperament, peer interaction, and puberty. In particular, the consistency of a child's "slow-to-warm-up" temperament or behavioral style should suggest his likely response to a new situation. The concept of gender identity as fixed and stable emerges at approximately 4 to 5 years of age and is unlikely to be a major issue at age 12 years for most children. Impulse control emerges as a developmental issue in the early preschool years (typically as the child learns to inhibit aggressive behaviors such as biting and hitting), but would not account for this child's cautious response to new situations. Synchrony refers to the reciprocal interactions between a newborn and parent. This child's pattern of cautious behavioral approach is not suggestive of acting-out behavior, which typically manifests as rejection of authority figures and alliance with peers.

The drive for autonomy typically is characterized by the child's strong desire to assume increasing responsibility for his own actions and resist parental suggestions and limit setting. A further manifestation of this drive for independence is the transferring of allegiance from the family to a peer group. A relative delay compared to peers in the onset of physical changes of puberty may cause concern on the part of the child or parents. During the school-age years, allowing the child to assume increasing responsibility for his actions may lessen family conflict and promote autonomy and positive self-regard. Competing with younger children would be unacceptable because it would be likely to lead to segregation among peers at a time when allegiance to a peer group is normal and important. Parental attempts to coerce the boy into participation, either directly or indirectly through friends, would likely be met with resistance. Neither the boy's "slow-to-warm-up" temperament nor his stage-related behavior indicates the need for a mental health referral, although pediatric counseling for the parents and child is indicated.

6. The answer is E (*III F 5*). Many infants display intermittent, unexplained crying, typically beginning in the first month of life and occurring during the late afternoon and evening hours. Although many theories have been proposed to explain colicky behavior, none of these theories has emerged as a singular cause for the majority of patients. Formula intolerance, constipation, teething, or illness usually do not account for such episodes. Spontaneous resolution usually occurs by 3 months of age.

7. The answer is E (*Figure 1-1 and Tables 1-2 and 1-3*). Mild to moderate systemic symptoms (including fever, fretfulness, or drowsiness) are predictable, usual reactions to diphtheria-tetanus-acellular pertussis (DTaP) immunization. These symptoms do not constitute contraindications to further immunization. The only true contraindications to DTaP immunization are anaphylaxis to the vaccine or anaphylaxis to a vaccine constituent, moderate or severe illness at the time of immunization (with or without fever), and encephalopathy within 7 days of administration of a previous dose of DTaP or DTP. Other severe reactions (including high fever, shock-like state, seizures, extreme irritability, or Guillain-Barré syndrome) are considered precautions against repeating pertussis vaccination, which mandate individual case-by-case weighing of the potential risks of immunization versus the risks of contracting the disease. If the child developed a high fever (> 105°F) and had a prolonged period of extreme irritability, administration of the diphtheria and tetanus toxoid vaccine with elimination of the pertussis component would be a reasonable approach at the age of 6 months. Td vaccine is only appropriate for children 7 years of age and older. Split doses should never be used because their efficacy is uncertain.

8. The answer is B (*III E 1 b, c, Table 1-4*). All breast-fed infants should receive supplementation with at least 200 IU of vitamin D, readily accomplished by daily administration of a liquid multivitamin. Fluoride supplementation should begin at 6 months of age for all infants drinking fluoride-deficient water, including exclusively breast-fed babies. Iron supplementation is not generally required for infants without risk factors for anemia. Iron supplementation may be necessary at 4 to 6 months of age if iron-containing foods are not added to the diet.

9–13. The answers are 9-E (*III B 3 a, E 5 a*), **10-C** (*IV B 3 a, III E 4, IV E 3*), **11-D** (*IV B 3 a, IV E 6*), **12-D** (*IV E 4, IV E 6*), **and 13-B** (*V E 7*). The state organization of the newborn is characterized by "predictable unpredictability." Thus, irregular feeding and sleeping schedules are to be expected. By 2 months of age, the infant's demands should become more regular.

Night awakening reflects the continuing importance of attachment. Reinforcing the awakening by holding or feeding the infant should be avoided. The behavior will resolve normally within several weeks if parents provide only brief, positive interaction and lovingly, but firmly, indicate that the child must sleep.

By 15 to 18 months of age, a child's negativism and resistant behavior dramatically reflect the struggle for autonomy, typified by temper tantrums. The child continually explores the limits of the environment while remaining dependent on adults. Distracting the child or ignoring the behavior (having first ensured his or her safety) is a reasonable approach to temper tantrums. Toilet training can also provide a forum for the struggle for independence. Toilet training is most successful when it is child oriented. Attempts at toilet training should therefore be deferred until the child's negativism and resistant behavior subsides.

The consistency of a child's style of behavior, or temperament, is predictive of the child's responses to certain situations. Slow adjustment to new situations, people, and places is typical of the slow-to-warm-up child. Entering school may pose particular difficulties for this child until he or she becomes more comfortable on repeated exposure.

chapter **2**

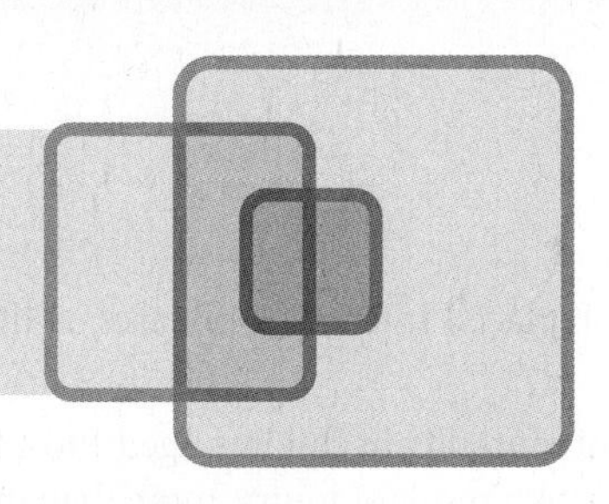

Injuries and Poisonings

ZOE CASEY • JAMES F. WILEY II

I GENERAL CONSIDERATIONS

A Definitions

1. **Injury** and **energy.** An injury refers to damage that is sustained to a person or thing. Injury results when a human being is exposed to excessive amounts of energy that surpass the body's ability to absorb or dissipate that energy without structural or functional damage. Energy may be mechanical (e.g., motor vehicle collision, falls, gunshot wounds, assault), thermal (e.g., scald burns), chemical (e.g., poisoning), electrical, or ionizing radiation. Injury also occurs from the absence of essential elements such as oxygen (e.g., choking, suffocation) and heat (e.g., hypothermia).

B Prevention: Public health approach

1. Injuries are often viewed as random acts of misfortune beyond one's control. Injuries should not be considered solely random acts of fate but rather events that can be understood, predicted, and often prevented. Asking and answering the following epidemiologic questions allows providers to move from treating the results of an injury to the preferred role of preventing the consequences of the injury:
   - **a.** What exactly is the problem?
   - **b.** Who has the problem and who is affected by it?
   - **c.** Why do they have it?
   - **d.** Where and when does it occur?
   - **e.** What can we do about it now and in the future?
2. **Primary** prevention to reduce injuries should employ three strategies:
   - **a.** Education (e.g., office-based counseling of the caregivers and child)
   - **b.** Engineering/environmental change (e.g., energy-absorbing surface in a playground, child-resistant cigarette lighters, smart airbags)
   - **c.** Legislation/enforcement (e.g., child safety seat laws, child-resistant medication and household cleaner containers)
3. **Injury prevention counseling priorities**
   - **a.** Counseled injuries should have documented epidemiologic significance.
   - **b.** Proven preventative methodologies should be recommended, particularly those with simple technologic implementation.
   - **c.** Counseling should be conducted in a developmentally appropriate manner based on injury risks specific to each developmental stage.
4. Four basic principles should be used in developing prevention strategies.
   - **a.** Passive strategies are more effective than those requiring repeated actions.
   - **b.** Specific advice is more effective than general information.
   - **c.** Injury control includes posttraumatic care and rehabilitation.
   - **d.** Particular attention should be focused on frequent injuries (e.g., motor vehicle crash, bicycle injury, house fires) to provide effective prevention strategies (e.g., car seats, bike helmets, smoke detectors).

C Epidemiology

1. Since 1950 injuries have replaced infectious diseases as the leading cause of death in children aged 1 to 19 years of age.
2. Injuries account for 48% of mortality in children aged 1 to 14 years in the United States. An average of 20 children die every day as a result of injury, more than die from all other diseases combined.
3. Around the world, injury is also the leading cause of pediatric deaths in every industrialized country.
4. **Death** and **morbidity** are two criteria by which the significance of childhood injuries can be measured. Although death is the worst outcome, injuries cause widespread morbidity, which results in the need for medical care as well as the inability to perform normal daily activities.
   a. For every injury-related death it is estimated that there are 19 hospitalizations, 233 emergency department visits, and 450 physician visits.
   b. Children under 15 years of age with nonfatal injuries represented 25% of emergency department visits.
      (1) An estimated 4.6 million males and 2.9 million females in this age group were evaluated in U.S. emergency departments.
      (2) Ninety-seven percent of the injuries are unintentional.
   c. Males consistently demonstrate a higher injury rate than females across all age groups with the difference increasing with age.
      (1) In children younger than 5 years, the injury rates were 33% higher in males than females.
      (2) Comparatively, the differential in the 10- to 14-year-old age group was 68%.
   d. In the United States, the annual cost of pediatric injuries is estimated at $224 billion.

D Relationship of child development to injuries

The types of injuries that children experience at different ages can be explained and even predicted by age-specific development and the mismatch between developmental level and the child's environment. Both motor and cognitive development play major roles.

1. **Infant: Birth to 1 year**
   a. **Motor development** is key. In the first 6 months, infants squirm and can fall from a changing table or adult bed even before they can roll over. The crib or playpen offers the safest environment.
   b. Child abuse (see Chapter 3) also is common in this age group
2. **Toddler: 1 to 2 years**
   a. Walking and then climbing allow toddlers mobility, reach, and speed. Fine motor control improves, so that containers and closets previously inaccessible can now be investigated. Ingestions occur frequently.
   b. Toddlers have no sense of danger; therefore, their motor activity is limited only by their physical ability. Falls, scald and contact burns, and drowning are all common injury mechanisms.
3. **Preschooler: 2 to 5 years**
   a. Running, climbing, and jumping are the mainstays of activity. Preschoolers can throw objects, ride tricycles, and interact with each other and their environment.
   b. Their thinking, however, remains illogical and egocentric. They are unable to appreciate cause and effect; thus, injury to themselves may not prevent similar episodes in the future. However, children can be taught in a way that can develop their skills and alter their behavior.
4. **School-age child: 5 to 10 years**
   a. Fine and gross motor skills become more refined. Organized games and rules are incorporated into play. Adventure and risk taking without appreciation of the consequences become the hallmarks of activity.
   b. Riding a bicycle becomes commonplace, as do its associated injuries.
   c. Children begin to assume increasing responsibility for their own safety, often out of the sight of their parents and teachers. Limitations in judging motor vehicle distance and speed result in unsafe street-crossing ability and frequent pedestrian injury.
5. **Preteen age and early teenage child: 10 to 14 years**
   a. Strenuous physical activity becomes common, and the incidence of sports-related injuries increases markedly. The use of bicycles, skateboards, roller blades, and other similar recreational devices is common.

b. Hobbies and scientific activities are begun.
c. Values and judgment become factors in decision making and risk taking.
d. Firearm-related injuries occur.

6. **Adolescent: Older than 14 years**
   a. Physical prowess is refined. Organized sports and part-time jobs make adolescents prone to sports- and work-related injuries. Resistance to the use of safety devices, such as bicycle helmets, is also common.
   b. Decision making becomes more logical but more abstract. Although there is knowledge of potential consequence, denial and a feeling of invulnerability often predominate in evaluating risks. Adolescents become drivers, and motor vehicle occupant injuries rise.
   c. Peer pressure and a need to feel comfortable in and accepted by a group may lead to substance- or alcohol-related injury, as well as assault and homicide.
   d. Difficulty in finding one's role in peer groups, family, school, and society in general may lead to depression or acting out, which sometimes culminates in suicide gestures or attempts.
   e. Dating is common, and some relationships are marked by verbal, physical, and sexual abuse.

II MOTOR VEHICLE INJURIES

A Epidemiology

In the United States motor vehicle injuries are the leading cause of death among children aged 1 to 19 years. A total of 1519 children died in motor vehicle crashes in 2005. This represents a decline of 8% and 58% compared to 2004 and 1975, respectively.

1. In 2005, the death rate was 28 per 1,000,000 for infants; 19.6 per 1,000,000 for 1- to 12-year-olds, and 178.7 per 1,000,000 for teenagers.
2. The occurrence of fatal motor vehicle crashes involving children is highest at the following times:
   a. Friday through Sunday
   b. The hours of 3 p.m. to 6 p.m.
   c. During the months of June through August
3. **Restraints.** The use of child safety seats and seat belts is the most important mechanism to prevent motor vehicle injury and death. Unfortunately, many child passengers are improperly secured.
   a. Child safety seats reduced the risk of death by 71% for infants and 54% for children 1 to 4 years of age.
   b. The LATCH system, introduced in 2002, was intended to standardize the way safety seats were anchored without utilizing the seat belts. A survey conducted in 2005 showed that only 40% of parents driving cars equipped with LATCH were using the system.
   c. Compared to the adult safety belt alone, the use of booster seats reduces fatal injury by 59% in the 4- to 7-year-old age group.
   d. In 2004, a survey of children younger than 12 years of age presenting to emergency departments revealed that 45% were either unrestrained or inappropriately restrained. The percentage of unrestrained children who were hospitalized was three times that of restrained children.
   e. As children get older, they are less likely to be restrained. In 2001, of children killed in motor vehicle crashes, 71% of children younger than 1 year were restrained compared to 44% of children aged 9 to 12 years.

B Populations at higher risk

1. **Children aged 4 to 8 years represent a special population,** as they have outgrown the safety seats designed for the younger population.
   a. They tend to be prematurely restrained solely by the adult seat belt or seated unrestrained.
   b. Nineteen of the 50 states in the United States allow children in this age group to ride unrestrained in the back seat of a motor vehicle.
2. **Alcohol-related incidents**
   a. One out of four of all occupant deaths among children younger than 14 years involves a drinking driver.
   b. The majority of children are unrestrained at the time of impact.

c. The drivers' survival rate was notably higher, suggesting that death may have been prevented if the child had been properly restrained.

d. Sixty percent of deaths occur during the hours of 6 A.M. to 9 P.M.

3. **Teen drivers.** Two of five deaths among U.S. teens are the result of motor vehicle crashes. The likelihood of a motor vehicle crash is highest in males and young (16- to 19-year-olds), inexperienced (< 1 year of driving) drivers.

a. In 2005, 61% of teenage passenger deaths occurred in vehicles driven by another teen.

b. Along with being inexperienced drivers, teens are more likely to perform risky activities such as exceed the speed limit, make illegal turns, ride unrestrained, or travel with an intoxicated driver. They are also more likely to underestimate or be unable to recognize dangerous situations.

c. At all levels of blood alcohol concentration, the risk of involvement in a crash is higher for teens than older drivers.

C Injury prevention

1. Children of all ages should always be appropriately restrained.
2. DUI and child restraint laws should be enforced, especially during times that fatal injuries occur with increased frequency.
3. Children younger than age 13 should be encouraged to ride in the backseat to reduce the injuries from air bags.
4. Booster seats should be used for children who are 4 to 8 years of age, heavier than 40 lbs, or under the height of 4 feet 9 inches.
5. Children should not be restrained by a seat belt alone until the lap belt fits flat across the hips (usually at 4 feet 9 inches tall).

III PEDESTRIAN INJURIES

A Epidemiology

Pedestrian injuries are a leading cause of both fatal and nonfatal injuries in children. Annually there are 68,000 nonfatal injuries with 12% of patients requiring hospital admission.

1. **Risk factors** for pedestrian injuries are multifactorial.

a. **Child.** Factors inherent to the child include small body size, inattentive behavior, and an inability to accurately judge vehicular distance and speed.

b. **Social and cultural factors.** Poor parental supervision and the presence of home stressors increase the likelihood of a child suffering pedestrian injuries.

c. **Physical environment.** The absence of play areas for children, increased housing density, and multifamily dwellings have been identified as risk factors for pedestrian injuries. Speed humps result in a safer living environment.

d. **Drivers.** Male drivers below the age of 40 years are most likely to strike a pedestrian. Other factors related to the driver include inattention, substance abuse, speeding, and disobeying traffic laws.

2. **Patterns of injury by age**

a. Infants and children younger than 5 years of age are typically struck as a vehicle is reversing out of the home driveway.

b. Younger school-age children tend to the injured as they dart out into traffic.

c. Adolescents are prone to injury especially when distracted, exhibiting lapses in judgment or using illicit substances.

B Injury prevention

1. Parents should be encouraged to provide continuous supervision while walking on the street or in parking lots.
2. Children younger than age 10 should not be allowed to cross the street alone.
3. Children should be encouraged to utilize sidewalks and pedestrian crossings.
4. The wearing of bright or reflective clothing, especially at night, should be advised.

IV BICYCLE INJURIES

A Epidemiology Annually, over 200 children are fatally injured while riding bicycles, with the number of injuries peaking in the 10- to 19-year-old age group.

1. Eighty-four percent of injuries occur in males.
2. Bicycle helmets reduce the risk of head injury by 85%.

B Injury prevention

1. Bicyclists should always wear properly fitting helmets.
2. Helmets that have been in a crash or are visibly damaged should be replaced.
3. As vehicle operators, cyclists should obey all road traffic signs and lane markings.
4. Cyclists should wear brightly colored clothing during the day and reflective clothing at dusk and nighttime. The bicycle should be fitted with a front light and rear reflector.
5. The brakes and tires should be checked before the cyclist mounts the bicycle.
6. The cyclist should be observant for irregularities in the road surface or other obstacles in the road.

V DROWNING/SUBMERSION INJURIES

A Definitions Drowning is defined as death that occurs within 24 hours of a submersion injury. Near-drowning is a submersion injury in which the person survives for at least 24 hours.

B Epidemiology Unintentional drowning is the second leading cause of injurious death in the 1- to 4-year-old age group and the third leading cause in the 5- to 15-year-old age group.

1. On average, there are three fatalities and five nonfatal submersion injuries daily.
2. Males represent 80% of the fatal drownings.
3. Drowning rates vary by area and tend to occur more in warmer climates.
4. Of the 1- to 9-year-old age group, drownings are most likely to occur in swimming pools, from 10 to 19 years of age, natural bodies of water are the most common locations for drowning.

C Pathophysiology

1. **Hypoxemia** and cellular acidosis are the major sequelae of submersion injury.
   a. Initially, voluntary apnea and a variable degree and duration of laryngospasm occur.
   b. Asphyxia results in a reduced level of consciousness, which permits relaxation of the airway and aspiration. This is referred to as wet drowning and is responsible for 85% of cases of drowning.
   c. Fifteen percent of drownings are referred to as dry drownings, where water in the larynx precipitates laryngospasm. The hypoxemia results in cardiac and respiratory arrest. In this circumstance no appreciable amount of fluid is aspirated.
2. **The morbidities** of drowning are hypoxic-ischemic encephalopathy and multiorgan system failure. The long-term neurologic disability may range from learning difficulties to a persistent vegetative state.

D Injury characteristics by age

1. **Infancy.** Drowning can occur in as little as a few inches of water, so water-filled containers such as buckets, toilets, and ice chests are hazardous. Bathtubs are the most common locale of drowning in the first year of life.
2. **Toddlers and school-age children.** Drownings typically occur in large bodies of water such as swimming pools, lakes, ponds, and oceans.
3. **Adolescence.** Alcohol use is involved in 25% to 50% of water-related deaths of adolescents. Intoxication affects balance and coordination, and also increases the likelihood of risk-taking behavior, such as not wearing a life jacket.

E Injury prevention

1. Children, regardless of their swimming ability, should not be left unattended in or near a body of water, even for a short time.
2. Flotation devices should be utilized but do not replace direct supervision as a safety measure.
3. Pool barriers include walls or fences, door alarms, and motorized pool covers.
   a. Studies evaluating pool-fencing interventions have shown that pool fencing significantly reduces the risk of drowning.
   b. Isolation fencing, which encloses the pool only, is superior to perimeter fencing, which encompasses the home and pool and thus allows access to the pool from the house.
   c. Pool enclosures should be at least 4 feet tall and have a secure self-closing and self-latching gate.
   d. Doors that open to the pool area should be fitted with alarms.
4. Toys should not be left in the pool as they may attract the child to the water.
5. School-age children should be taught how to swim (most children start lessons about age 3 and some people advocate training younger).
6. Parents, especially those who live close to bodies of water, should be trained in cardiopulmonary resuscitation (CPR).

VI BURNS AND FIRES

A Epidemiology

Unintentional fires and burns are the third and second leading causes of injury and death, respectively, in the 1- to 4-year-old and 5- to 9-year-old age groups.

1. Over 150,000 children were seen in emergency departments for injuries related to fires and burns with 4% requiring admission.
2. Relative to adults, children have thinner skin and subsequently suffer more severe injuries at lower temperatures.
3. Burns may be caused by thermal, radiation, chemical, or electrical contact.
4. Of children age 4 and younger hospitalized for thermal burns, 65% suffered scald burns and 20% flame or contact burns.
5. Most residential fire deaths occur at nighttime and during the winter months.

B Flame burns

1. Children younger than 5 years of age are 56% more likely than a young adult to die in a residential fire.
2. Injuries occur most frequently as a result of residential fires with heating equipment such as space heaters and wood-burning stoves as the leading cause.
3. Of fatal fires initiated by children playing, 70% involve the child igniting clothing, mattresses, bedding, or upholstery.
4. By 2002, the number of residential child-playing fires had declined by 50% since 1994, when the child-resistant lighter standard went into effect.
5. **Injury mechanism.** Seventy percent of deaths are the result of smoke or toxic gasses. The closer the victim is to the fire origin, the greater the likelihood of burns to cause death.

C

Scald burns from hot tap water cause more deaths and injuries than any other hot liquid. Children aged 6 months to 2 years of age are typically burned by hot foods or liquids spilled during food preparation.

D Fire prevention

1. **Smoke alarms.** Data from 2004 revealed that 96% of homes surveyed had at least one smoke alarm.
   a. Homes with smoke alarms have a death rate that is 40% to 50% less than homes without them.

   b. The likelihood of fatality is reduced by providing occupants with an early warning.
   c. Smoke detectors should be installed on each floor and the battery checked at least once a year.
2. **Sprinkler systems** react very quickly and dramatically reduce the heat, smoke, and flames produced by a fire.
   a. The mortality rate from fire in homes equipped with systems has been reduced by 50% to 75%.
   b. Sprinkler systems are increasingly being required in all new one- and two-family dwellings.
3. **Fire extinguishers** should be used for contained fires that are not growing rapidly. A multipurpose extinguisher should be selected.
4. **Sleepwear**
   a. Flame-resistant garments are manufactured from flame-resistant fibers or are treated with a flame retardant, which is designed to no longer burn when removed from direct contact with a small flame.
   b. Sleep wear, even if not flame resistant, should be snug fitting as it is less likely to come into contact with a flame and does not ignite as easily or burn as rapidly as there is little air under the garment to feed a fire.
5. **Emergency plan.** With the children parents should practice two escape routes from every room in the house, and teach them to stop, drop, and roll if their clothes catch on fire.
6. Lighters or matches should never be used as a source of amusement for children.
7. If a child expresses curiosity about fire or has been playing with fire, parents should calmly but firmly explain that matches and lighters are tools for adults only.
8. Only lighters designed with child-resistant features should be used.
9. Young children should be taught to inform an adult if they see matches or lighters.

E Burn prevention

1. The water heater thermostat should be set to 120°F or below. Antiscald devices can be placed on water faucets and shower heads.
2. Parents should check the water temperature before placing a child in bath water.
3. Preferentially the back burners on a stove should be used and pot handles kept turned away from the edge of the stove.
4. When cooking, parents should ensure that children remain in a safe area such as a high chair or play pen.
5. A child should never be carried while one is carrying a hot drink or hot food.
6. Tablecloths or place mats can be pulled by young children, which can spill hot food or drinks.
7. Irons, curling irons, and other heat appliances and their cords should be kept out of a child's reach.
8. Children should not be allowed to handle fireworks.

VII FIREARMS

A Epidemiology In 2004, there were 2852 firearm deaths among children age 0 to 19 years of age. Ninety-five percent of these injuries occurred in the 10- to 19-year-old age group. Intentional injuries predominate in the 10- to 19-year-old age group.

1. **Unintentional injuries.** Approximately one third of families with children keep one or more guns in the home for hunting and recreation (40%) or protection (60%). Guns intended for protection are likely to be stored loaded and unlocked.
2. **Family and individual risk factors for intentional injuries include:**
   a. Learning disorders, attention deficits, or a history of emotional problems
   b. Substance abuse, school failure, or association with delinquent peers
   c. Exposure to violence and conflict in the family
   d. Low emotional attachment to parents or caregivers

e. Low parental education and income
f. Social rejection by peers

B **Injury prevention** Educating children about gun safety and reducing the accessibility of firearms in the home is paramount to preventing firearm-related death and injury in children.

VIII CHOKING

A **Epidemiology** Mechanical suffocation is a leading cause of injury-related death in children younger than 1 year of age. One hundred and sixty choking deaths and 17,000 nonfatal choking episodes occur annually.

1. During infancy, mobility and dexterity improve; subsequently, objects can be quickly and efficiently placed in the mouth.
2. Death occurs most commonly in the first year of life.
3. Food is implicated in 60% of cases.

B **The acute management** of airway obstruction depends upon whether the obstruction is complete, gauged by the ability of the child to cough, breathe, or speak.

1. A blind finger sweep should not be performed.
2. If the child is able to phonate or cough, no further emergency intervention need be performed.
3. When complete airway obstruction is suspected, rapid initiation of basic life support for foreign body as taught by the American Heart Association may be life saving.
4. **Morbidity.** Mechanical airway obstruction and subsequent cerebral anoxic injury may result in death or disability.

C **Injury prevention**

1. Parents should keep a watchful eye on their children when they are eating and playing, and avoid hard, smooth foods in children younger than 4 years of age (e.g., peanuts, M&Ms, popcorn).
2. Play or talking during meals should be discouraged.
3. Age-inappropriate toys, foods, and all household items should be kept out of reach.
4. Parents should learn how to provide early treatment for children who are choking.

IX ALL-TERRAIN VEHICLES

A **Epidemiology** It is estimated that children younger than 16 years of age account for 14% of all all-terrain vehicle (ATV) riders; however, this age group represents one third of all deaths related to ATVs. Thirteen percent of children killed are younger than 12 years old. Annually, there are 40,000 visits to emergency departments with injuries related to ATV use.

B **Vehicle types**

1. ATVs are available as three- or four-wheeled motorized cycles designed for off-road use on a variety of terrains.
2. Factors contributing to a lack of safety include a high center of gravity, poor or absent suspension, and the ability to attain speeds of 30 to 65 mph.

C **Mechanisms of injury** Typically, injuries occur as the driver loses control and the vehicle rolls over or strikes a solitary object.

1. Off-road vehicles are particularly dangerous for children younger than 16 years who may have immature judgment and motor skills.
2. Injuries frequently occur to passengers.

D **Injury prevention**

1. ATVs should not be operated by children under the age of 16.

2. All riders should wear helmets, eye protection, and protective reflective clothing. Appropriate helmets are those designed for motorcycle (not bicycle) use, and should include safety visors/face shields for eye protection.
3. Riding double should not be permitted.
4. Parents should never permit the street use of off-road vehicles, and nighttime riding should not be allowed.
5. Flags, reflectors, and lights should be used to make vehicles more visible.
6. Drivers of recreational vehicles should not drive after drinking alcohol.

X FALLS

A Epidemiology Falls are the leading cause of nonfatal injury for children aged 14 years and younger.

1. These injuries are responsible for 2.3 million emergency department visits each year.
2. Fifty percent of cases occur in children 5 years of age and younger.
3. Annually, 120 fall-related deaths occur.
4. The severity of injuries is related to the height of the fall and the landing surface.
5. Head injuries are responsible for the majority of cases resulting in death or severe injury.

B Fall injury characteristics by age

1. **Infants** tend to have fall injuries related to stairs, baby walkers, or climbing on furniture.
2. **Toddlers** are at risk for window-related falls.
3. Eighty percent of children are under the age of 4 years.
4. Falls in older children occur due to sports injury and from playground equipment.

C Baby walker injuries

1. Each year, an estimated 14,000 children are seen in emergency departments with injuries related to baby walkers.
2. Falls down stairs represent the more severe and the majority of injuries.
3. Wheeled baby walkers allow for increased mobility and speed of the infant beyond the infant's developmental capability to control the consequences.
4. Other injuries such as burns and poisonings occur as objects that would be otherwise out of reach become accessible.

D Window falls

1. These injuries are responsible for over 4000 injuries and 18 deaths per year.
2. Typically the injured child is male, under the age of 5 years, and playing unsupervised at the time.
3. Children living in apartment buildings in areas with low-income housing have a higher incidence of window-related falls.

E Playground falls

1. Annually 2000 injuries are evaluated in emergency departments and 15 fatalities occur.
2. Seventy percent of injuries involve falls to the ground and 10% onto equipment.
3. Of these injuries, 41% are fractures, with the upper extremity injured most commonly.
4. Lacerations represent 22% of injuries subsequent to falls in the playground.

F Injury prevention

1. Window guards that can be readily released in the event of a fire should be installed.
2. Parents should visit playgrounds that have protective surfacing under and around equipment.
3. The use of mobile walkers is strongly discouraged.
4. Self-closing safety gates should be placed both at the top and bottom of stairs.

XI POISONING

A Epidemiology

1. Poisoning refers to a toxic exposure that results in adverse effects for the patient. Toxic exposure encompasses all forms of contact (ingestion, inhalation, intravenous, intramuscular, rectal, vaginal, or topical) that MAY lead to adverse clinical effects.
2. According to the Centers for Disease Control and Prevention, up to 4 million toxic exposures occur annually in the United States. In 2007, regional poison control centers (PCCs) handled over 2.4 million telephone calls involving human exposures. Children younger than 5 years of age account for over 50% of calls, and boys are more likely to be exposed in this age group. The typical exposure for young children involves the unintentional ingestion of a single toxic substance. In contrast, more females than males are exposed in the teenage years. These exposures are frequently intentional and express suicidal intent, poor impulse control, or recreational use.
3. Children under 6 years of age are often exposed to over-the-counter medications, household chemicals, nutraceuticals, and plants. In addition to these toxins, adolescents and adults are commonly exposed to prescription medicines, especially sedative hypnotics, antipsychotics, antidepressants, and cardiovascular drugs.
4. Poisoning is the second leading cause of death due to injury in the older adolescent, comprising 7 deaths per 100,000 population. Carbon monoxide inhalation is the most common cause of death due to a specific poison by virtue of its contribution to all fire-related deaths.

B Pathophysiology

Toxic exposures represent an interplay of factors similar to the infectious disease model of host, environment, and vector.

1. Hosts vary by their behavioral and developmental susceptibility to toxic exposure.
   a. All toddlers have innate curiosity that leads them to explore their environment using hands and mouth. Some have pica, excessive ingestion of nonfood items, especially patients with nutritional deficiency (e.g., iron poisoning, vitamin B_{12} deficiency) and developmental delay.
   b. Factors described for toddlers may persist for school-age children with behavioral and developmental abnormalities (e.g., autism). Intentional ingestion due to depression or as an expression of child abuse also occurs in this age group.
   c. In adolescents, intentional ingestion as an expression of depression or other psychiatric illness often occurs. In addition, substance abuse is common, as is unintentional exposures related to occupation.
2. Social setting (environment)
   a. Disruption in the home environment or introduction of the high-risk host (toddler) into a new and less safe setting creates a high-risk environment. Common scenarios include:
      (1) A young child ingests leftover drinks after a holiday party.
      (2) Elderly relatives leave out or drop prescription medications that are ingested by a toddler.
   b. Chronic deficit in oversight by the child's parent or guardian may occur in situations where the caretaker is overburdened, negligent, or abusive.
3. Toxin (infectious organism)
   a. Poisons vary in degree of toxicity. As little as a single adult dose or one swallow (1/2–1 teaspoon) of some poisons can cause life-threatening effects in a 10-kg toddler (Table 2-1).
   b. Toxic substances may be easily accessible because of improper storage, disabling of child-proof caps, use of medicine organizers without child-resistant features, or mixing of multiple medicines together in the same medicine bottle.

C Prevention

Passive prevention efforts have had the greatest impact on reducing serious poisonings in children.

1. Enacted in 1970, the Poisoning Prevention Act mandates safety packaging for pharmaceuticals. A significant drop in the frequency of poisoning and death due to poisoning in children followed passage of this legislation.
2. Anticipatory guidance varies by age:
   a. Parents of toddlers and developmentally/delayed children need to know proper storage of potential household toxins, appropriate use of child-proof caps on prescription medications,

TABLE 2-1 Medications That Are Deadly in a Single Dose for a 10-kg Toddler

Benzocaine	Methyl salicylate (oil of wintergreen)
Camphor	Oral hypoglycemics
Chloroquine	Quinidine
Clonidine	Propranolol
Cyclic antidepressants	Theophylline
Diphenoxylate/atropine (Lomotil)	Thioridazine
Lindane	Verapamil
Methadone (and other opioids)	

high-risk poisons, and social situations that promote toxic exposures, and should not refer to medicines as "candy." Of note, prescribing of syrup of ipecac at the 1 year well-child visit is no longer recommended by the American Academy of Pediatrics (AAP) because of its lack of efficacy in mitigating poisoning and because of its potential misuse by teenagers with eating disorders.

b. Parents of school-age children and adolescents need to be able to recognize signs of depression and drug abuse. In addition, parents should be encouraged to educate themselves and their children about the dangers of recreational drug use while their child is school aged.

3. Active surveillance
   a. Regional PCCs contribute to a centralized database that is utilized to identify severity of toxic exposures by specific agent or brand and class of agents. New trends in intentional and unintentional poisonings are regularly identified and shared among the regional poison centers, as well as with federal regulatory agencies. This surveillance informs decisions about drug safety and has led to withdrawal of prescription medications from the U.S. market.
   b. Regional PCCs also provide surveillance for suspected biologic and chemical exposures that are of a criminal nature and report to local law enforcement, FBI, and Department of Homeland Security (*see XI E 2 e*).

D Regional poison control centers The nearest PCC can be reached by calling toll-free: 1-800-222-1222.

1. The first PCC opened in 1953 in response to an AAP report estimating that 50% of all serious childhood injuries were due to poisoning.
2. Regional PCCs have strict requirements with respect to constant availability, onsite availability of comprehensive toxicology resources, training of personnel, written medical treatment guidelines, documentation of phone calls, performance improvement, research, and education. Phone calls are typically answered by certified poison specialists (RN or PharmD) or physicians who have extensive training in the assessment and management of poisoning.
3. In addition to guiding management of acute human poisonings, poison specialists provide drug information, drug and toxin identification, environmental exposure treatment, and exposure management for animal poisoning.
4. PCCs are able to manage up to 85% of pediatric poisoning calls without sending the patient to a health care facility.
5. When calling the PCC, be ready to provide the following information:
   a. Age and weight of the child
   b. What the suspected toxin(s) is/are (exact name of the substance or identifying features such as color of pill, pill number, and markings)
   c. Where the exposure occurred
   d. When the exposure occurred
   e. Clinical findings and treatment given
6. PCC consultation should be sought for all exposures requiring medical intervention. PCC advice is superior to attempting to interpret online poison references, especially when the patient has significant clinical abnormalities or when antidote administration is considered.

E Approach to the poisoned pediatric patient

1. Most pediatric patients come to medical attention with known exposure. Sudden onset of lethargy, coma, seizures, cardiac dysrhythmias with shock, or respiratory distress in a previously well child should raise suspicion for possible poisoning.
2. **Primary survey and stabilization of the poisoned patient**
   a. Most toxins do not have specific antidotes, and patient outcomes after poisoning depend on good supportive care of the airway, breathing, and circulation.
   b. During stabilization, history should focus on the exact toxin(s), type and amount of exposure, allergies, current medications, pertinent past medical history, and key events leading up to the poisoning.
   c. Patients should undergo external decontamination with warm water (wet decontamination) if they are exposed to toxic agents that can be absorbed through the skin. Rapid drying, clean clothes, and a warm ambient environment will avoid hypothermia in children after wet decontamination. Members of the medical team should don personal protective equipment to protect themselves from toxic exposures in the course of patient care.
   d. Vital signs, mental status, pupil size, and other physical findings such as cardiac rhythm, bowel sounds, or odors may demonstrate typical patterns following poisoning with certain toxins. These "toxidromes" may help guide presumptive management during stabilization of the poisoned patient (Table 2-2).
   e. Exposure to biologic or chemical warfare agents also requires prompt recognition during stabilization (Table 2-3). These exposures may present with nonspecific findings of flu-like symptoms, rapidly progressive pneumonia, paralysis, vomiting, diarrhea, coma, or seizures. Clustering of similar clinical presentations among several victims is an important feature pointing to an intentional release of these agents.
   f. Gastrointestinal (GI) decontamination refers to therapeutic measures that prevent absorption of toxins. Administration of 1 g/kg (maximum 50–100 g) of activated charcoal (AC) within 1 hour of a potentially serious ingestion is currently recommended for most toxic ingestions. AC should not be given to comatose patients prior to endotracheal intubation, patients with GI bleeding, or those who have ingested caustic substances or aliphatic hydrocarbons. Certain substances (e.g., iron, lead, other heavy metals) do not bind to AC. Syrup of ipecac is no longer recommended in the emergent management of the poisoned patient. Gastric lavage requires orogastric or nasogastric intubation followed by repeated instillation and

TABLE 2-2 Common Toxidromes

Toxin Classification	Vital Signs	Pupils	Mental Status	Other
Opioids	↓HR ↓RR ↓T ↓BP	↓↓	Coma	↓ Bowel sounds
Sympathomimetics[a]	↑T ↑HR ↑BP	↑↑	Hallucinations, delirium, seizures	↑ Bowel sounds; cool, clammy diaphoretic skin
Anticholinergic[b]	↑T ↑HR ↑BP	↑↑	Delirium, seizures	↓ Bowel sounds; flushed, dry, warm skin
Sedative hypnotics	↓HR ↓RR ↓T ↓BP	↓	Coma	↓ Bowel sounds; nystagmus
Ethanol	↓HR ↓RR ↓T	↓	Coma	Nystagmus, flushed skin, sickly sweet breath odor
Serotonin excess	↑↑T ↑HR ↑BP	↑	Seizures	Diaphoresis, lower extremity rigidity with clonus
Cholinergic crisis[c]	↓HR ↓RR ↓BP	↓↓	Seizures	Bronchorrhea, bronchospasm, salivation, lacrimation, vomiting, diarrhea

BP, blood pressure; HR, heart rate; RR, respiratory rate; T, temperature.
[a]Refers to mixed α- and β-sympathomimetics (cocaine, amphetamines, LSD). Pure α-adrenergic agents (phenylpropanolamine, pseudoephedrine) cause a reflex bradycardia in overdose.
[b]In addition to anticholinergic findings, cyclic antidepressants cause coma and ventricular tachydysrhythmias.
[c]Often seen in conjunction with nicotinic symptoms of muscle weakness, fasciculations, and paralysis after exposure to organophosphate pesticides.

TABLE 2-3 Clinical Findings Caused by Biologic and Chemical Warfare Agents

Agent	Clinical Findings
Biologic	
Anthrax	Pneumonic form: Fever, dyspnea, cough, and pneumonia with widened mediastinum, respiratory failure, and hemodynamic collapse Cutaneous form: Pruritic, vesicular papule progressing to painless ulcer with black eschar over several days with lymphadenopathy and lymphangiitis
Pneumonic plague	Fever, dyspnea, cough, hemoptysis, and fulminant bronchopneumonia
Inhalational tularemia	Fever, dyspnea, and cough with fulminant pleuropneumonitis
Botulism	Descending paralysis marked by bulbar cranial nerve abnormalities leading to diplopia, blurred vision, dysarthria, dysphagia, and respiratory muscle weakness
Hemorrhagic fever	Fever, myalgia, headache, cough, chest pain, vomiting, and diarrhea (flu-like presentation) progressing to shock with coagulopathy manifested by petechiae, ecchymoses, and hemorrhage
Smallpox	Fever and myalgias followed by development of vesicular/pustular rash on the face and extremities, with lesions in the same stage of development
Chemical	
Chorine gas	Burning of eyes, nose, and throat; early laryngeal and pulmonary edema
Phosgene gas	Early mild irritation of eyes and upper respiratory tract with delayed severe damage with pulmonary edema
Cyanide gas	Coma, seizures, tachypnea, tachycardia, dyspnea, metabolic acidosis, and sudden death
Blister agents (mustards, Lewisite)	Erythema and blistering of skin, eye irritation and burns, vomiting, cough, dyspnea, and acute, severe pneumonitis with respiratory failure; bone marrow suppression 3–5 d after exposure
Nerve agents	Cholinergic syndrome (see Table 2-2); also, lethargy, coma, seizures, and generalized weakness, paralysis, and respiratory arrest. Nicotinic stimulation: Mydriasis, fasciculations, tachycardia, and hypertension
Riot control agents (tear gas)	Blepharospasm, tearing, eye and upper respiratory tract irritation, and bronchospasm that resolves with decontamination and supportive care
Incapacitating agents	BZ (3-quinuclidinyl benzilate): Anticholinergic toxidrome (see Table 2-2) Opioids: Opioid toxidrome(see Table 2-2)

removal of warmed isotonic saline in attempts to remove toxin. It is reserved for those patients who can receive this therapy within 1 hour of ingestion and who have obvious signs of serious poisoning. Whole bowel irrigation (WBI) involves administration of large amounts of polyethylene glycol in order to push toxins through the GI tract. WBI has been successfully employed after ingestion of iron, lead, other heavy metals, sustained-release products, and illicit drugs packaged in latex condoms.

g. Most poisonings (96% of all PCC calls) do not require antidotes. Dextrose and naloxone are the antidotes most commonly used during resuscitation of pediatric poisoned patients. Table 2-4 lists poisons and potential antidotes.

3. Secondary survey and definitive care. A comprehensive history and physical examination will identify the potential toxin in up to two thirds of poisoned patients.

a. Parents often feel guilty and need to be questioned in an objective and empathetic fashion. It is important to ask what prescription medications are used by household members and to inquire about alternative medications and nutraceuticals. Discussion of poisoning prevention should occur after physiologic stabilization of the child.

b. General diagnostic testing including 12-lead electrocardiogram (ECG) with rhythm strip, rapid serum glucose, electrolytes, blood gas determination, and measured serum osmolality is a useful adjunct to history and physical examination. Serum ethanol level, urine pregnancy testing in females, and urine assay for drugs of abuse are indicated for adolescent patients. Specific drug levels may be helpful but only if they are rapidly available (within 2–4 hours) and will dictate a specific treatment such as antidote therapy or extracorporeal drug removal.

TABLE 2-4 Poisons and Potential Antidotes

Poison	Antidote
Acetaminophen	N-acetylcysteine
Anticholinergic agents (antihistamines, anticholinergic plants and mushrooms)	Physostigmine
Benzodiazepines	Flumazenil
β-Adrenergic blocking agents (propranolol, atenolol)	Glucagon
Calcium channel blocking agents (verapamil, diltiazem)	Insulin with glucose
Carbon monoxide	Hyperbaric oxygen
Cholinesterase inhibitors (organophosphate pesticides, nerve gas)	Atropine, pralidoxime, benzodiazepines
Cyanide	Sodium nitrite and sodium thiosulfate or hydroxocobalamin alone
Cyclic antidepressants	Sodium bicarbonate
Digoxin, digitoxin	Digoxin-specific antibody fragments (Fab)
Insulin	Dextrose, glucagon
Iron	Deferoxamine
Isoniazid	Pyridoxine
Lead	2,3-Dimercaptosuccinic acid (Succimer), $CaNa_2$-EDTA, dimercaprol (BAL)
Methemoglobinemia	Methylene blue
Methotrexate	Folinic acid (leucovorin)
Opiates	Naloxone
Oral hypoglycemic medications	Dextrose, octreotide
Snake venom (snake bite)	Antivenom
Toxic alcohols (ethylene glycol, methanol)	Fomepizole
Valproic acid	L-carnitine

BAL, British AntiLewisite; EDTA, ethylenediaminetetraacetic acid.

4. **Disposition.** PCC consultation is advisable to assist with disposition of toxic exposures in children. In general, the clinician should (a) admit patients who are symptomatic, require antidote therapy, or ingested a drug with a long half-life and potential for delayed toxicity (e.g., oral hypoglycemic medications); (b) admit or observe intentional ingestions, even if asymptomatic, until psychiatric evaluation occurs; and (c) discharge patients who ingested nontoxic substances or who remain asymptomatic past the time that peak effects would be expected.

F Emergency management for selected poisonings

1. **Acetaminophen**
   a. **Toxicity and pathophysiology.** Acetaminophen is the drug most commonly administered to children. Toxicity may occur in an acute dose of 150 mg/kg (ten times the therapeutic dose of 10–15 mg/kg) but can also occur after repeated ingestions of as little as 20 to 30 mg/kg/dose or a total daily dose of 160 mg/kg (approximately two times the therapeutic dose).
   b. **Clinical findings.** Acetaminophen poisoning has three stages:
      (1) Stage I (1/2–24 hours postingestion): Often asymptomatic, occasionally nausea, vomiting, diaphoresis, pallor
      (2) Stage II (24–48 hours postingestion): Nausea, vomiting, right upper quadrant pain, elevation of aspartate aminotransferase (AST), alanine aminotransferase (ALT), bilirubin, and alkaline phosphatase
      (3) Stage III (72–96 hours postingestion): Fulminant hepatic failure with thrombocytopenia, prolonged prothrombin time, and hepatic encephalopathy. Renal failure and cardiomyopathy may occur. If the patient survives, complete resolution of liver abnormalities occurs.
   c. **Diagnostic studies.** An acetaminophen level at 4 to 24 hours postingestion can predict the potential for toxicity and determine the need for antidote administration when plotted on the

Rumack-Matthew nomogram. Diagnosis requires a low threshold for suspicion since most patients are asymptomatic. All patients who attempt suicide require an acetaminophen level. Frequently, acetaminophen is overlooked as a coingestant with cough/cold preparations.

d. Management

(1) **GI decontamination.** Activated charcoal does bind acetaminophen and may be useful to administer within 1 hour of ingestion to prevent a toxic amount of acetaminophen from being absorbed.

(2) **Antidote.** All patients with acetaminophen levels that fall within the potential toxicity area on the Rumack-Matthew nomogram require administration of N-acetyl cysteine. N-acetyl cysteine is most effective when given within 12 hours of ingestion, though it still has efficacy at any time in seriously poisoned patients.

(3) **Supportive care.** Repeated testing every 12 to 24 hours for liver damage, liver function, and renal function accompanies antidote administration. Supportive care as appropriate for liver failure may be necessary.

2. Iron

a. Toxicity and pathophysiology. Iron acts as a gastrointestinal mucosal irritant and as an inhibitor of oxidative phosphorylation in the mitochondria. Iron ingestions are categorized by the amount of *elemental* iron ingested. Serious toxicity occurs with ingestions over 100 mg/kg of elemental iron. One 325-mg ferrous sulfate tablet contains 65 mg of elemental iron. Iron preparations are commonly prescribed for pregnancy and iron deficiency anemia. Frequently, parents do not regard iron as a "drug" and fail to include iron as a possible ingestant. Iron poisoning was the most common cause of pediatric death from acute unintentional pharmaceutical ingestion from 1983 to 1990.

b. Clinical findings. Iron poisoning has an early phase consistent with GI irritation and marked by nausea, vomiting, diarrhea, abdominal pain, melena, and hematemesis occurring 0 to 6 hours after ingestion. Patients who ingest large amounts of iron ($>$ 150 mg/kg elemental iron) may also have lethargy, coma, tachycardia, and hypotension. GI perforation with life-threatening hemorrhage can occur. In some patients, the initial GI symptoms subside and the patient appears well for the next 6 to 24 hours. This quiescent phase is then interrupted by recurrent hematemesis and melena accompanied by coma, cardiovascular collapse, pulmonary edema, and hepatic failure with chemical signs of hepatic necrosis presenting 12 to 48 hours after ingestion. Some patients may progress from early symptoms directly into recurrent signs without an intervening quiescent phase.

c. Diagnostic studies. An abdominal flat-plate radiograph can confirm iron ingestion and give an impression of the amount of unabsorbed iron. However, a negative radiograph does not exclude iron ingestion, particularly more than 2 hours after ingestion since dissolved or absorbed iron is *not* radio-opaque. A stat serum iron level 3 to 4 hours postingestion that is $>$ 500 μg/dL confirms iron poisoning.

d. Management

(1) **Decontamination.** Perform gastric emptying if spontaneous emesis has not occurred. Consider whole bowel irrigation if the patient displays signs of serious iron poisoning and there are no contraindication to its use such as ileus or GI perforation. Activated charcoal does *not* bind iron. Gastric concretions of iron tablets may require endoscopy or gastrostomy.

(2) **Antidote.** Patients with clinical symptoms and an iron level over 500 μg/dL should receive deferoxamine, an iron chelator. Asymptomatic patients with retained iron tablets and a level over 350 μg/dL may also benefit.

(3) Supportive care should focus on fluid resuscitation during the early phase followed by management of respiratory, cardiovascular, and hepatic toxicity during the recurrent phase. Patients who suffer serious iron poisoning should undergo an upper GI radiograph to look for strictures 3 to 4 weeks after ingestion.

3. Hydrocarbons

a. Toxicity and pathophysiology. Hydrocarbons include the aliphatic (kerosene, mineral seal oil), aromatic (benzene, toluene), halogenated (trichloroethylene, carbon tetrachloride), and terpene (turpentine, pine oil) groups. The most common ingestion in children involves aliphatic hydrocarbons (e.g., kerosene), which have the potential for aspiration and pneumonitis but few systemic effects. High volatility, low viscosity, and low surface tension favor aspiration and dispersal of the hydrocarbon throughout the lung with disruption of surface tension, alveolar collapse, atelectasis, and bronchospasm. Severe hypoxemia and respiratory failure may result.

b. Clinical findings. Hydrocarbons frequently cause gastric irritation and emesis with subsequent aspiration. The majority of patients are asymptomatic at initial evaluation after aliphatic hydrocarbon ingestion. Respiratory distress may develop 4 to 6 hours after exposure, necessitating a judicious observation period, and pulmonary injury may progress up to 48 to 72 hours after ingestion. Pneumonitis is suggested by tachycardia, retractions, cough, fever, or hypoxemia.

c. Diagnostic studies. Up to 91% of patients who develop pneumonitis will have an abnormal chest radiograph 4 hours postingestion.

d. Management

(1) Decontamination. Emesis should not be induced nor gastric lavage attempted after ingestion of an aliphatic hydrocarbon. Activated charcoal does not bind hydrocarbons and should not be used.

(2) Supportive care. Patients with signs of respiratory distress or abnormal chest radiographs should be admitted. Close attention to oxygenation, supplemental oxygen, and mechanical ventilation for signs of respiratory failure is needed to ensure a good outcome. Bronchospasm requires treatment with β_2 agonists. Epinephrine may induce cardiac dysrhythmias after hydrocarbon ingestion and should be avoided. Most patients recover fully if given proper supportive care. Patients who develop severe, unremitting pulmonary failure may be salvaged with extracorporeal membrane oxygenation.

4. Caustic ingestions

a. Toxicity and pathophysiology. One may divide caustic agents into alkalis (NaOH, KOH, NH_3), commonly used as drain cleaners, oven cleaners, and automatic dishwasher detergents, and concentrated ammonia products and acids (HCI, H_2SO_4), commonly used as toilet bowel cleaners and drain cleaners. Damage from alkali typically depends on pH > 12, concentration, amount ingested, and contact time (crystals > liquid). Damage from acids depends on pH < 2, concentration, and amount. Alkali cause liquefaction necrosis with saponification of membranes and spreading of injury after exposure. Acids cause coagulation necrosis with eschar formation, which impedes further injury. Alkali account for most corrosive ingestions, but acids account for the most mortality after a caustic ingestion. Most soaps, bleaches, and detergents (except dishwasher detergents) are nontoxic.

b. Clinical findings. Burns of exposed surfaces, including skin, eyes, oral mucosa, upper airway, and GI tract, occur after alkaline or acid poisonings. In terms of GI tract exposures, alkalies tend to injure the esophagus more than the stomach, and acids tend to injure the stomach more than the esophagus. Aspiration causes chemical pneumonitis. Patients can have significant GI burns without overt symptoms of caustic ingestion. Determination of extent of injury requires endoscopy within the first 24 to 48 hours.

c. Diagnostic studies. Chest radiography may be indicated if esophageal perforation is suspected.

d. Management

(1) Decontamination. Exposed skin and eyes should receive vigorous irrigation with water/normal saline. Assess the pH of the area after irrigation. Alkaline eye exposure may require prolonged irrigation. Do *not* induce vomiting. Dilution of small exposures with milk or water is acceptable as a first aid measure. One should not neutralize the ingestion (give alkalies to acid ingestions or visa versa) since further damage may occur from an exothermic reaction. Activated charcoal does *not* bind caustics and will impede subsequent endoscopy. Early nasogastric lavage of *large* acid ingestions may prevent gastric perforation and death.

(2) Supportive care. Perform endoscopy within 24 to 48 hours to assess degree of injury. Watch for signs of upper airway burns (chemical epiglottitis), especially common after ingestion of dishwasher detergents. Studies suggest no role for prophylactic steroids or antibiotics. Serious acid or alkaline eye exposures require urgent ophthalmology consultation and management. Watch for acidosis after large acid ingestions. Watch for signs of esophageal or gastric perforation.

TABLE 2-5 Lead Poisoning Toxicity in Children

Clinical Manifestations	Expected Blood Lead Level (μg/dL)
Severe	
CNS: Lead encephalopathy (coma, seizures with cerebral edema), ataxia, incoordination, developmental delay, bizarre behavior	> 70
GI: Vomiting	
Hematologic: Anemia with basophilic stippling	
Symptomatic	
CNS: Irritability ("difficult child"), decreased activity	50–70
GI: Abdominal pain, poor appetite, occasional vomiting	
Asymptomatic (chronic effects)	
CNS: Decreased intelligence, behavioral problems (impulsivity, attention deficit disorder with or without hyperactivity), impaired coordination	0–49

CNS, central nervous system; GI, gastrointestinal.

5. **Lead poisoning**
   a. **Toxicity and pathophysiology.** Lead is a heavy metal that is readily absorbed through the GI tract in young children and through inhalation at all ages. It causes multisystem toxicity by binding sulfhydryl, phosphate, and carboxyl groups on enzymes and interfering with calcium, zinc, and iron homeostasis. Leaded paint and dust from deteriorated lead paint in houses built before 1978 are the primary sources of lead exposure in children.
   b. **Clinical findings.** Symptoms correlate with whole blood lead levels (Table 2-5). The majority of chronically exposed children are asymptomatic. Children with low-level lead poisoning have measurable and statistically significant declines in intelligence.
   c. **Diagnostic studies** (see Chapter 1). Whole blood lead performed by atomic mass spectroscopy is the gold standard test. An abdominal flat plate radiograph is useful for identifying retained gastrointestinal leaded objects and leaded paint chips.
   d. **Management**
      (1) **Decontamination.** Removal of the child from the source of lead and abating that source is the key intervention. Children with retained gastrointestinal lead by radiograph may benefit from whole bowel irrigation if the lead is diffuse and located beyond the stomach or by endoscopy and removal if there is a leaded foreign object in the stomach.
      (2) **Antidote.** Children with a lead level over 45 μg/dL should undergo chelation therapy. The treatment varies by blood lead level and may include oral treatment with 2,3-dimercaptosuccinic acid (Succimer), oral penicillamine, intravenous $CaNa_2$-ethylenediaminetetraacetic acid (EDTA), or intramuscular dimercaprol (British AntiLewisite).
      (3) **Supportive care.** In addition to chelation, children with lead encephalopathy require meticulous supportive care that focuses on the management of increased intracranial pressure and seizure control.

BIBLIOGRAPHY

Arena J: The pediatrician's role in the poison control movement and poison prevention. *Am J Dis Child* 137: 870–873, 1983.

Centers for Disease Control and Prevention. Recognition of illness associated with the intentional release of a biologic agent. *MMWR Wkly* 50(41):893–897, 2001.

Consumer Product Safety Commission. The NEISS sample: design and implementation. The National Electronic Injury Surveillance System-All Injury Program (NEISS-AIP). Edited by Kessler E, Schroeder T. Washington, DC, Consumer Product Safety Commission, 2000. http://www.cdc.gov/mmwr/preview/mmwrhtml/mm5522a2.htm. Accessed.

Durbin DR, Chen I, Smith R, et al.: Effects of seating position and appropriate restraint use on the risk of injury to children in motor vehicle crashes. *Pediatrics* 115:305–309, 2005.

Durbin DR, Elliott MR, Winston FK: Belt-positioning booster seats and reduction in risk of injury among children in vehicle crashes. *JAMA* 289(14):2835–2840, 2003.

Felitti V, Anda R, Nordenberg D, et al.: Relationship of childhood abuse and household dysfunction to many of the leading causes of death in adults. *Am J Prev Med* 14(4):245–258, 1998.

Henretig FM, Cieslak TJ, Eitzen E Jr: Biological and chemical terrorism. *J Pediatr* 141:311–326, 2002. http://www.iihs.org/research/fatality_facts/children.html

Jenny C, Hymel KP, Ritzen A, et al.: Abusive head trauma: an analysis of missed cases. *JAMA* 281:621–626, 1999.

Lai MW, Klein-Schwartz W, Rodgers GC, et al.: 2005 annual report of the American Association of Poison Control Centers' National Poisoning and Exposure Database. *Clin Toxicol* 44:803–932, 2006.

Osterhoudt KC: The toxic toddler: drugs that can kill in small doses. *Contemp Pediatr* 17:73–88, 2000.

Osterhoudt KC, Burns Ewald M, Shannon M, et al.: Toxicologic emergencies. In: *Textbook of Pediatric Emergency Medicine,* 5th ed. Edited by Fleisher GR, Ludwig S, Henretig FM. Philadelphia, Lippincott Williams & Wilkins, 2006.

Thompson R, Choonara I, Hewitt S. Age and sex of drivers associated with child pedestrian injuries. *J Child Health Care* 7(3):184–190, 2003.

Wazana A, Krueger P, Raina P. Review of risk factors for child pedestrian injuries: are they modifiable? *Inj Prev* 3(4):295–304, 1997.

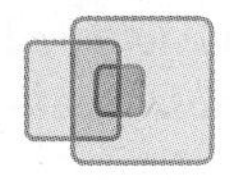

Study Questions

Directions: *Each of the numbered items or incomplete statements in this section is followed by answers or completions of the statement. Select the ONE lettered answer or completion that is BEST in each case.*

1. A 16-year-old is found unresponsive, restrained in the driver seat of his car. He was involved in a head-on collision with another car and there is significant front-end damage. Which of the following preventative interventions is most likely to reduce mortality from frontal impact in automobile collisions?

A Padded dashboards
B Driver side airbags
C Seat belts
D Driver's education
E Graduated driver licensing system

2. You are at a park walking your dog and hear a mother screaming for help. Upon arriving at her location you see her kneeling next to her child, who appears to be approximately 5 years of age. He is sitting against the bench, his eyes are open very wide, and he has his hands around his throat. He seems to be trying to cough but you do not hear any noise. His mother screams, "Help us; he is choking." Which of the following is the most appropriate action for you to take?

A Ask him to open his mouth and perform a finger sweep in an attempt to retrieve the object
B Have him lie supine and perform abdominal thrusts
C Lay the child over your lap and alternate back blows with chest thrusts
D Kneel behind the child and perform the modified Heimlich technique
E Leave the family to activate alert emergency medical services

3. A 9-year-old girl with asthma drinks from a water bottle that was being used to store red lamp oil containing kerosene. After ingestion, she coughs for several minutes and vomits once. She arrives in the emergency department 1 hour later with an odor of petroleum distillates on her breath. Vital signs show normal temperature with a respiratory rate of 24 breaths per minute, heart rate of 100 beats per minute, blood pressure of 90/60 mm Hg, and pulse oximetry of 92%. Her physical examination is remarkable for diffuse wheezing in all of her lung fields. Which of the following is the most appropriate next step in management?

A Oral administration of syrup of ipecac
B Oral administration of activated charcoal
C Oral administration of corticosteroids
D Epinephrine 1:1000, subcutaneously
E Albuterol by nebulized inhalation

4. A 2-year-old boy has a lead level of 45 μg/dL (normal < 10 μg/dL) on routine screening. An environmental investigation is initiated, and he is started on chelation therapy with dimercaptosuccinic acid. Which of the following is the most likely source of his lead poisoning?

A Art supplies at his day care
B Household water supply
C Airborne lead from gasoline
D Leaded solder in canned goods
E Dust containing leaded paint

***Directions:** Each set of matching questions in this section consists of a list of 4 to 6 lettered options followed by several numbered items. For each numbered item, select the ONE lettered option that is most closely associated with it. Each lettered option may be selected once, more than once, or not at all.*

QUESTIONS 5–8

For the each of the following patients, select the most likely substance ingested

- A Acetaminophen
- B Ethanol
- C Imipramine
- D Iron
- E Lye

5. An 18-month-old female is found with vomiting, lethargy, ataxia, hypoglycemia, and sickly sweet odor on the breath.

6. A 2-year-old presents with hematemesis, tachycardia, and poor perfusion after ingesting his pregnant mother's medication.

7. A depressed teenager is noted to have jaundice and signs of liver failure 2 days after transfer to a psychiatric facility.

8. A 3-year-old is found in the garage with red, swollen lips, drooling, and stridor after drinking a liquid stored in a soda bottle.

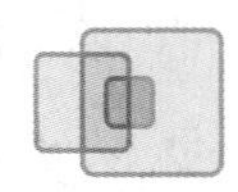

Answers and Explanations

1. The answer is C (*II A 3*). Proper use of lap and shoulder belts has the greatest effect in reducing the severity of injury. Analysis of the injuries sustained in relation to the average crash severity from which they resulted has demonstrated that for frontal impacts, the use of seat belts has had a major protective effect in reducing injury severity. The risk of moderate to serious injury to front-seat passengers is reduced by 45% to 55% and mortality decreased by 40% to 50%. Airbags require no active participation by the occupant but they must be used in conjunction with seat belts in order to decrease the severity of injury. Padded dashboards were introduced in the 1960s and are intended to reduce facial and torso trauma of the front-seat passenger. A learner's permit generally requires students to take a driver's education class that includes both classroom time and driving time with an authorized instructor. Graduated driver's licensing eases younger drivers into driving through a phased approach. In an ideal system, learner's permit holders may not drive unless accompanied by a licensed driver who is at least 21 years old.

2. The answer is D (*VIII B*). Pediatric Advanced Life Support outlines an algorithm for the management of choking victims. If the child is able to cough or speak, he should be encouraged to continue to cough to remain calm. Blind finger sweeps should never be performed as the object may be pushed further down into the airway. If the patient loses consciousness, back blows and chest thrusts are indicated for the infant and abdominal thrusts for the unresponsive child.

3. The answer is E (*XI F 3 d*). Aliphatic hydrocarbons, like kerosene, cause toxicity when they are swallowed and then aspirated into the lung. Chemical pneumonitis often results. The patient in this vignette has a history of coughing and vomiting that makes pulmonary aspiration of the lamp oil a significant concern. This patient has symptoms of tachypnea, wheezing, and decreased pulse oximetry on initial evaluation. Treatment with albuterol inhalation using an oxygen-driven nebulizer will treat bronchospasm and provide supplemental oxygen. Both syrup of ipecac and activated charcoal administration increase the potential for more vomiting that could lead to additional aspiration of hydrocarbon from stomach contents. Corticosteroids are not indicated in the treatment of aliphatic hydrocarbon poisoning. Subcutaneous epinephrine can precipitate life-threatening ventricular dysrhythmias after hydrocarbon ingestion.

4. The answer is E (*XI F 5*). Leaded paint dust remains the most common source of environmental lead. The risk is highest in communities with a high proportion ($> 27\%$) of housing built before 1978. Art supplies used for children are generally nontoxic, although important recalls of foreign chalk and crayons have occurred because of lead contamination. Water is the second most common source of lead in the environment and is present due to leaching from leaded solder from copper pipes. Very old houses (18th or 19th century) may have lead pipes as the prime feeder from a water main. Gasoline no longer contains lead in the United States. Leaded solder can be a hazard of foreign canned foods but is banned for foods canned in the United States.

5–8. The answers are: 5-B (*Table 2-2*), **6-D** (*XI F 2*), **7-A** (*XI F 1*), **and 8-E** (*XI F 4*). Ethanol causes life-threatening hypoglycemia in addition to typical findings of inebriation in young children because it inhibits gluconeogenesis and the ability of glycogen stores to be mobilized from the liver. Iron is commonly prescribed to pregnant women and in the early stages of toxicity can cause vomiting, gastrointestinal hemorrhage, and shock. Acetaminophen overdose causes delayed hepatotoxicity and can be overlooked if not sought for because the patient may be asymptomatic for the first 24 to 48 hours after ingestion. Finally, lye or sodium hydroxide is a highly basic caustic substance that can cause severe mucosal burns of the upper airway and esophagus after ingestion.

chapter 3

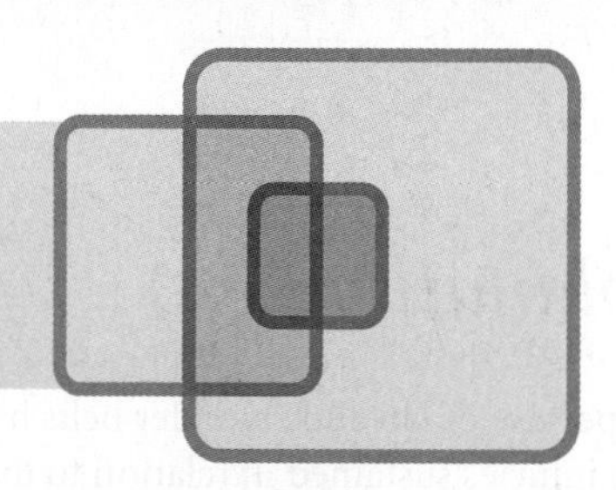

Psychosocial Pediatrics

PATRICIA JOYCE

I INTRODUCTION

This chapter addresses those aspects of child and adolescent health that are primarily influenced by the social and psychological status of the child and caregivers. There is considerable overlap with developmental and behavioral pediatrics (Chapter 4), with adolescent medicine (Chapter 5), and with the prevention aspects of health supervision (Chapter 1); psychosocial issues presenting in those domains are identified below. Prevailing social issues including violence, poverty, and the influence of media exposure are explored, and the role of the pediatrician in advocating for children's health is addressed.

In every situation, the physician should approach the patient problem/encounter with a working understanding of the developmental, behavioral, societal, and cultural norms in effect. Effective, respectful communication with the child and caregiver is key to eliciting information about sensitive issues. Supportive listening may be as beneficial as active intervention for many issues.

From a developmental standpoint, key psychosocial issues include:

A **Newborn** caregiver issues

1. Physical and emotional health/substance use and dependence
2. Family violence
3. Failure to thrive

B **Infant/toddler** caregiver issues

1. Family violence
2. Failure to thrive

C **School-aged child**

1. Bullying
2. School avoidance
3. Violence exposure/family violence
4. Caregiver issues
5. Media exposure
6. Chronic illness or disability

D **Adolescence**

1. Bullying
2. Violence exposure/family and intimate partner violence
3. Risk behaviors/substance use
4. Media exposure
5. Chronic illness or disability

II CAREGIVER STATUS

In all circumstances, a careful evaluation of the health of the primary caregiver(s) should be made, with emphasis on:

A Physical health—ability to physically meet the child's needs

B Mental health

C Substance use/dependence

D Family violence

The early identification of caregiver risk factors will allow the physician to implement primary prevention of many psychosocial problems.

III FAILURE TO THRIVE

A Failure to thrive (FTT) applies to the following:

1. A rate of weight gain significantly below that of other children of the same age and sex
2. Height or weight less than the third to fifth percentile on two or more occasions
3. Height or weight falling two or more percentiles on growth charts

These values must be assessed over time.

B **Facts**

1. Up to 10% of children present with FTT in the primary care setting.
2. Poverty is the greatest single risk factor for developing FTT.
3. FTT may inhibit permanent growth potential.
4. FTT may permanently inhibit cognitive development in children younger than 5 years of age.
5. Psychosocial failure to thrive is more common in females.

C **Causes** There is a broad array of specific causes of failure to thrive, but all share the same common pathways:

1. Poor caloric intake (e.g., feeding problems, neglect, caregiver or patient depression)
2. Poor absorption or utilization of calories (e.g., celiac disease, renal tubular acidosis, cystic fibrosis)
3. Overutilization of calories (e.g., thyroid disease, chronic illness, recurrent infections, malignancy)

D **Evaluation**

1. **History**
   a. Diet history with focus on caloric intake (food diary)
   b. Breastfeeding versus formula and formula preparation
   c. Voiding and stooling patterns
   d. Mealtime situations and behaviors
   e. Perinatal problems (exposures, illnesses)
   f. Associated signs and symptoms (bowel habits, changes in skin or hair, fevers, vomiting or reflux, poor feeding, developmental delay, acute illnesses, travel)
   g. Family situation/caregiver status
2. **Physical exam.** A full physical examination should be conducted, with special attention to the following:
   a. General appearance
   b. Affect and the interaction of the persons present
   c. Growth parameters over time

d. Vital signs
e. Hair and skin changes
f. Anatomic or mucous membrane abnormalities of the oral cavity
g. Signs of chronic infection
h. Heart and lung sounds
i. Abdominal masses
j. Organomegaly and/or lymphadenopathy
k. Musculoskeletal abnormalities (e.g., bowing of the lower legs)
l. Neurodevelopmental status

3. **Laboratory.** Specific laboratory evaluation should be driven by the findings of the history and physical examination. When no specific cause is determined through history and physical examination, the physician may choose to defer laboratory testing. However, many physicians will choose to investigate broad categories of disease with a few laboratory tests:
   a. **Complete blood count** (CBC) to look for evidence of infection, inflammation, or malignancy as a cause, and anemia as a result
   b. **Erythrocyte sedimentation rate (ESR) or C-reactive protein (CRP)** as markers of inflammation
   c. **Electrolytes/blood urea nitrogen (BUN)/creatinine** to look for evidence of renal disease. A **urine pH** should be obtained simultaneously with the electrolytes, to look for renal tubular acidosis.
   d. **Stool for ova and parasites**
   e. **Stool fat** to look for evidence of malabsorption
   f. **Thyroid studies, liver function tests (LFTs), sweat chloride, purified protein derivative (PPD), and human immunodeficiency virus (HIV) antibody** if there are known risk factors, regardless of symptoms
   g. **Prealbumin** as a marker for nutrition status
4. **Evaluation of family interaction/home situation**
   a. In over 80% of cases without an identifiable organic cause, an interactional problem may be identified.
   b. An interdisciplinary approach, with expertise in home health care, social work, nutrition, behavioral and developmental problems, psychology and/or psychiatry, and occupational or physical therapy (for physical feeding problems and feeding aversions), should be utilized whenever possible.
   c. Hospitalization is warranted when FTT is severe, when close observation outside the home situation is necessary, or when the primary caregiver is unable or unwilling to cooperate in the evaluation plan. During hospitalization, the child's behaviors are carefully observed and an accurate daily caloric intake measured. A child who gains weight during hospitalization, without any active interventions, has psychosocial failure to thrive.
5. **Management**
   a. Management will be tailored to the identifiable cause.
   b. When psychosocial failure to thrive is diagnosed, the primary intervention will be with the caregiver. Support of the caregiver's physical, emotional, and mental health should be initiated, often in concert with the caregiver's physician. Additional supports to the child, such as developmental services and occupational and physical therapy, should also be implemented. Most of these services will be home based. Child Protective Services can help the parents achieve success in the necessary interventions.
   c. Frequent measurements of the child's growth parameters should occur, as well as ongoing developmental surveillance.
   d. When a safe, nurturing environment for the child cannot be achieved in the child's home, Child Protective Services *must* be notified. The child may need to undergo placement into foster care until the home situation can be improved, or until a more permanent out-of-home placement can be arranged.
   e. Remember that FTT is often multifactorial. Even those cases with identifiable organic causes may have associated caregiver stress and might benefit from a multidisciplinary approach.

IV CHILD ABUSE AND NEGLECT

A Definitions

1. The federal government defines child abuse and neglect as:
   a. Any recent act or failure to act on the part of a parent or caretaker that results in death, serious physical or emotional harm, sexual abuse, or exploitation
   b. An act or failure to act that presents an imminent risk of serious harm
2. Generally, the broader term ***child maltreatment*** encompasses the following:
   a. **Physical abuse** is physical injury such as bruising, skeletal fracture, or blunt trauma incurred as a result of an adult intentionally striking a child. Also included in this category is abusive head trauma, or "shaken baby syndrome," which refers to intracranial injuries sustained when an adult intentionally shakes a child, usually an infant.
   b. **Neglect** refers to the failure of the responsible adult to provide for a child's basic needs, such as food, clothing, shelter, medical care for identified problems, education, and supervision. Such failure is deemed to occur if it results in harm to the child or risk of harm to the child.
   c. **Sexual abuse** includes both contact offenses, such as fondling and oral, anal, or genital penetration, and noncontact offenses, such as indecent exposure and sexual solicitation or exploitation.
   d. **Emotional abuse** or neglect occurs when a caregiver's behaviors convey to a child a sense of worthlessness or of being unwanted. Emotional neglect in infants and toddlers is frequently associated with failure to thrive.
   e. **Münchhausen syndrome by proxy** (also named **factitious disorder by proxy**) refers to a caretaker's fabrication of symptoms of illness in a child for the purpose of the caretaker's gratification, causing the child to undergo unnecessary tests or procedures for diagnosis or treatment. The caretaker may exaggerate the report of real symptoms or may actively induce symptoms in the child. The caretaker receives gratification from receiving sympathy and praise from others in caring for the "sick" child.

B Facts

1. In 2004, there were 872,000 reports of child victimization (or 11.9 per 1000 children) substantiated in the United States.
2. Of these cases, 62% represented neglect, 18% physical abuse, 10% sexual abuse, 7% emotional abuse, and 2% medical neglect.
3. Repeat victims accounted for 25% of cases.
4. The rate of victimization was inversely related to the age of the child, with the highest rate, 10%, occurring in children under the age of 1 year.
5. The leading cause of injury death in infants is homicide. In 84% of victim cases, the perpetrator was a parent acting alone or with another person.
6. Domestic violence is the risk factor most associated with child abuse fatalities.

C Risk factors for physical abuse and neglect

Risk factors for physical abuse and neglect are virtually identical. They pertain to characteristics of the perpetrator, the victim, and the situation.

1. **Perpetrator risk factors**
   a. Young parental age at time of first child
   b. Single parent
   c. Social isolation
   d. Lack of resources—money, education, social support
   e. Domestic violence
   f. Substance abuse
   g. Parental psychiatric illness
   h. Parental history as victim of abuse
2. **Victim risk factors**
   a. Age younger than 3 years
   b. Prematurity
   c. Chronic illness/disability

3. **Situational risk factors**
   a. Social isolation
   b. Lack of resources—social, educational, financial
   c. Domestic violence
4. **Clinical clues.** In addition to identifying risk factors, the physician should be alert to several clinical clues to abuse or neglect. They include:
   a. Pattern injuries
   b. Repeated injuries
   c. Discrepancies in history—chronologic, developmental, and those between persons and between the history and the physical exam
   d. Delay in seeking care
   e. Symptoms without explanation
   f. Failure to thrive
   g. Poisonings
   h. Absenteeism
   i. Absence of new problems while in a protective setting

D Injuries

1. **Pattern injuries** and their differential diagnoses are summarized in Table 3-1. They include:
   a. **Bruising.** Most "normal" bruises in children occur on the lower legs, as a result of minor bumps and falls. Inflicted bruises are more likely to occur on parts of the body usually covered by clothing, such as the buttocks, upper thighs, and back. Bruises with well-defined borders or shapes may outline the implement with which the child was struck. It is not possible to estimate the age of a bruise by the color of the lesion, as the color progression is determined by too wide a variety of factors, including extrinsic (how much force) and intrinsic (skin color, vascularity, patient age). Illnesses such as Henoch-Schönlein purpura (HSP) and idiopathic thrombocytopenia (ITP), bleeding diatheses (hemophilia, von Willebrand disease), and skin lesions (blue slate patches) can be mistaken for bruising and should be ruled out. Connective tissue diseases such as Ehlers-Danlos can cause skin to be easily friable and may lead to an overestimate of the traumatic force delivered. Some cultural healing practices, such as coining, cupping, and moxibustion, leave ecchymoses on the skin and, while leaving a clear pattern mark, should not be mistaken for inflicted injury.
   b. **Bites.** A common injury among toddlers, bites can be inflicted by adults as well as by playmates. The bite arc should be measured and compared to normative data if an adult-inflicted bite is suspected.
   c. **Burns.** These require a careful assessment of whether the physical distribution of the burn is consistent with the history. Most concerning are burns in a stocking or glove distribution

TABLE 3-1 Pattern Injuries and Differential Diagnoses

Pattern	Appearance	Do Not Confuse With
Bruising	Areas usually hidden by clothing Well-defined borders (outline of implement used)	Blue slate patches Cultural healing methods (coining, cupping, moxibustion) Disorders of clotting and coagulation (idiopathic thrombocytopenia, Henoch-Schönlein purpura, hemophilia) Connective tissue diseases (Ehlers-Danlos)
Burns	Stocking/glove Buttocks/perineum Grid pattern Location	Cultural healing methods (moxibustion) Skin conditions/infections (bullae)
Bites	Bite arc consistent with adult dentition	Bites from children
Fractures	Multiple, in different stages of healing Large bone spiral fractures (humerus, femur)	Bone disease (osteogenesis imperfecta) Congenital syphilis (metaphysitis)

(involving the whole hand or foot, with a well-demarcated transition to normal skin), as these are most likely to have been accomplished by forced immersion in hot liquid. Burns to the buttocks and perineum may also represent forced immersion. Burns yielding a grid pattern indicate contact with a hot solid object for a period of time. Splash burns may be either accidental or inflicted; accidental burns may represent neglect of adequate supervision.

d. Fractures. Unexplained fractures, repeated fractures, multiple fractures in different states of healing, and fractures attributed to feats beyond the developmental level of the child should all raise concern. Most fractures in preambulatory infants are inflicted, and frequently involve the ribs, metaphysis, and skull. Torsion or spiral fractures of a large bone such as the humerus or femur should also raise suspicion, as children are rarely able to generate the torque force for these. Spiral fractures of the tibia, in contrast, may frequently be seen in the normally active, uncoordinated toddler. Diseases affecting bone (osteogenesis imperfecta, rickets, congenital syphilis) must be considered in the child with unusual or multiple fractures.

2. Additional signs of inflicted injury

a. Retinal hemorrhages. These occur secondary to ruptured retinal vessels due to abusive head trauma. They are often visible in infants suffering from "shaken baby syndrome," where a frustrated or angry caretaker shakes a young infant, causing intracranial bleeding, usually as a subdural hematoma. Infants may also have other injuries, such as rib and metaphyseal shear fractures.

b. Blunt trauma. This may be inflicted on any part of the body, but the abdomen is the most frequent target. Typical clinical findings include ruptured viscera (intra-abdominal bleeding, free air in the peritoneum), obstruction due to hematoma, or the creation of a pancreatic pseudocyst.

E **Evaluation**

1. History should be obtained from all pertinent parties—patient and caregiver(s), interviewed separately if necessary (and possible).
2. A careful, thorough physical exam that evaluates all skin surfaces should be performed.
3. Photographs of suspicious injuries should be obtained.
4. The chart should include a thorough recounting of the history, using quotes as appropriate, and a detailed description of the distribution, shape, color, size, and pattern of any visible injuries.

F **Laboratory** In addition to any studies performed to evaluate the identifiable injury (radiograph of injured limb, cranial computed tomography [CT] scan for suspected head trauma), the following should be considered in the further evaluation:

1. Prothrombin time (PT)/partial thromboplastin time (PTT)/platelets/von Willebrand factor to rule out a clotting or coagulation disorder
2. Skeletal series of long bones in children under 2 years old, to identify old or hidden fractures
3. Radionucleotide bone scan, which may be an adjunct to skeletal series in evaluating old or hidden fractures

G **Sexual abuse**

1. Facts

a. Characteristics of both victims and perpetrators cross all demographic groups.

b. By age 18 years, up to one in three females (heightened risk in adolescence) and up to one in five males will become a victim.

c. Perpetrators of child sexual abuse are most often persons known to the child; it is only rarely a crime of strangers.

d. Physical signs and symptoms are not always present.

e. When signs and symptoms are present, they include vaginal discharge, abdominal pain, secondary enuresis, genital trauma and lesions, and pregnancy.

f. Associated behavioral signs and symptoms include sexualized behavior, excessive crying, sleep disturbances, aggression, school failure, and school avoidance.

g. Childhood sexual abuse is associated with an increased risk of developing posttraumatic stress disorder and other psychiatric disorders, and with subsequent substance abuse.

H Evaluation

1. History yielding suspicion should be obtained. The child and accompanying adult should be interviewed separately whenever possible. It is important to identify the child's language for the involved body parts and to use these words in interviewing the child. It is important to determine the following:
   - a. What type of contact took place (Is there a risk of sexually transmitted infection or pregnancy?)
   - b. The identity of the perpetrator and whether the perpetrator has ongoing access to the child
   - c. When the most recent occurrence took place—if within the past 72 hours, a modified rape evaluation may be performed for forensic purposes
2. For cases in which the history indicates a possibility of sexually transmitted infection, the physician should obtain the appropriate cultures from the appropriate orifices, and serum for rapid plasma reagin (RPR), HIV, and hepatitis testing.
3. When a special sexual abuse investigation program is available, referral to that program should be made immediately to complete the evaluation. This permits the child to be interviewed by a single, trained interviewer and for the physical examination to be done in a controlled circumstance that allows visual recording of the findings.

I Role of the physician for all cases of child maltreatment

1. In addition to the roles of interviewer and examiner, the physician is also a **"mandated reporter."** This means that the physician is required by law to notify the local child protection agency about any situation where the physician has a reasonable suspicion that a child has been harmed or is at risk of harm.
2. Additionally, the physician should utilize available resources to provide support for the child and family in question.
3. For cases of sexual abuse, it is vital to begin counseling as quickly as possible.
4. Primary prevention should be the goal of every physician. To reduce the risk of physical abuse and neglect, the physician should identify those families at high risk and refer to local parenting support programs.
5. Primary prevention of sexual abuse can occur at every health supervision visit, by educating parents about the need for vigilance, and by teaching children about their rights to privacy and personal integrity—"good touch, bad touch."

V FOSTER CARE

A Facts

1. In the United States, over 500,000 children are in foster placement at any given time.
2. Approximately one in four of them are eligible for and awaiting adoption.
3. Most children adopted from foster care are older than 4 years old.
4. About 50% of children spend at least 3 continuous years in foster placement before either reunification or adoption; about 25% spend at least 5 continuous years waiting.
5. The majority of children exiting foster care return to their birth parents.
6. Children who experience multiple successive foster placements, or who return to the biologic family and again to foster care, are more likely to experience functional disabilities in attachment and emotional development.

B Common health problems of children in foster care

Children entering the foster care system have usually suffered prolonged neglect, or repeated or severe physical or sexual abuse. They present a disproportionate array of mental, physical, and emotional health problems, as well as developmental delay. Some of the problems more commonly seen are as follows:

1. Anxiety/depression
2. Attachment disorders

3. Behavioral disorders
4. Chronic illness, poorly treated or controlled
5. Congenitally acquired infections (e.g., HIV)
6. Dental caries
7. Developmental delay
8. Direct effects of abuse (fractures, head trauma, sexually transmitted illnesses)
9. Effects of prenatal substance exposure (e.g., cocaine, opiates, alcohol)
10. Failure to thrive
11. Immunization delay

C Role of the physician Although the child welfare agency has legal responsibility for the removal and subsequent out-of-home placement of each child, the physician has a role in advising the legal system about the identification and treatment of each child's specific needs. This begins with a comprehensive assessment of the physical, developmental, emotional, and mental health of the child. Special needs that are identified should be explained, as well as the interventions necessary to meet them, including developmental services, specialty medical services, mental health care, and special nurturing needs. The physician may also advise on the extent and frequency of contact with the child's biologic family, including siblings and supportive relatives.

VI ADOPTION

A Background

1. Adoption of an infant or child is a varied experience. Each circumstance has its own set of legal issues, many of which are being actively debated and/or changed at any given time.
2. Adoptions may:
   a. Be "open" (biologic and adoptive parents known to each other) or "closed"
   b. Occur through:
      (1) The child welfare system
      (2) International contacts
      (3) Private persons or agencies
   c. Be sought by:
      (1) Stepparents
      (2) Single male or female parents
      (3) Heterosexual couples or same-sex couples
      (4) Married or unmarried couples

B Facts

1. In the United States, 1.5 million children are adopted.
2. Nearly half of those adoptions are by a stepparent.
3. International adoptions have doubled since 1990.
   a. Most of these children are infants.
   b. Most are female.
4. Children adopted as young infants have more successful transitions.
5. Most children adopted from foster care are over 4 years old.

C Common health problems of adoptees Children who are adopted through the child welfare system share the commonly seen health problems of foster children. Internationally adopted children may have additional risks associated with their place of origin, and with the effects of institutionalization. These incude:

1. Attachment disorders
2. Birth defects
3. Congenital infections (HIV, syphilis)

4. Delayed, absent, or unknown immunizations
5. Developmental delay
6. Hepatitis A, B, or C
7. Inadequate or absent past medical and family histories
8. Parasites
9. Prenatal substance exposure (fetal alcohol syndrome)
10. Sensory integration disorders
11. Tuberculosis

D Role of the physician In the preadoption period, the physician can help the family identify potential health risks and conditions. For international adoptions, it is especially important for the adoptive parent to gather as much information as possible while abroad, and the physician can offer direction about the type of information needed. After the adoption, the physician should schedule a visit with the newly formed family as soon as possible to identify specific health risks and needs, and to offer support. Adoption, while joyful, can also be stressful for the adoptee, the parent(s), and any other children already in the household. The physician should assist the entire family in recognizing and treating stress to accomplish a healthy transition. In the special circumstance of international adoption, the physician will need to become acquainted with the health risks of the population from which the child comes, and arrange for specific health, behavioral, and developmental screenings and interventions.

VII DIVORCE AND SEPARATION

A Facts

1. Divorce affects over 1 million children annually.
2. Nearly half of those children will not have subsequent contact with their father.
3. Nonmarried parental separation raises the number of children affected considerably.
4. Divorce and separation contribute significantly to childhood poverty.

B Effects of divorce and separation

1. Parental conflict leading up to separation produces tension in the household.
2. Separation subsequently occurs, not just from the departing parent, but often from a home, neighborhood, friends, school, and lifestyle. Parents, suffering through their own separation issues, may not be able to recognize or acknowledge these effects on their children.
3. A child's reaction to separation and divorce depends largely on his or her developmental level and temperament, as well as the coping success and mental health of the caregiver.
   a. **Infants and toddlers** may display irritability, heightened separation anxiety, and regression in development.
   b. **Preschoolers**, engaged in magical thinking, may also feel responsible for the discord.
   c. **School-aged children** may develop poor academic performance, become withdrawn or aggressive, and struggle with conflicted feelings of disloyalty to one or both parents.
   d. **Adolescents** may additionally seek to cope by becoming more autonomous, physically and emotionally, at an accelerated pace; consequent difficulty with substance abuse, premature or dysfunctional sexual relationships, and school and career planning may ensue.
   e. **Children of all ages** may present with psychosomatic complaints as signs of sadness and depression.

C Role of the physician At every health supervision visit, and whenever a psychosomatic origin to complaints is suspected, the physician should inquire about the child's relationships with all family members (including a nonmarried parent's "significant other") and about any stressors within or outside of the family. When discord is uncovered, the pediatrician should assess the current or potential effects on the child, based on the child's developmental level and emotional and temperamental status, and advise the parents accordingly. The physician facilitates the family's receiving counseling or therapy support as necessary. The physician may also offer the court an expert opinion on how the child's needs should be met.

VIII SCHOOL ISSUES

Children struggling with learning and behaving in school may have a variety of precipitants to these problems (see Chapter 4). Circumstances related to the social environment within and outside of school contribute to both learning and behavioral dysfunction.

A **School avoidance** can be due to:

1. Problems occurring at or on the way to school (bullying, community violence)
2. Unwillingness or fear of leaving home (parental illness, domestic violence)
3. Underlying psychiatric disorder (anxiety disorders, obsessive-compulsive behaviors)
4. Poor interactions with fellow students or teachers
5. Fear of failing an educational task

B **School avoidance may manifest** with physical symptoms such as headache and abdominal pain. These sensations may be real but exist as manifestations of underlying stress, or they may be invented. School avoidance can also be more overt, such as the child who simply refuses to leave the house, or who travels to school but then does not enter. Parents may or may not be aware of the latter.

C **Role of the physician**

1. School avoidance is essentially a stress-induced response to a life situation. A well-performed history and physical examination will usually suffice to determine that the child does not have a serious medical condition; if so, no additional testing is in order.
2. It is important that neither the physician, the parent, nor the school minimize the child's actual complaint. Rather, the physician should help the parent and school to understand that the child may really be experiencing symptoms, but those symptoms are not indicative of organic dysfunction. Parents can help the physician identify the child whose temperament increases his or her likelihood of a stress response to even minor concerns. A daily diary of the complaint will often illuminate a pattern of occurrence that can then be related to circumstances in the child's life, helping the patient, parent, school, and physician to better understand this complex phenomenon. Circumstances in every aspect of the child's life, and in every environment the child frequents, should be explored. Counseling may assist with identification of the child's concerns, and with helping the child develop healthy coping responses.

IX VIOLENCE

A **Background**

1. Violence exposure may occur in the home, school, or neighborhood environments; it is nearly pervasive in media. For children and youth, the experience of violence, whether as a victim or a perpetrator, is a more prevalent health risk than infectious disease, cancer, or congenital disorders.
2. Violence, whether experienced as a victim or as a witness (other than via media), has been associated with health risk behaviors such as:
   a. Increased and earlier substance use (tobacco, alcohol, and marijuana)
   b. A greater incidence of substance abuse
   c. Becoming sexually active at a younger age
   d. High-risk sexual behaviors (not using condoms, multiple partners)
   e. The concomitant risks of pregnancy and sexually transmitted infections
   f. Aggression
3. Adolescents who have experienced violence in several ways have the highest risk.
4. School-associated violence includes those acts of threatening, bullying, and physical attacks that occur within the school building, on the school grounds, and during travel to and from school.

Children and youth who have been victims of such violence, or those who have witnessed it, may exhibit school avoidance behaviors.

B Bullying

1. **Definition.** Bullying occurs when a person uses a position of power to humiliate, frighten, or cause harm to another person. It can take on physical aspects (actual or threatened physical injury), verbal aspects (teasing, insults, slurs), or social aspects (isolation, exclusion from activities).
2. **Facts**
   a. **About bullying**
      (1) U.S. Department of Justice statistics indicate an increase in reported incidents of bullying during the years 1999–2003, with the highest rates in the middle-school years. It is unclear if this reported increase reflects a heightened awareness of the problem (or reporting requirements) or an actual increase in events.
      (2) Bullying can lead to psychosomatic complaints in victims, and is associated with school avoidance.
      (3) Many of the most recent incidents of fatal school shootings have come at the hands of children who were bullied, seeking revenge.
   b. **About bullies**
      (1) Bullies tend to have difficulty with empathy, to frustrate more easily, to have difficulty following rules, and to have a positive attitude toward violence.
      (2) Students who are bullies are more likely to carry a weapon to school (as are their victims, to a lesser degree).
      (3) Children who are bullied at home, by a primary caretaker or other household member, or who witness violence in the home are more likely to become bullies.
   c. **About victims**
      (1) Children with an obvious disability, mental impairment, or physical flaw (short stature, obesity, dermatologic conditions) are at higher risk of becoming victims of bullies.
      (2) Children who are insecure or timid by nature may also be at higher risk, and are less likely to assert themselves the first time an incident occurs, leading to an increased likelihood of subsequent incidents.
      (3) Children who are victims of bullies often report being in frequent fights and may, in turn, become bullies to those who are younger or weaker.
      (4) Children who are chronic targets of bullying may become resentful and may themselves become violent.
3. **Role of the physician.** The physician has a role in identifying both the bully and the victim. Whenever risk factors such as disabilities, psychosomatic complaints, or school avoidance are reported, specific history should be obtained about bullying. At a routine health supervision visit, the physician should always inquire about home and school behavioral issues, perceived personal safety, and exposure to violence. Many states have enacted legislation to address the problem of school-based bullying. Physicians should be familiar with the legislation and policies in effect where they are practicing and establish a communication pathway with the school the child attends. Where no such protections exist, physicians should advocate for their development.

C Family/domestic/intimate partner violence

1. **Background.** Violence occurring within the home or within intimate relationships can take many forms. Verbal abuse, threats, intimidation, and actual physical violence can all be equally harmful to those victimized as well as to those witnessing it. Common terms used in describing such situations include **family violence, domestic violence,** and **intimate partner violence.**
2. **Facts**
   a. Exposure to domestic violence has been associated with bullying, aggression, and antisocial behavior in children.
   b. Children in such settings may also exhibit anxiety, depression, somatic complaints, sleep disorders, regressive behaviors, learning problems, and school avoidance.

c. More than 50% of homes where domestic violence occurs include children under 12 years of age; 30% to 60% of those children may become victims of child abuse.
d. Intimate partner violence in the parental relationship is a major risk factor for fatality from child abuse.
e. Risk factors for being in a violent intimate relationship include being a victim of abuse as a child, substance abuse (by victim or perpetrator), being divorced or separated, or being young.
f. The highest rates of intimate partner violence are experienced by young women, ages 16 to 24.

3. **Role of the physician.** Each health supervision visit should include an explicit inquiry as to the presence of domestic violence in the home. Questions might include: When disagreements occur at home, does anyone ever physically fight? Are you ever afraid? (Remember that intimidation through the threat of violence does not leave a physical mark.) Physicians should also include an assessment for intimate partner violence in their exploration of risks with adolescent patients. At each encounter, the physician should be alert to any associated behavioral and physical signs and symptoms exhibited by both the child and parent, and explore the possibility of domestic violence. As mandated reporters, physicians should notify Child Protective Services whenever ongoing domestic violence is reported as occurring in a household where children also live.

X MEDIA EXPOSURE

A Background Children between the ages of 2 and 18 years experience 4 to 6 hours of combined media input daily. This input includes television programming, movies and videos, computers, video and computer games, audio recordings, and print media. The content and influence of such media presence are important factors for physicians and parents to monitor.

B Facts

1. Children and youth who are heavy viewers of violent media often become desensitized to violence.
2. Violence depicted through media has been associated with an increased pattern of aggression and violence as a means of conflict resolution; such behaviors extend into adulthood.
3. This is especially true when the violence is perpetrated by a character with whom the child or youth identifies.
4. Other associated problems include depression, sleep disturbances such as nightmares, and posttraumatic stress disorder.
5. Sexual innuendo or inference is present even in "family hour" television at a rate of up to eight instances per hour. Few of these sexual references deal with abstinence, contraception, or the physical or emotional consequences of sex.
6. Exposure to sexual content in media has been associated with the initiation of intercourse at an earlier age.
7. Increased exposure to advertising for alcohol has been associated with adolescent drinking; the average teen in the United States sees approximately 2000 alcohol-related commercials per year.
8. Children and youth who watch more than 4 hours of television daily are five times more likely to initiate smoking than those who watch fewer than 2 hours daily.
9. Smoking in movies is a risk factor for adolescent smoking.
10. Each hour of television viewed daily at age 4 years increases the risk of subsequent bullying behavior.
11. Children and youth focused on body image in media may be at higher risk of developing eating disorders.
12. Excessive television viewing is associated with obesity.

C Role of the physician

1. Health supervision visits should include an assessment of media use and exposure. When excessive exposure is identified, an assessment of associated behaviors (fear, aggression, sleep disturbance) should be made. Conversely, when a patient presents with associated symptoms, the physician should inquire about media-related habits. For all patients, physicians should advise parents to:
   a. Limit screen time to 1 to 2 hours daily, with strong parental supervision of content

b. Keep all media located in a central, supervised area, and not in the child's bedroom
c. Know and understand the rating system for the media used by their children
d. Review and discuss media content with their children
e. Encourage non–media-related activities
f. Become "media literate"—that is, to understand the process and purpose of media and advertising, to recognize the potential effects of media, and to develop a plan to counteract undesired effects
g. Help their children to develop media literacy

2. On a community level, physicians can advocate for responsible media production, and clear and universal rating systems.

XI POVERTY

A Background Because of the complexity of the problem and the myriad ways in which it imposes limits on opportunities for improvement, living in poverty proves to be the strongest predictor of diminished health and well-being for children. Conversely, while poverty is associated with a lower standard of living, children living in poverty do not necessarily have a lower quality of life.

B Facts

1. Poverty is a risk factor for the following:
   a. Child abuse
   b. Adolescent pregnancy
   c. Low birth weight, prematurity
   d. Failure to thrive
   e. Violence victimization and exposure
   f. Chronic health problems
   g. School failure
   h. Depression
   i. Substance use and abuse
   j. Poor health outcomes
2. In general, families with children tend to be poorer than those without.
3. Women, adolescent parents (both sexes) and their children, and single-parent (usually women) households are also more likely to be poor.

C Adverse health issues

1. Access to health care or ability to adhere to a prescribed regimen may be limited by lack of insurance, or by high deductibles and required copayments. Transportation to appointments may be difficult to access or afford. Low literacy may contribute to parents and children being unable to follow directions about planned treatments.
2. Overcrowding in homes may contribute to chronic illness effects (e.g., asthma), to recurrent/recalcitrant infectious diseases, and to poor nutrition practices.
3. Behavior and mental health problems may be precipitated or exacerbated by stressful home situations, including unsafe neighborhoods, homelessness (including shelter housing), overcrowding, and lack of resources such as furniture and utilities.
4. A delay in seeking health care may lead to overutilization of emergency care, increased hospitalization, decreased immunization rates, and decreased utilization of early intervention services.

D Role of the physician

1. At each health supervision visit, the physician should inquire about the home situation, including household members, housing conditions, stressors, and supports. At every visit, the physician should inquire about barriers to accomplishing the plan of action. When a patient has missed one or more appointments, the physician or office should inquire about barriers to access at that time. For all circumstances, the physician or office should have knowledge of available support services and how to help patients connect to them. Whether supporting a family in

accessing transportation, in keeping utilities connected, in acquiring subsidized housing (i.e., Section 8, Housing Choice Voucher Program), or in adhering to a medical regimen, the physician can function as a strong individual patient and family advocate.

2. It is important to differentiate willful neglect of a child from that imposed by poverty. Child welfare agencies may be able to assist a family in crisis, but will not be able to resolve the long-term lack of resources. It is also important for the physician to recognize that those living in poverty may lack the stamina to identify and make initial contact with resources.
3. On a public policy level, the physician is uniquely positioned to articulate to the larger community the detrimental effects of poverty on children and families. Education of legislators, the judiciary, and the electorate is imperative to effecting change.

XII CHRONIC ILLNESS AND DISABILITY

A Background In addition to direct health effects, chronic illness and disability can greatly affect the accomplishment of normal social and emotional development in children and adolescents.

1. By limiting the time and/or scope of activities in which those afflicted are able to participate, chronic illness and disability limit opportunities for social interaction.
2. Children may feel isolated, lack self-confidence, or suffer poor self-image and self-esteem.
3. Adolescents normally develop a heightened concern about body image; this may be exaggerated with illness or disability.
4. Adolescents may choose to rebel by failing to comply with medication or other treatment regimens.
5. Adolescents may also have delayed achievement of independence, in part due to their own fear of assuming responsibility, but also in part due to the reluctance of their caretakers to relinquish responsibility.

B Role of the physician

1. Children with chronic illness or disability should receive coordinated primary care in a medical home setting. The primary care physician should learn the priorities of the child and family, and help them to make lifestyle decisions accordingly. Anticipating the social and emotional needs of the child/adolescent, as well as the ways in which the health problem will affect them, will allow the physician to guide the family to appropriate resources. The physician should work with the child's school to develop a program that suits the child's intellectual, physical, and social needs.
2. Children with chronic conditions require repeated education about the nature of the condition, with information consistent with their current developmental level. The physician should assess the child's understanding and readiness to assume responsibility for aspects of their own care. The physician should also work with the parents to effect this transition of responsibility.
3. The chronic illness of one family member affects all members of the family. The physician should be alert to stress, guilt, and diminished coping capacities in family members. Support services, including respite care, should be identified and families encouraged in their use.

XIII ADVOCACY

Advocacy is achieved on both an individual and a population basis, through individual encounters, through community-based interventions, and through the establishment of public policy. Examples of advocacy on various levels are summarized in Table 3-2.

A A physician advocates for an individual patient by identifying specific health risks and concerns, providing care, and connecting the patient to necessary resources.

B When a problem is pervasive within a population, or when the necessary resources are not available, the physician may advocate on a community basis by documenting the need and/or by working with others in the community to design and implement the intervention.

C When a broader societal change is necessary, the physician may bring the problem to the attention of policy makers, providing witness and expertise regarding the problem and possible solutions.

TABLE 3-2 Examples of Advocacy Occurring on Different Levels

Problem	Individual	Community Based	Public Policy
Asthma	Screening/diagnosis/treatment	Neighborhood and housing assessments Education	Insurance coverage for metered dose inhaler spacers and outreach
Violence	Risk assessment/identification/ counseling	Education Alternative activities	Legal consequences Gun control legislation
Motor vehicle accidents	Risk assessment/seat belt use	Driver education	Graduated licensing laws for teens
Media exposure	Risk assessment/parental supervision	Alternative activities "TV-free month"	Rating systems
Obesity	Risk assessment/nutrition counseling	Education After-school activities	Removal of unhealthy snacks from schools. Insurance coverage for weight loss and physical fitness programs
Poverty	Risk assessment/medication samples	Soup kitchen Food pantry	Food stamps/WIC Minimum wage increase

BIBLIOGRAPHY

American Academy of Pediatrics Committee on Early Childhood, Adoption and Dependent Care: Developmental issues for young children in foster care. *Pediatrics* 106(5):1145–1150, 2000.

Bethea L: Primary prevention of child abuse. *Am Fam Physician* 59(6):1577–1585, 1591–1592, 1999.

Block R, Krebs N, the American Academy of Pediatrics Committee on Child Abuse and Neglect and the American Academy of Pediatrics Committee on Nutrition: Failure to thrive as a manifestation of child neglect. *Pediatrics* 116(5):1234–1237, 2005.

Botash A: Foster care: health concerns of children in foster care. http://www.childabusemd.com/foster/health-concerns.shtml. Accessed February 16, 2007.

Brooks-Gunn J, Duncan GJ: The effects of poverty on children. *The Future of Children: Children and Poverty.* 7(2):55–71, 1997.

Child Welfare League of America: National fact sheet. http://www.cwla.org/advocacy/nationalfactsheet06.htm. Accessed February 16, 2007.

Christian CW: Assessment and evaluation of the physically abused child. *Clin Fam Pract* 5(1):47–56, 2003.

The Evan B. Donaldson Adoption Institute: Foster care facts. http://www.adoptioninstitute.org/FactOverview/foster.html. Accessed February 16, 2007.

Goodman P: The relationship between intimate partner violence and other forms of family and societal violence. *Emerg Med Clin North Am* 24:889–903, 2006.

Grube JW, Waiters E: Alcohol in the media: content and effects on drinking beliefs and behaviors among youth. *Adolesc Med Clin* 16:327–343, 2005.

Hogan MJ: Adolescents and media violence: six crucial issues for practitioners. *Adolesc Med Clin* 16:249–268, 2005.

Lyznicki JM, McCaffree M, Robinowitz CB: Childhood bullying: implications for physicians. *Am Fam Physician* 70(9):1723–1728, 2004.

McDonald KC: Child abuse: approach and management. *Am Fam Physician* 75(2):221–228, 2007.

Schulte E, Springer S: Health care in the first year after international adoptions. *Pediatr Clin North Am* 52:1331–1349, 2005.

Strasburger VC: Adolescents, sex, and the media: ooooo, baby, baby—a Q & A. *Adolesc Med Clin* 16:269–288, 2005.

Strasburger VC: Risky business: what primary care practitioners need to know about the influence of the media on adolescents. *Primary Care Clin Office Pract* 33:317–348, 2006.

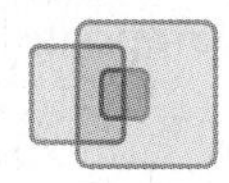

Study Questions

Directions: *Each of the numbered items or incomplete statements in this section is followed by answers or completions of the statement. Select the ONE lettered answer or completion that is BEST in each case.*

1. A 4-year-old boy is brought to the office with symptoms of gastroenteritis. As the physician is examining him, he has a bout of diarrhea. Once his mother removes his soiled clothes, the physician notes linear bruises on his posterior thighs and a loop mark on his abdomen. Which of the following is the appropriate management for the physician to comply with the legal requirement as a mandated reporter?

- A Interview all caretakers to determine how these injuries may have occurred
- B Admit the child to the hospital to ensure his safety
- C Perform clotting studies to determine whether the child bruises easily
- D Ask the mother to bring her other children in for evaluation
- E Report a reasonable suspicion of child abuse to Child Protective Services

2. You are called in for a consultation by an emergency department physician at your local community hospital. He is seeing an 18-month-old boy, brought in by both parents. They report that he tripped on a throw rug and fell. A radiograph of his leg reveals a spiral fracture of the femur. He would like your advice as to what other evaluations he should perform. Which of the following is the most appropriate study for the emergency department physician to order to further evaluate this child?

- A PT, PTT
- B Platelets
- C CT scan of the head
- D Skeletal series of the long bones
- E Genetic testing for osteogenesis imperfecta

3. A mother presents to the office with her 5-month-old son. She reports being a bit stressed as she has been the sole caretaker for the child during the past 2 weeks while her husband has been away on a business trip. The baby has a purple mark that resembles a bruise on his left leg. The mother reports that he fell while crawling up the stairs 4 days ago. Which of the following elements of history or physical examination most confirms that you should be suspicious that this child's injury is consistent with child abuse?

- A A bruise that is 4 days old should be yellow/green in color
- B Mothers are the most common perpetrators of child abuse
- C A typical 5-month-old is unable to crawl
- D The child should not have had access to stairs
- E The mother has been the sole caretaker for her son in the past 2 weeks

4. A 15-month-old girl who had been growing and gaining weight steadily was not brought in for her 9-month or 12-month visits. At her 15-month visit, a significant weight loss is noted, but she has maintained adequate linear growth. No specific organic cause is indicated by history or physical examination. Which of the following is the most appropriate next step in management?

- A Hospital admission for observation and medical evaluation
- B Extensive outpatient laboratory investigation
- C High-calorie diet with outpatient weight check in 1 week
- D Referral to a pediatric gastroenterologist
- E Referral of the family for home-based nutrition and social service evaluation

5. In early fall, an 8-year-old boy presents to your office complaining of abdominal pain for the past 3 weeks. It occurs most mornings, and is gone by noon. It does not seem to have affected his appetite, and there is no association with particular foods or meals. There is no associated nausea, vomiting, diarrhea, or constipation. He has missed or been late for school six times because of this pain. His weight is tracking and his physical examination is entirely normal. Which of the following is the most appropriate next step in his assessment?

- A Request a daily log of symptoms, diet, and activities
- B Order stool for *Helicobacter pylori* antigen
- C Order serum for gliadin antibody
- D Order a complete blood count with erythrocyte sedimentation rate
- E Obtain stool for ova and parasites

6. A 7-year-old boy is brought in by his mother for a health supervision visit. He's doing well in the first grade and has had no behavior problems in the past. His mother expresses concern that he has become very aggressive toward his younger brother since starting school. Which of the following is the MOST LIKELY cause of this child's new onset of aggressive behavior toward his younger sibling?

- A He is developing a conduct disorder
- B He has attention deficit hyperactivity disorder (ADHD)
- C He has a learning disability
- D He is being bullied at school
- E He has sibling rivalry

7. A 6-year-old girl is brought in by her mother for a 2-day history of vaginal discharge. There is no history of dysuria, contact irritant exposure, or known trauma. The child nods when asked if she was touched in the genital area. Which of the following is the most appropriate next step for evaluation/management by the physician?

- A Call Child Protective Services
- B Call the local sexual abuse evaluation center
- C Obtain further history (Who? When? Where?)
- D Perform a genital exam
- E Perform a complete physical exam

8. You receive a call from the emergency department about one of your patients, a 17-year-old boy who has presented with "bizarre behavior." The emergency department toxicology screen is positive for methamphetamine. You realize this is the third such call you've received about patients in your practice during the past 4 months. What of the following is your most effective response?

- A Refer the teens for drug counseling/rehabilitation
- B Obtain permission from the teens to discuss the problem with their parents
- C Contact the police to advise them of the local methamphetamine problem
- D Contact the local middle and high schools about developing a drug resistance program
- E Include a question about drug use in your health supervision visits

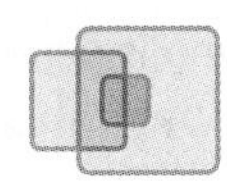

Answers and Explanations

1. The answer is E (*IV I*). In every patient encounter, the physician is responsible for obtaining a clear, detailed history. When a child presents with unexplained bruising, the history includes an inquiry as to how the injuries occurred, which may necessitate speaking with several different individuals. When bruises may have been acquired accidentally, the physician may choose to perform clotting studies to determine if the child has a clotting disorder. In this case, however, since the child has linear bruises and loop marks, the injury is clearly nonaccidental. The physician working with limited information in the clinical setting cannot be certain about the child's safety once that child has left this setting. As a mandated reporter, the physician is obligated to notify the appropriate legal body, usually Child Protective Services, of the reasonable suspicion of inflicted injury in this child. Child Protective Services will then perform a home assessment, and evaluate the child, siblings, caretakers, and the environment, to best ensure the safety of minors in the household.

2. The answer is D (*IV F 2*). A spiral fracture of a large bone such as the femur or humerus is generally pathognomonic for child abuse, as a young child cannot generate enough torque force to produce this type of injury accidentally. Therefore, the physician in this case should have a strong suspicion that this is an inflicted injury. When these types of skeletal injuries occur in very young children, who have limited or no verbal ability, or who simply cannot recall a prior injury, a full skeletal series of all long bones is recommended, which seeks evidence of other, perhaps prior, older, fractures. A radionucleotide bone scan may serve as an adjunct study, as it may demonstrate residual remodeling that is not visible on a plain radiography. Clotting studies are appropriate when investigating unexplained bruising, but not for fractures. A cranial CT scan is not indicated unless there are neurologic concerns. Osteogenesis imperfecta can present with unexplained fractures, but does not present with spiral fractures.

3. The answer is C (*IV C 4*). A physician should be alert to the possibility of child abuse when there is a discrepancy in the history reported for the injury. Such discrepancies may occur between two persons' reports, between reports from the same person provided at different times, between the appearance of the injury and the history, or between the child's developmental capabilities and the history. In this case, the most concerning aspect of the history is the attribution of advanced developmental capability (crawling) to a 5-month-old infant. Anyone under significant stress may become a perpetrator of abuse, women as well as men. The time an injury occurred cannot be determined by the color of the bruise; the color is determined by a wide a variety of factors, including the patient's age and skin condition and the force applied.

4. The answer is E (*II, III D 4*). This child is failing to thrive. In the absence of significant findings in the history or physical examination, the likelihood of an organic cause is minimal; therefore, neither extensive laboratory evaluation nor referral to medical specialty services is in order. The most helpful information in such a situation is likely to come from psychological evaluation of the caregiver and child, and an assessment of the home. Hospitalization for observation and intervention may eventually be necessary, but should only be considered in severe or recalcitrant cases. A high-calorie diet may well be implemented, but when a family has already demonstrated a failure to attend scheduled health care visits, "close outpatient follow-up" should not be the foundation of the care plan.

5. The answer is A (*VIII A–C, IX B*). Psychosomatic symptoms, such as recurrent abdominal pain, are genuine sensations not attributable to organic causes. In children, such symptoms are frequently seen as part of a pattern of avoidance behavior, such as school avoidance. In a well-appearing child with no concerning findings in the history or physical examination, an organic cause of disease is unlikely, and laboratory evaluation may be postponed. A prospective history of symptoms, with additional recording of daily events, can yield information that is helpful to both patient and physician. When school avoidance is suspected, the physician should explore concerns within the home environment, such as domestic violence or parental illness; within the school environment, such as performance anxiety or bullying; or in the transition between home and school, such as community violence.

6. The answer is D (*IX B*). Children who are bullied often cope by themselves becoming bullies to those who are younger or weaker than they are. A child who displayed no evidence of ADHD symptoms before age 7 years will not meet the criteria for this diagnosis. A learning disability is unlikely in a child who is performing well in school. A child with a conduct disorder is unlikely to have symptoms only in the home setting. Sibling rivalry may never totally resolve, but is far less likely in a child of 7 years than in a toddler.

7. The answer is C (*IV H*). The physician should ascertain information about the nature of the contact and the time of the last contact. For protection purposes, the physician should also inquire about the identity of the alleged perpetrator and the access that person has to the child. When this information is obtained, it should be forwarded immediately to Child Protective Services. A child who presents with a history of possible sexual abuse should undergo both a forensic interview and a forensic physical examination. Sexual abuse evaluation centers offer trained professionals to conduct these types of histories and physical examinations, and should be utilized whenever available. However, the timing of the forensic evaluation may be driven by the likelihood of recovery of physical evidence. If the sexual contact has occurred within the prior 72 hours, the forensic evaluation should take place immediately, as physical evidence may be recovered. Laboratory testing for sexually transmitted infections is not indicated unless there has been contact between adult genitalia and the child. If a sexual abuse evaluation service is not available, the physician may conduct the physical examination of the child; in this circumstance, a full physical examination should be conducted. This may alleviate some anxiety in the child who has had such complete physicals in the past, and also allows the physician to identify other signs of trauma.

8. The answer is D (*XIII*). The physician should always assess individual risk and should always play the role of advocate for each individual patient. But when a problem becomes pervasive within the community, the physician should seek a community-based solution or public policy intervention. In the case of substance abuse, where public policy mandates already exist, the most effective solution is likely to be a community-based education intervention. Working with professionals from other disciplines, the physician can identify the population at highest risk, the most effective time and venue for intervention, and the type of educational technique that is most likely to be effective.

chapter **4**

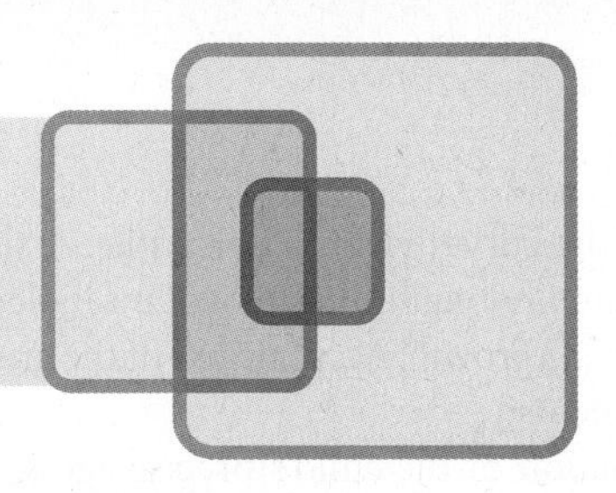

Growth, Developmental Disorders, and Behavioral Problems

FREDERICK J. BOGIN

I INTRODUCTION

The foundation of pediatric care rests on the monitoring and promotion of healthy growth, development, and behavior. This chapter will provide an overview of normal growth and development, common behavioral themes, and the approach to detecting significant deviations in any of these three areas.

II GROWTH

A Normal patterns

1. **Birth.** At birth, the final outcome of intrauterine growth can be assessed by plotting weight, length, and head circumference (HC) on a standard newborn growth curve. The growth plot places the newborn in one of three categories:
   a. **Appropriate for gestational age (AGA)** defined as birth weight between 10% and 90% for gestational age. Length and HC should also plot in this "normal range" on the corresponding curves.
   b. **Small for gestational age (SGA)** babies fall below the 10th percentile. It is informative to note whether HC is normal while weight alone (or weight and length) are below the 10th percentile. This pattern of growth restriction (normal HC, low weight) is referred to as **asymmetric** and reflects milder prenatal insults of shorter duration. This is in contrast to **symmetric** growth restriction, in which all three parameters plot below the 10th percentile, suggesting a more long-term or severe insult (e.g., intrauterine infection occurring early in the pregnancy).
   c. **Large for gestational age (LGA)** babies plot above the 90th percentile. The birth of an LGA baby should alert one to the possibility of gestational diabetes (with attendant risk for neonatal hypoglycemia) (see Chapter 6).
   d. **Newborns** routinely lose weight (as much as 10% of birth weight) for the first 2 to 3 days of life. Term newborns are expected to regain their birth weight by 10 to 14 days of life. Return to birth weight typically takes longer in premature infants.
2. **Growth curves**
   a. The key to monitoring growth and detecting deviations from normal is the regular, longitudinal plotting of growth points (routinely done at well-child visits) (see Chapter 1) on the appropriate age- and gender-specific growth curve. A 2000 revision of the growth curves from the National Center for Health Statistics (NCHS) is utilized. These curves can be viewed and printed on the Centers for Disease Control and Prevention (CDC) Web site (www.cdc.gov). The following curves are available:
      (1) **Birth to 36 months:** Weight, length, HC, and a curve plotting weight for height
      (2) **2 to 20 years:** Height, weight, weight for height, and body mass index (BMI)
      (3) Special growth curves exist for children with **Down syndrome, Turner syndrome,** and **achondroplasia** (see Chapter 8).

b. Each growth point on the curves yields a percentile. A single growth point is a "snapshot" of growth at one point in time. A longitudinal plot of multiple growth points over time yields a more complete picture of a child's growth. Accurate use of the growth curves depends on the following:
   (1) Accurate measurement
   (2) Accurate determination of the child's precise age (e.g., a child presenting for the 2-year health supervision visit may be 27 months of age and must be plotted accordingly). When plotting growth of children born prematurely, one should correct for prematurity (i.e., subtract the number of weeks prior to full term [40] from the chronologic age, then plot) until 18 months of age for HC, 24 months for weight, and 40 months for height.

3. **Infancy:** The first 12 months of life
   a. **Weight.** The infant is weighed naked or wearing only a diaper.
      (1) In the first 3 months of life, babies gain an average of approximately 1 ounce (30 grams) per day.
      (2) This drops to an average of 17 to 18 grams per day in months 3 to 6.
      (3) Average weight gain from the 6th to 12th months ranges from 9 to 13 grams per day.
      (4) Infants typically **double** their birth weight by 5 months of age and **triple** it by 1 year.
   b. **Length**
      (1) Length is measured in the recumbent position until 2 years of age.
      (2) Infants grow approximately 10 inches in the first year of life.
   c. **Head circumference.** This is obtained by carefully measuring the largest fronto-occipital diameter and plotting it on the NCHS Birth to 36 Month curves.
      (1) The average HC at birth is 35 cm.
      (2) The approximate rate of head growth is:
         (a) 2 cm per month for the first 3 months
         (b) 1 cm per month for months 4 to 6
         (c) 0.5 cm per month for months 6 to 12
      (3) HC reflects **brain growth** in the normal infant.
      (4) **Microcephaly** is defined as HC > 2 standard deviations (SDs) (some authorities say 3 SDs) below the mean for age. In the newborn, this generally reflects abnormal growth due to genetic, infectious, or teratogenic forces. It is often, but not always, associated with developmental delay.
      (5) **Macrocephaly** is defined as HC > 2 SD above the mean for age on the standard curve. It is important to determine HC of both parents in order to interpret this finding. A common etiology is benign familial macrocephaly. However, one must also consider the possibility of pathologic conditions such as hydrocephalus.
      (6) HC should be measured and plotted on the standard curve at each well-child visit until 18 to 24 months of age.

4. **Toddler** growth
   a. A common parental concern in the second year of life is expressed as, "He/she just doesn't eat anything!" This phenomenon can be understood in the context of two principles of toddler growth and development:
      (1) The **rate of growth** in the second year of life is dramatically slower than that seen in the first 12 months of life. Average weight gain in the first year is approximately 14 lbs (6.3 kg) versus an average gain of roughly 5 lbs (2.3 kg) from 12 to 24 months. Length typically increases by 10 inches (25.4 cm) during the first year, which is double the growth rate seen in the second year.
      (2) A principal developmental theme of the second year of life, the drive for **autonomy,** often manifests in parent-child struggles over eating. Toddlers have final say over what food does or does not enter their mouths!

5. **Growth** in **preschool** and **school-aged** children
   a. The key to monitoring the growth of children ages 3 years and older is proper use of the NCHS growth curves.
   b. **Weight.** From age 2 years to puberty, there is a progressive increase in the rate of weight gain in normally growing children, as follows:
      (1) **Preschoolers** gain approximately 2 kg per year.
      (2) **Early school-aged** children approach 3 kg per year.
      (3) **Children ages 9 to 12 years** gain in the range of 4 kg per year.

c. **Height**
   (1) **Preschoolers'** height growth is approximately 3 inches per year.
   (2) From **early school age** to **puberty,** the rate drops to approximately 2 inches per year.
   (3) The longitudinal plotting of height on the NCHS growth curve will reflect any significant deviation from normal growth patterns. After 2 years of age, height percentiles should be fairly consistent. In the first 12 to 15 months of life, one can see growth points crossing several major percentiles due to **genetic channeling.** This normal phenomenon represents the "equilibration" from birth size (which is not related to parental size) to anticipated height, which is genetically determined.
   (4) Simple formulas for predicting ultimate height are:
      (a) For **boys:** (mother's height + 5 inches [13 cm] + father's height)/2
      (b) For **girls:** (mother's height + father's height − 5 inches [13 cm])/2

B Abnormal growth patterns

1. **Failure to thrive** (see Chapter 3).
   a. A not uncommon problem encountered in pediatric practice, particularly during the first 2 to 3 years of life, is inadequate growth. There is no universally agreed upon definition of failure to thrive, but two commonly used parameters are weight below the fifth percentile on the NCHS curves, or weight dropping across two percentiles (e.g., from 50% to below 10%). Children with height and weight below the fifth percentile may have nutritional, genetic, or endocrine causes for their small size, whereas children with normal height but inadequate weight gain are not receiving or absorbing adequate calories/nutrition to meet their requirements for normal growth.
   b. The **differential diagnosis** for failure to thrive is extensive, including organic and psychosocial factors (see Chapter 3).
2. **Short stature**
   a. **Genetic (familial) short stature.** In children with familial short stature, one or both parents are short, growth in the early years is normal, puberty is not delayed, bone age is normal (see below), pubertal growth is in the lower end of the normal range, and adult height is short.
   b. **Constitutional delay in growth.** In this condition, growth rate is often diminished in the first 2 years of life, bone age is delayed, onset of puberty is delayed, and often one or both parents had delayed puberty (see Chapter 17). Growth continues past an age where most peers have stopped growing and ultimate height can be in a normal range (consistent with midparental height).
   c. Constitutional delay and familial short stature are considered variants of normal growth and represent the most common causes of short stature after the first 2 years of life.
   d. **Bone age** is determined from a radiograph of the **left hand and wrist** interpreted according to an atlas compiled by Greulich and Pyle. The bone age is particularly helpful in distinguishing familial short stature from constitutional delay as well as pathologic causes of short stature including hypothyroidism, growth hormone deficiency, or chronic disease (e.g., inflammatory bowel disease) (see Chapter 17).
3. **Obesity.** Obesity is the most prevalent nutritional disorder in children in the United States. In two decades, the prevalence has doubled in 6- to 11-year-olds and tripled in adolescents. Approximately one third of American children are either overweight or at risk of becoming overweight.
   a. The 0- to 36-month growth curves include a plot of weight for height. In this age group one can identify **overweight** as children plotting above the 95th percentile mark on the weight for height curve.
   b. From age 2 to 20 years, the most commonly employed tool to detect overweight/obesity is the use of the **BMI.** BMI is derived from the body weight divided by the height squared.
      (1) BMI calculators are available online. BMI calculation "wheels" are also available. Unlike adults, in children the BMI must be interpreted as a percentile.
      (2) Once the BMI is determined, it is plotted at the appropriate percentile for age and gender.
      (3) There exists some difference of opinion regarding terminology:
         (a) The CDC defines children with BMIs between 85% and 95% as **at risk for overweight** and > 95% as **overweight.**
         (b) The Institute of Medicine considers 85% to 95% as overweight and > 95% as **obese.**
         (c) Many prefer to drop the term obese because they feel that it is demeaning.

(d) The key point is that children with a BMI > 85% are **at risk** and should be managed accordingly (see Chapter 17).

III DEVELOPMENTAL DISORDERS

A Overview Monitoring development is best accomplished through a longitudinal process described as **developmental surveillance** (see Chapter 1). Developmental milestones and themes of normal child development are reviewed in Chapter 1. In this chapter, we review some of the major conditions impacting development and learning.

B Specific developmental disabilities

1. **Developmental delay.** A challenge for child health supervision is the early identification of children with significant developmental delay (see Chapter 1). An excellent way to facilitate that process is by beginning a visit with the question, "Do you have any concerns about how your child is developing, learning, or behaving?" Parental concerns must always be taken seriously. Additional "red flags" regarding development can arise from the process of developmental surveillance/screening. A child may experience delays in one or multiple developmental domains. Parent opinions and concerns may be efficiently and effectively solicited through the use of tools such as the Ages and Stages Questionnaires and the Parents Evaluation of Developmental Status (PEDS).
   a. **Language delay**
      (1) Speech-language delays are the most common form of developmental delay in children (affecting as many as 10% of preschool children).
      (2) Language ability correlates well with cognitive development.
      (3) Underlying conditions resulting in delayed speech and/or language include hearing loss, global developmental delay/mental retardation (MR), autism spectrum disorders, developmental language disorder, and environmental deprivation.
      (4) **Absence** of the following language "benchmarks" indicates the need for further evaluation:
         (a) Responsive cooing (by 4–6 months)
         (b) Consonant sounds (e.g., bababa, gagaga) and turns when name called (by 9 months)
         (c) Jargon (babbling with intonation), points at objects, and follows one-step commands (by 12 months)
         (d) Five words plus jargon (by 18 months)
         (e) Rapid growth of vocabulary, beginning of two-word phrases, points at pictures in a book, and follows two-step commands (by 2 years)
         (f) Three-word phrases, small sentences, and knows one color (by 3 years)
         (g) Uses pronouns and speech fully understandable by a stranger (by 4 years)
      (5) All children with suspected speech-language delays **must** have formal hearing **(audiologic)** evaluation.
   b. **Motor delay.** Indications for further motor evaluation include:
      (1) Rolling over before 3 months
      (2) Poor head control at 3 months
      (3) Persistent primitive reflexes (see Chapters 1 and 18) after 6 months
      (4) Not sitting independently by 7 months
      (5) Lack of parachute response by 12 months
      (6) Hand dominance established before 18 months
   c. **Global developmental delay.** Children with delays in all developmental domains may ultimately be diagnosed with mental retardation. However, before the age of 5 years, the term *developmental delay* is generally used to indicate current level of functioning, as opposed to predicting future performance. In evaluating children, it is always most useful to describe current strengths and concerns and determine appropriate intervention. Predicting future function during early childhood is generally not reliable or helpful.

2. **Cerebral palsy** is a disorder of movement and posture caused by a defect or lesion in the brain (see Chapter 18).

3. **Autism spectrum disorder (ASD)**
   a. **Definition**
      (1) Autism spectrum disorders are characterized by profound impairment in social interaction (e.g., lack of eye contact, poor peer relationships); restricted, repetitive, and stereotyped

patterns of behavior (e.g., unusual preoccupations, inflexibility, stereotyped motor movements); and altered communication (verbal and nonverbal) ranging from no speech to jargon, echolalia, and "pedantic speech."

(2) **Clinical subtypes**

(a) **Autism**—as defined above

(b) **Asperger syndrome.** Children who have this disorder meet criteria for ASD but are said to have normal cognition and language, although they often have difficulty with the social aspects of language (pragmatics).

(c) **Pervasive developmental disorder-not otherwise specified** (PDD-NOS). Children are given this diagnosis if they meet many but not all the criteria for autism. Currently, the term *autism spectrum disorder* is preferred by many clinicians.

b. Etiology. Autism is recognized as a **neurobiologic disorder.** It may be associated with specific genetic disorders (e.g., Fragile X syndrome), prenatal insults (e.g., congenital rubella), and central nervous system (CNS) structural abnormalities (e.g., agenesis of the corpus callosum). Genetic factors clearly play a role (as demonstrated by twin studies). However, the majority of cases have no identifiable etiology.

c. Assessment

(1) Children with impaired language/communication should be screened for problems in social interaction (e.g., poor eye contact, lack of joint attention, preference for solitary activity, lack of pointing to objects, failure to show objects to adults) and restricted interests and play (e.g., lack of symbolic play at 18 months, lack of imitation, perseverative activities).

(2) Screening tools such as the **Modified Checklist for Autism in Toddlers (M-CHAT)** are an excellent aide to early identification. Children suspected of ASD on the M-CHAT or by parent/provider concerns should be referred to an appropriate resource for a full evaluation. Children suspected of possible ASD should be referred as close to 18 months of age as possible.

(3) All children with possible ASD should have a formal **audiologic** evaluation.

(4) Differential diagnosis of ASD includes global developmental delay/mental retardation, hearing loss, developmental language disorder, Landau-Kleffner syndrome (rare), and severe social-emotional deprivation.

(5) Laboratory evaluation should include DNA testing for Fragile X and routine chromosome analysis. Other laboratory (e.g., metabolic testing) or imaging studies should only be done if indicated by findings on history or physical exam.

4. Mental retardation

a. Definition. Mental retardation is defined as significantly subaverage intellectual functioning existing concurrently with deficits in adaptive behavior (e.g., communication, self-care, self-direction) and manifested during the developmental period (i.e., before age 18 years).

b. Incidence. Between 1.5% and 3% of the population is affected.

c. Classification. Four subgroups of retardation have been designated.

(1) **Mild—IQ levels of 55 to 70** (2–3 SDs below the mean of 100). This group represents 80% of the retarded population. As adults, these people are able to live independently, marry, and be employed, and they have functional reading and writing skills. Their major deficits are in judgment.

(2) **Moderate—IQ levels of 40 to 55** (3–4 SDs below the mean). This group represents 12% of the retarded population. These people do not necessarily require custodial care, but they do require continuous supervision and economic support. They are capable of self-care and employment in a sheltered setting.

(3) **Severe—IQ levels of 25 to 40** (4–5 SDs below the mean). This group represents approximately 7% of the retarded population. These people are totally economically dependent and require close supervision. They may acquire language and can be trained in elementary self-care skills.

(4) **Profound—IQ levels of < 25.** This group represents 1% of the retarded population. These people have limited communication and self-care skills and often have associated complex medical needs. They require a highly structured environment, with continuous care and supervision.

d. A more recent system of classification has moved beyond the traditional classification based solely on IQ and utilizes the categories of **intermittent, limited, extensive,** or **pervasive** to reflect the level of services and supports required by an individual with mental retardation. A newer, preferred term for mental retardation is **cognitive-adaptive disabilities.**

e. Etiology. The conditions associated with mental retardation are varied and represent a wide variety of biologic and environmental factors. Only a minority of cases of mental retardation can be attributed to known biologic factors. Mild retardation is more prevalent among lower socioeconomic groups and is rarely explained by biologic causes. Moderate and severe retardation are more evenly distributed throughout all socioeconomic groups and more frequently tend to have a biologic explanation.

f. Assessment

(1) History. The family's pedigree and details of pregnancy, delivery, and the immediate postnatal period are critical.

(2) Physical examination. Attention should be given to the head circumference, dysmorphic features and associated anomalies that might suggest a syndrome (see Chapter 8), and the neurologic exam (see Chapter 18).

(3) Diagnostic testing. The diagnosis of mental retardation can be made only with the use of standardized psychometric testing administered by a qualified examiner. Testing includes both measures of intellectual function (e.g., Wechsler Intelligence Scale for Children [WISC]) and measures of adaptive function (e.g., Vineland Adaptive Behavior Scale). Diagnosis cannot be made with screening instruments, and it rarely is made in young children below 5 years of age because of the lack of stability of the test scores. Medical evaluation of children with cognitive-adaptive disabilities includes hearing and vision testing, routine chromosome analysis, and DNA testing for Fragile X syndrome. Magnetic resonance imaging (MRI), metabolic studies, and newer genetic tests (e.g., fluorescence in situ hybridization [FISH] studies) should be performed when suggested by history or physical examination.

5. Learning Disabilities

a. Definition

(1) As defined by federal legislation, the term ***learning disabilities*** refers to a heterogeneous group of disorders manifest by significant difficulties in the acquisition and use of listening, speaking, reading, writing, reasoning, or mathematical abilities. These disorders are intrinsic to the individual and presumed to be due to central nervous system dysfunction. Even though a learning disability may occur concomitantly with other handicapping conditions or environmental influences, it is not the direct result of these conditions or influences.

(2) This definition is based on a recognized discrepancy between a child's academic performance and potential. This discrepancy is presumed to be secondary to subtle central nervous system dysfunction or subtle human variation.

(3) These disabilities can be described by reference to the **academic function** they affect (e.g., dyslexia for difficulty reading, spelling, and/or writing) or by the **psychological process** that is weak (e.g., deficits in auditory processing, visual-motor integration, sequential memory, or higher-order cognitive [executive] function).

(4) Learning disabilities are found in 3% to 15% of school-age children.

b. Assessment

(1) History. Elements of the history should include:

(a) A review of the past medical history looking for **risk factors** (e.g., pre- or perinatal insults, CNS infection, seizures, or trauma)

(b) History of other family members with learning problems

(c) A review of school functioning

(2) Physical examination

(a) Hearing and vision should be screened.

(b) Evidence of possible genetic syndromes (e.g., dysmorphic features), markers of neurocutaneous disorders (e.g., café au lait spots for neurofibromatosis [see Chapter 18]) and the presence or absence of "hard" neurologic findings (e.g., spasticity) are noted.

(c) Ears are checked for evidence of middle ear disease and head circumference is measured and plotted looking for macrocephaly or microcephaly.

(3) Laboratory investigation is not called for unless there is a specific suggestion on history or physical exam. Imaging studies (computed tomography [CT] or MRI) and electroencephalography (EEG) also require a specific indication.

TABLE 4-1 Selected Symptoms Associated with Attention Deficit Hyperactivity Disorder

Symptoms Associated with Inattention
- Often makes careless mistakes
- Problems sustaining attention in school and at play
- Problems with organization and forgetfulness
- Lack of follow-through on schoolwork and chores
- Easily distracted

Symptoms Associated with Hyperactivity/Impulsivity
- Often fidgets, squirms, or is out of seat
- Often "on the go" and frequently running
- Excessive talking
- Often blurts out answers or interrupts others
- Problems awaiting a turn

Adapted from the *Diagnostic and Statistical Manual of Mental Disorders*, 4th ed. Washington, DC, American Psychiatric Association, 1994.

(4) **Psychoeducational assessment** includes a battery of tests of intellectual functioning (IQ tests) as well as specific academic tests to profile a child's strengths and weaknesses. Usually these tests are performed by the public schools, which are mandated to test the child under the Individuals with Disabilities Education Act (Public Law 101-476, IDEA, 1990). The psychoeducational profile is the basis on which an individualized educational plan is constructed. Amendments to IDEA extend the mandate for special education assessment to the 3- to 5-year-old age group.

6. **Attention deficit hyperactivity disorder (ADHD)** (Table 4-1)

a. **ADHD** is a behavioral syndrome characterized by inadequate attention span, impulsivity, and hyperactivity. The syndrome gives rise to challenges in academic performance, behavior, and social functioning. Diagnostic criteria for ADHD are outlined in the *Diagnostic and Statistical Manual of Mental Disorders,* 4th ed. *(DSM-IV).* Incidence figures suggest that 4% to 6% of U.S. children may be affected, which makes ADHD the most common disorder of school-age children. Boys are affected more frequently than girls.

b. **Assessment**

(1) **History.** Essentials of the history include:

(a) History of medical "risk factors" for CNS insult

(b) Child's early temperament

(c) Detailed preschool and school history

(d) Family history of attention/activity problems, learning difficulties, psychiatric history, and history of substance abuse

(e) Early childhood history looking for evidence of hyperactivity (e.g., precocious gross motor milestones)

(2) **Physical examination.** Behavioral observations of the child during the physical examination should be cautiously interpreted, because anxiety may increase or decrease inattention/hyperactivity. The same components of the physical and neurologic exam as outlined in the learning disabilities section (*5 b 2* above) are pertinent.

(3) **Hearing and vision assessment**

(4) **Behavioral observation** (e.g., parent and teacher measures such as the Vanderbilt Assessment Scales or Conners' Rating Scales). Communication with parents, teachers, and other observers of the child is essential, as the diagnosis of ADHD requires that the symptoms be present in more than one setting.

c. **Differential diagnosis.** A number of different factors or conditions can give rise to the symptomatology of ADHD. These include:

(1) Hearing loss

(2) Cognitive limitations (e.g., mild MR or "slow learner")

(3) Learning disabilities. These can coexist with ADHD, but frustration in school due to undetected or untreated learning problems can cause secondary inattention and/or hyperactivity.

(4) Psychiatric issues (e.g., anxiety, depression, bipolar disorder, posttraumatic stress disorder [PTSD])
(5) Toxins such as lead poisoning (see Chapter 2)
(6) Family-social stresses such as chronic chaos in the home (see Chapter 3)
(7) Temperament (the difficult child)
(8) Inappropriate parent/teacher expectations

d. A **comprehensive assessment** of children suspected of having ADHD should include a search for the above factors (i.e., hearing test, lead testing, cognitive and educational evaluations, family-social history, and psychological evaluation, as indicated).

IV BEHAVIORAL PROBLEMS

A Infants

1. The **transactional model** of development underscores the contribution of both the **infant** and the **parent/caregiver** to developmental-behavioral outcomes. **Attachment** is a key concept within this model (see Chapter 1).
2. **Colic**
   a. A late afternoon, early evening fussy period is very common in many babies between 2 weeks and 3 to 4 months of life. Generally these babies respond to soothing by the parent.
   b. Colic can be defined as > 3 hours of crying per day for more than 3 days in a week. This can be viewed as an exaggerated form of the normal fussy period described above. In colic, the crying episodes are more intense, of longer duration, and less responsive to the parent's attempt to soothe. The age interval tends to be the same (2 weeks to 3 or 4 months).
   c. History and physical exam should rule out feeding problems (under- or overfeeding), medical conditions (e.g., gastroesophageal reflux), or other causes of pain (e.g., hair tourniquet).
   d. Some interventions that have been attempted (with mixed success) include removal of cow's milk protein and/or soy protein from diet, swaddling, white noise, or vibrating devices.
3. **Sleep**
   a. Sleep patterns established in infancy often have long-term consequences.
   b. An important topic for anticipatory guidance is the goal of putting an infant into the crib partially awake and allowing the infant to soothe him- or herself to sleep (see Chapter 1).
   c. If infants are nursed, bottle-fed, or rocked to sleep, then placed into the crib, they may come to depend on the external stimulus to initiate sleep.
   d. There are physiologic, brief awakenings during sleep. Infants unable to soothe themselves back to sleep will tend to cry for the external stimulus at these times.

B Toddlers

1. The healthy toddler, having formed a secure attachment in the first year of life, is now ready to venture forth and begin to explore. Important developmental-behavioral themes of the toddler stage include **mastery, autonomy, negativism,** and the use of **transitional objects** (see Chapter 1).
2. **Feeding problems**
   a. Parental concerns about decreased food intake in toddlers is extremely common (*see II A 4 2*).
   b. Power struggles over feeding reflect the toddler's emerging mastery (desire to feed self) and autonomy (having control over what foods he or she will accept).
   c. Anticipatory guidance around the underlying reasons for this phenomenon can help avert power struggles, which generally aggravate the problem.
3. **Temper tantrums**
   a. Tantrums are normative behavior in the toddler age range. They include crying, screaming, hitting, kicking, and throwing self to floor.
   b. Tantrums are an expression of acute frustration, often in response to a parental "no" or the child's inability to master a specific skill or task.
   c. Parental response can unwittingly reinforce tantrum behavior, either by "giving in" (i.e., changing "no" to an "OK") or by providing negative attention (e.g., yelling and screaming at the child), which can also serve as a reward.
   d. Some potential "red flags" that tantrums are beyond the normative range include:

(1) Frequent, prolonged tantrums (more than three times a day or longer than 15 minutes)
(2) Occurring before 1 year of age or after age 4
(3) Excessive emotional response (e.g., anger, guilt) by parent to the tantrums
(4) Injury to self or others (parents should remove child to a safe location and not allow child to hit the parent or anyone else)

e. Distracting children from milder tantrums and ignoring more intense tantrums (until the child has started to calm down) are helpful responses.

4. Toilet training

a. Toilet training represents one of the major developmental challenges/achievements of the toddler years.

b. The vast majority of children in the United States achieve daytime continence by age 3 and nighttime continence by 4.

c. Anticipatory guidance regarding toilet training is an appropriate discussion point for the 18-month well-child visit (see Chapter 1).

d. The American Academy of Pediatrics (AAP) has outlined the following as indicating a toddler's readiness for toilet training: Child stays dry for at least 2 hours, has regular bowel movements, follows simple instructions, walks to and from bathroom and helps undress, is uncomfortable with dirty diapers, asks to use the toilet or potty, and asks to wear "big girl" or "big boy" underwear.

e. The goals of the toilet-training process are to avoid power struggles, accept the inevitability of regressions, and frame the process as a show of mastery to be celebrated.

C Preschool years

1. Prominent behavioral themes are described in Chapter 1. These include moving from parallel play to **interactive, cooperative play** (a notable lack of interactive play should trigger further developmental evaluation). Other themes include **fantasy, imagination, fears and nightmares, imaginary friends, and magical thinking.**

2. **Lying** at this age is generally not a cause for concern, as the preschooler does not yet have a firm grasp on the distinction between fantasy and reality.

3. **Aggression,** which is normative in the 18-month-old toddler, should be greatly diminished in the preschool years. Persistent aggressive behavior in a preschooler is an indication for both behavioral and developmental assessment.

D School-age years

1. Behavioral concerns in the school-aged child can present as **academic difficulties** (e.g., due to attentional weakness), **social concerns,** and/or **disruptive behaviors.**

2. Behavioral screening by the pediatric provider may identify areas of concern before the school has detected such problems. One useful tool for such screening is the Pediatric Symptom Checklist (PSC). The checklist includes 35 behavioral symptoms, which are scored as never, sometimes, or often by the parent. It can be used for children age 4 through 16 years. Cut-off scores indicate the need for mental health referral.

3. **Depression** and **anxiety disorders** are important psychiatric concerns confronting the school-age child. Anxiety disorders are the most common mental health disorder in children, affecting as many as 13% of children and adolescents. Moderate to severe depression is felt to exist in 2% of school-age children. A number of common features apply to anxiety and depression in children. They are both underdiagnosed. They have different clinical presentations than seen in older adolescents and adults. For example, symptoms of inattention and overactivity can be seen in children with anxiety, depression, or both. Such children are at risk for being mistakenly diagnosed and treated for ADHD. Evidence supports the view that both anxiety and depression often result from the impact of environmental factors on individuals with a genetic predisposition for these disorders. An important defining feature of both diagnoses is significant interference with function (academic, social, behavioral) of the child. Given the central role of school in the lives of children, it is not surprising to find that learning, attention, or social challenges can all give rise to depression and anxiety disorders. Problems with sleep, concentration, mood/irritability, somatic complaints, and school avoidance can all be seen in both disorders.

4. Attention deficit hyperactivity disorder (*see III B 6*) and the autism spectrum disorders (*see III B 3*) have been reviewed previously.

V COMMON RECURRENT PAIN SYNDROMES

A Introduction and definition Recurrent pain occurs frequently in children. The emphasis in this section is on those entities that are not caused by organic disease—**functional gastrointestinal disorders** (e.g., dyspepsia and functional abdominal pain) (see also Chapter 11), **headache** (e.g., tension type) (see also Chapter 18), and **musculoskeletal pain** (growing pains and widespread musculoskeletal pain, commonly known as fibromyalgia). These pains typically occur at least monthly for a 3-month period, during which no organic pathology is found; during the interval between episodes, the child is well. Because of similarities in the approach to assessing and treating these entities, they are discussed here as a group.

B Incidence Functional gastrointestinal disorders occur in 22% of school-age children. Musculoskeletal pains occur in 22% of school-age children. Headache occurs in 23% of school-age children. These pain syndromes have a marked increase in prevalence by 8 years of age, reaching a peak incidence around 14. Children with these conditions often report multiple pain sites and this tendency increases with age.

C Etiology Purely organic or purely emotional etiologic explanations account for only a minor percentage of recurrent pain. Current thinking regarding recurrent pain refutes the previous dichotomy of either an organic or a psychological explanation for these problems. Pain may result neither from pathophysiology nor obvious psychopathology, but may be the result of mild individual differences in physiology. These physiologic differences make the child vulnerable to pain and stress-induced exacerbations. Research has shown that individuals with headache, abdominal pain, and musculoskeletal pain often have disordered sensory processing. This results in an increased sensitivity to pain, both peripherally and centrally.

D Assessment

1. **History.** Essentials include the following:
   a. Characteristics of the pain must be noted, such as onset, frequency, duration, and associated symptoms.
   b. Evidence of obvious psychopathology must be sought in both the parents and the child, and major stressors on the family and the child should be identified. It is also important to identify whether other family members have symptoms similar to those of the patient.
   c. A review of pertinent social/educational concerns such as learning disorders, ADHD, and bullying is needed.
2. **Physical examination** to rule out obvious organic explanations for the symptoms is essential. Normal growth and development are unlikely in the face of chronic organic disease.
3. **Laboratory investigation.** Complete blood count, erythrocyte sedimentation rate, and urinalysis represent a good screening. Further investigation should take place only if suggested by the history and physical examination.

E General principles of chronic pain management

1. If **organic disease** is identified, it should be treated appropriately.
2. Labels such as psychogenic or psychosomatic are usually inaccurate and unhelpful.
3. Treatment should be multimodal from the outset.
   a. Demystify the problem—share with the child and family our current understanding of chronic pain problems.
   b. Encourage normal activity. Parents should not be overly solicitous or apologetic.
   c. Offer pharmacologic interventions if appropriate for pain, sleep, and fatigue.
   d. Physical therapy should emphasize graded exercise.
   e. Provide cognitive behavioral strategies/psychological support.
4. Attention to sleep, school attendance, and social functioning is critical and often a more sensitive indicator of success than pain ratings.

VI ENURESIS

A Definition Enuresis is the involuntary discharge of urine at an age after continence has been reached by most children. Typically, this is 5 years of age in girls and 6 years of age in boys. Approximately 5% to 8% of school-age children are enuretic. Overall, the incidence decreases with age to 1% of 18-year-olds. Two subclassifications of enuresis are important.

1. **Primary versus secondary**
   a. Children with **primary** enuresis have never been continent for a period of time lasting at least 3 to 6 months.
   b. Children with **secondary** enuresis have had a prolonged period of bladder control but have resumed enuretic behavior.
2. **Nocturnal versus diurnal**
   a. **Nocturnal** enuresis occurs only at night and affects approximately 85% of all enuretic children.
   b. **Diurnal** enuresis occurs during the day and affects approximately 5% of enuretic children.
   c. Approximately 10% of enuretic children have a **mixed-type** (nocturnal and diurnal) enuresis.

B Assessment

1. **History.** Essential elements of the history include:
   a. **Family history** of enuresis
   b. **Pattern** of enuresis (primary vs. secondary; nocturnal vs. diurnal)
   c. Defining **urinary habits** (frequency, urgency, dysuria, dribbling)
   d. Inquiring about history of **constipation**
   e. Identifying **psychological stressors**
2. **Physical examination.** Essential elements include:
   a. **Height and weight**
   b. **Blood pressure**
   c. A thorough **neurologic examination** emphasizing lower spinal vertebral function
   d. Examination of the **external genitalia** for abnormalities such as hypospadias
   e. **Rectal examination** for constipation
3. **Laboratory and radiographic investigation**
   a. A **urinalysis** should be obtained and should include specific gravity as well as determinations of glucose, protein, blood, and white blood cells. A **urine culture** should also be obtained.
   b. Routine radiographic studies are not indicated for enuretic children who have normal urinalysis results, negative findings from physical examination, and no evidence of neurologic disease. Children who have diurnal enuresis may require more extensive evaluation.

C Therapy

1. **Behavioral approaches** include counseling, charting, hypnosis, bladder stretching exercises, night awakening by parents 1 hour after sleep onset, and use of a buzzer alarm, which is the most successful treatment currently available. In this system, a moisture-sensitive buzzer alarms when the child voids, which has the effect of eliminating bedwetting in 70% of children within 2 months.
2. **Pharmacologic management:** Drugs for enuresis should be considered for short-term relief of symptoms to prevent embarrassment (camp, overnights, vacations).
   a. **Desmopressin** intranasal formulations are no longer indicated for the treatment of primary nocturnal enuresis.
   b. **Tricyclic antidepressants** (e.g., imipramine) may be successful in reducing enuretic episodes, but the relapse rate on discontinuation is high. In addition, there are potentially serious side effects and marked toxicity with overdosage.

VII ENCOPRESIS

A Definition Encopresis is involuntary fecal soiling at an age beyond which continence should have been achieved, which in most children is age 4 years. Approximately 1.5% of 7-year-old children have encopresis.

1. **Primary versus secondary**
   a. Primary encopresis occurs in children who have never been completely toilet trained.
   b. Secondary encopresis occurs in children who have had at least 3 to 6 months of fecal continence.
2. **Retentive versus nonretentive**
   a. **Retentive.** Most encopretic children suffer from chronic stool retention, with subsequent overflow incontinence.
   b. **Nonretentive** encopretic children (i.e., nonconstipated children who have encopresis) tend to have neurogenic sphincters or significant psychiatric illness.

B Assessment

1. **History**
   a. A detailed bowel history—including the age of the child at toilet training, the frequency of bowel movements, any history of constipation, and a description of the stools—is necessary to adequately assess encopresis.
   b. Also, gaining insight into the child's and the family's functioning can help determine if there are predisposing factors for encopresis.
2. **Physical examination.** Essentials include:
   a. Assessing **growth patterns**
   b. A **neurologic examination** evaluating lower extremity deep tendon reflexes
   c. An **abdominal examination**
   d. A **rectal examination** evaluating sphincter tone and the presence of stool in the rectal ampulla, which is indicative of constipation
3. **Laboratory and radiographic investigation**
   a. Thyroid testing should take place if deemed necessary from physical findings.
   b. An abdominal radiograph to determine the extent of fecal retention may be helpful if there is no response to initial therapy.
   c. If Hirschsprung disease is suspected (see Chapter 11), anal manometry or rectal biopsy is indicated.

C Therapy

1. **Initial treatment**
   a. **Discussion** should remove blame from the child and parent and demystify the origins of the problem.
   b. **Initial catharsis** with a series of enemas and laxatives or stool softeners will remove retained stool.
2. **Maintenance therapy**
   a. Mineral oil (1–2 tablespoons twice daily; the typical course is a gradual decrease of mineral oil with discontinuation after approximately 4–6 months)
   b. Bowel retraining by sitting on the toilet after meals to take advantage of the gastrocolic reflex
   c. Dietary changes, which should emphasize increased roughage and liquid and decreased milk and milk products

BIBLIOGRAPHY

American Psychiatric Association: *Diagnostic and Statistical Manual of Mental Disorders*, 4th ed. Washington, DC, American Psychiatric Association, 1994.

Dixon S, Stein M: *Encounters with Children, Pediatric Behavior and Development*, 3rd ed. St. Louis, Mosby, 2000.

Feldman H: Developmental-Behavioral Pediatrics. In: *Atlas of Pediatric Physical Diagnosis*, 4th ed. Edited by Zitelli B, Davis H. Philadelphia, Mosby, 2002, pp 58–86.

Parker S, Zuckerman B, Augustyn M: *Developmental and Behavioral Pediatrics*, 2nd ed. Philadelphia, Lippincott Williams & Wilkins, 2005.

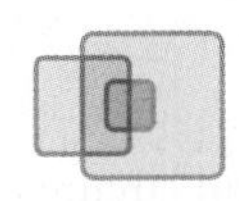

Study Questions

Directions: *Each of the numbered items or incomplete statements in this section is followed by answers or completions of the statement. Select the ONE lettered answer or completion that is BEST in each case.*

QUESTIONS 1 AND 2

1. Bill is a 7-year-old boy who has a lifelong history of bedwetting. He wets almost every night, but has no daytime wetting or incontinence. He has never had more than 1 or 2 consecutive dry nights. He has no history of dribbling and findings on physical examination including measurements, blood pressure, and neurologic and external genitalia exam are normal. Which of the following is the most appropriate term to classify this child's enuresis?

- A Dysfunctional voiding
- B Nocturnal enuresis
- C Mixed pattern enuresis
- D Primary nocturnal enuresis
- E Urinary urgency-frequency syndrome

2. Which of the following evaluations is the most appropriate first step for Bill?

- A Renal ultrasound
- B Voiding cystourethrogram (VCUG)
- C Urinalysis and urine culture
- D 24-hour urine collection
- E Urodynamic study

QUESTIONS 3 AND 4

Amy is a 9-year-old who has recent onset of school failure and inattention. She had been a marginal student until the third grade, with no prior report of obvious attentional or behavioral problems either at home or in school. In third grade, she reports that the work has become too difficult for her. She has normal findings on neurologic examination and no major stressors other than school. Vision and hearing screens are normal.

3. Which of the following is the most likely diagnosis for Amy's difficulties in school?

- A ADHD
- B Mental retardation
- C Learning disability
- D Seizure disorder
- E Oppositional-defiant disorder

4. Which of the following is the most appropriate next step in terms of diagnostic evaluation for Amy's school problems?

- A MRI
- B EEG
- C Speech-language evaluation
- D Psychoeducational assessment (i.e., cognitive and educational testing)
- E Psychological evaluation

QUESTIONS 5 AND 6

A 9-month-old boy is seen by his pediatrician for a routine health supervision visit. His head circumference, which plotted at the 85th percentile at age 6 months, is now slightly above the 95th percentile. Neurologic exam is normal. He is babbling, sits independently, pulls to stand, and looks for a ball of yarn that is dropped away from his sight. His father has long-standing difficulty finding hats that fit.

5. Which of the following is the most likely diagnosis for this child's macrocephaly?

- A Hydrocephalus
- B Developmental delay
- C Familial macrocephaly
- D Posterior fossa tumor
- E Pseudotumor cerebri

6. Which of the following is the most appropriate initial diagnostic test for this child?

- A Ultrasound of the head
- B CT scan of the head
- C Lumbar puncture to measure cerebrospinal fluid pressure
- D MRI
- E EEG

QUESTIONS 7 AND 8

You are evaluating a 5-year-old boy for the first time. At today's visit, his height plots just below the 5th percentile. The parents brought his previous growth curves, which reveal that since age 9 months, his length/height has followed a curve parallel to, but just below, the fifth percentile. His mother's height is 5 feet 1 inch and his father's height is 5 feet 4 inches. History and physical examination are otherwise entirely normal.

7. Which of the following is the most likely diagnosis for this child's short stature?

- A Constitutional delay in growth
- B Growth hormone deficiency
- C Noonan syndrome
- D Familial short stature
- E Hypothyroidism

8. Which of the following is the most useful test that would support the correct diagnosis for short stature in this child?

- A Skull radiograph
- B Bone age radiograph
- C Thyroxine (T_4) and thyroid-stimulating hormone (TSH)
- D Chromosome analysis
- E Growth hormone assay

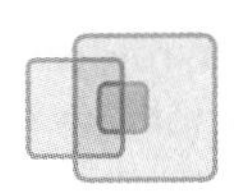

Answers and Explanations

1. The answer is D (*VI A*). By definition, a child with lifelong bedwetting, with no prolonged periods of dryness and no daytime wetting, has primary nocturnal enuresis. Dysfunctional voiding relates to abnormal bladder function resulting in both daytime and nighttime wetting. Nocturnal enuresis tells us that the child has only nighttime wetting, but does not clarify if it is primary (lifelong) or secondary (recurrence of enuresis following a prolonged dry period). Secondary enuresis raises the question of possible medical (e.g., urinary tract infection) or psychosocial (e.g., victim of bullying) etiologies. Mixed pattern enuresis indicates both diurnal and nocturnal wetting. Urinary urgency-frequency syndrome is characterized by the apparent pressing need to void frequently with no medical explanation. It is generally seen in the preschool age group and does not result in bedwetting.

2. The answer is C (*VI B 3*). In a child with primary nocturnal enuresis and no evidence of neurologic abnormalities or other difficulties, evaluation is appropriately limited to a urinalysis and culture. Imaging studies are not indicated, nor is a 24-hour urine collection. Renal ultrasound is commonly performed as part of the evaluation of a young child with a urinary tract infection (UTI). VCUG is also part of the UTI workup, looking for evidence of reflux and also used to rule out posterior urethral valves in a young male infant. Twenty-four-hour urine collection is utilized in the evaluation of proteinuria and other renal conditions. Urodynamic studies assess abnormal bladder function.

3. The answer is C (*III B 5 a*). It is unlikely that attention problems would present de novo in the third grade without prior history of similar difficulties (the diagnostic criteria for ADHD calls for onset of symptoms prior to age 7 years). Although mental retardation cannot be ruled out by the information supplied, it is likely that this problem would have been identified prior to the third grade. There is no evidence to suggest that Amy has a seizure disorder (e.g., brief episodes of staring) or oppositional defiant disorder (very challenging behavior). More than likely, she has a learning disability. Learning disabilities frequently present in mid/elementary school, when the work becomes increasingly difficult and individuals who had barely been able to keep up with the work are no longer able to do so.

4. The answer is D (*III B 5 b 4*). With a normal neurologic exam and no evidence of a seizure disorder, neither an MRI nor an EEG is warranted. While a speech-language evaluation might be of interest, the most high-yield investigation would be psychoeducational testing, looking at both cognitive ability and academic performance. Cognitive testing might reveal one of three significant findings: Mental retardation (unlikely in our case as explained above), gifted child (also unlikely in the case vignette), and, perhaps, slow learner (IQ in the 70–80 range, creating substantial educational challenges for the child). There is no information presented that suggests the need for psychological evaluation.

5. The answer is C (*II A 3 c 5*). While the jump in percentile for head circumference should prompt consideration of the possibility of hydrocephalus, the history of a father with a large head, coupled with a normal neurologic exam and normal developmental milestones, suggests that familial macrocephaly is the most likely diagnosis. He has not demonstrated any symptoms or signs of increased intracranial pressure, which would suggest tumor or pseudotumor cerebri.

6. The answer is A (*II A 3 c*). Assuming the anterior fontanelle is still patent, an ultrasound of the head can be performed, which will assess ventricular size looking for evidence of hydrocephalus. Ultrasound is the preferred initial test and would avoid exposure to radiation from a CT scan. There is no indication for a lumbar puncture. MRI would not be the initial test of choice due to expense and the need for sedation. An EEG would not be relevant to the child in question. If the anterior fontanelle is no longer patent, then a CT or MRI would be indicated. One of these imaging studies would also be appropriate if the ultrasound result is abnormal or equivocal.

7. The answer is D (*II B 2 a*). The child's normal growth velocity combined with the family history of short stature strongly suggests that familial short stature is the most likely diagnosis. With constitutional delay in growth, one or both parents typically have a history of delayed onset of puberty and usually demonstrate normal adult stature. Growth hormone deficiency and acquired hypothyroidism would be expected to present with significant fall-off in growth velocity. Physical exam does not reveal any evidence of Noonan syndrome or hypothyroidism.

8. The answer is B (*II B 2 a, d*). A bone age radiograph will help to distinguish constitutional delay in growth (delayed bone age) from familial short stature (normal bone age). A skull radiograph would not be informative. Thyroid function testing would be indicated if short stature was accompanied by obesity and pertinent findings on exam (e.g., so-called "hung up" or diminished return phase of Achilles deep tendon reflexes). Chromosome analysis would be indicated if Noonan syndrome was suspected on exam. Growth hormone testing is not indicated based on the growth pattern.

chapter **5**

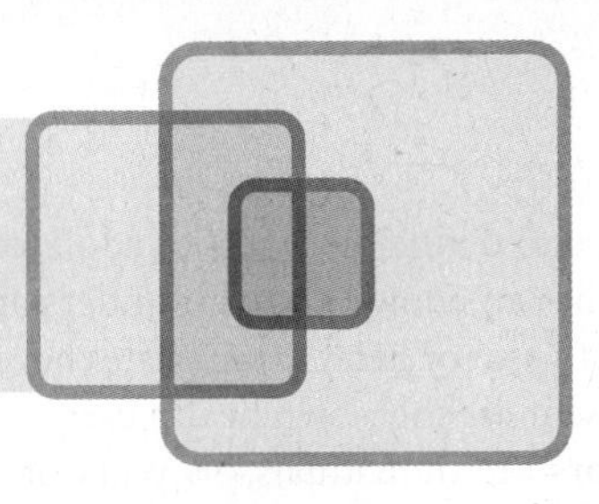

Adolescent Health

ARIC SCHICHOR

I OVERVIEW OF ADOLESCENT HEALTH CARE

A Objectives Adolescence is a time of physical growth and personality development. This transition from childhood to adulthood may be a confusing and turbulent period for adolescents, parents, and health care providers. Adolescent health should focus on more than strictly medical issues; it also should consider the issues that affect a teenager's day-to-day well-being. Health care providers are required to:

1. Deal with acute health needs
2. Provide comprehensive health care, including:
   a. General medical care
   b. Care in high-risk health areas (e.g., sexual activity, substance abuse, depression, suicide, injuries, violence)
   c. Anticipatory guidance (e.g., peer relationships, school progress, home environment, relationship with parents)
3. Provide health education
4. Promote independence in health-seeking behavior
5. Support and counsel parents
6. Educate, assist, and work with other adults in the community

B Adolescent health concerns

1. Leading causes of mortality (ages 10–17) in the United States are unintentional (14.3 per 100,000) and intentional (5.7 per 100,000) injuries. Motor vehicle crashes (see Chapter 2) are the leading cause of unintentional injuries (40% associated with the use of drugs or alcohol). Suicide (2.9 per 100,000) and homicides (2.8 per 100,000) are the other leading causes, with homicide surpassing suicide in the larger inner-city populations.
2. Leading causes of morbidity include survivors of automobile crashes and homicide or suicide attempts, drug and alcohol abuse, sexually transmitted diseases, behavioral and mental health issues, and obesity and eating disorders.

C Approach to the adolescent

1. **Setting the stage** during the initial adolescent health visit is essential. This visit allows the health provider, in partnership with the parents, to begin to help the adolescent take control of her or his own health care. The goal is that by the time the adolescent is 17 or 18 years old, he or she will be capable and comfortable in taking care of his or her own health care needs. Efforts are needed to not alienate the parent from this process.
2. **Confidentiality** is a central concept for adolescent health care. The adolescent needs to be informed that confidentiality may be breached when life is at risk.
   a. **State laws** vary regarding the right of adolescents to receive care without parental consent. In many states, adolescents may be treated for drug abuse and sexually transmitted diseases (STDs) and may receive mental health counseling as well as family planning and pregnancy counseling without parental consent. The right to an abortion without parental or legal consent is now limited to only two states (Connecticut and Maine) and the District of Columbia.

b. **Common terms** are used to define the rights of adolescents.
   (1) **Mature minor** defines an adolescent who understand the risks and benefits of the services being provided to him or her. Certain states have a mature minor law that allows adolescents to give consent for their own health care.
   (2) **Emancipated minors** are individuals, 16 years of age or older, who are married, have joined the armed forces, or have proved in a court of law that they are living on their own and managing their own financial affairs. Emancipated minors are allowed to give consent for their own health care. Adolescent females who have children have the right to give consent for health care for their children but may not have the right to give consent for their own health care.
   (3) **Adult status** is confirmed at age 18 along with the ability to vote.

3. **Hearing both sides of the story** is also essential. Parents need to have input about acute concerns, conditions at home, the adolescent's performance at school, the adolescent's relations with peers, and other private concerns.
4. **The physician's office** should be adolescent friendly: Waiting area decorated for adolescents, exam room equipped with gynecologic examination table, and support staff comfortable in working with adolescents.
5. **Family involvement** can result in support for adolescents, increased adolescent health care adherence, and improved relationship with parents.

D Maximizing the adolescent health care visit

1. **Why do adolescents come for health care?** Most adolescents come because they require completion of a physical exam form or because they are acutely ill and they typically expect a visit to last for 10 to 15 minutes. It may be helpful to inform the adolescents what will be accomplished in the visit and how long it will take. If the adolescent or family is unable to stay for the required amount of time, then plans need to be made to complete the visit at another time.
2. **Finding the real reason for the visit.** The adolescent may have a specific concern other than the stated reason for coming in. For example, the adolescent may report a cold but is really concerned about the possibility of having a sexually transmitted disease. An effort should be made to elicit other concerns as time permits.
3. **Making the time to ask the questions.** Follow-up visits for such issues as acne and birth control may provide enough time to consider issues identified but not addressed in earlier visits.
4. **Using questionnaires.** Questionnaires are another way to obtain information and save time. Such questionnaires are available from the American Academy of Pediatrics (www.brightfutures.aap.org) and the American Medical Association (Guideline to Adolescent Preventive Services [GAPS]).

II HEALTH SUPERVISION ISSUES

A History

1. **Goals** of the patient history include:
   a. Determining the specific concerns of the adolescent
   b. Obtaining information about high-risk behaviors, especially those that may lead to intentional or unintentional injuries
   c. Identifying the uniqueness of each adolescent
2. **Methods**
   a. A **variety of approaches** to asking questions should be used:
      (1) **Direct approach** (e.g., "Have you ever been in a hospital overnight?")
      (2) **Indirect approach** (e.g., "Some people who get down or depressed sometimes think of ending it all or killing themselves.... Have you ever had such thoughts?")
      (3) **Open-ended approach** (e.g., "What do you do for fun? What three things would you change to make your life better? On a scale of 1 to 5, with 1 being poor, 3 being average, and 5 being great, how would you rate your general health?")
   b. **Follow-up** to such questions should focus on what changes could be made to improve the situation and which changes the adolescent would like to pursue.

3. **Using the HEADSS approach for the history**
   a. **Home:** Level of support, safety, privacy, and communication. What could be changed to make things better?
   b. **Education and Employment:** Level of performance, future plans, safety at school, missed days from school, suspensions, detentions, level of support at school
   c. **Activities:** After-school activities, hobbies, special interests, friends adolescent can talk to about personal issues
   d. **Drugs** (see below)
   e. **Sexual activity** (see below)
   f. **Suicide and depression** (see below)
4. **Midhistory assessment.** There should be increased concern where there is little parental communication or support, lack of privacy or safety at home, poor school performance, significant number of days missed from school, no clear future plans, no structured after-school activities, and no real friends.
5. **Asking the harder questions**
   a. **Drugs,** alcohol, and cigarette use (substance use)
      (1) **Looking in.** Ask about exposure to substance use at school and in the neighborhood, and exposure to gangs who may be selling drugs. Ask about substance use at home.
      (2) **CRAFFT.** The CRAFFT questionnaire (Table 5-1) was specifically formulated to assess substance abuse by adolescents. One positive answer means the adolescent is at risk for substance use; two positive answers means he or she has substance abuse problem.
   b. **Sexual activity**
      (1) **Talking at the same level.** Make sure that both the provider and adolescent are talking about the same thing. Define sexual activity as having oral, vaginal, or rectal intercourse.
      (2) **Determine sexual preference**
      (3) **Type of sexual involvement.** Does adolescent have sex with a romantic (love) interest or with a friend ("friend with benefits")?
      (4) **Risk assessment.** Determine the number of partners and forms of protection used (against STDs and pregnancy). Encourage safe sex for all adolescents, regardless of sexual preference. Dental dams should be used with oral sex and condoms should be used with rectal sex.
      (5) **Encourage communication.** Encourage the adolescent to talk to his or her partner about the use of protection. Females in a heterosexual relationship need to insist on the use of a condom.
      (6) **Sexual safety.** Inquire about forced sexual activity.

TABLE 5-1 CRAFFT Questionnaire

	Yes	No
1. Have you ever ridden in a **C**ar driven by someone (including yourself) who was high or had been using alcohol or drugs?	____	____
2. Do you ever use alcohol or drugs to **R**elax, feel better about yourself, or fit in?	____	____
3. Do you ever use alcohol or drugs while you are by yourself, **A**lone?	____	____
4. Do you ever **F**orget things you did while using alcohol or drugs?	____	____
5. Do your **F**amily or **F**riends ever tell you that you should cut down on your drinking or drug use?	____	____
6. Have you ever gotten into **T**rouble while you were using alcohol or drugs?	____	____

Scoring: Two or more positive items indicate the need for further assessment.

c. **Suicide,** homicide, and depression
  (1) Past and present episodes of being depressed, having suicidal ideation, or attempting suicide: Positive history requires additional information about mental health supports. Active suicidal ideation requires more in-depth mental health assessment.
  (2) Past and present episodes of feeling angry enough to want to kill someone or having tried to kill someone: Positive history of homicidal ideation or attempt requires additional information about violence prevention skills and supports. Active homicidal ideation requires more in-depth mental health assessment.

B **Review of systems** Specific issues for adolescents include:

1. Assume that the adolescent is a **concrete thinker**. For example, ask about bumps on the face rather than problems with skin. Provide closer health supervision. For example, monitor new starts on birth control pills in 2 to 3 weeks, rather than in 2 to 3 months.
2. **Vegetative symptoms.** Ask about sleeping at night and appetite level.
3. **Body image.** How comfortable is the adolescent with her or his body? What would the adolescent like to change about her or his body?
4. **Vision.** Adolescents may refuse to wear glasses because they don't like the way they look and may not be able to afford contact lenses.
5. **Dental care.** What is the frequency of brushing and flossing? When was the last dental appointment? Adolescents often resist going for dental care because of the fear of having a painful experience.
6. **Diet history.** Document meals and snacks. Many adolescents do not eat breakfast and have snacks that are high in fat and calories. Morning school performance may have a strong correlation to what is eaten for breakfast. Monitor calcium input. Review snacks and drinks that are low in fat and calories.
7. **Menarche, menses, and dysmenorrhea.** Determine age of menarche, regularity and length of menses, and level of dysmenorrhea. Menses may not be regular during the first year or two after menarche.

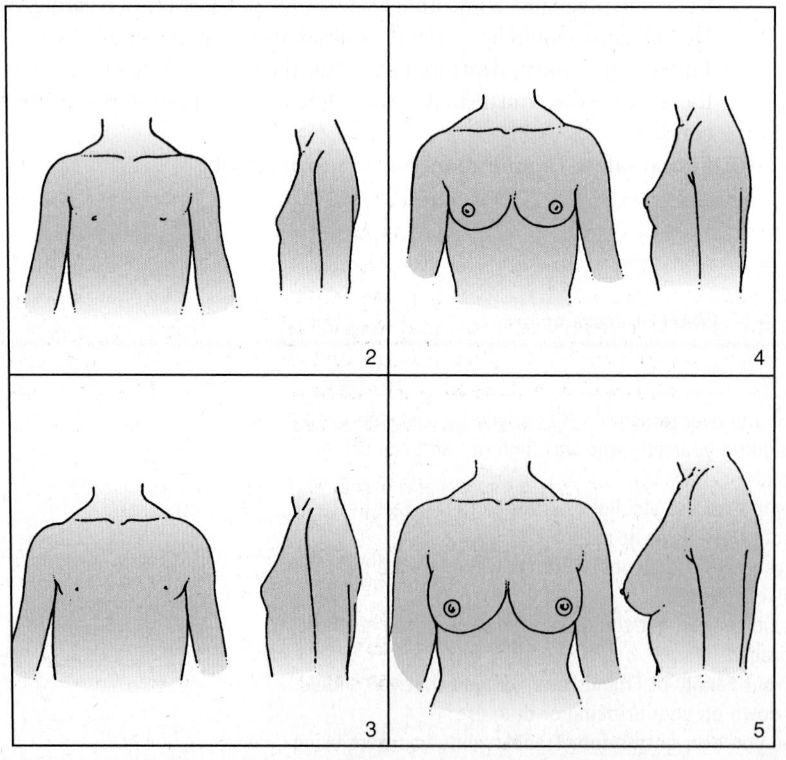

FIGURE 5-1 Sex maturity rating (SMR) for breast development. SMR 1 (not shown): Prepubertal—elevations of papilla only. SMR 2: Breast buds appear; areola is slightly widened and projects as small mound. SMR 3: Enlargement of the entire breast, with no protrusion of the papilla or nipple. SMR 4: Enlargement of the breast and projection of areola and papilla as secondary mound. SMR 5: Adult configuration of the breast, with protrusion of the nipple. Areola no longer projects separately from the remainder of the breast. (From Daniel WA, Paulshock BZ: A physician's guide to sexual maturity rating. *Patient Care* 13:129, 1979. Illustration by Paul J. Singh-Roy.)

8. **Musculoskeletal.** Focus questions on types of physical activities or sports in which the adolescent is involved. Review past or recent injuries and how these have been resolved. How does the adolescent keep in shape?

C **Physical examination** provides an opportunity to teach health maintenance, especially routine self-examination of breasts or testicles.

1. **Maximize comfort.** Promote privacy with gowns and sheets as needed. Communicate with the adolescent during the exam. Use a chaperone for breast, testicular, or pelvic exam.
2. **Areas requiring special focus**
   a. **Hair.** Note whether there is the presence of **tinea capitis.**
   b. **Skin.** Note the presence and degree of acne. Presence of facial and axillary hair implies the later half of pubertal development (sex maturity rating [SMR] 4; see Figures 5-2 and 5-3.
   c. **Dentition.** Evaluate level of hygiene, and review the development of the third set of molar teeth (wisdom teeth).
   d. **Neck.** Evaluate the size of the thyroid gland.
   e. **Breasts.** Examine for developmental stage (Figure 5-1), tenderness, erythema, dimpling, asymmetric masses, significant size difference, discharge, and axillary adenopathy.
   f. **Heart sounds** may be accentuated because of a thin chest wall, and functional and other murmurs may become more apparent.
   g. **Male genitalia.** Examine for developmental stage (Figure 5-2), urethral discharge, scrotal masses, testicular size, inguinal adenopathy, and presence of inguinal hernia. Check for

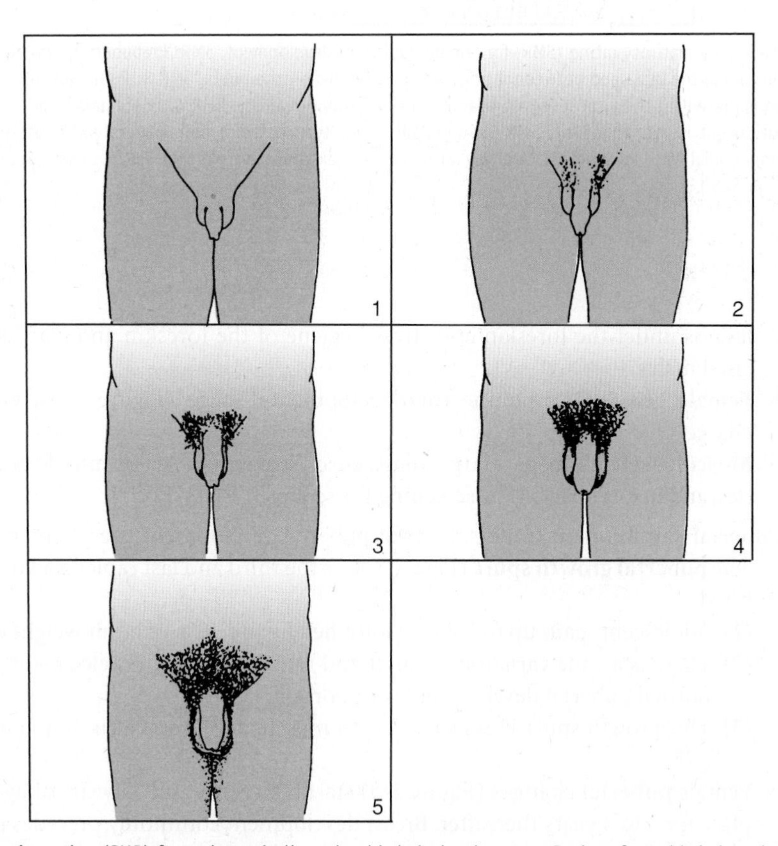

FIGURE 5-2 Sex maturity rating (SMR) for male genitalia and pubic hair development. Ratings for pubic hair and genital development can differ in a typical boy at any given time because pubic hair and genitalia do not necessarily develop at the same rate. SMR 1: Prepubertal—no pubic hair; genitalia unchanged from early childhood. SMR 2: Light downy hair develops laterally and later becomes dark. Penis and testes may be slightly larger. Scrotum becomes more textured. SMR 3: Pubic hair has extended across the pubis. Testes and scrotum are further enlarged. Penis is larger, especially in length. SMR 4: More abundant pubic hair with curling. Genitalia resemble those of an adult. Glans penis has become larger and broader. Scrotum is darker. SMR 5: Adult quantity and pattern of pubic hair, with hair present along the inner border of the thighs. Testes and scrotum are adult in size. (From Daniel WA, Paulshock BZ: A physician's guide to sexual maturity rating. *Patient Care* 13:129, 1979. Illustration by Paul J. Singh-Roy.)

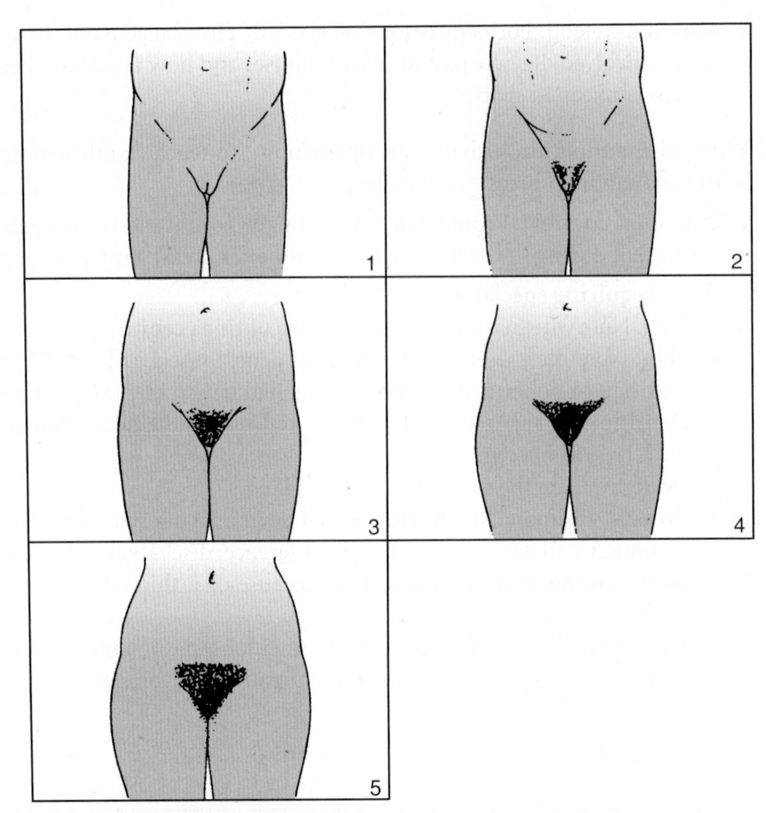

FIGURE 5-3 Sex maturity rating (SMR) for female pubic hair development. SMR: Prepubertal—no pubic hair. SMR 2: Straight hair extends along the labia and between ratings 2 and 3, begins on the pubis. SMR 3: Pubic hair has increased in quantity, is darker, and is present in the typical female triangle but in smaller quantity. SMR 4: Pubic hair is more dense, curled, and adult in distribution but is less abundant. SMR 5: Abundant, adult-type pattern; hair may extend onto the medial aspect of the thighs. (From Daniel WA, Paulshock BZ: A physician's guide to sexual maturity rating. *Patient Care* 13:129, 1979. Illustration by Paul J. Singh-Roy.)

lesions under the foreskin and stress hygiene of the foreskin and glans penis in uncircumcised males.

h. Female genitalia. Examine for developmental stage (Figure 5-3), vulvar rash, or discharge.

i. Musculoskeletal. Inspect large joints, check strength of major muscle groups in all extremities, and inspect back. (For screening for scoliosis, *see IV D 1.*)

3. Pubertal development (for disorders of pubertal development, see Chapter 17)

a. The pubertal growth spurt (Figure 5-4) is the third and last rapid growth stage during childhood.

(1) Adolescents gain up to 25% of adult height and 50% of adult weight during this period.

(2) There is a wide variation in onset and rate of pubertal development. Reassurance about normal pubertal development is important.

(3) This growth spurt is associated with muscle development in boys and fat deposition in girls.

b. Female pubertal changes (Figure 5-5) start between 8 and 13 years of age, and changes take place for 3 to 4 years thereafter. Breast development commonly precedes pubic hair development. Peak height spurt occurs midway through puberty (SMR 3). Menarche occurs after the peak height spurt is reached.

c. Male pubertal changes (Figure 5-6) start between 9.5 and 13.5 years of age, and changes occur for approximately 3 to 3.5 years thereafter. Testicular enlargement is usually the first sign of male pubertal development. Peak height spurt occurs in the latter half of puberty (SMR 4).

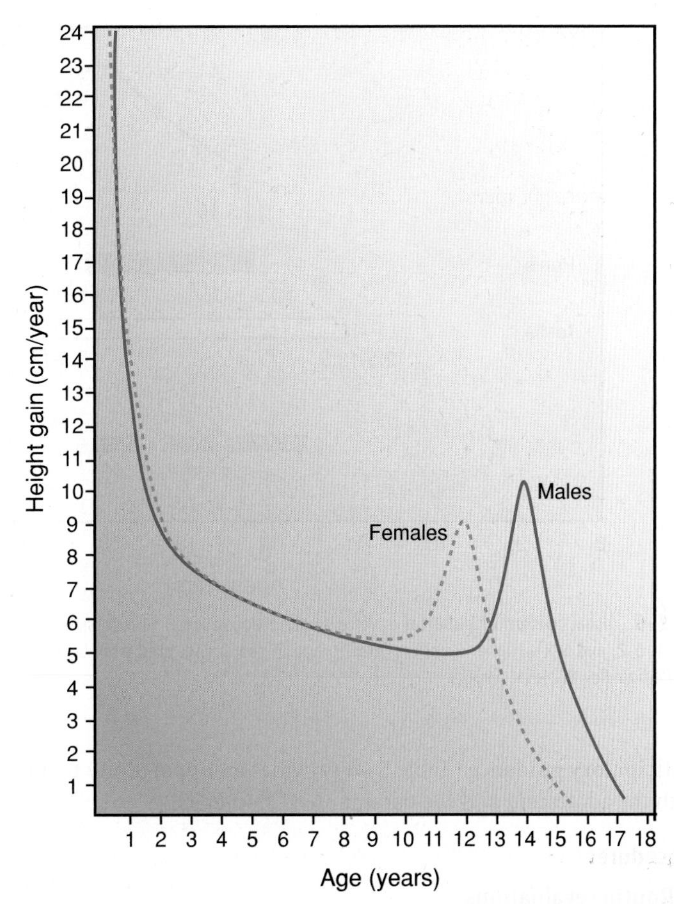

FIGURE 5-4 Graph showing the height gain (postnatal and pubertal growth spurts) in males and females between birth and age 18 years. (Reprinted from Tanner JM, Whitehouse RH, Takaishi M. Standards from birth to maturity for height, weight, height velocity, and weight velocity in British children, 1965. *Arch Dis Child* 41:454–471, 1965.)

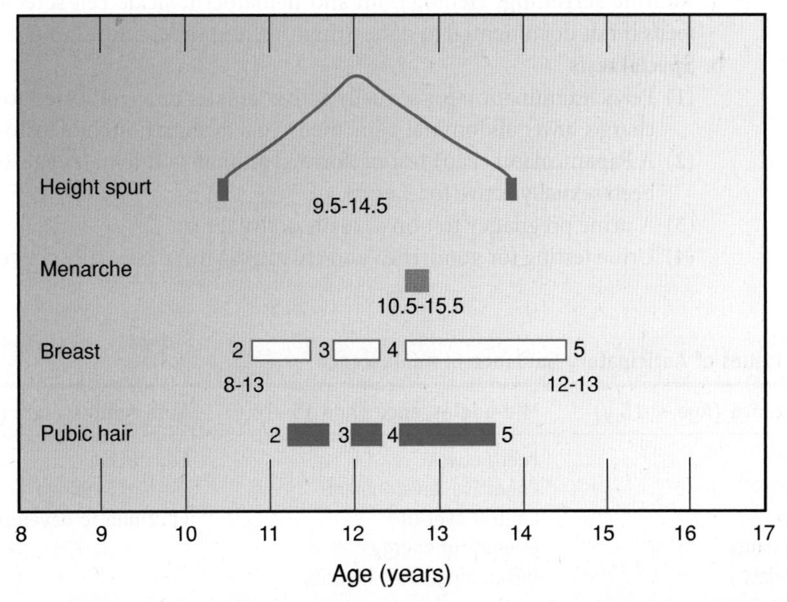

FIGURE 5-5 Usual pattern of pubertal development in normal girls. Lower numbers refer to sex maturity rating (SMR) rating (see Figures 5-1, 5-2, and 5-3). Higher numbers refer to age in years. (Adapted from Copeland KC: Variations in normal sexual development. *Pediatr Rev* 8(2):53, 1986.)

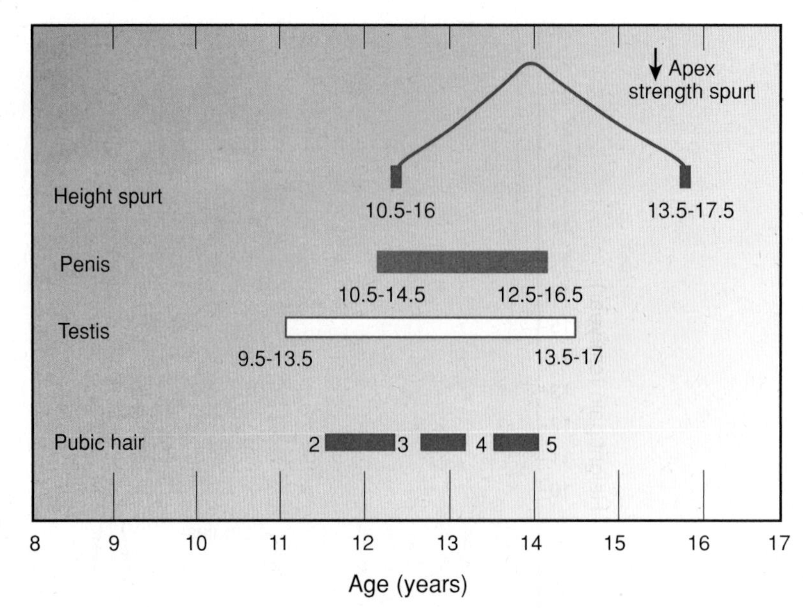

FIGURE 5-6 Usual pattern of pubertal development in boys. Lower numbers refer to sex maturity rating (SMR) rating (see Figures 5-1, 5-2, and 5-3). Higher numbers refer to age in years. (Adapted from Copeland KC: Variations in normal sexual development. *Pediatr Rev* 8(2):51, 1986.)

D **Anticipatory guidance** (Table 5-2) provides an opportunity to address developmental issues with both the adolescent and the parents (see Chapter 1).

E Procedures

1. **Routine evaluations**
   a. **Height, weight,** and **blood pressure** should be measured and plotted on the appropriate charts. A body mass index should also be calculated and plotted.
   b. **Vision, hearing,** and **immunizations** (see Chapter 1) should be checked. Immunizations specific for early and midadolescents include meningococcus, human papilloma virus, and TdaP. Late adolescents who are missing any of these immunizations should be brought up to date.
2. **Laboratory studies**
   a. **Routine screening:** Hemoglobin and hematocrit, sickle cell screen for black and Hispanic teens if not documented to date, urinalysis, and tuberculin skin test for high-risk teens
   b. **Special tests**
      (1) Pelvic examination for sexually active females or as indicated for an unusual vaginal discharge, lower abdominal pain, menstrual dysfunction, or a history of exposure to an STD
      (2) A Papanicolaou (Pap) test performed annually on females age 21 and above or who have been sexually active for 3 years
      (3) A urine pregnancy test on sexually active females
      (4) Urine testing for gonorrhea and chlamydia for all sexually active adolescents

TABLE 5-2 Issues of Anticipatory Guidance in Adolescence

Early Adolescence (Age < 15 y)	Mid-adolescence (Age 15–16 y)	Late Adolescence (Age ≥ 17 y)
Puberty	Peer network	Separation
Privacy	Cognitive development	Decision making
Independence	Control over life	Continue to develop adult identity
Peers as confidants	Bundles of energy	
Adult role models	Developing adult identity	
Mood swings		
School transition		

(5) Cholesterol (nonfasting) level on initial visit and as indicated by dietary/family histories. If the level is elevated (above 190 mg/dL), then fasting lipid profile should be measured (see Chapter 1).

(6) Testing for other sexually transmitted disease such as human immunodeficiency virus (HIV), syphilis, and hepatitis C.

III PREPARTICIPATION SPORTS EXAMINATION

A Objectives

1. Identify medical problems that may result in **life-threatening complications** such as hypertrophic cardiomyopathy, aortic rupture associated with Marfan syndrome, mitral valve prolapse, cardiac arrhythmias, syncope, sickle cell disease, and persistent hypertension.
2. Identify medical problems that may **limit sports participation** such as asthma, allergic rhinitis, febrile illness, insulin-dependent diabetes, eating disorders, and use of drugs and alcohol.
3. Identify previous **musculoskeletal injuries** and review plan for continued rehabilitation of these injuries as well as plan for ongoing **fitness training** related to the selected sport.
4. Review and update any past restrictions on sports participation.

B Timing of evaluation

1. Preparticipation examination is recommended at the start of middle or junior high school, high school, and college. This examination is not meant to take the place of the annual comprehensive physical examination.
2. Examination should be completed at least a month prior to the start of the sport to allow for appropriate planning for rehabilitation and fitness training.
3. Yearly review of any physical changes and injuries coupled with a focused physical examination is helpful to ensure safe continued sports participation. Health information should be obtained from the adolescent and the parent.

C History

1. Obtain a detailed family medical history related to factors that can lead to life-threatening complications from sports participation.
2. Obtain a detailed history of any past physical injuries, physical limitations, and health concerns. Focus questions specifically on the parts of the body most involved with the sport.
3. Inquire about head injuries and syncope as well as chest pain, palpitations, and dyspnea with exercise.

D Physical examination

1. The adolescent needs to be undressed to allow most of the musculoskeletal system to be visualized.
2. **Special features of examination**
   a. **Body symmetry.** Look at shoulders, hips, arms, legs, and hands.
   b. **Range of motion.** Check range of motion at all major joints starting with the neck and working down.
   c. **Muscle strength and reflexes.** Check muscle strength in all extremities and hands. Check deep tendon reflexes.

E Recommendation

Information should be shared with both the parents and the adolescent.

1. **Cleared for participation:** No physical limitations noted
2. **Cleared for participation with limitations:** Able to participate but not up to full level, such as in a case of a resolving injury
3. **Excluded from participation pending further evaluation:** In case where physical finding may place the adolescent at significant risk

IV COMMON HEALTH ISSUES

A **Acne** is the major skin problem in adolescents.

1. **Pathophysiology.** Acne is caused by increased sebum production stimulated by androgens during puberty. Sebum is a mixture of follicular keratin and secretions of the sebaceous glands. Bacteria (*Propionibacterium acnes*) in the follicles use substrate from the sebum to stimulate a white blood cell response. This response releases a variety of hydrolytic enzymes, causing a local inflammatory reaction, and may lead to scarring.
2. **Definition of terms**
   a. A **comedo** is hyperkeratosis of the follicular epithelium and is the initial observable change in acne. **Whiteheads** are closed comedones that appear as slightly elevated papules in the skin. **Blackheads** are a later stage of enlarged comedones containing melanin that may open and cause inflammatory responses.
   b. **Cystic acne** is not actually composed of cysts but of **nodules** formed during the inflammatory reaction; these nodules develop into **erythematous papules (pimples)** or **pus-filled papules (pustules).**
3. **Therapy** is aimed at reducing sebum production and decreasing bacterial activity.
   a. **Comedolytic** and **antikeratolytic agents** include topical retinoic acid and benzoyl peroxide (also noted to have an antibacterial effect) and systemic isotretinoin.
   b. **Antibacterial agents** usually consist of topical or systemic antibiotics.
   c. **Sebaceous gland inhibitor agents** include systemic isotretinoin and agents that decrease or counteract androgen production (e.g., birth control pills, dexamethasone).
   d. Other methods include **surgical removal** of comedones, use of **exfoliating agents** (e.g., ultraviolet light, cryotherapy), and use of **anti-inflammatory agents** such as steroids.
   e. The use of water-based instead of oil-based cosmetics is helpful.
   f. Diet manipulation has not proved effective.

B Genitourinary and reproductive health issues

1. **Pregnancy**
   a. **General considerations.** The pregnancy rate in the United States for 15- to 19-year-olds has dropped significantly between 1982 and 2002 from 110 to 75 per 1000. The rate is higher for African American (134 per 1000) and Hispanic (132 per 1000) teens than for non-Hispanic White (42 per 1000) teens. Teenage mothers have a 20% to 40% chance of becoming pregnant again 1 to 2 years after the initial delivery.
   b. **Medical complications** of teenage pregnancy include toxemia and anemia. Infants born to mothers who are younger than 15 years of age have a higher mortality rate and a high incidence of low birth weight compared to infants of older adolescents.
   c. **Causes of teenage pregnancy**
      (1) **Concrete operational stage** (see Chapter 1). Teenagers deny their ability to get pregnant, are unable to think of events 9 months in the future, and exhibit poor compliance with contraception.
      (2) **Family influence.** Mother or a sibling became a parent as a teenager. Decreased support and supervision because of lack of an extended family, families in which both parents work, or single-parent families may be contributing factors.
      (3) **Gradually decreasing age of menarche** has made pregnancy possible at an early age.
      (4) **Situational stress** (e.g., school performance, family relations, pressure from a sexual partner or peer group)
      (5) **Societal influences.** Lack of positive role models, lack of opportunities in the job market, increased emphasis on sex in the media, and relaxation of moral codes contribute to teenage pregnancy.
      (6) **Desire to become pregnant.** Teenagers may feel that becoming a parent will give them someone to take care of, provide them with unconditional love, and offer them a way to become independent.
      (7) **Often the males involved are older** and desire to have children.

d. Evaluation for possible pregnancy

(1) **History.** Correlate sexual activity and menstrual cycle. Symptoms of pregnancy include swelling of the breasts, nausea and vomiting, fatigue, and urinary frequency.

(2) **Physical examination.** Check the size and color of the cervix as well as the size and consistency of the uterus.

(4) **Clinical studies.** Urine evaluation for human chorionic gonadotropin (hCG) can determine a pregnancy within 10 days of conception. Blood analysis for hCG can quantitate the duration of the pregnancy.

e. Decision making for a pregnant teenager. Review options. Encourage adolescent to involve parents and partner in the discussion. It may be helpful to talk to other teens who have been through this experience.

(1) **Options.** Options include keeping the baby, putting the baby up for adoption, placing the baby in foster care (thus allowing for a later decision), and terminating the pregnancy.

(2) **Factors influencing the decision.** Consequences of parenthood such as decreased personal freedom, increased financial and physical responsibility, need for a support system, change in lifestyle, and delay in achieving career goals need to be balanced with the positive feelings associated with parenthood.

f. Care and support for a pregnant teenager. The provider needs to link the adolescent to early prenatal care, facilitate continuation of school, and help develop a support system, especially for future parenting.

2. Contraception

a. Oral contraceptive pill. This is the form of contraception most commonly used by adolescent females. It has a failure rate of 2% to 4%. This rate may go up to 18% in certain adolescent populations.

(1) Parental involvement in the adolescent's decision to start a birth control method is associated with increased compliance. Adolescents should be encouraged whenever possible to share such decisions with their parents.

(2) **Mechanism of action.** It suppresses ovulation, decreases the likelihood of implantation of the fertilized egg, and makes the cervical mucus more hostile to sperm.

(3) **Types of pills**

(a) **Combination pill** contains both estrogen and progesterone and may have fixed doses of each (monophasic pills) or may vary the dose of these hormones through the cycle (multiphasic pills).

(b) **Progesterone-only pill** works in a manner similar to the combination pill except that it may not regularly prevent ovulation. The failure rate is higher partly because the pill causes irregular menstrual periods, which results in users stopping these pills from fear that they may be pregnant. This pill is reserved for females who cannot tolerate estrogen.

(c) **Emergency contraception** ("morning-after pill") is a progesterone preparation used up to 5 days after unprotected intercourse to prevent pregnancy.

(4) **Common side effects** of the pill are listed in Table 5-3.

(5) **Advantages** of the pill are listed in Table 5-3.

b. Barrier methods of contraception (aside from condoms) are used regularly by less than one fifth of the adolescent population who use any form of contraception. The failure rate varies from 10% to 20%, depending on the form of barrier contraceptive being used. Condom use by high school students during the last episode of sexual intercourse has increased from 46% to 63% from 1991 to 2003 and has remained at that level through 2005. The **failure rate** for condoms is approximately 10%.

(1) **Mechanisms of action.** Barrier methods prevent sperm from entering the uterus or kill sperm while they are in the vagina.

(2) **Types of barrier contraceptives**

(a) **Diaphragm:** A circular rubber dome that, when properly placed, is an effective barrier between the vagina and cervix

(b) **Cervical cap:** A firm plastic cap held in place by suction at the cervical opening

(c) **Female condom:** A soft polyurethane liner for the vagina

TABLE 5-3 Advantages and Disadvantages of Birth Control Methods

Type	Advantages	Disadvantages
Oral contraceptive pills	Decreased menstrual bleeding Decreased dysmenorrhea No interference with intercourse Improvement of acne	Weight gain Bleeding between periods Nausea Headaches Having to take a pill each day Mood changes Period of anovulatory cycles after the pill is stopped
Barrier methods Diaphragm Cervical cap Female condom Spermicides Condom	No systemic effects No contraindications for use Easily available without prescription Helps prevent passage of STDs, including HIV Used only at the time of intercourse	Interfere with spontaneity Has to be inserted into vagina May decrease sensation Irritation or allergic reactions Are considered messy Interrupt lovemaking
Injectable progesterone	Lasts for 3 mo Works independently	Need for shot every 3 mo Irregular or absent menses Weight gain
Patch	Transdermal delivery Level serum concentration Less frequent dosing	Dependent on application technique Delivery varies by placement site Need to remember to change patch Similar to pill
Ring	Ease of use Rapid onset of action Lower hormone doses	Unintended bleeding Vaginitis Device-related issues Need to place in vagina
Intrauterine device (IUD)	Long-term contraceptive Decreases ectopic pregnancy Works independently	Heavy menses (copper IUD) Uterine perforation Dysmenorrhea (copper IUD) Vaginal discharge Expulsion Difficult to remove

HIV, human immunodeficiency virus; STD, sexually transmitted disease.

(d) **Spermicides:** Foams, jellies, or suppositories

(e) **Condoms** are an effective barrier method of contraception. A combination of a condom and a spermicide is almost as effective as the pill but with fewer side effects. Condoms serve as the most effective deterrent to HIV transmission.

(4) **Advantages and disadvantages** of barrier contraceptives are listed in Table 5-3. Toxic shock syndrome can occur when the diaphragm is left in the vagina for an extended period of time.

c. **Intrauterine devices (IUDs)** are available in two forms: Copper or progestin based. Past data associating IUDs with increased STDs have been challenged by more recent studies.

(1) **Mechanism of action** is not clearly understood. The IUD blocks the implantation of a fertilized egg in the lining of the uterus, either by causing a mild endometritis or affecting endometrial enzymes.

(2) **Side effects** include pelvic infection, uterine perforation, ectopic pregnancy, and subsequent infertility.

d. **Injectable progesterone** (medroxyprogesterone acetate) is popular because of its high level of effectiveness and the need to take it only once every 12 weeks.

(1) **Mechanism of action** is similar to the progesterone-only pill but is more effective in the suppression of ovulation.

(2) **Side effects** are similar to those seen with the progesterone-only pill and are listed in Table 5-3.

e. The **patch** is a transdermal method of delivery of estrogen and progesterone used for 1 week at a time for a 3-week period. Menses occur in the fourth, patch-free week.

(1) **Mechanism of action.** Unlike the birth control pill, where hormone is delivered in a burst at the time that the pill is taken, the patch delivers hormone on a constant rate throughout the 24 hours. The patch works in a similar manner to the pill.

(2) **Side effects** are similar to the pill.

f. The **ring** is made of a soft, flexible, transparent polymer containing both estrogen and progesterone. It is placed in the vagina for 3 weeks and then removed for 1 week to allow for the menstrual period.

(1) **Mechanism of action** is similar to the patch with a constant release of hormone over 24 hours.

(2) **Side effects** are similar to those seen with the pill, in addition to vaginal discomfort and vaginitis.

(3) **Orientation** is needed to promote the use of the ring. Adolescents who use tampons during their periods may be more receptive to this method.

g. **Continuous contraception** is a method used by women who desire to decrease their number of menstrual periods. This is accomplished by skipping the hormone-free week when on the pill, patch, or ring.

h. **Quick start** focuses on beginning contraception as soon as possible. The method may be started immediately if the adolescent's pregnancy test is negative and she denies unprotected intercourse within the prior 2 weeks.

3. **STDs** (Table 5-4) are acquired by sexual contact and intercourse (including genital, rectal, and oral penetration). These diseases are most common in the adolescent and young adult population (15–24 years of age).

a. **Agents of specific STDs**

(1) ***Chlamydia trachomatis*** is the cause of the most common nonviral STD in the United States. It is an intracellular bacterium (inclusion body) found in columnar lining cells of the cervix, uterus, fallopian tubes, liver capsule, urethra, rectum, pharynx, and skin. *C. trachomatis* is the most common cause of **nongonococcal urethritis** in men, as well as **lymphogranuloma venereum, epididymitis,** and **inclusion conjunctivitis.** It is the leading cause of infertility in females.

(2) ***Neisseria gonorrhoeae*** is an intracellular, Gram-negative diplococcus found in a distribution similar to that of *C. trachomatis.* Joint involvement can lead to arthritis.

(3) **HIV** is acquired through sexual transmission or intravenous spread from blood products or illicit drug use (see Chapter 9).

(4) ***Ureaplasma urealyticum*** is the second most common cause of nongonococcal urethritis in men. It is a T-strain mycoplasma with genital and pelvic distribution similar to that of *C. trachomatis.*

(5) ***Treponema pallidum,*** the cause of **syphilis,** is a less common cause of infection in adolescents compared to adults. It is seen more regularly in association with other STDs and in adolescents who use illicit drugs. It is a motile spiral microorganism 5 to 20 mm long that can start in the genital area with a skin lesion called a chancre, or occur in other parts of the body.

(6) ***Haemophilus ducreyi,*** the cause of chancroid, should be considered in the differential diagnosis of a painful genital ulcer often accompanied by tender inguinal lymphadenopathy.

(7) **Herpes simplex virus (HSV)** infection has increased in incidence to more than 1 million cases per year in the United States. HSV is a DNA virus causing ulcer-like lesions in the genital region (HSV type 2).

(8) **Human papillomavirus (HPV)** is a DNA virus causing venereal warts and changes leading to cervical cancer. HPV is the most common STD found in adolescents.

(9) **Molluscum contagiosum** is a poxvirus infection found in any part of the body, but it is usually present in greater concentration in the genital area when sexual transmission is involved.

(10) ***Trichomonas vaginalis*** is a flagellate protozoan present most commonly in the vagina but also found near the urethra of both sexes.

(11) ***Phthirus pubis*** (pediculosis pubis, crab lice) is a parasite that is < 4 mm long, found in pubic hair and causing pruritus.

TABLE 5-4 Sexually Transmitted Diseases in Adolescents

Agent	Clinical Features	Diagnosis
Chlamydia trachomatis	Cervical ectopy and friability Mucoid cervical discharge with ↑ leukocyte count Dysuria (in men may not be accompanied by discharge) Pelvic tenderness in women Pharyngitis Rectal irritation/tenderness	Cell culture or rapid urine test
Neisseria gonorrhoeae	Similar clinical features as with chlamydial infection	Gram-positive diplococci in male urethral discharge, culture or rapid urine test
	Infection in men more likely to include purulent urethral discharge	Gram-negative diplococci in male urethral discharge
Human immunodeficiency virus (HIV)	Different from adult presentation: Lower male-to-female ratio More prevalent in Black/Hispanic urban youth Higher percentage of heterosexual transmission	Specific blood assay for HIV virus (see Chapter 9)
Ureaplasma urealyticum	Similar characteristics to chlamydial infection	Culture
Treponema pallidum (syphilis)	Stage of disease: Primary (10–40 d): Chancres, regional lymphadenopathy Secondary (2–6 mo): Generalized malaise, lymphadenopathy, skin changes/alopecia Late (2–10 y): Central nervous system changes, cardiovascular changes, musculoskeletal involvement	Darkfield examination or direct fluorescent antibody tests of lesion Serologic tests: Nontreponemal Treponemal
Haemophilus ducreyi (chancroid)	Painful genital ulcer Tender inguinal lymphadenopathy	Culture Clinical picture
Herpes simplex virus	Vesicles/ulcers on external genitalia, in vagina, on cervix, and around rectal area Tender inguinal lymphadenopathy Dysuria Dyspareunia	Viral culture Tzanck test
Human papillomavirus	Sexually transmitted warts such as condyloma acuminatum and cervical changes that may result in cancer	Clinical appearance and DNA typing done with the Pap smear Biopsy
Molluscum contagiosum	Small papule with umbilical centers	Clinical appearance Potassium hydroxide smear of contents Biopsy
Trichomonas vaginalis	Presence of flagellate protozoan Malodorous yellow-green vaginal discharge Vaginal irritation	Microscopic identification of organism
Phthirus pubis (pediculosis pubis, crab lice)	Pruritus in pubic hair Tan egg cases in pubic hair	Crab lice or egg cases in pubic hair

b. Therapy for STDs should include all exposed individuals, whenever possible. The specific treatment depends on accurate identification of the causative organism; the choice of antibiotic must take into consideration the organism's sensitivity and the patient's age and history of allergies. Two general treatment recommendations should be taken into consideration:

(1) Whenever possible, treat the STD with a single dose of medication right on the spot to ensure compliance. This is possible for gonorrheal, chlamydial, and trichomonal infections. The latest treatment guidelines for STDs are published by the Centers for Disease Control and Prevention (see the Bibliography).

(2) If either gonorrhea or chlamydial infection is suspected, treatment should be given for both diseases.

(3) Reduction of the prevalence of HPV is now possible with a vaccine.

c. Prevention includes abstinence; proper use of condoms can eliminate the risk of transmitting most STDs except HPV and HSV.

d. Pelvic inflammatory disease (PID) is the spread of an infection from the vagina to the cervix, uterus, fallopian tubes, and peritoneum, potentially resulting in endometritis, salpingitis, parametritis, perihepatitis, and peritonitis. Such infections may cause subsequent infertility.

(1) **Clinical features** include significant abdominal pain, as well as adnexal and cervical motion tenderness. Infection commonly starts during the menstrual period and may be associated with fever and a history of recent or past exposure to an STD. The erythrocyte sedimentation rate (ESR) is elevated. A pelvic ultrasound may show increased fluid outside these organs or formation of an abscess.

(2) **Etiology.** The most common causes of PID are *N. gonorrhoeae* and *C. trachomatis.* Other organisms include *Mycoplasma hominis, Staphylococcus aureus, Streptococcus* species, *Escherichia coli,* and anaerobic bacteria, such as *Bacteroides* species. PID is often caused by multiple organisms.

(3) **Therapy.** PID needs to be treated quickly and aggressively. Adolescents with significant abdominal pain and fever should be hospitalized for IV antibiotics and stabilization. Refer to the 2006 Centers for Disease Control and Prevention guidelines for the latest recommendations (see Bibliography).

4. Dysmenorrhea is menstrual pain (usually in the lower abdomen).

a. Primary dysmenorrhea, which accounts for 75% of all cases of dysmenorrhea, is not associated with any other pelvic abnormality, and lasts from a few hours to 2 to 3 days.

(1) Symptoms include nausea, vomiting, headaches, back pain, and dizziness.

(2) The exact cause of the pain is unclear, but it may be related to increased myometrial activity (contractions of the smooth muscle coat) of the uterus associated with increased production of prostaglandin.

b. Secondary dysmenorrhea is caused by a definable pelvic abnormality such as inflammation, structural abnormalities, adhesions, endometriosis, tumors, polyps, ovarian cysts, and IUDs.

c. Evaluation

(1) **History.** Determine the relation of pain to the menstrual cycle, the duration of pain, associated symptoms and degree of dysfunction, and familial history of similar pain. Level of sexual activity and exposure to an STD are helpful. Systemic disease (e.g., gastroenteritis, urinary tract infection) should be ruled out.

(2) **Pelvic examination** is indicated when the patient is in severe pain that lasts longer than 3 days and does not respond to treatment for primary dysmenorrhea.

(3) **Laboratory evaluation** should be considered for cases that do not fit the definition of primary dysmenorrhea. Tests include a complete blood count and ESR to check for pelvic infection, vaginal wet smear, tests for STDs, ultrasound of the pelvis for ovarian cysts, and laparoscopy for severe, unresolved cases.

(4) **Therapy**

(a) **Mild pain** with no limitation of activity may not need any treatment or may respond well to aspirin or a prostaglandin inhibitor (e.g., ibuprofen).

(b) **Moderate pain** that causes some limitation of activity but does not result in reduced school attendance may be eased by regular use of an over-the-counter prostaglandin inhibitor.

TABLE 5-5 Stages of Substance Abuse

Stages	Description
Stage 1: Experimentation	Usually starts with peer pressure Few if any behavioral changes User struggles between the euphoria achieved and associated guilt
Stage 2: To relieve stress	Use is more than occasional and in nonsocial situations Supply of the substance is maintained, and peer group develops around substance abuse Exhibits mood swings and a decline in school performance
Stage 3: Regular abuse	Becomes involved with drug-oriented culture Most, if not all, peers use drugs Behavioral problems are chronic, may include problems with the law Depression when not using drugs Must raise money to support habit
Stage 4: Dependence	Drug is used to prevent depression May drop out of school and become involved in destructive family dynamics Physical changes may include weight loss, fatigue, blackouts, and chronic cough

(c) **Severe pain** that causes the adolescent to miss school may be relieved by a prescription-strength prostaglandin inhibitor or a trial of oral contraceptives.

C Substance abuse

1. **Overview**
   a. **Definition.** Substance abuse is consumption of cigarettes, alcohol, or drugs to the point of compromising health or causing dysfunctional behavior (Tables 5-5 and 5-6). Chronic substance abuse causes arrest of psychosocial development.
   b. **Annual prevalence** (proportion of adolescents reporting use of illicit drug in past 12 months) continues to **decrease** from the peak rates seen in the 1990s. Rates in 2006 were 15% for 8th graders (down 33%), 29% for 10th graders (down 25%), and 37% for 12th graders (down 12%).
   c. **Laboratory studies.** Confirm drug abuse through urine or blood tests and check for changes in liver and pulmonary functions.
   d. **Therapy** includes ambulatory care for first and second stages (Table 5-5) of involvement, and hospitalization for third and fourth stages. Many substance abusers do not realize or do not admit that they have a problem.
2. **Tobacco** is the most commonly used substance and strongly correlates with use by parents and peers. Daily cigarette use in 2006 was 4% for 8th graders, 7.6% for 10th graders, and 12.2% for 12th graders, an overall drop of 50% from 1990 levels. Using smokeless tobacco (snuff) has also decreased by about 50% with rates of ever used in 2006 being 10.2% for 8th graders, 15% for 10th graders, and 15.2% for 12th graders.
3. **Marijuana,** the most prevalent illicit drug, is now being used more frequently than alcohol by certain adolescent populations. Marijuana use reported in 2006 as one or more times in the past 30 days was 6.5% in 8th graders (down 36%), 14.2% in 10th graders (down 30%), and 18.3% in 12th graders (down 23%). The active ingredient, tetrahydrocannabinol (THC), is metabolized in the liver but is also stored in body fat, resulting in a long half-life.
4. **Alcohol** is the second most commonly used substance after tobacco. In 2006, reported alcohol use of one or more times in the past 30 days was 17.2% in 8th graders (down 33%), 33.8% in 10th graders (down 17%), and 45.3% in 12th graders (down 14%).
5. **Hallucinogens.** The rate of hallucinogens ever been used decreased, with 2006 data showing 3.4% in 8th graders (down 42%), 6.1% in 10th graders (down 42%), and 8.3% in 12th graders (down 38%). The most common hallucinogens are **lysergic acid diethylamide (LSD),** derived

TABLE 5-6 Hazards Associated with Drug and Alcohol Abuse

Substance	Hazards
Tobacco	Altered lung function Chronic symptoms such as productive cough and chest pain Decrease in performance endurance Lung cancer, coronary heart disease
Snuff	Associated with development of oral squamous carcinoma
Marijuana	Lung impairment greater than with cigarettes Short-term memory and learning changes Decreased reaction time, coordination, visual perception
Alcohol	Decreased reaction time, coordination, visual perception Acute illness (hangover) Liver changes leading to cirrhosis Chronic depression Withdrawal syndrome if used long term
Hallucinogens	Self-inflicted physical harm "Bad trips," "flashbacks" Chronic CNS changes Overdose
Stimulants	Depression Cardiovascular impairment Psychosis Overdose Rapid addiction Slurred speech Ataxia Impulsive behavior Respiratory depression Severe withdrawal reaction
Narcotics	Complications from injectable drugs Addiction Overdose
Inhalants	Nasal and bronchial irritation Systemic effects such as liver and renal toxicity, cardiac arrhythmias, and CNS changes
Anabolic steroids	Impaired excretion by liver Hypertension Impaired glucose tolerance Aggressive behavior
Club drugs	Increased heart rate, temperature, blood pressure Insomnia, anxiety, tremors, sweating Memory problems Cognitive defects Coma Seizures Hallucinations Impaired motor functions Kidney failure Respiratory failure

CNS, central nervous system.

from rye fungus; **mescaline,** derived from a cactus; **psilocybin (PCP),** derived from the mushroom *Psilocybe mexicana;* and **phencyclidine,** a drug initially developed as a general anesthetic.

6. **Stimulants.** Amphetamines and cocaine are the most frequently used stimulants. Crack cocaine, a smokable form of the drug, became popular in the 1980s and continues to be very dangerous.

7. **Depressants.** The most commonly abused depressants are barbiturates and tranquilizers.
8. **Narcotics**
   a. The most commonly abused narcotics are **heroin, methadone, meperidine,** and **propoxyphene.**
   b. **Naloxone** is effective in counteracting the effects of narcotics.
9. **Club drugs** include **Ecstasy** (MDMA, or 3-4 methylenedioxymethamphetamine), **GHB** (γ-hydroxybutyrate), **ketamine,** and **Rohypnol** (flunitrazepam). These drugs are used in nightclubs, raves, and trance events that may last most of the night. They can cause intoxicating highs that are said to deepen the trance or rave experience.
10. **Inhalants** usually have depressant and sedative effects. They are more commonly used by younger adolescents.

D Musculoskeletal disorders

1. **Scoliosis** is lateral curvature of the spine involving the thoracic and lumbar vertebrae. **Incidence** is 3% to 5% of the pediatric population. Etiology is unknown in 75% of cases. Scoliosis occurs more frequently in females when onset is in adolescence.
   a. Known **causes** include congenital failure of spinal development, musculoskeletal disease (e.g., cerebral palsy), neurofibromatosis, Marfan syndrome, juvenile rheumatoid arthritis, trauma (e.g., fracture and destruction of vertebrae, severe burns), and structural defects (e.g., different leg lengths).
   b. **Evaluation** includes examination of the back with the patient in an erect and a bent-at-the-hips position looking at vertebral, scapular, and muscular asymmetry. Check leg lengths and symmetry at the hips and shoulders. Obtain radiographs of the spine to quantitate degree of curve in more advanced cases.
   c. **Therapy** depends on the degree of back curvature and ranges from monitoring and back exercises to bracing and surgical intervention.
      (1) Because scoliosis progresses more quickly during the pubertal growth spurt, it should be checked every 3 months if the curvature is 15 to 20 degrees.
      (2) Curvature $\geq$ 20 degrees should be referred to an orthopedic surgeon for additional evaluation.
   d. **Sequelae** may include deformity of the chest, limitation of lung function leading to polycythemia and pulmonary hypertension, and compromise in cardiac function from pressure on the chest cavity.
2. **Slipped capital femoral epiphysis** is a displacement of the femoral head, usually posteriorly and medially off the femoral metaphysis. It occurs most often in males and is associated with obesity during the pubertal growth spurt.
   a. **Evaluation.** History should inquire as to any pain in the hip or the knee, antalgic gait, and obesity. Physical examination may reveal few positive findings except a limitation in the range of motion of the hip. Radiography shows femoral head changes.
   b. **Therapy** is surgical correction.
3. **Osgood-Schlatter disease** causes stress changes in the tibial tuberosity at the attachment of the patellar tendon. This typically occurs during the pubertal growth spurt and is more common in males who are active in sports.
   a. **Evaluation** includes a history of tenderness around the tibial tuberosity. **Physical examination** may identify swelling and point tenderness at the tibial tuberosity.
   b. **Therapy** includes supportive care, pain relief, and reduced physical activity when pain is severe. Bracing may become necessary if supportive care is not sufficient.

E **Mental health issues** (see also Chapter 4)

1. **Depression.** More than half (60%) of teenagers surveyed while receiving routine health care indicated that they feel down or depressed as frequently as once a month to daily. Females experience depression more commonly than do males.
   a. **Etiology.** A number of factors may lead to depression, including:
      (1) **Changes in peer relationships** (e.g., loss of a boyfriend or girlfriend, exclusion from the peer group, lack of peer group support, inability to be with peers)

(2) **Family influences** (e.g., lack of independence, poor communication, decreased availability of parents, problems between the parents). Adolescents who do not feel that their parents are supportive are at greater risk for depression.
(3) **School experiences** (e.g., poor performance, conflict with teachers, peer conflict or pressure, unrealistically high expectations from parents)
(4) **Poor self-image** (e.g., dissatisfaction with one's physical appearance, lack of self-confidence, a hopeless vision of the future)

b. Clinical features

(1) **Recurrent somatic complaints** (e.g., headaches; chest, abdominal, or back pains; and changes in eating habits, sleep patterns, and levels of activity)
(2) **Mood swings** (manifested as restlessness; withdrawal from peers and family; decreased ability to function on a day-to-day basis; and acting-out behavior such as violence, substance abuse, risk taking, and little or no recognition of authority)
(3) **A decline in the level of school performance**
(4) **Apathy** (e.g., a loss of interest in sports, hobbies, and community-related activities)

c. Therapy. Counseling programs associated with health services, school-based support services, and intervention in parent-adolescent conflict should be available. The 24-hour telephone availability of a health network can provide reassurance.

2. Suicide. Data from the 2005 Youth Risk Behavior Survey showed that 16.9% of adolescents considered attempting suicide, 13% had made a suicide plan, and 8.4% completed a suicide attempt. Suicide attempts outnumber successful suicides by as much as 200 to 1. Females make more attempts than males, but successful suicide is four times more common in men. More than half (60%) of teenagers who commit suicide have attempted suicide previously.

a. Methods. Most frequent methods in order of occurrence are firearms, hanging, and drug overdose. Females most frequently commit suicide by drug overdose and males by guns.

b. Attempts to prevent suicide should include the following steps:

(1) **Questioning.** All adolescents should be asked about suicidal thoughts and suicide attempts, not just those who seem depressed.
(2) **Assessment of risk.** If the adolescent has suicidal thoughts, the level of risk should be evaluated by identifying any history of suicide attempts and level of familial support.
  (a) **Degree of depression.** A severely depressed teenager may be unable to mobilize to commit suicide, but a teenager who is recovering from depression may be more at risk for suicide.
  (b) **Danger signs** include getting affairs in order, giving away favorite possessions, withdrawing from friends, social and school activities, and a history of suicide or alcohol abuse in the family.
  (c) Look for **precipitating event** such as a breakup with a girlfriend or boyfriend, a conflict with peers, pregnancy, and, most frequently, a conflict with parents.
(3) **Therapy** involves a team approach, including the services of a physician, a social worker, and a consulting psychiatrist.

3. Eating disorders

a. Anorexia nervosa

(1) **Definition**
  (a) **Refusal to maintain appropriate body weight** for height, resulting in a weight that is 85% or less than expected for the given height
  (b) Intense **fear of gaining weight** or being fat
  (c) **Disturbed body image,** such as feeling fat when one is actually almost emaciated
  (d) Absence of at least three consecutive **menstrual cycles** in females
(2) **Occurrence.** Anorexia nervosa is most commonly seen in middle to late adolescence, traditionally in approximately 1% of white females of higher socioeconomic groups. More recently, this disorder has been seen in younger adolescents and other socioeconomic groups. Males make up $< 10\%$ of the patient population.
(3) **Etiology and contributing factors**
  (a) Exact etiology is unknown.
  (b) Norms that promote thinness as beautiful are pervasive cultural influences.

(c) The patient often displays obsessive, overachieving, and controlling personality traits.
(d) There are often disordered family relationships.
(e) There is often a family history of mental health problems, substance abuse, and eating disorders.

(4) **Evaluation**

(a) **History**

(i) Understand the patient's body: What is acceptable, what is too fat, and what is too thin.
(ii) Document the chronology of the weight loss, and dietary history.
(iii) Ask about vomiting, excessive exercise, laxative abuse, and willingness to eat with friends and family.
(iv) Identify and explore relationships with family and friends.
(v) Review of systems should consider chronic illness or pain, menstrual history, signs of depression, and assessment of level of self-esteem.

(b) **Physical examination** should include accurate vital signs, weight with only a dressing gown, and body temperature. Skin may have a dry, mottled appearance with signs of lanugo (fine hair) and lack of subcutaneous fat. There may be a weak pulse. Muscle tone may be decreased with generalized weakness.

(c) **Laboratory studies**

(i) Routine laboratory test findings such as hemoglobin, ESR, urinalysis, electrolyte levels, calcium, phosphorus, and serum protein are usually negative. Blood urea nitrogen (BUN) may be elevated when dehydration is present.
(ii) **Special studies.** Levels of triiodothyronine, luteinizing hormone, and follicle-stimulating hormone may be low, whereas cholesterol, cortisol, and endorphin levels may be elevated. An electrocardiogram should assess for bradycardia, decreased QRS amplitude, nonspecific ST-segment and T-wave changes, and prolonged QT interval.
(iii) A computed tomography (CT) scan should be obtained in boys who are initially seen with weight loss because the incidence of brain tumor is higher. It also may be possible to document cerebral atrophy.

(5) **Therapy** involves making an initial decision whether to treat on an ambulatory basis or in a hospital. Greater than 20% weight loss associated with electrolyte, cardiovascular, or neurologic signs suggests the need for hospitalization, as does failure to gain weight in an ambulatory program.

(a) **Medical management**

(i) Nutritional support ranging from high-caloric diet to replacement by nasogastric tube or hyperalimentation, if necessary
(ii) Vitamin supplements as indicated
(iii) Estrogen supplement to reinitiate menses

(b) **Psychological management**

(i) **Behavior modification.** A system of privileges is often established, depending on the patient's intake.
(ii) **Psychotherapy,** both individual and family, is essential.
(iii) **Psychopharmacology.** Antidepressant agents may be helpful.
(iv) **Goals of therapy** include weight gain up to 10% of expected body weight, associated with a contract to maintain this weight gain and enrollment in a comprehensive program that deals with nutritional, medical, and psychological needs.

(6) **Prognosis** is variable, with mortality as high as 20%. Early identification and comprehensive care can reduce the mortality rate to as low as 2%.

b. **Bulimia**

(1) **Definition**

(a) Repetitive binge eating involving rapid consumption of a large amount of food over a short period of time

(i) Feeling of lack of control over eating during binge episodes
(ii) Minimum of two binge episodes per month for 3 months

(b) Weight loss by vomiting, use of laxatives or diuretics, fasting, or vigorous exercise
(c) Overconcern with body shape and weight

(2) **Prevalence.** Bulimia is seen mainly in **older teenagers** (average age is 18 years), with a rate of 4% in a college population and a female-to-male ratio of 10 to 1.

(3) **Clinical features** include poor self-image associated with depression (especially after a binge episode); thoughts about suicide; substance abuse; antisocial behavior (e.g., stealing); and self-mutilation.

(4) **Medical complications** may include esophagitis, gastric dilatation and possible rupture, aspiration, cardiac arrhythmia, pancreatitis, metabolic alkalosis associated with hypochloremia and hypokalemia, swelling of the parotid and submandibular glands, and dental problems such as erosion of dental enamel and dentin and loss of teeth.

(5) **Evaluation**

(a) **History.** Ask about eating patterns and food intake history, purging behavior, past weight fluctuations, body image, level of depression, risk-taking behavior, and family dynamics.

(b) **Physical examination** includes assessment of vital signs for possible hypovolemia, assessment of dentition, and evaluation of cardiac function. Abdomen should be palpated for tenderness or distention. Hands should be checked for scars from repeated induced vomiting.

(c) **Laboratory studies** should evaluate electrolyte level, hydration, and cardiovascular status.

(6) **Therapy** should stabilize the patient's medical condition. The focus of treatment is to normalize the metabolic state and encourage the adolescent to become involved in counseling. Antidepressant medication may be helpful in specific cases.

V ADOLESCENTS WITH SPECIAL HEALTH CARE NEEDS

A There are over 12 million children with special health care needs (about 18% of all children). About **2 million are adolescents** with disabilities or chronic health conditions that limit their daily activities.

B Potential implications on development and health

1. **Delayed pubertal development** as seen in sickle cell disease and cystic fibrosis
2. **Decreased peer interactions** as seen in adolescents with mental health or musculoskeletal limitations
3. **Decreased compliance** with use of medications or recommended health procedures as seen with asthma and insulin-dependent diabetes
4. **Delay in achievement of independence**
5. **Development of coping mechanisms** may vary. Adolescents may use different mechanisms at different times. Positive mechanisms include acceptance of the disease or disability and compensation in ways to better deal with the impact. Negative mechanisms include denial of the disability, acting out, or showing regressive behavior.

C Approach to health care

1. **Important issues** to consider include the adolescent's mental health, physical and psychological development, and level of family support.
2. An **important goal** is to enable the adolescent to become as self-sufficient and independent as possible.
3. A **multidisciplinary team approach** is important, in which the adolescent has access to the multiple services needed to deal with the disability. Team members should also be able to provide educational and vocational support and help with transition to adult health care.
4. **Link the adolescent with support groups** where available.

BIBLIOGRAPHY

Centers for Disease Control and Prevention: 2006 guidelines for treatment of sexually transmitted diseases. *MMWR* 47(RR-1):1–94, 2006.

Choice of contraceptives. *Treatment Guidelines from the Medical Letter.* 2(24):55–62, 2004.

Emans SJ, Laufer MR, Goldstein DP: *Pediatric and Adolescent Gynecology,* 5th ed. Philadelphia, Lippincott Williams & Wilkins, 2005.

Green M, ed. *Bright Futures. Guidelines for Health Supervision of Infants, Children, and Adolescents,* 2nd ed, revised. Washington, DC, National Center for Education in Maternal and Child Health, 2002.

Guidelines for Adolescent Preventive Services (GAPS). Chicago, American Medical Association, 1997.

Knight JR, Sherritt L, Shrier LA, et al.: Validity of the CRAFFT substance abuse screening test among adolescent clinic patients. *Arch Pediatr Adolesc* 156(6):607–614, 2002.

Neinstein LS: *Adolescent Health Care: A Practical Guide,* 5th ed. Philadelphia, Lippincott Williams & Wilkins, 2007.

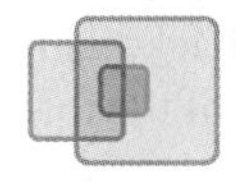

Study Questions

Directions: *Each of the numbered items or incomplete statements in this section is followed by answers or completions of the statement. Select the ONE lettered answer or completion that is BEST in each case.*

1. A 15-year-old girl with type I diabetes mellitus requests to start oral contraceptive pills. She has not had sexual intercourse to date, but feels that she may become sexually active in the near future. Which of the following is the most likely side effect she would experience from oral contraceptive pills?

A Hair loss
B Decreased control of her diabetes
C Bleeding between periods
D Dysmenorrhea
E Longer menstrual periods

2. You have a 17-year-old son at home who is busy making college plans. You know that he will be leaving for college in another year and a half. You believe that spending a summer as a counselor at an overnight camp will be good preparation for him before he goes off to college. Which of the following developmental tasks of adolescence would be addressed and thus would be the most important benefit to this 17 year-old from spending a summer as a counselor in an overnight camp?

A Promoting independence
B Developing a peer network
C Helping to form adult role models
D Separation
E Taking responsibility

3. You are completing a history on a 17-year-old female. She reports that things are not going very well at school. She received a "C" in math instead of her usual "B," and several weeks ago had a brief physical altercation with another girl in her grade who accused her of flirting with the girl's boyfriend. The patient is sexually active and uses condoms but on one recent occasion, the condom "broke." She also tells you that her parents are not very supportive. Before you begin the physical examination, you note that she gained 2 lbs in the past year. After listening to the history, you are concerned about the possibility of depression in this patient. Which of the following items reported to you in the history is most concerning regarding possible depression in this young woman?

A Math grade of "C" instead of usual "B"
B Physical altercation with a peer at school
C Recent condom failure
D Two-pound weight gain during the past year
E Parents perceived as unsupportive

4. A 17-year-old female comes to your office and tells you that she is very upset. She has been told that she has a sexually transmitted disease and that it might interfere with her ability to have children in the future. She has no complaints of abdominal pain. On pelvic examination, there is a mucoid discharge without vulvar lesions and moderate friability of the cervix. There is no cervical motion tenderness or adnexal tenderness. Which of the following sexually transmitted diseases is most likely to be present in this patient?

A Human papillomavirus
B Syphilis
C Herpes
D Chlamydia
E Trichomonas

5. The school nurse referred a 15-year-old female to you for evaluation of scoliosis. The note from the nurse indicates that on a routine scoliosis screening the left scapula was noted to be higher than the right. The adolescent tells you that she has had her period for 2 years and that she has no back pain. Physical exam shows back curvature that measures about 8 degrees with a scoliometer. Which of the following is the best approach to management for this patient's scoliosis?

- [A] Reassure and follow up as needed
- [B] Refer to orthopedics for further evaluation
- [C] Prescribe back exercises and follow up in 6 months
- [D] Order back radiograph to better document the degree of scoliosis
- [E] Recommend bracing to halt the progression of scoliosis

6. A 17-year-old female comes in for evaluation of a 2-day history of lower abdominal pain. She just finished her menstrual period. She is sexually active and claims to use a condom every time that she has intercourse; she does admit one break of a condom 1 week ago. Patient's temperature is 102°F. Pelvic examination reveals tenderness on movement of the cervix and in adnexa bilaterally. Normal saline preparation of the cervical discharge shows numerous white cells. Which of the following is the most appropriate next step in management of this patient?

- [A] Order a STAT pelvic ultrasound
- [B] Request a consultation from surgery
- [C] Treat for sexually transmitted disease (STD) and follow up in 2 days
- [D] Admit to the hospital
- [E] Order a STAT abdominal CT scan

7. You are an adolescent medicine clinician for a large inner-city population. Which of the following is the most appropriate strategy to reduce the mortality for the leading cause of death in this population?

- [A] Substance abuse prevention programs
- [B] School-based depression screening programs
- [C] Raise minimum driving age and increase restrictions on teenage drivers
- [D] Community-based outreach gang rivalry intervention programs
- [E] Mandatory smoke alarms for all rental units with surveillance programs

8. You are performing an adolescent health supervision visit and after discussing adolescent confidentiality you need to obtain history about sexual activity. Which of the following topics should you cover first in order to maximize the potential for productive history taking and patient education?

- [A] Ask about sexual preference
- [B] Ask about having sex and make certain to define your terms
- [C] Ask about ever having sex
- [D] Ask about using protection
- [E] Ask about date rape

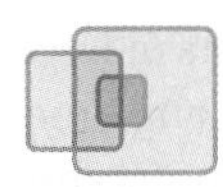

Answers and Explanations

1. The answer is C (*Table 5-3*). Birth control pills may affect glycemic control in patients with type I diabetes mellitus, but these effects are usually minor and easily corrected. Bleeding between periods, or breakthrough bleeding, is one of the most common side effects of oral contraceptive pills. This effect usually resolves after the second or third cycle of pills. Hair loss can occur but is much less common. Birth control pills usually reduce dysmenorrhea and the length of the menstrual period.

2. The answer is D (*Table 5-2*). Going to college is associated with late adolescence when separation is one of the major developmental issues. At this point adolescents not only think that they are independent in their own minds, but they are often also physically living under a separate roof than their parents for the first time in their lives. In actuality, the transition to college is much easier than the transition of leaving home to set out entirely on one's own. Independence, peer networking, and finding adult role models are typically more important issues during early and mid-adolescence, which may continue to be important during late adolescence.

3. The answer is E (*IV E 1 a [2]*). An adolescent's perception that he or she lacks parental support is the strongest marker for depression identified in data derived from histories obtained during annual physical examinations. Adolescents who perceive that they have good parental support tend to be more resilient in dealing with other at-risk behaviors. An adolescent who has been involved in a physical fight at school needs violence prevention skills, at the very least. An adolescent who has had a condom failure needs counseling for prevention of pregnancy and sexually transmitted diseases.

4. The answer is D (*IV B 3 a [1]*). Chlamydia is the leading cause of infertility for women. This infection is often asymptomatic. The carrier may not seek treatment until the infection passes to the fallopian tubes. Salpingitis may occur causing lower abdominal pain and eventual scarring of the tube. Unfortunately, such changes can occur without pain. Human papillomavirus, the leading cause of cervical cancer in women, can present as external genital warts or as a silent infection that is identified through HPV changes noted on a Pap smear. Trichomonas is associated with a frothy, irritating vaginal discharge caused by motile organisms seen under the microscopic in a wet prep of the discharge. Herpes is associated with painful, ulcerlike pustular lesions that can occur on the vulva, vagina, and cervix. Syphilis is a systemic disease that may start with cutaneous lesions.

5. The answer is A (*II C 3 b, IV D 1*). This adolescent is 2 years past onset of menarche and therefore has achieved most of her maximal pubertal growth. Further additional significant progression in the degree of back curvature is unlikely (although not impossible) to occur. Referral for orthopedic evaluation should generally be considered as curvatures begin to approach 20 degrees. Measurement of the degree of back curvature is more accurate by radiography than by scoliometer. While back exercises can be useful for all adolescents since the back is a body part that rarely gets exercised on a regular basis, there are no data that demonstrate effectiveness of exercise on altering the progression of a scoliosis curve. Patients who are prepubertal or in very early puberty need to be monitored much more closely than their counterparts in late puberty, because of the increased likelihood of curve progression with decreased skeletal maturity.

6. The answer is D (*IV B 3 d*). The combination of lower abdominal pain, cervical motion tenderness, and adnexal tenderness strongly suggests a pelvic infection. The presence of fever and adnexal tenderness confirms systemic involvement of the infection and need for aggressive therapy. Hospitalization for further evaluation and intravenous antibiotic therapy to cover for both gonorrhea and chlamydia is the most appropriate next step in management. Pelvic ultrasound is recommended to rule out an abscess but is usually performed only if there is no response after 1 to 2 days of intravenous antibiotic therapy. Surgical consultation and/or a STAT abdominal CT scan are generally reserved for cases in which the source of the pain remains unclear after a pelvic infection has been ruled out. Patients who have very mild cervical motion tenderness without adnexal tenderness and minimal to no fever can be initially treated on an outpatient basis with oral antibiotics and observation for 1 to 2 days. If the pain does not resolve, hospital admission and intravenous antibiotic therapy are indicated.

7. The answer is D (*I B 1*). Homicide continues to be the leading cause of death for adolescents in large inner-city populations. This often happens when an adolescent is at the wrong place at the wrong time. Many of these deaths are related to intergang rivalry. Automobile accidents are the most common cause of death for all adolescents. Drug overdoses are common forms of suicide attempts, many of which may not be lethal but are cries for help.

8. The answer is B (*II A 5 b [1]*). It is most helpful to begin by clarifying that you and your adolescent patient are using the same terms and talking about the same things. "Having sex" means having vaginal, oral, or rectal intercourse. Some adolescents who are having oral intercourse may not consider themselves to be sexually active. It is also useful to determine an adolescent's sexual preference early in the discussion, although not before relevant words/terms are explicitly defined.

chapter 6

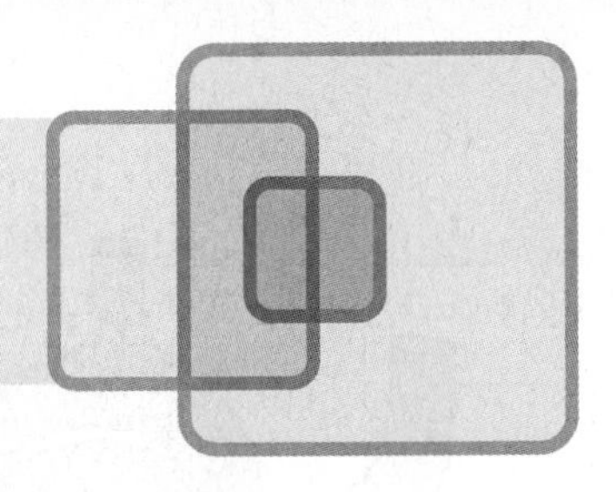

Neonatology

JOHN CASEY • TED S. ROSENKRANTZ

I GENERAL PRINCIPLES

Many problems that arise in the newborn are discussed in detail in other chapters. This chapter emphasizes those problems that are unique to the perinatal period. In this section, some general concepts are introduced, which are amplified in subsequent sections.

A Definition of terms

1. The normal human **gestational period** is 280 days, or 40 weeks, calculated from the first day of the mother's last menstrual cycle.
   a. **Preterm gestation** refers to delivery at < 37 weeks' gestation.
   b. **Term gestation** refers to delivery at 37 to < 42 weeks' gestation.
   c. **Postterm gestation** refers to delivery at or after 42 weeks' gestation.
2. The **neonatal period** is defined as the first 28 days (4 weeks) of life for term infants, although, from a practical standpoint, it is extended in the case of a prematurely delivered infant.

B Major concepts and concerns inherent to the neonatal period

1. **Transition from fetal to neonatal life.** Changes in body and organ function occur as the fetus adapts to extrauterine life and begins to function independently. Organs mature at different rates and times during gestation. A preterm or complicated delivery may alter the normal sequence of these events. Some major changes occur in the following organ systems during the transition from fetal to neonatal life.
   a. **Cardiovascular system** (see Chapter 12)
      (1) **Prenatal circulation** (Figure 6-1)
         (a) Oxygenation of the blood occurs in the **placenta**—an organ of low vascular resistance—and the oxygenated blood returns to the fetus via the **umbilical vein,** which enters the liver at the porta hepatis.
         (b) Blood passes through the **ductus venosus** to the inferior vena cava. Preferential shunting allows this oxygenated blood to be predominantly shunted through the **foramen ovale** to the left atrium and left ventricle and on to the coronary, carotid, and cerebral arteries. This allows for the most highly oxygenated blood to reach the cerebral and cardiac circulations.
         (c) Desaturated blood of the inferior and superior venae cavae travels to the right atrium and right ventricle and on to the pulmonary artery. Due to the high vascular resistance in the lung, 90% of the pulmonary artery blood bypasses the lung and is shunted through the **ductus arteriosus,** which enters the descending aorta.
         (d) Blood in the descending aorta, which is intermediately deoxygenated, supplies the remainder of the systemic circulation and is returned to the placenta by way of the **umbilical arteries.**
      (2) **Postnatal circulation**
         (a) At birth, upon clamping of the umbilical cord, the low-resistance vascular bed in the placenta is removed causing an overall rise in systemic vascular resistance.
         (b) With exposure of the pulmonary vascular bed to oxygen and mechanical expansion in the first few breaths, pulmonary vascular resistance decreases considerably (to 80% of normal), and pulmonary blood flow increases dramatically.

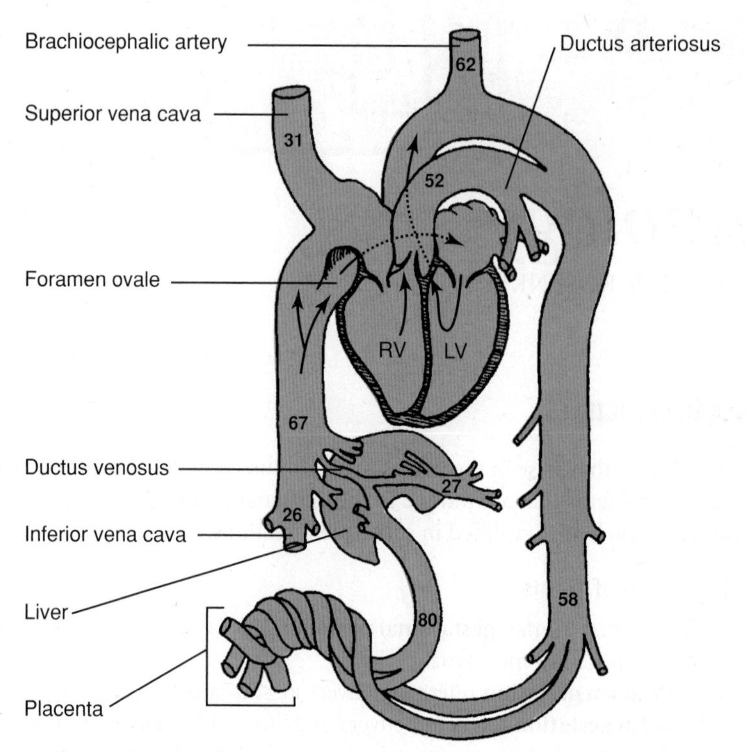

FIGURE 6-1 Knowledge of the human fetal circulation is based on fetal animal studies, such as the fetal lamb. The fetal lamb circulation is diagramed here, with numbers representing the percent oxygen saturation in various segments. These values are believed to correspond closely to those in the human fetus. LV, left ventricle, RV, right ventricle. (Reprinted from Born GVR, Dawes GS, Mott JC, et al.: Changes in the heart and lungs at birth. *Cold Spring Harbor Symp Quant Biol* 19:102, 1954.)

(c) As a result of increased blood return to the left ventricle from the pulmonary artery, the foramen ovale closes; concurrently the ductus arteriosus begins to constrict. These processes allow all deoxygenated blood returning to the right ventricle to go on to the lung and become oxygenated.

b. **Pulmonary system** (see Chapter 13)

(1) By the end of gestation, the major airways and alveoli are filled with fluid that contains large amounts of **surfactant.**

(2) At birth, the negative pressure created by the first breaths draws air into the lungs, and an air-fluid interface is formed. The surfactant spreads along the epithelial lining of the alveoli and decreases surface tension at the end of expiration.

c. **Hepatobiliary system.** Prenatally, bilirubin conjugation in the liver is suppressed. In the first days of life, increased **glucuronyl transferase** activity results in conjugation and elimination of bilirubin, via reduction products, in the stool.

d. **Nutrition and gastrointestinal system** (see Chapter 11). In utero, the placenta continuously transports nutrients to the fetus. Intestinal absorption is thought to be minimal. Due to discontinuation of this system at birth and a relatively minimal amount of oral nutrition in the first 24 to 48 hours of postnatal life, endogenous factors must be activated. Important examples are the deposition of fat during the third trimester and the end-organ utilization of fat via lipolysis and ketones as oxidative fuel. Despite this, organs such as the brain and red blood cells are considered obligate glucose users. The approximately 6-hour storage pool of glycogen in a full-term neonate is readily accessed in response to the catecholamine burst at delivery through glycogenolysis. Glucose homeostasis is further maintained by gluconeogenesis.

e. **Renal system** (see Chapter 14). Glomerular function, which is relatively low in fetal life as reflected by the glomerular filtration rate (GFR), increases with gestational age as well as postnatal age. Tubular function also improves with age, which has important consequences for the elimination of many drugs from the body.

f. **Temperature regulation.** In utero, a neutral thermal environment is constant and places few demands on the growing fetus. Upon transitioning to the extrauterine environment, the neonate is at a distinct disadvantage with respect to thermoregulation. Heat loss is increased (i.e., four times) relative to adults, due to decreased epidermal and dermal thickness and increased surface area-to-body weight ratio (i.e., three times greater than adults). Furthermore, an immature nervous system is often unable to adequately modulate peripheral vasoconstriction as another potential source of loss. However, the neonate has developed a mechanism referred to as "nonshivering thermogenesis," which leads to heat production via oxidation of brown fat. It is a catecholamine-mediated process and does lead to an increased metabolic rate and increased oxygen consumption.

2. **Growth.** The growth rate of the fetus is greater than that of the infant or older child. Growth slows just before birth, limited by placental substrate transport, and a loss of body weight occurs in the first few days after birth due to loss of extracellular water and inadequate nutritional intake. As the newborn acclimates to the extrauterine environment and improves behavioral organization, feeding improves and growth accelerates again. Adequate nutrition along with control of possible hyperbilirubinemia or infection is crucial to normal growth and development in the newborn. (*See IV B 1, 2* for further discussion of growth and the nutritional needs of the newborn.)

II DELIVERY ROOM MANAGEMENT OF THE NEWBORN

A Goals The goals of delivery room management are to assess and promptly attend to the immediate needs (e.g., oxygenation, ventilation) and potential problems (e.g., serious anomalies) of the newborn.

B Preparation for delivery

1. **Obtaining perinatal information.** The pediatrician must have specific information concerning the mother and fetus to prepare for routine care of the mother and newborn as well as treatment of specific problems related to a particular delivery.
   a. **Obstetric history** should include all information that may be pertinent to the immediate fetal (newborn) condition. The information is best obtained from the obstetrician and the medical chart and by direct communication with the parents. Important items are listed in Table 6-1.
   b. **Labor history** should be obtained (Table 6-2).

C Assessment of the newborn and **the Apgar score.** The goal of the initial assessment is to determine the newborn's state of oxygenation and ventilation. This is usually done by performing an Apgar evaluation (Table 6-3).

1. The Apgar score was devised as a means of assessing the oxygenation, ventilation, and degree of asphyxia in a uniform manner that quickly communicates information to all persons involved in

TABLE 6-1 Essential Parts of Obstetric History

Maternal age
Medical and previous obstetric history
Length of gestation
Blood group incompatibilities
Maternal infection (e.g., syphilis, gonorrhea, rubella, herpes, human immunodeficiency virus, hepatitis)
Maternal drug use
Ultrasound evaluation of fetal growth and amniotic fluid volume, as well as for the possibility of congenital anomalies
Signs of chorioamnionitis, including prolonged rupture of the fetal membranes, maternal fever, and leukocytosis on complete blood count
Results of other fetal evaluations, including lecithin/sphingomyelin ratio (*see V A 1 b 1 b*), nonstress test, and biophysical profile

TABLE 6-2 Essential Parts of Labor History

Fetal heart tracing
Duration of fetal membrane rupture
Evaluation of amniotic fluid (color and quantity)
Progress of labor
Fetal scalp blood pH

the resuscitation of the newborn. The Apgar evaluation is routinely performed at 1 and 5 minutes after birth, with continuation at 10 and 20 minutes in the case of a score of < 7. Five signs—heart rate, respiratory effort, muscle tone, reflex irritability, and skin color—are examined and assigned a score of 0, 1, or 2. The Apgar score is obtained by adding all individual scores.

a. A **score of 8 to 10** reflects good oxygenation and ventilation and indicates no need for vigorous resuscitation.

b. A **score of 5 to 7** indicates a need for stimulation and supplemental oxygen.

c. A **score of** $<$ **5** indicates a need for assisted ventilation and possible cardiac support (*see II D 2*).

2. The Apgar score is a useful method of communicating the well-being of the newborn. However, urgently needed resuscitation should not be delayed while a full examination is performed. Bradycardia or a poor respiratory effort alone indicates a need for immediate resuscitation.

3. The Apgar score at 5 minutes reflects the adequacy of resuscitation and the potential degree of perinatal asphyxia.

D Resuscitation

1. The primary purpose of resuscitation is to reoxygenate the central nervous system (CNS) of the newborn by providing oxygen, establishing ventilation, and ensuring an adequate cardiac output. Although it may be difficult to differentiate primary apnea from secondary apnea, a quick assessment of the newborn's skin color, respiratory activity, and heart rate should allow prompt institution of appropriate resuscitation (Figure 6-2).

2. **Routine procedures.** The evaluations and procedures that constitute the resuscitation of the newborn are listed in the order in which they should be initiated.

a. **Maintenance of body heat.** The infant should be dried and provided with radiant heat to maintain body temperature. It is important to avoid hypothermia, which will increase the newborn's oxygen consumption.

b. **Establishment of an airway.** Immediately after delivery, the infant's head should be placed in a neutral or slightly extended position and an airway established by clearing the mouth, nose, and pharynx of thick secretions or meconium (*see V A 3 c*). Deep and frequent oropharyngeal suctioning should be avoided because it will increase vagal output, causing apnea and bradycardia.

TABLE 6-3 Apgar Evaluation of the Newborn

	Score		
Sign	0	1	2
Heart rate	Absent	$<$ 100 beats per min	$>$ 100 beats per min
Respiratory effort	Absent	Weak, irregular	Strong, regular
Muscle tone	Flaccid	Some flexion	Well flexed
Reflex irritability (response to catheter in nostril)	No response	Grimace	Cough or sneeze
Skin color	Blue, pale	Body pink, extremities blue	Entire body pink

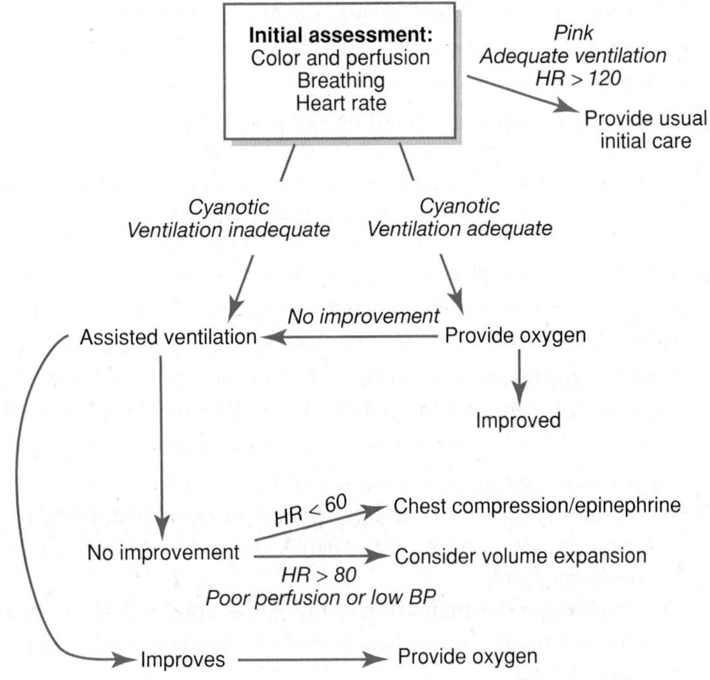

FIGURE 6-2 Scheme for assessment and resuscitation of the newborn. BP, blood pressure; HR, heart rate (given in beats per minute).

c. **Ventilation.** The adequacy of air exchange in the newborn must be assessed. In most cases, drying off, suctioning, and tactile stimulation (e.g., gentle flicking of the feet or rubbing of the back) are adequate to induce effective spontaneous ventilation (see Figure 6-2).
   (1) If ventilation is adequate, **supplemental oxygen** may be given to improve heart rate or skin color.
   (2) If supplemental oxygen does not improve heart rate or skin color, or if ventilation is inadequate, **mechanical ventilation** should be initiated, using mask and bag ventilation.
      (a) If spontaneous ventilation improves, mechanical ventilation should be stopped and supplemental oxygen resumed.
      (b) If the response is poor or if airway obstruction occurs, an endotracheal tube should be inserted and mechanical ventilation continued.

d. **Circulation.** If mechanical ventilation does not improve the heart rate or skin color, one of the following steps is taken:
   (1) **If heart rate is < 60 beats per minute,** or between 60 and 80 beats per minute and not improving, **cardiac compression** is initiated; if heart rate does not improve, **epinephrine** is administered via an umbilical venous catheter or endotracheal tube.
   (2) **If heart rate is 80 beats per minute or greater** but there is poor perfusion or weak pulse, a plasma volume-expanding agent is administered at a dose of 10 to 15 mL/kg.

e. **Drug support.** The following medications may be useful during resuscitation:
   (1) **Sodium bicarbonate** should be reserved until it is clear that a metabolic acidosis exists.
   (2) **Naloxone** may be helpful for poor spontaneous respiratory effort secondary to maternal narcotic use during labor. Naloxone is contraindicated in an infant born to a mother who is addicted to narcotics.

III GENERAL ASPECTS OF NEWBORN HEALTH SUPERVISION

A Goals

1. Assess wellness of the newborn, and screen for congenital anomalies, birth trauma, or acquired medical problems.
2. Assess the newborn for gestational age and appropriateness of size for gestational age.

3. When appropriate, confirm infant's normality to parents.
4. When appropriate, demystify and reassure parents about common, benign variations in newborn physical examination characteristics or behavior.
5. Foster early infant-parent bonding and parental self-confidence.

B History Maternal health and current pregnancy history, family health history, and family psychosocial history are reviewed. Details about labor, delivery, and neonatal condition are added.

C Goals of the **newborn physical examination** are to identify major and minor congenital anomalies, sequelae of birth trauma, and neonatal medical problems, as well as determine gestational age and appropriateness of size for gestational age (see Chapter 1).

1. **General appearance.** Important observations include body proportions, activity, quality of cry, skin color, gross abnormalities, unusual features, and signs of respiratory distress. Weight, length, and head circumference measurements are obtained and recorded.
2. **Skin. Color** may suggest cyanosis, pallor, or jaundice.
   a. Manifestations of **normal peripheral vascular instability** include skin mottling, perioral cyanosis, and cyanosis of the hands and feet, with lips, mucous membranes, and nail beds remaining pink.
   b. **Cracking or desquamation** of the skin is normal in the term and postmature infant. In the term infant, fine downy hair known as lanugo covers the skin, particularly the shoulders and upper back.
   c. **Jaundice** in the neonate is first visible on the face and, as the serum bilirubin level rises, the jaundice progresses caudally to include the rest of the body and the sclerae. Natural sunlight should be used to inspect the skin for the extent of jaundice.
   d. Common **birthmarks** that are visible at birth include flat vascular nevi (i.e., salmon patch nevus and port wine stains) and mongolian spots (*see III C 8*). Raised vascular nevi usually become apparent several weeks after birth (i.e., a capillary hemangioma [also known as strawberry hemangioma] or cavernous hemangioma).
   e. Benign **rashes** are common.
      (1) **Erythema toxicum neonatorum** has a "flea-bite" appearance with scattered erythematous macules that may contain papulopustular centers filled with eosinophils. This rash typically changes distribution from day to day.
      (2) **Milia** are fine, pinpoint, yellow-white papules caused by retained sebum that typically cover the bridge of the nose, chin, and cheeks. These are transient.
      (3) **Neonatal pustular melanosis** consists of small vesiculopustules that are present at birth and rupture within a few days, leaving transient pigmented macules with scaly borders.
3. **Head and neck.** The head and face frequently exhibit sequelae of the birth process, including bruises and asymmetries. Most of these sequelae resolve spontaneously. Facial features should be carefully inspected for size, placement, and symmetry.
   a. Palpation of the skull determines contour, extent of separation or overriding of sutures, and size of the fontanelles.
      (1) **Molding** of the head shape into an elongated or asymmetric contour occurs secondary to intrauterine pressure or forces on the skull during delivery.
      (2) **Cephalohematoma** is a subperiosteal hemorrhage manifested by a unilateral scalp swelling.
      (3) **Caput succedaneum** is edema of the scalp due to the pressure caused during labor and delivery. In contrast to cephalhematomas, these swellings extend beyond suture lines.
   b. **Eyes.** Dimming the room lights, talking to the baby, or cradling the occiput in the examiner's hand to lift the baby's head off the mattress may stimulate the baby to open his or her eyes.
      (1) Conjunctival or scleral hemorrhages resolve spontaneously and are usually of no clinical significance.
      (2) The presence of a **red reflex** excludes the presence of lens opacities (e.g., cataracts) and retinoblastoma.
      (3) Up to the age of 3 months, the eyes may normally appear to cross intermittently. However, a fixed eye misalignment is always abnormal.

c. **Ears.** Patency of the canal should be determined. Malformed or low-set ears may be associated with auditory or renal abnormalities. A tympanic membrane examination is unnecessary in a healthy newborn.

d. **Nose.** Newborns are nose-breathers. Obstruction of the nasal passages results in respiratory distress.

e. The **mouth** should be examined by inspection and palpation. Common minor anomalies include small, white **epithelial pearls** along the gum margins; small, white cysts termed **Epstein pearls** along the median raphe of the hard palate; and small, hard tumors within the gingiva, termed **epulis.** Palpation may reveal a submucosal bony cleft of the palate.

f. The **neck** must be hyperextended to inspect adequately for masses. Congenital masses include **goiter, cystic hygroma, branchial cleft cysts,** and **thyroglossal duct cysts.** A webbing of the neck is seen in a variety of syndromes, the most common of which is Turner syndrome (see Chapter 8).

4. **Chest**

a. The **clavicles** are palpated for signs of fracture, including irregularities or crepitations, most often resulting from a difficult delivery.

b. **Respiratory rate, pattern,** and the presence of **chest asymmetry, retractions, grunting,** and **nasal flaring** must be determined. In some healthy infants, transient crackles may be auscultated during the first few hours after birth, unaccompanied by signs of respiratory distress. The clinician may observe a normal pattern of periodic breathing—with pauses up to 10 to 15 seconds—that is unaccompanied by bradycardia or changes in color and tone.

c. An abnormality in **cardiac location** is screened for by determining that the heart sounds are loudest in the left chest. Soft systolic heart murmurs are commonly heard in the first 24 hours of life, probably because of a closing ductus arteriosus or normal changes in pulmonary vascular resistance. These murmurs usually disappear within 48 hours after birth.

5. The **abdomen** is convex and moves prominently with respiration.

a. A normal **liver edge** may be palpated 1 to 2 cm below the right costal margin, and the tip of the normal spleen may be palpated at the left costal margin.

b. Because the most common **abdominal masses** in the newborn involve the genitourinary tract, palpation of the kidneys is especially important. The kidney may be palpated with fingertips pressing deeply onto the lower lateral aspect of the abdomen, with the opposite hand resting under the baby's back at a level just superior to the iliac crest.

6. **Inguinal region and genitalia**

a. Femoral pulses must always be palpated because diminished pulses suggest coarctation of the aorta.

b. Examination of **male genitalia** should include location of the urethral meatus, palpation of the testes, and a search for a bulge in the groin or scrotum, which suggests a hernia or hydrocele.

c. Examination of the **female genitalia** should ascertain the presence of urethral and vaginal openings as well as a normal-sized clitoris to exclude ambiguous genitalia, imperforate hymen, and vaginal atresia. In normal infants, a transient swelling of the labia minora or a vaginal discharge that is mucoid or bloody results from the influence of maternal hormones.

d. The **anus** is inspected for patency and placement.

7. **Extremities.** Temporary flexion contractures at the elbows, hips, and knees are seen in the term newborn as a result of intrauterine pressure effects. Approximately 5% of all newborns have more significant limb deformities, either **deformations** caused by positional abnormalities and intrauterine posture or true **malformations** (see Chapter 8).

a. **Developmental dysplasia** of the hip occurs in 1 in 1000 live births and is much more common in girls and breech deliveries. Asymmetries in lower limb length, placement of medial thigh and gluteal folds, or degree of hip flexion should raise suspicion for unilateral hip dislocation. When the hips are flexed to 90 degrees, the legs normally can be abducted fully to touch the examining table. "Telescoping" of the femoral head with the subluxation (Barlow) maneuver or a palpable "thump" with the Ortolani maneuver suggests dislocation.

b. Trauma to the cervical nerves during delivery may result in asymmetric or diminished arm movements, which indicates **Erb palsy** (C5 and C6 nerve roots) or **Klumpke palsy** (C8–T2 nerve roots).

c. **Metatarsus adductus** is a condition in which the forepart of the foot is adducted and usually supinated. It may result from intrauterine positional compression.

8. **Back.** The spine is inspected and palpated for sinus tracts or overlying lesions such as lipomas, hairy tufts, or hemangiomas, any of which may be signs of a covert neural tube defect. Gray-blue macular birthmarks called mongolian spots are most commonly seen over the lower spine and buttocks but are also found on the upper back and shoulders. These spots have no clinical significance.

9. **Neurologic examination.** Overall state of consciousness and the ease with which the infant makes transitions from walking to sleeping or fussing to calming, as well as strength of cry, should be noted. Cranial nerves, primitive reflexes, and tone should also be assessed.

10. **Gestational age** and appropriateness of **size** for gestational age

a. Gestational age can be determined prenatally in many ways: Date of last menstrual period, ultrasound examination, and date of first reported fetal activity.

(1) **Classification.** All newborns are classified by gestational age and birth weight. Gestational age is categorized as preterm, term, and postterm as described earlier. Weight can be further classified.

(a) **Small for gestational age (SGA):** Defined as 2 standard deviations below the mean weight for gestational age or below the 10th percentile (see Chapter 4)

(b) **Appropriate for gestational age (AGA)** (see Chapter 4)

(c) **Large for gestational age (LGA):** Defined as 2 standard deviations above the mean weight for gestational age or above the 90th percentile (see Chapter 4)

b. Methods of determining postnatal gestational age

(1) **Delivery room assessment.** A rapid evaluation in the delivery room can prove to be a useful, if not precise evaluation of maturity:

(a) Creases in sole of foot: Increase in density and coverage with increasing gestational age

(b) Breast nodules: Increase in size with increasing gestational age

(c) Scalp hair: Coarsens with increasing gestational age

(d) Ear lobe: Stiffens with increasing gestational age

(e) Testes and scrotum: Testes descend and scrotum develops rugae with increasing gestational age

(2) The **new Ballard score** (Figure 6-3) is an exam consisting of six neuromuscular criteria and six physical criteria. It is useful in determining gestational age in infants from 20 to 44 weeks' gestation. Its accuracy is considered to be within 2 weeks of gestational age if performed at < 12 hours of life in < 26-week-gestation infants and < 96 hours of life in others.

(a) It is administered twice by two separate examiners.

(b) The six separate neuromuscular and six separate physical criteria scores are totaled. This score can then be converted to estimate gestational age.

D Procedures

1. **Prophylaxis of gonococcal ophthalmia** is recommended for all newborns. Either a 1% silver nitrate solution in single-dose ampules or a sterile ophthalmic ointment containing 1% tetracycline or 0.5% erythromycin in single-use tubes is an acceptable regimen. Unfortunately, this regimen is not effective in preventing the most common cause of conjunctivitis in the newborn, which is *Chlamydia trachomatis.*

2. Every newborn should receive a single parenteral dose of 0.5 to 1.0 mg of natural **vitamin K oxide** (phytonadione) within 1 hour of birth to prevent vitamin K-dependent hemorrhagic disease and coagulation disorders.

3. **Metabolic screening.** Before discharge, a blood sample should be obtained from every neonate for screening for the presence of the **hyperphenylalaninemias** (including **phenylketonuria** [PKU]) and congenital **hypothyroidism.** In many states, screening is also performed for other inborn errors or diseases such as **homocystinuria, maple syrup urine disease, histidinemia, galactosemia, cystic fibrosis,** and **sickle cell anemia.** Cost effectiveness is greatly improved by a screening program that encompasses multiple disorders (e.g., the PKU and hypothyroidism screening is performed through state laboratories). This screening must be part of a comprehensive program ensuring effective treatment for problems that are disclosed.

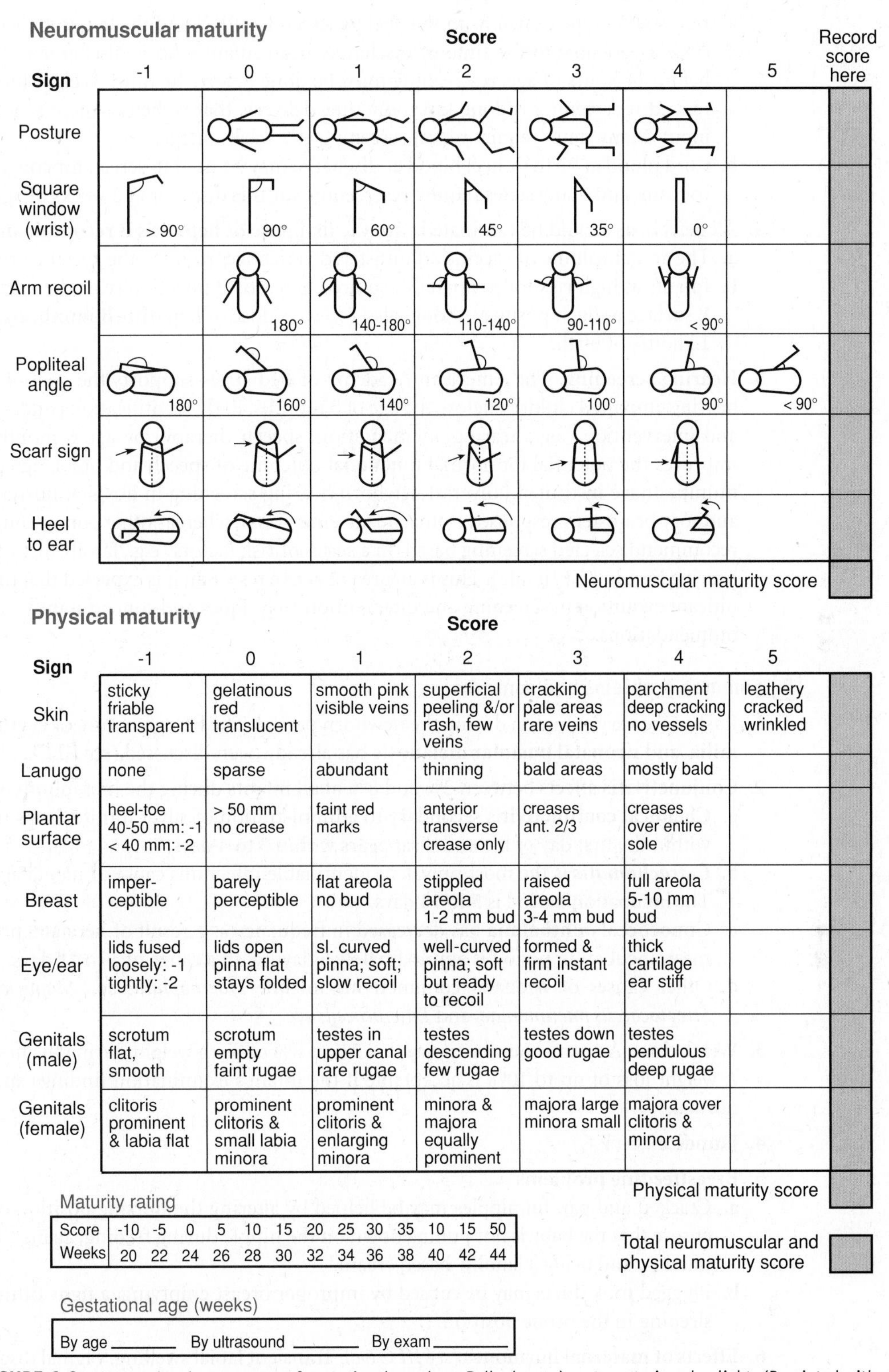

Neuromuscular maturity

Sign	Score -1	0	1	2	3	4	5	Record score here
Posture								
Square window (wrist)	> 90°	90°	60°	45°	35°	0°		
Arm recoil		180°	140-180°	110-140°	90-110°	< 90°		
Popliteal angle	180°	160°	140°	120°	100°	90°	< 90°	
Scarf sign								
Heel to ear								

Neuromuscular maturity score

Physical maturity

Sign	Score -1	0	1	2	3	4	5	Record score here
Skin	sticky friable transparent	gelatinous red translucent	smooth pink visible veins	superficial peeling &/or rash, few veins	cracking pale areas rare veins	parchment deep cracking no vessels	leathery cracked wrinkled	
Lanugo	none	sparse	abundant	thinning	bald areas	mostly bald		
Plantar surface	heel-toe 40-50 mm: -1 < 40 mm: -2	> 50 mm no crease	faint red marks	anterior transverse crease only	creases ant. 2/3	creases over entire sole		
Breast	imper-ceptible	barely perceptible	flat areola no bud	stippled areola 1-2 mm bud	raised areola 3-4 mm bud	full areola 5-10 mm bud		
Eye/ear	lids fused loosely: -1 tightly: -2	lids open pinna flat stays folded	sl. curved pinna; soft; slow recoil	well-curved pinna; soft but ready to recoil	formed & firm instant recoil	thick cartilage ear stiff		
Genitals (male)	scrotum flat, smooth	scrotum empty faint rugae	testes in upper canal rare rugae	testes descending few rugae	testes down good rugae	testes pendulous deep rugae		
Genitals (female)	clitoris prominent & labia flat	prominent clitoris & small labia minora	prominent clitoris & enlarging minora	minora & majora equally prominent	majora large minora small	majora cover clitoris & minora		

Physical maturity score

Maturity rating

Score	-10	-5	0	5	10	15	20	25	30	35	10	15	50
Weeks	20	22	24	26	28	30	32	34	36	38	40	42	44

Total neuromuscular and physical maturity score

Gestational age (weeks)

By age ______ By ultrasound ______ By exam ______

FIGURE 6-3 Maturational assessment of gestational age (new Ballard score). ant., anterior; sl., slight. (Reprinted with permission from Ballard JL, Khoury JC, Wedig K, et al.: New Ballard score, expanded to include extremely premature infants. *J Pediatr* 119:417–423, 1991; and Ross Laboratories, Columbus, Ohio, 1991.)

a. Blood should be drawn from the heel to screen for PKU and the hyperphenylalaninemias as close as possible to the time of discharge. If an infant who is discharged early is screened before 24 hours of age, rescreening must be done before the third week of life. Cases may be missed if screening is done too soon after delivery, that is, before there is adequate protein input. Many states require repeat screening at 2 weeks of age.
b. Cord blood at birth or heel blood at discharge may be used to screen for congenital hypothyroidism, and many states require rescreening for this disorder at 2 weeks of age.

4. All newborns should be vaccinated with the first dose of **hepatitis B recombinant vaccine.**
   a. The actual volume of vaccine administered varies according to the specific product.
   b. Infants at high risk for perinatally acquired hepatitis B infection (e.g., the mother is hepatitis B surface antigen positive) should also receive a dose of **hepatitis B immunoglobulin** within 12 hours of birth.
5. **Hearing screening.** The American Academy of Pediatrics supports the goal of identifying all hearing-impaired children before the age of 3 months. Early identification (under age 3 months) and intervention (e.g., hearing augmentation, speech therapy) by age 6 months significantly improves the potential for normal functional outcome of speech and oral language. Most communities have instituted universal newborn hearing screening in hospital nurseries (e.g., using auditory brainstem response or otoacoustic emissions), whereas other communities continue to recommend selected screening based on a series of risk factors (e.g., family history of hereditary hearing loss, low birth rate). This is an area of active research; it is expected that there will be significant evolution in screening and intervention techniques and concomitantly in screening recommendations.

E Common problems and concerns

1. **Rashes** are very common during the newborn period. The benign nature of **erythema toxicum, milia,** and **neonatal pustular melanosis** has already been discussed (*see III C 2 e*).
2. **Conjunctivitis** affects between 2% and 8% of all infants during the first month of life.
   a. **Chemical conjunctivitis** secondary to administration of silver nitrate drops usually appears within the first day of life and disappears within 3 to 4 days.
   b. ***C. trachomatis*** is the most prevalent identifiable infectious cause of neonatal conjunctivitis. The incubation period is 5 to 14 days.
   c. **Gonococcal ophthalmia** has decreased in frequency as a result of neonatal prophylaxis. The mean incubation period is approximately 6 days, with a range of 1 to 21 days.
   d. Other causes of neonatal conjunctivitis include *Haemophilus* sp., *Staphylococcus aureus, Streptococcus pneumoniae,* and *Enterococcus* sp.
3. **Weight loss.** A normal newborn may lose 5% to 8% of birth weight during the first 3 days of life. A weight loss of up to 10% is acceptable if the infant's examination findings and behavior are normal.
4. **Jaundice** (*see V C*)
5. **Breastfeeding problems**
   a. Cracked and painful nipples may be helped by altering the nursing position of the infant to ensure that the baby is not pulling down on the nipple during feeding, airing the nipples after nursing, and using a lanolin-based cream.
   b. Plugged milk ducts may be caused by improper breast emptying, a tight-fitting brassiere, or sleeping in the prone position.
6. **Effects of maternal hormones** *(see III C 6 c).* Transient labial swelling, vaginal discharge, or vaginal bleeding may result from the influence of maternal hormones. For the same reason, breasts of both sexes may demonstrate transient swelling, reddening, and discharge of a milky substance.

F Anticipatory guidance

Areas for discussion with parents during the postpartum period include the following:

1. **Physical status.** During the immediate postpartum period, concerns for the baby's well-being are of highest priority for parents.

2. **General care.** Issues include bathing, dressing, skin care, and cord care.
3. **Feeding**
   a. **Breastfeeding** is facilitated by a hospital rooming-in policy, which permits a demand-feeding schedule of 8 to 12 feedings per 24 hours. No dietary supplementation with either formula or water should be provided unless there is a medical indication. Nursing and medical staff must provide consistent, accurate advice about breastfeeding. This advice is best reinforced by skilled personnel periodically observing the feeding process during the first several postpartum days.
   b. Commercial **infant formula** is a satisfactory substitute for human milk. For most newborns, a lactose-containing modified cow's milk formula is well tolerated. Rarely, infants who are intolerant of lactose or cow's milk protein may require a formula containing alternative carbohydrates (e.g., sucrose, dextrose, maltose, dextrins) or an alternative protein source (e.g., soy isolate, casein hydrolysate). Commercial infant formulas for normal infants contain 20 calories per ounce of liquid. After the first few days of life, the normal infant usually requires approximately 100 to 110 kcal/kg/day, or 150 mL/kg/day of formula for adequate growth (see Chapter 1).
4. **Elimination.** Infants vary considerably in their patterns of elimination. A pattern of urinating six times within 24 hours suggests adequate fluid intake. Infants may have a bowel movement as frequently as after every feeding or as infrequently as once every 4 to 5 days. Breast-fed babies tend to have loose stools with small curds, and the bowel movements may be explosive.
5. **Behavioral and developmental issues** (see Chapter 1)
   a. **State organization.** The normal variability in infant behavior is vividly demonstrated by the newborn's frequent changes in state of consciousness. The newborn is able to shut out disturbing aspects of the new environment and has the capacity to choose to respond to certain stimuli.
   b. **Synchrony.** From the outset, the nature of the parent-infant relationship is one of mutual awareness, with parents and newborn each responding to one another via cues.
   c. **Attachment.** The unique relationship between parent and child is being established as early as the postpartum period.
   d. **Temperament.** Individual differences in behavior style are evident as early as the newborn period.

IV SPECIFIC ASPECTS OF NEWBORN CARE

In this section, some specific aspects of newborn physiology, pathophysiology, and therapy are reviewed.

A **Fluid** and **electrolyte requirements** (see Chapter 14). Water represents 94% of the fetal weight at 3 months' gestation. At term, water content has declined to 80% of the birth weight of the newborn.

1. **Fluid loss** and **replacement**
   a. **Fluid loss**
      (1) During the first week of life, the extracellular fluid space contracts, resulting in a large reduction in body water. This water loss is responsible for 5% of the weight loss observed in term infants. The preterm infant may lose up to 10% to 15% of his or her birth weight.
      (2) Water loss through evaporation from the skin and expired air is referred to as **insensible water loss.** Water loss through the urine and stool is referred to as **sensible water loss.** Stool accounts for a small amount of sensible water loss.
   b. **Fluid replacement** is based on fluid loss and is calculated as the sum of insensible and sensible water losses. Initial parenteral fluid replacement should be accomplished with a 10% dextrose solution.
      (1) Insensible water loss varies with gestational age and factors related to the nursing environment, such as the heat source, humidity, and use of phototherapy (for treatment of hyperbilirubinemia).
      (2) In addition to water lost in the urine, other sensible losses such as gastric secretions (i.e., vomitus) should be included in the calculation of total water loss.

c. **Fluid balance** is monitored by examining:
(1) Urine output
(2) Change in body weight
(3) Serum sodium concentration
(4) Urine specific gravity

2. **Electrolyte loss** and **replacement**

a. **Sodium, potassium,** and **chloride** are the principal salts that are lost through the urine and should be replaced accordingly. Assuming an adequate urine output, replacement is begun 24 hours after birth at the following rates:
(1) **Sodium:** 1 to 3 mEq/kg/day
(2) **Potassium:** 1 to 2 mEq/kg/day
(3) **Chloride:** 1 to 3 mEq/kg/day

b. **Calcium.** A decrease in serum calcium concentration frequently occurs during the first week of life. Total serum calcium concentrations below 7 mg/dL are considered hypocalcemic.
(1) **Early neonatal (physiologic) hypocalcemia.** Nearly all infants experience a small decline in total serum calcium levels during the first few days of life due to intrauterine parathyroid hormone suppression. Early neonatal hypocalcemia rarely requires treatment except in preterm infants, infants of diabetic mothers, and asphyxiated infants.
(2) **Late neonatal (nonphysiologic) hypocalcemia** is seen at the end of the first week of life. Causes include:
(a) Increased phosphate ingestion, as occurs in infants who are fed cow's milk or high-phosphate rice cereal
(b) Hypomagnesemia
(c) Hypoparathyroidism
(3) **Therapy** usually consists of calcium replacement with calcium gluconate and treatment of any underlying cause of the hypocalcemia.

c. **Other required minerals** include:
(1) Phosphorus
(2) Magnesium
(3) Iron
(4) Trace metals

B Nutritional requirements Adequate caloric intake with the correct balance of carbohydrate, protein, and fat is needed for homeostasis and growth. The specific nutritional requirements of the newborn are reviewed here.

1. **Fetal** and **neonatal growth**

a. **Fetal growth.** The fetal growth rate is 5 g/day at 14 to 15 weeks' gestation, 10 g/day at 20 weeks, and 30 g/day at 32 to 34 weeks. The growth rate slows after 36 weeks' gestation.
(1) During the first trimester, growth parameters (i.e., weight, length, head circumference) are fairly uniform in all fetuses.
(2) Variability in fetal growth during the last trimester is the result of several factors, including genetic endowment, fetal nutrition, and multiple gestation (fetal growth rate declines at 31 weeks' gestation in twins and at 29 weeks' gestation in triplets).

b. **Neonatal growth**
(1) After birth, there is a loss of weight due to a loss of extracellular water and suboptimal caloric intake. Term infants lose 5% of their birth weight; preterm infants lose up to 15% of their birth weight.
(2) Term infants regain their birth weight by the end of the first week of life, and thereafter gain 20 to 30 g/day.

2. **Nutritional considerations.** The composition of the nutritional solution and the route of delivery depend on the gestational age, general medical condition, and possible special nutritional needs of the newborn.

a. **Enteric nutrition**
(1) **Route of feeding**
(a) The **term infant** can be bottle-fed or breast-fed on demand, as long as attention is paid to intake and fluid balance.

(b) The otherwise healthy **preterm infant who is between 34 and 38 weeks' gestational age** should be fed every 3 to 4 hours by bottle, breast, or gavage, depending on the infant's strength and alertness.

(c) The **preterm infant who is < 34 weeks' gestational age** does not have a well-coordinated suck-and-swallow reflex, and therefore should be fed via a feeding tube. The feedings may be gastric bolus every 2 to 3 hours, except in infants weighing < 1000 g, where continuous feeding regimens are frequently considered.

(2) **Feeding solution.** The composition of the feeding solution depends on the presence or absence of special protein, carbohydrate, or fat requirements or intolerances, which, in turn, depend on gestational age, gastrointestinal motility status, and the possibility of intestinal enzyme deficiencies, protein allergy, or other metabolic disorders (e.g., PKU).

(a) **Term infants who do not have complicating metabolic problems.** All of the water, calorie, protein, and vitamin requirements of the normal term infant are met by human milk or 20 kcal/ounce cow's milk-based formula. The specific nutritional needs of these infants for normal growth are as follows:

(i) The normal term infant needs 100 to 120 kcal/kg/day to meet basal and growth requirements.

(ii) This infant also needs 2 to 3 g/kg/day of protein for cellular growth, which represents approximately 10% of the total daily calorie intake.

(iii) In addition, 40% of the daily calorie requirements should be derived from carbohydrates, with the remainder provided by dietary fats.

(b) **Preterm infants** have decreased gastric motility and intestinal lactase activity as well as increased calcium and phosphorus requirements, among other nutritional problems. As positive nitrogen balance is achieved, the infant may be advanced to a formula that is high in calcium, phosphorus, and protein, or to fortified human milk. A 24 (or greater) kcal/ounce formula is reserved for infants whose water intake must be restricted, who cannot tolerate adequate feeding volumes, or who have increased caloric requirements.

(c) **Infants with special metabolic needs.** Special formula solutions are available for infants who have selected intestinal enzyme deficiencies (e.g., sucrase-isomaltase deficiency) or metabolic diseases (e.g., PKU).

(3) **Vitamins** and **minerals.** Commercially available formulas are now fortified with vitamins, minerals, and trace elements. Therefore, formula-fed term infants do not routinely require vitamin or mineral supplementation.

(a) **Special vitamin needs**

(i) Infants who are fed human milk may receive a multiple-vitamin supplement containing vitamins A, D, and C.

(ii) Due to small body stores and inadequate feeding volumes, preterm infants should routinely receive a multiple-vitamin supplement containing the fat-soluble vitamins (A and D) and the water-soluble vitamins (B and C). In addition, the preterm infant who is < 36 weeks' gestational age should receive vitamin E to prevent hemolytic anemia.

(b) **Special mineral and trace element needs**

(i) **Iron.** All infants require iron supplementation, which may be obtained via iron-fortified formula or through a separate supplement. Iron supplementation may be delayed in the preterm infant until enteric feedings are tolerated. Because of the increased bioavailability of iron in human milk, iron supplementation in term breast-fed infants may await the introduction of iron-fortified cereal at 4 to 6 months of age.

(ii) **Calcium** and **phosphorus.** The needs of the growing term infant are met by either commercial formula or human milk (see Chapter 1). Due to rapid bone growth, the calcium and phosphorus requirements of the preterm infant are greater and necessitate special fortified formulas or supplementation if human milk is fed.

b. Total parenteral nutrition. Preterm and other sick infants may require total parenteral nutrition because of gastrointestinal disorders (e.g., neonatal necrotizing enterocolitis) as well as nongastrointestinal disorders (e.g., respiratory disease, sepsis). An intravenous solution of dextrose, amino acids, fat, vitamins, and minerals can be administered by either peripheral or central venous access. Appropriately used, total parenteral nutrition can provide adequate calories and protein to support the basal needs and growth of the sick infant.

V SPECIAL MANAGEMENT PROBLEMS IN THE NEWBORN

Many of the disorders mentioned in this section are covered more extensively in other chapters of this book. However, their clinical presentation and management warrant special consideration in the newborn.

A Disorders of the respiratory system The newborn may have a variety of respiratory disturbances, which may be developmental in origin or may originate at birth or soon after. Specific respiratory disorders of the newborn are reviewed here, after a brief overview of prenatal respiratory system development.

1. **Prenatal development of the respiratory system**
   a. **Anatomic development** begins at 3 weeks' gestation, with the division of the foregut into the esophagus and trachea. Major bronchial branching occurs by 4 weeks' gestation. With premature birth, the two final stages of development may evolve following delivery.
      (1) The **canalicular stage of lung development** (16–25 weeks) is characterized by formation of terminal alveolar sacs, capillary approximation with the alveolar sacs, and differentiation of types I and II alveolar cells.
      (2) The **alveolar,** or **terminal sac, stage** (26–40 weeks) is characterized by a progressive increase in the number of alveolar sacs, which creates a greater surface area for gas exchange. Surfactant is also produced during this stage of development.
   b. **Biochemical development.** An important prenatal event is the production of surfactant by type II alveolar cells. Table 6-4 outlines factors that accelerate or retard this production.
      (1) **Function and composition of surfactant**
         (a) The major function of surfactant is to decrease alveolar surface tension and increase lung compliance. Surfactant prevents alveolar collapse at the end of expiration and allows for opening of the alveoli at a low intrathoracic pressure.
         (b) The group of phospholipids comprising surfactant is also referred to as lecithin. The ratio of **lecithin (L)** to **sphingomyelin (S)** in the amniotic fluid is a reflection of the amount of intrapulmonary surfactant and lung maturity. An **L/S ratio** of 2:1 or greater usually indicates biochemical lung maturity. The presence of phosphatidylglycerol as well as a critical number of lamellar bodies in the amniotic fluid is an additional indicator of biochemical maturity.
2. **Developmental disorders**
   a. **Hyaline membrane disease (respiratory distress syndrome of the newborn)** is a respiratory disorder that primarily affects preterm infants who are born before the biochemical maturation of their lungs.

TABLE 6-4 Factors That Affect Fetal Lung Surfactant Production

Increase Production	Decrease or Delay Production
Maternal steroid administration in the presence of a female fetus	Combined fetal hyperglycemia and hyperinsulinemia as observed in maternal diabetes
Prolonged rupture of the fetal membranes	Acute hypoxia
Maternal narcotic addiction	
Preeclampsia	
Chronic fetal stress (i.e., placental insufficiency)	
Thyroid hormone (i.e., a long-acting thyroid stimulator-associated maternal hyperthyroidism or hypothyroidism with secondary fetal hyperthyroidism)	
Theophylline	

(1) **Pathophysiology.** The lungs are poorly compliant due to a deficiency of surfactant, resulting in the classic complex of progressive atelectasis, intrapulmonary shunting, hypoxemia, and cyanosis. The hyaline membrane that forms and lines the alveoli is composed of protein and sloughed epithelium—the result of oxygen exposure, alveolar capillary leakage, and the forces generated by the mechanical ventilation of these infants.

(2) **Clinical features.** Affected infants characteristically have tachypnea, grunting, nasal flaring, chest retraction, and cyanosis in the first 3 hours of life. There is decreased air entry on auscultation.

(3) **Clinical course.** The natural course is a progressive worsening over the first 48 to 72 hours of life.

(a) After the initial insult to the airway lining, the epithelium is repopulated with type II alveolar cells.

(b) Subsequently, there is increased production and release of surfactant, so that there are sufficient quantities in the air spaces by 72 hours of life. This results in improvement in lung compliance and reduction of the respiratory distress. It is important to note that this favorable course is often altered or reversed in moderate to severe cases, requiring aggressive ventilatory management.

(4) **Diagnosis** is confirmed by a chest radiograph that reveals a uniform ground-glass pattern and an air bronchogram that is consistent with diffuse atelectasis.

(5) **Therapy** and **prognosis**

(a) Conventional therapy for the affected premature infant includes supportive care as well as the administration of **oxygen.** It may also be necessary to increase the mean airway pressure by use of continuous positive airway pressure, intermittent assisted **ventilation,** or high-frequency oscillation. Outcome with conventional therapy is good.

(b) **Exogenous surfactant replacement therapy** with animal-derived surfactant has become an important intervention for those infants who have severe surfactant deficiency. Alveolar opening and improvement in oxygenation and ventilation occur almost immediately.

(6) **Prevention.** When amniotic fluid assessment reveals fetal lung immaturity and preterm delivery can be delayed but not prevented, administration of corticosteroids to the mother 48 hours before delivery can induce or accelerate the production of fetal lung surfactant.

(7) **Complications** associated with hyaline membrane disease are a result of organ immaturity associated with asphyxia and mechanical ventilation. Common complications and associated findings include pneumothorax, patent ductus arteriosus, intraventricular hemorrhage, necrotizing enterocolitis, bronchopulmonary dysplasia, and retinopathy of prematurity.

b. Transient tachypnea of the newborn is thought to result from decreased lymphatic absorption of fetal lung fluid. It most commonly occurs in infants born near term by cesarean section, without preceding labor.

(1) **Clinical features.** The tachypnea is quiet or mild and usually not associated with retractions. The infant appears comfortable and is rarely cyanotic.

(2) **Diagnosis** is based on the delivery history and a chest radiograph, which characteristically reveals fluid in the major fissure, prominent vascular markings, increased interstitial markings, and hyperinflation. Auscultation may reveal rales.

(3) **Therapy** is supportive. The tachypnea should resolve within 72 hours. Supplemental oxygen may be required.

c. Persistence of the fetal circulation, or **persistent pulmonary hypertension of the newborn,** is usually a disease of term infants who have experienced acute or chronic in utero hypoxia. It is seen frequently in infants who have meconium aspiration syndrome (*see V A 3 c*).

(1) **Pathophysiology.** The primary abnormality is a failure of the pulmonary vascular resistance to fall with postnatal lung expansion and oxygenation.

(a) Normally at birth the systemic vascular resistance rises as a result of cessation of blood flow through the placenta, and pulmonary vascular resistance falls with the first breaths.

(b) With persistence of the fetal circulation, the pulmonary vascular resistance continues to be high, and may in fact be higher than the systemic resistance. This results in shunting of the deoxygenated blood, which is returning to the right side of the heart, away from the lungs. The right-to-left shunt can occur at both the atrial level (foramen ovale) and through the ductus arteriosus. Because the lungs are bypassed, the blood is not oxygenated and hypoxemia ensues.

(2) **Clinical features.** These infants have rapidly progressive cyanosis associated with mild to severe respiratory distress. There is a varied response to oxygen administration, depending on the size of the shunt.

(3) **Diagnosis**

(a) The diagnosis is suggested by a history of perinatal hypoxia and clinical cyanosis at birth combined with negative findings from both the cardiovascular examination and chest radiograph, although parenchymal disease may coexist (e.g., group B streptococcal pneumonia, hyaline membrane disease, meconium aspiration syndrome).

(b) Echocardiography should be used to establish the diagnosis and should demonstrate:

(i) The absence of cyanotic heart disease

(ii) Increased pulmonary vascular resistance

(iii) The presence of a right-to-left shunt at the foramen ovale, ductus arteriosus, or both

(4) **Therapy** is both supportive and oriented to lowering the pulmonary vascular resistance and includes supplemental oxygen, mechanical ventilation, hyperventilation, support of systemic blood pressure, maintenance of an alkalotic pH, and administration of pulmonary vasodilators such as inhaled nitric oxide.

(5) **Prognosis.** The overall mortality rate associated with this disease is moderate. Extracorporeal membrane oxygenation likely improves the outcome in certain patients.

3. Acquired disorders

a. Pneumonia

(1) **Etiology.** Pneumonia is often associated with chorioamnionitis and may be caused by aspiration of infected amniotic fluid. The infectious agent may also cross the placenta, enter the fetal circulation, and spread to the lungs. Sepsis is often present (*see V E 2*).

(2) **Clinical features.** The infant has signs of respiratory distress, including tachypnea, cyanosis, and retractions. Auscultation may reveal rales, rhonchi, or diminished breath sounds. Other signs of systemic infection may be noted, including poor perfusion, hypotension, acidosis, and leukopenia or leukocytosis.

(3) **Diagnosis** is confirmed by a chest radiograph that reveals any one of a variety of patterns, including diffuse or patchy infiltrates or consolidation. The process may be unilobar or multilobar. A tracheal aspirate may also reveal bacteria and an increased number of neutrophils.

(4) **Therapy** and **prognosis.** Treatment includes administration of appropriate antibiotics (*see V E 2 f*), supplemental oxygen, and mechanical ventilation, if needed. The outcome is usually good.

b. Pneumothorax is the presence of free air in the pleural space. The air is often under tension (i.e., at greater than atmospheric pressure), and in this setting is referred to as tension pneumothorax.

(1) **Incidence** and **etiology.** Asymptomatic, spontaneous pneumothorax occurs in 1% to 2% of otherwise healthy newborns at birth. Symptomatic pneumothorax more commonly occurs in the infant who is receiving mechanical ventilation or who has underlying lung disease (e.g., hyaline membrane disease, pulmonary interstitial emphysema, meconium aspiration pneumonia).

(2) **Clinical features.** Symptoms and signs include cyanosis, tachypnea, and elevation of the affected hemithorax. Auscultation reveals diminished breath sounds on the affected side.

(3) **Diagnosis**

(a) The diagnosis is made by a chest radiograph that demonstrates a dense, partially collapsed lung surrounded by a large area of radiolucent air within the hemithorax. Depending on the degree of tension and lung compliance, the mediastinal structures are shifted toward the opposite side of the chest.

(b) Transillumination of the thorax may aid in the diagnosis of pneumothorax in emergencies; positive evidence is the transmission of light through the affected side.

(4) **Therapy** varies with the severity of the symptoms.

(a) If no other lung disease exists and there is minimal respiratory distress, supplemental 100% oxygen (nitrogen washout technique) for several hours is usually sufficient.

(b) If a significant degree of tension, respiratory distress, or some other lung disease exists, the air should be evacuated by aspiration with a syringe and needle or by insertion of a chest tube. Constant suction should be applied to the chest until the air leak resolves.

c. **Meconium aspiration syndrome** is a multiorgan disorder with perinatal asphyxia as the underlying cause. It most commonly occurs in postterm infants and infants who are small for gestational age due to intrauterine growth retardation. Both have placental insufficiency as a common pathway for fetal hypoxia.

(1) **Pathophysiology.** The fetal hypoxia triggers, via a vagal reflex, the passage of thick meconium into the amniotic fluid. The contaminated amniotic fluid is swallowed into the oropharynx and aspirated prior to or at birth with the initiation of breathing. Other organs affected by the perinatal hypoxia include the brain, heart, gastrointestinal tract, and kidneys.

(2) **Diagnosis** is established by the presence of meconium in the trachea or amniotic fluid combined with symptoms of respiratory distress and a chest radiograph that reveals a pattern of diffuse infiltrates with hyperinflation.

(3) **Therapy.** Because most episodes of aspiration occur with the initiation of respiration, the most effective therapy is prevention. This consists of removal of the meconium before the initiation of ventilation. The meconium is removed from the infant's airway as follows:

(a) The oropharynx is suctioned before both delivery of the thorax and initiation of breathing, and again when the infant is on the warmer bed.

(b) The vocal cords are visualized using a laryngoscope, and a large endotracheal tube is passed through the vocal cords and into the lower airway.

(c) Direct wall-unit suction (at a pressure of 80 cm H_2O) is applied to the tube as it is removed. The procedure is repeated if significant meconium is recovered. **Only after the trachea is cleared of any meconium should spontaneous or artificial ventilation be initiated.**

(d) If aspiration has occurred and the infant is in distress, therapy consists of administration of oxygen and mechanical ventilation.

(e) Persistent pulmonary hypertension may also coexist and should be vigorously treated.

d. **Bronchopulmonary dysplasia** (see Chapter 13). This is a chronic pulmonary disease of infants that can result from oxygen and mechanical ventilation therapy for hyaline membrane disease in a preterm infant. It is characterized by the need for oxygen therapy beyond 28 days of life. A characteristic series of changes is seen on radiography.

4. Breathing disorders

a. Regulation of breathing

(1) **Initiation of breathing.** The fetus has periodic breathing movements in utero. It is not until after birth that breathing becomes regular and sustained. It is still not clear what mechanism initiates the infant's first breath.

(a) With the first breath, the pulmonary stretch receptors do not cause complete exhalation; instead, a second inhalation follows. This is called **Head's paradoxic reflex.** It never occurs again throughout life.

(b) Before birth, the alveoli are only minimally distended with lung fluid, and surface tension is high. The first few breaths must create a large negative intrathoracic pressure to open and distend the alveoli.

(c) The first few breaths also allow dispersion of surfactant, which prevents alveolar collapse at the end of expiration by lowering the surface tension. Therefore, minimal negative pressure must be created by subsequent breaths to re-expand the alveoli.

(2) **Maintenance of breathing.** Normal function of the respiratory center in the brain results in rhythmic inhalation and exhalation. The respiratory rate and depth of each breath are

TABLE 6-5 Causes of Apnea

Infection	Pulmonary Edema
Intracranial hemorrhage	Metabolic disturbances (e.g., hypoglycemia, hypocalcemia, hyponatremia)
Airway obstruction	Inappropriate environment temperature (hot or cold)
Gastroesophageal reflux	
Seizures	
Hypoxia	

modulated by the **Hering-Breuer reflex,** carotid bodies, diaphragmatic strength, and cerebrospinal fluid (CSF) pH.

b. Apnea (see Chapter 13) is the cessation of breathing for > 20 seconds. Apnea often occurs in preterm infants (**apnea of prematurity**) and reflects immaturity of the respiratory control mechanisms in the brainstem.

(1) **Clinical features.** Bradycardia (i.e., heart rate < 80 beats per minute) is often associated with apnea. Apnea of prematurity is characterized by periodic breathing and intermittent hypoxia, which further diminish respiratory drive.

(2) **Diagnosis** of apnea of prematurity is made after excluding other reasons for the apnea (Table 6-5).

(3) **Therapy**

(a) **Apnea of prematurity.** Treatment measures include tactile stimulation, maintenance of the neutral thermal zone and core body temperature, supplemental oxygen, and administration of respiratory stimulants (e.g., theophylline, caffeine). It also may be necessary to increase the mean airway pressure by use of continuous positive airway pressure or intermittent assisted ventilation.

(b) **Other causes of apnea.** Treatment of the underlying disorder usually leads to cessation of the apneic episodes.

B **Neonatal necrotizing enterocolitis** refers to a spectrum of varying degrees of acute intestinal necrosis usually following ischemic injury of the bowel, with secondary bacterial invasion and devitalization of the bowel wall.

1. Incidence. This is a serious and common problem, affecting 1% to 5% of all newborns admitted to intensive care units. Affected infants most commonly are premature, asphyxiated, and suffering from other medical problems. Necrotizing enterocolitis is rarely observed in healthy term infants.

2. Etiology and pathogenesis

a. Bowel ischemia secondary to preceding perinatal asphyxia is generally regarded as the cause of bowel wall injury. The introduction of formula or human milk then provides the substrate for bacterial overgrowth. Bacterial invasion of the bowel wall, often with gas production (**pneumatosis intestinalis**), leads to tissue necrosis and perforation.

b. Other predisposing factors include:

(1) Systemic hypotension
(2) Patent ductus arteriosus
(3) Placement of an umbilical artery catheter
(4) Exchange transfusion
(5) Previous treatment with systemic antibiotics
(6) Use of hyperosmolar formula
(7) Rapid advancement of the feeding volume

3. Clinical features and **diagnosis**

a. Signs and **symptoms** are usually noted during the first 2 weeks of life, shortly after enteric feeding has begun (Table 6-6).

b. Laboratory findings

(1) Suggestive blood findings include:

(a) Leukocytosis or neutropenia
(b) Thrombocytopenia

TABLE 6-6 Signs and Symptoms of Necrotizing Enterocolitis

Gastric residuum, which often is bile stained	Poor perfusion, with hypotension or shock
Abdominal distention	Abdominal wall discoloration
Blood in stool (occult or gross)	Unstable temperature
Apnea	Hyperglycemia
Lethargy	Metabolic acidosis

(2) Suggestive findings on abdominal radiography include:
(a) Dilated, thickened bowel loops
(b) Pneumatosis intestinalis, which often starts in the right lower quadrant
(c) Perforation, with free abdominal air and portal vein air

4. **Clinical course.** Two distinct clinical patterns are noted.
   a. Most infants follow a course characterized by feeding intolerance, abdominal distention, occult blood in the stool, and dilated bowel loops on radiography. These infants improve rapidly with therapy.
   b. The other group of infants has severe, progressive symptoms, including gross blood in the stool, extreme abdominal tenderness, hypotension, disseminated intravascular coagulation (DIC), and sepsis. Pneumatosis intestinalis and perforation frequently occur in this setting.
5. **Therapy**
   a. Treatment should begin with discontinuation of enteric feeding, gastric drainage, and administration of intravenous fluids.
   b. Once cultures have been taken, broad-spectrum systemic antibiotics (e.g., ampicillin, gentamicin, clindamycin) should be given. Also, any accompanying disorders (e.g., DIC) should be treated.
   c. Surgical resection of the necrotic bowel segment is indicated for infants who have had a progressive downhill course and for those in whom intestinal perforation has occurred.
6. **Prognosis.** The mortality rate associated with necrotizing enterocolitis, which is highest in the most premature infants, is approximately 30%.

C **Neonatal hyperbilirubinemia** is a condition characterized by an excessive concentration of bilirubin in the blood. There are two types of hyperbilirubinemia: **Unconjugated,** which can be physiologic or pathologic in origin, and **conjugated,** which always stems from pathologic causes. Both types may lead to **jaundice.** Neurotoxic concentrations of unconjugated bilirubin can cause **kernicterus.**

1. **Normal bilirubin metabolism.** Bilirubin is a bile pigment formed from the degradation of heme and is mainly derived from red blood cell (RBC) destruction (75%), but also from ineffective RBC production (25%).
   a. The intermediary product of hemoglobin degradation—**biliverdin**—is converted to bilirubin through a reduction reaction.
   b. Fat-soluble bilirubin normally circulates in plasma bound to albumin, from which it is transported into hepatocytes.
   c. Conjugation with glucuronide converts bilirubin to a water-soluble product, which is excreted into the bile.
2. **Unconjugated** or **indirect hyperbilirubinemia** may occur because of excessive bilirubin production (hemolysis), defective bilirubin clearance from the blood, or defective bilirubin conjugation by the liver. The most common cause in the neonatal period is a physiologic delay in the ability of the liver to clear, metabolize, and excrete the relatively large bilirubin burden at birth. At extremely high levels, fat-soluble unconjugated bilirubin enters the brain and causes neuronal dysfunction and death.
   a. **Clinical manifestations**
      (1) **Jaundice** occurs in 50% of all newborns and reflects an accumulation of unconjugated bilirubin in the blood and other tissues. Jaundice can be clinically observed at blood

concentrations of 5 mg/dL or greater. Unconjugated hyperbilirubinemia or jaundice may be the result of physiologic or nonphysiologic causes.

(a) **Physiologic jaundice** refers to the increased serum concentration of unconjugated bilirubin that is observed during the first few days of life.

(i) **Causative factors** include delayed activity of glucuronyl transferase, increased bilirubin load on hepatocytes, and decreased bilirubin clearance from the plasma.

(ii) **Clinical features.** Physiologic jaundice is associated with an umbilical cord serum bilirubin concentration of < 2 mg/dL, a peak serum bilirubin level of < 12 to 15 mg/dL on the third day of life, and a return to normal levels by the end of the first week of life. In preterm infants, bilirubin levels are usually higher and the physiologic jaundice lasts longer. Breast-fed infants have higher bilirubin levels compared to those fed a commercial formula.

(b) **Nonphysiologic jaundice** refers to hyperbilirubinemia that is secondary to a pathologic process. Specific causes of nonphysiologic indirect hyperbilirubinemia include:

(i) Hemolytic diseases of immune cause (e.g., fetomaternal blood group incompatibilities) as well as nonimmune cause (e.g., spherocytosis, hemoglobinopathy, enzyme deficiency [see Chapter 15])

(ii) Extravascular blood loss and accumulation (e.g., due to cephalhematoma)

(iii) Increased enterohepatic circulation (e.g., due to intestinal obstruction)

(iv) Breastfeeding associated with poor intake

(v) Disorders of bilirubin metabolism (e.g., Lucey-Driscoll syndrome, Crigler-Najjar syndrome, Gilbert syndrome)

(vi) Metabolic disorders (e.g., hypothyroidism, panhypopituitarism, galactosemia)

(vii) Bacterial sepsis

(2) **Kernicterus** is a severe neurologic condition associated with very high levels of unconjugated bilirubin in the blood (generally > 20 mg/dL in term infants). Kernicterus is characterized by yellow staining of the basal ganglia, hippocampus, and cerebellum, which is accompanied by widespread cerebral dysfunction.

(a) **Causes.** Kernicterus occurs when free bilirubin crosses the blood-brain barrier and enters the brain cells.

(i) Normally, unconjugated bilirubin is bound tightly to albumin, which prevents bilirubin from crossing the blood-brain barrier. Free bilirubin exists when the amount of unconjugated bilirubin exceeds the binding capacity of albumin.

(ii) **Bilirubin also may enter the brain at low concentrations** due to the following: Displacement from the albumin-binding site by another compound (e.g., sulfa drug), which leads to an increased free bilirubin concentration; disruption of the blood-brain barrier by sepsis, asphyxia, acidosis, or infusion of hyperosmolar solutions; or a more permeable blood-brain barrier associated with prematurity.

(b) Kernicterus causes a complex of **neurologic symptoms,** including lethargy or irritability, hypotonia, opisthotonos, seizures, mental retardation, and hearing loss.

b. Diagnosis

(1) **Physiologic jaundice** is present if underlying pathologic causes of the hyperbilirubinemia can be excluded. As the most common causes of unconjugated hyperbilirubinemia are physiologic and hemolytic, the initial evaluation should include:

(a) Complete blood count with peripheral smear and reticulocyte count

(b) Determination of maternal and infant blood types

(c) Coombs test (indirect and direct)

(d) Determination of direct and indirect concentrations of bilirubin

(2) **Nonphysiologic jaundice** should always be suspected when the umbilical cord serum bilirubin concentration is elevated, the clinical appearance of jaundice is within the first 24 hours of life, or the conjugated fraction of the serum bilirubin concentration exceeds 2 mg/dL.

c. Therapy consists of treatment of any underlying causes of hyperbilirubinemia and the prevention of kernicterus.

(1) **Treatment modalities**

(a) **Phototherapy** converts unconjugated bilirubin into several water-soluble photoisomers that can be excreted without conjugation. **Lumirubin,** a structural isomer, is the major excretory product.

(b) **Exchange transfusion** is used principally in hemolytic disease or when the bilirubin concentration is very high. This procedure directly removes the bilirubin from the intravascular space. Unbound antibodies that initiate the hemolytic process are also removed.

(2) **Specific indications for the use of phototherapy** and **exchange transfusion** are discussed in detail in most neonatology texts. The specific bilirubin concentration that requires treatment varies with gestational age, the cause of the jaundice, and the presence of medical complications (e.g., sepsis, acidosis).

3. **Conjugated** or **direct hyperbilirubinemia**

a. **Clinical manifestations.** Jaundice associated with conjugated hyperbilirubinemia is always pathologic in origin.

b. **Causes**

(1) TORCH infections (toxoplasmosis, rubella virus, cytomegalovirus, herpes simplex virus; see Chapter 10)

(2) Metabolic disorders (e.g., galactosemia)

(3) Bacterial sepsis

(4) Obstructive jaundice (e.g., due to biliary atresia; see Chapter 11)

(5) Prolonged administration of intravenous protein solutions

(6) Neonatal hepatitis (see Chapter 11)

c. **Diagnosis** is based on a conjugated fraction of the serum bilirubin concentration that exceeds 2 mg/dL. Further evaluation should be directed to possible underlying causes of the direct hyperbilirubinemia.

d. **Therapy** is directed to the underlying causes of the hyperbilirubinemia.

D Hematologic disorders

1. **Anemia** (see Chapter 15). In the newborn, anemia is defined as a hematocrit $< 40\%$. Normally, the hematocrit at term gestation is 50% to 55%.

a. **Etiology.** The principal causes of anemia in the newborn can be divided into those associated with acute blood loss, chronic blood loss, and impaired red blood cell production (Table 6-7). The most frequent cause—**hemolytic disease of the newborn**—is discussed first in somewhat more detail than the other causes.

(1) **Hemolytic disease of the newborn** (erythroblastosis fetalis) usually results from blood group incompatibility between the mother and the fetus. Hemolysis occurs when maternal antibodies to a blood group antigen on the fetal red blood cell cross the placenta. These antibodies bind to fetal RBCs, which are then destroyed in the spleen.

(a) ABO blood group antigens are most common, although they rarely cause sufficient hemolysis to result in severe anemia.

(b) Before the use of Rh_o(D) immune globulin (human), the most commonly involved antigen was **Rh_o(D)**—from the Rh blood group system. Rh incompatibility is associated with **extravascular hemolysis.**

(c) Rarely, hemolytic disease of the newborn is caused by other blood group incompatibilities (e.g., c, E, Kell), a congenital defect or deficiency in enzymes (e.g., glucose-6-phosphate dehydrogenase [G6PD]), a membrane defect, infection, or vitamin deficiency (e.g., vitamin E).

(d) In utero, if the anemia is severe (usually involving Rh incompatibility), the fetus (infant) will exhibit the signs and symptoms of **hydrops fetalis** with severe edema, anasarca, and hypoproteinemia.

(2) Anemia can be caused by a number of other problems. Table 6-7 lists the symptoms and related causes.

b. **Diagnosis.** The specific cause of the anemia is established on the basis of information collected from the following sources:

(1) History

TABLE 6-7 Causes and Clinical Features of Anemia

Anemia Associated With	Causes	Clinical Features
Acute blood loss	Placenta previa Placental abruption Fetomaternal transfusion Fetoplacental transfusion Cord rupture Internal hemorrhage	Acute distress Shallow, rapid respirations Tachycardia Weak to absent pulse Hypotension Absence of hepatosplenomegaly Low blood volume
Chronic blood loss	Hemolytic disease Twin-to-twin transfusion (monochorionic) Fetomaternal transfusion Chronic phlebotomy	Pallor disproportionate to the degree of distress Weak to normal pulse Normal blood pressure Signs of congestive heart failure Hepatosplenomegaly Normal blood volume
Impaired red blood cell production	Diamond-Blackfan syndrome (congenital hypoplastic anemia)	Pallor (see Chapter 15)

(2) Complete blood count with peripheral smear and reticulocyte count
(3) Evaluation of maternal and infant blood for Rh or ABO incompatibility
(4) Coombs test
(5) Other tests (e.g., Kleihauer test [to identify and quantify fetal RBCs], hemoglobin electrophoresis, G6PD evaluation)

c. **Therapy**

(1) **Hemolytic disease of the newborn.** Therapy is indicated when the hemoglobin and hematocrit are low enough to compromise the oxygen-carrying capacity of the blood, which can cause congestive heart failure, respiratory distress, acidosis, poor perfusion, and hypotension. The blood volume is usually normal. Therefore, the anemia is corrected by performing a partial exchange transfusion with packed RBCs.
(2) **Acute blood loss** should be treated rapidly. Therapy includes restoration of blood volume and red cell mass and elimination of the cause of blood loss, if it is still present.
(3) **Chronic blood loss.** Depending on the clinical condition and cause of blood loss, therapy varies and may consist of packed RBC transfusion, partial exchange transfusion with packed RBCs, iron therapy, or no intervention.

2. **Polycythemia** occurs in 2% to 5% of all newborns and is defined as a hematocrit of 65% or greater when a freely flowing blood sample is taken from a large vein. **Hyperviscosity** of the blood almost always exists in association with polycythemia.

a. **Etiology.** Polycythemia has been associated with the following conditions:

(1) Fetoplacental transfusion associated with birth asphyxia or delayed cord clamping
(2) Twin-to-twin transfusion
(3) Chronic intrauterine hypoxia secondary to placental insufficiency (e.g., pregnancy-induced hypertension with fetal growth retardation) or increased fetal metabolism (e.g., with maternal diabetes)
(4) Endocrine disorders (e.g., hyperthyroidism)
(5) Genetic disorders (e.g., Down syndrome, Beckwith-Wiedemann syndrome)

b. **Pathophysiology**

(1) Many of the problems associated with polycythemia were originally thought to be caused by organ ischemia and hypoxia secondary to an increase in blood viscosity. It is now known that most of the blood flow reduction is the result of increased oxygen content in the arterial blood. This reciprocal relationship of decreased blood flow and increased arterial oxygen content results in a normal or increased delivery of oxygen to most organs.

TABLE 6-8 Organisms Responsible for Transplacental Infections Before Birth

Cytomegalovirus	Rubella virus
Treponema pallidum (the agent of syphilis)	*Toxoplasma gondii*
Human immunodeficiency virus, the agent of acquired immune deficiency syndrome	Echovirus
	Listeria monocytogenes

TABLE 6-9 Abnormalities Associated With Infection Acquired in the First Trimester

Congenital malformation	Hydrocephalus
Intrauterine growth retardation	Stillbirth
Microcephaly	

(2) Therefore, most of the problems associated with polycythemia are more likely the result of the perinatal events (i.e., acute or chronic hypoxia) that are also responsible for the development of the polycythemia, rather than any flow disturbances attributable to the polycythemia itself.

c. **Clinical features**

(1) **Symptoms** and **signs** associated with polycythemia include:

(a) Tachypnea and cyanosis
(b) Jitteriness and seizures
(c) Hypoglycemia
(d) Renal dysfunction
(e) Necrotizing enterocolitis

(2) **Complications.** Polycythemia is associated with an abnormal long-term neurologic outcome.

d. **Therapy** is generally supportive. Reduction of the hematocrit by partial exchange transfusion may be helpful in alleviating respiratory distress, renal dysfunction, and hypoglycemia, but this measure may increase the risk of necrotizing enterocolitis. No study has shown a beneficial effect of partial exchange transfusion on long-term neurologic outcome.

E **Infection** continues to be a major cause of neonatal morbidity and mortality despite advances in therapy. Although perinatally acquired bacterial infections are the most common, infections that are acquired in utero remain an important source of long-term disability.

1. **General considerations**

a. **Predisposing factors.** The newborn is particularly susceptible to infection due to immaturity of immune system mechanisms, including:

(1) Neutrophil chemotaxis
(2) Neutrophil phagocytosis
(3) Bactericidal activity
(4) Humoral components

b. **Timing** and **route of infection.** The causative organism and abnormalities associated with neonatal infections vary with the time and route of infection.

(1) **Organisms responsible for transplacental infections before birth** are listed in Table 6-8. Abnormalities associated with infection acquired in utero are listed in Tables 6-9 and 6-10.

(2) **Perinatal infections** include infections acquired through the fetal membranes, ascending infections acquired after rupture of the fetal membranes, and infections acquired via the birth canal. Common **causative organisms** are listed in Table 6-11, and **associated abnormalities** are listed in Table 6-12.

TABLE 6-10 Abnormalities Associated With Infection Acquired Later in Pregnancy

Microcephaly	Intracranial hemorrhage
Hydrops fetalis	Hepatosplenomegaly
Disseminated intravascular coagulation	Jaundice
Anemia	Skin and eye lesions
	Stillbirth

TABLE 6-11 Organisms Responsible for Perinatal Infections

Group B β-hemolytic streptococcus	Herpes simplex virus
Escherichia coli	*Chlamydia trachomatis*
Klebsiella species	*Neisseria gonorrhoeae*
Streptococcus pneumoniae	*Neisseria meningitidis*

TABLE 6-12 Abnormalities Associated With Perinatal Infections

Respiratory distress	Thrombocytopenia
Temperature instability	Meningitis
Septic shock	Death
Neutropenia	

TABLE 6-13 Common Organisms Involved in Postnatal Infections

Staphylococcus aureus	*Klebsiella pneumoniae*
Staphylococcus epidermidis	*Clostridia* species
Pseudomonas aeruginosa	*Bacteroides* species
Candida albicans	Enterococcus
Escherichia coli	

(3) **Postnatal infections** most often are acquired as a result of nosocomial or community exposures. Hospitalized newborns who are premature or require instrumentation are particularly susceptible. Common **causative organisms** are listed in Table 6-13, and **associated abnormalities** are listed in Table 6-14.

2. **Bacterial infection** and **neonatal sepsis.** Bacterial infections most frequently are acquired via the birth canal or nosocomially. The infection is almost always bacteremic (often with seeding of the meninges by way of the blood) and associated with systemic symptoms—a condition referred to as **neonatal sepsis.**
   a. **Incidence.** Neonatal sepsis is common in premature infants. Approximately 1% to 4% of these infants have at least one episode of sepsis during their hospitalization. Sepsis in term infants is rare, occurring in $< 1\%$.
   b. Risk factors for early neonatal sepsis include:
      (1) Premature labor
      (2) Prolonged rupture of the fetal membranes
      (3) Low birth weight
      (4) Chorioamnionitis
      (5) Maternal fever
   c. **Etiology.** The most common causative organisms include:
      (1) Gram-positive cocci, especially group B β-hemolytic streptococci, but also *Staphylococcus aureus* and *Staphylococcus epidermidis*
      (2) Gram-negative rods, especially *Escherichia coli* and *Klebsiella pneumoniae*
      (3) Gram-positive rods (e.g., *Listeria monocytogenes*)
   d. **Clinical features**
      (1) **Signs** and **symptoms** of bacterial infection include:
         (a) Unexplained respiratory distress
         (b) Unexplained feeding intolerance
         (c) Temperature instability
         (d) Hypoglycemia or hyperglycemia
         (e) Apnea
         (f) Lethargy
         (g) Irritability
      (2) **Laboratory findings** include:
         (a) Abnormal white blood cell count, including neutropenia or neutrophilia
         (b) Prolonged prothrombin time (PT) and partial thromboplastin time (PTT)
         (c) Tracheal aspirate containing bacteria and neutrophils

TABLE 6-14 Abnormalities Associated With Postnatal Infection in the Newborn

Respiratory distress	Disseminated intravascular coagulation
Feeding intolerance	Hypoglycemia or hyperglycemia
Apnea	Temperature instability
Anemia	
Shock	

e. **Diagnosis.** In addition to the physical examination, the laboratory evaluation for neonatal sepsis should include:
   (1) Complete blood count (neutropenia [< 1800/mm3] or an elevated ratio of immature to total neutrophils suggests sepsis)
   (2) Blood cultures
   (3) Lumbar puncture
   (4) Culture and counterimmunoelectrophoresis or latex agglutination testing of the urine
   (5) Gram stain and culture of a tracheal aspirate, if the infant is intubated
   (6) Chest radiograph
   (7) Gastric aspirate (at the time of delivery) for neutrophil count, Gram stain, and culture

f. **Therapy**
   (1) Empiric antibiotic therapy should begin after the diagnostic workup and consist of a broad-spectrum penicillin (usually ampicillin) and an aminoglycoside (usually gentamicin). Once culture data are available, therapy should be tailored to the specific organism.
   (2) The initial choice of antibiotics for nosocomial infection depends on nursery, community, and individual patient exposure information.
   (3) The duration of therapy is usually 7 to 10 days, except for invasive infections (e.g., meningitis, osteomyelitis), which require longer courses of antibiotic therapy.
   (4) Other complications (e.g., DIC) should always be investigated and treated.

3. **Viral infection** is uncommon in the newborn but can be devastating. Viral infections can be divided into those acquired prenatally and those acquired perinatally or postnatally.

a. **Prenatal viral infections**
   (1) **Common agents** include rubella virus, cytomegalovirus, echovirus, herpes zoster virus, and human immunodeficiency virus (see Chapter 10).
   (2) **Clinical features** are listed in Table 6-15.

b. **Perinatal** and **postnatal viral infections**
   (1) **Common agents** are listed in Table 6-16.
   (2) **Clinical features**
      (a) **Herpes virus infections.** Symptoms do not appear until at least 3 to 7 days and up to 4 weeks after birth. These infections manifest as vesicular skin eruptions, DIC, shock, pneumonia, and encephalitis.
      (b) **Respiratory syncytial virus** infections manifest as temperature instability, respiratory distress, apnea, clear nasal discharge, and poor feeding.

c. **Diagnosis** begins with a high index of suspicion and is based primarily on infant culture data, cord immunoglobulin M level, changing infant serum antibody titers, results of rapid antigen or antibody tests, maternal medical history and culture data, and time of the year.

d. **Therapy** is available for herpes virus and respiratory syncytial virus infections.
   (1) Herpes virus infections are treated systemically with vidarabine or acyclovir and ophthalmologically with vidarabine ointment.
   (2) Respiratory syncytial virus infections are occasionally treated with aerosolized ribavirin.
   (3) Congenital cytomegalovirus (CMV) infection may be treated with ganciclovir. Efficacy for this therapy is being established.

TABLE 6-15 Clinical Features Associated With Prenatal Viral Infection

Intrauterine growth retardation	Hepatosplenomegaly
Congenital anomalies	Ocular lesions
Skin lesions	Coagulopathy
Central nervous system defects	Hearing loss

TABLE 6-16 Common Viruses Responsible for Perinatal and Postnatal Infection

Herpes simplex virus	Echovirus
Herpes zoster virus	Coxsackievirus
Hepatitis A and B viruses	Cytomegalovirus (vertical transmission from mother or via blood transfusion)
Respiratory syncytial virus	

TABLE 6-17 Prenatal Risk Factors for Asphyxia

Extremes in maternal age (i.e., < 20 y or > 35 y)	Fetal bradycardia
Placental abruption	Malpresentation
Placenta previa	Multiple gestation
Preeclampsia	Prolonged rupture of the fetal membranes
Preterm gestation	Maternal diabetes
Postterm gestation	Maternal use of illicit drugs
Meconium-stained amniotic fluid	

TABLE 6-18 Complications Associated With Perinatal Asphyxia

Hypotension	Adrenal hemorrhage and necrosis
Hypoxic encephalopathy and seizures	Hypoglycemia
Persistent pulmonary hypertension	Polycythemia
Hypoxic cardiomyopathy	Hypocalcemia
Ileus and necrotizing enterocolitis	Disseminated intravascular coagulation
Acute tubular necrosis	

F **Neurologic disorders** generally result in abnormalities of tone, strength, and state of consciousness. The most common neurologic problems occurring in newborns are briefly reviewed here.

1. **Asphyxial brain injury** is the most common neurologic abnormality in the neonatal period.
   a. **Risk factors for perinatal asphyxia** are summarized in Table 6-17.
   b. **Pathophysiology**
      (1) During mild to moderate perinatal asphyxia, blood flow to the brain is preserved due to redistribution of the cardiac output.
      (2) During severe perinatal asphyxia, cerebral hypoxia and ischemia occur, initially in the cerebral cortex and eventually in the cerebellum and brainstem.
   c. **Clinical features** are summarized in Table 6-18.
   d. **Therapy**
      (1) Treatment is primarily supportive (i.e., ventilation with oxygen and maintenance of cardiac output) while awaiting spontaneous recovery, especially with a mild insult.
      (2) Severely asphyxiated infants may require more extensive support of neurologic function as well as respiratory, cardiac, and renal function.
      (3) Anticonvulsants are helpful in controlling seizures, although the seizure activity is usually self-limited.
      (4) Cooling therapy to reduce cerebral edema or lower the cerebral metabolic rate is currently being evaluated and may show promise in certain circumstances.
   e. **Prognosis** is variable and sometimes difficult to predict. Mild asphyxia is almost always associated with a good outcome, whereas severe asphyxia is frequently associated with significant morbidity and mortality. The electroencephalogram (EEG) in the neonatal period and time to recover normal neurologic function are predictive of long-term outcome.
2. **Seizures** (see Chapter 18) are not uncommon in the neonatal period. Subtle seizures—which manifest as rhythmic eye deviation or blinking, lip smacking, "bicycling," or apnea—are the most common form, followed by generalized tonic, multifocal clonic, focal clonic, and myoclonic seizures.
   a. **Etiology.** Underlying causes of seizure activity include:
      (1) Asphyxia
      (2) Brain anomalies (e.g., holoprosencephaly)
      (3) Intracranial hemorrhage, particularly within the brain parenchyma
      (4) Systemic metabolic disorders (e.g., hypoglycemia, hyponatremia, hypocalcemia, hypernatremia, hyperammonemia) and inborn errors of amino acid and organic acid metabolism
      (5) Meningitis and encephalitis
      (6) Pyridoxine dependency
   b. **Diagnosis.** The following evaluations should be made in an effort to pinpoint the cause of the seizure activity:
      (1) Neurologic examination
      (2) EEG

(3) Ultrasound, computed tomography, or magnetic resonance scanning, especially in the presence of lateralization of the seizure or EEG

(4) Screening for metabolic disorders (e.g., involving glucose, calcium, or sodium), inborn errors of metabolism (e.g., involving amino acids or organic acids), and pyridoxine dependency

(5) Lumbar puncture (in the absence of increased intracranial pressure) and evaluation of the CSF for sepsis

c. **Therapy** should be promptly initiated. Phenobarbital is the drug of choice. Pyridoxine dependency should be considered in term infants who show no clear cause for the seizure activity and who do not respond to routine therapy.

d. **Prognosis** varies with the underlying cause.

3. **Periventricular leukomalacia (PVL)** refers to the cystic lesions in the cerebral cortex, lateral to the lateral ventricles. These lesions can be contiguous with the ventricles and extend far into the cortex. PVL is an injury of preterm infants thought to be due to cerebral ischemia.

4. **Hydrocephalus** (see Chapter 18) refers to an excessive collection of CSF within the ventricular system due to imbalanced production and absorption of CSF.

5. **Hypotonia,** a condition characterized by diminished tone of the skeletal muscles, is the most common neurologic motor disorder of the neonatal period. An evaluation must be performed to determine at which level in the progression of nerve impulse to muscular contraction the defect exists. Table 6-19 lists common causes.

6. **Myelomeningocele** (see Chapter 18) is the most common congenital anomaly of the nervous system. It results from failure of the neural tube to close. The risk of developing myelomeningocele is greatly reduced by administration of the B vitamin folate to the mother before conception and throughout the first trimester.

G **Hypoglycemia** is defined as a plasma glucose concentration < 30 mg/dL during the first 24 hours of life and < 45 mg/dL thereafter. Hypoglycemia is very common in infants of diabetic mothers as well as in infants who are born after various perinatal complications, including prematurity, intrauterine growth retardation, and asphyxia (see Chapter 17).

1. **Pathogenesis.** The pathogenesis varies depending on the clinical setting and the associated conditions affecting the infant.

a. **Maternal diabetes.** The hypoglycemia in infants of diabetic mothers is the result of a hyperinsulinemic state that persists after the umbilical cord is cut and the maternal supply of glucose is interrupted.

b. **Prematurity.** Preterm infants become hypoglycemic due to diminished glycogen stores and immaturity of gluconeogenic enzymes.

c. **Growth retardation.** Growth-retarded infants frequently are depleted of hepatic glycogen and quickly become hypoglycemic.

d. **Perinatal asphyxia** forces the fetus (infant) to use anaerobic metabolism, which quickly depletes stored glycogen and results in hypoglycemia.

e. **Cold stress** increases oxygen consumption as well as glucose consumption. It may also increase free acids and result in hypoglycemia.

f. **Sepsis** may cause hypoglycemia, although hyperglycemia is also observed, which presumably is caused by insulin insensitivity.

TABLE 6-19 Common Causes of Hypotonia
Asphyxia (brain defect)
Werdnig-Hoffman disease (spinal cord defect)
Congenital myasthenia gravis (neuromuscular junction defect)
Muscular dystrophy (muscle defect)
Myotonic dystrophy (muscle defect)
Hypothyroidism (metabolic defect)

g. **Beckwith-Wiedemann syndrome** is characterized by hypoglycemia, visceromegaly, macroglossia, and omphalocele. Hyperinsulinism secondary to pancreatic islet cell hyperplasia is responsible for the hypoglycemia.

h. **Nesidioblastosis** and **pancreatic islet cell adenoma** are associated with hyperinsulinemia and hypoglycemia.

i. **Metabolic disorders,** such as galactosemia and panhypopituitarism, are also associated with hypoglycemia.

2. **Clinical features.** Infants who have hypoglycemia are not always symptomatic. However, the following symptoms may occur:
   a. Hypotonia or jitteriness
   b. Apnea or tachypnea
   c. Seizures

3. **Diagnosis.** Screening for hypoglycemia may be done using any of a number of bedside reagent strips. The diagnosis is confirmed by the actual measurement of the plasma glucose concentration by the clinical laboratory.

4. **Therapy**
   a. Primary therapy is intravenous glucose. Bolus infusions of hypertonic glucose should be avoided because they may result in a rebound hypoglycemia.
   b. Hypoglycemia that is secondary to hyperinsulinemia and resistant to intravenous glucose should be treated with corticosteroids or diazoxide. If drug treatment fails, pancreatectomy should be performed.

H Disorders associated with maternal diabetes The pregnancy of a diabetic woman is one that is associated with multiple complications affecting both mother and fetus. The key to an optimal outcome is consistent euglycemia in the mother.

1. **Diabetic embryopathy**
   a. **Caudal regression,** or underdevelopment of the lower spine (bony and neurogenic tissue), is a congenital anomaly that is specifically associated with infants of diabetic mothers. It is clearly related to maternal hyperglycemia during organogenesis.
   b. **Other anomalies** also occur at an increased rate. In the United States, congenital anomalies of the heart and CNS are the most common.

2. **Prenatal growth abnormalities.** Glucose easily crosses the placenta, whereas insulin does not; therefore, maternal hyperglycemia causes fetal hyperglycemia and a reactive fetal hyperinsulinemia. This combination results in increased somatic growth of the fetus due to cellular hyperplasia and hypertrophy. The large size of the fetus often results in dystocia. The brain is the only organ whose growth is not affected by the fetal hyperglycemia and hyperinsulinemia.

3. **Late fetal death** occurs more frequently in the poorly controlled diabetic pregnancy than in the normal pregnancy or euglycemic diabetic pregnancy.

4. **Preterm delivery** is common and the result of fetal distress or a planned early delivery. Effective production of surfactant is delayed in these infants; therefore, an L/S ratio should always be determined before an elective delivery to indicate the level of lung maturity (*see V A 1 b 1 b*).

5. **Hypoglycemia** is very common in infants of diabetic mothers and is related to the mother's overall glycemic control as well as the intrapartum glucose levels (*see V G*).

6. **Other metabolic disturbances** seen in infants of diabetic mothers include hypocalcemia and hyperbilirubinemia.

7. **Polycythemia** associated with elevated erythropoietin levels is observed and probably reflects chronic fetal hypoxia.

8. **Alterations in normal neonatal behavior** are commonly observed. Abnormalities include lethargy, hypotonia, and poor feeding. A cause is not clear.

9. **Large body size.** Those infants who are large for gestational age are more likely to continue to be large for age beyond infancy.

I Intrauterine drug exposure Studies have documented fetal exposure to numerous drugs, including antibiotics, caffeine, nicotine, alcohol, aspirin, and antihistamines. Over the past decade, the use of illicit drugs (e.g., heroin, cocaine, marijuana) by pregnant women has also grown. The intravenous use of illicit drugs is associated with a high risk for preterm birth as well as a significant risk of hepatitis and acquired immune deficiency syndrome in both the mother and infant. The drug-seeking behavior of these mothers often makes it difficult for them to care for their infants. The following are some commonly used drugs that may have major effects on the developing fetus and newborn.

1. **Nicotine** is absorbed through the lungs from cigarette smoke and is accompanied by the diffusion of carbon monoxide across the alveoli into the mother's blood. Nicotine is a vasoconstrictor that may limit uterine blood flow, and carbon monoxide decreases the arterial oxygen content. Together the two substances reduce the transfer of oxygen and nutrients from mother to fetus. The result is decreased intrauterine growth and chronic hypoxia.
2. **Alcohol** is a well-established teratogen. Fetal exposure may result in a spectrum of effects ranging from mild reduction in cerebral function to classic **fetal alcohol syndrome** (see Chapter 8).
3. **Heroin and methadone**
   a. Narcotic use by the mother is associated with intrauterine growth retardation, infant narcotic withdrawal syndrome, and increased risk of sudden infant death. There is accelerated maturation of several fetal organs, including the liver and lung (surfactant production).
   b. Many of these infants will experience **narcotic withdrawal syndrome,** which is characterized by irritability, poor sleeping, high-pitched cry, diarrhea, sweating, sneezing, seizures, poor feeding, and poor weight gain. Naloxone should never be given to such infants in the delivery room because it precipitates acute withdrawal.
   c. The long-term neurologic consequences of fetal narcotic exposure have not been investigated completely.
4. **Cocaine** use by pregnant women has increased dramatically over the past decade. Such use is associated with congenital anomalies, intrauterine growth retardation, intracranial hemorrhage, placental abruption, and preterm birth. Infants may undergo withdrawal (irritability, poor feeding). Studies have demonstrated abnormalities in control of respiration and an increased risk for sudden infant death.

VI CARE OF THE PARENTS

Whether the parents have the happy experience of bonding to a healthy newborn or the tragic experience of mourning a dying infant, it is the pediatrician's role to provide the parents with support and information and answer their questions.

A Parent-infant bonding

1. Bonding, or the process of psychological attachment of the parents to the newborn, appears to begin during pregnancy and intensify as the fetus begins to move inside the uterus and react to external stimuli. During this period, the parents often form a mental image of what the infant will look like at birth.
2. At the time of delivery, it is thought that the mother experiences a unique psychological state or "window." This close contact with the infant in the delivery room fosters ideal bonding and promotes optimal future mother-infant interactions. Although every effort should be made to ensure parent-infant bonding in the delivery area, medical problems (e.g., hypothermia, respiratory distress) must take precedence.
3. The process of bonding continues for hours and days after birth. Even if the delivery room bonding experience does not occur, it has been shown that strong mother-infant ties will be established if the mother and infant are given long periods of contact together over the next few days.

B Support for the parents of a malformed infant

The birth of a malformed infant is a tragedy that creates a complex challenge for the pediatrician who must care for the child and help the parents through the disappointment and period of adjustment.

1. **Stages of parental reaction.** Parents go through four stages in reacting to their malformed infant, starting with mourning the loss of the expected healthy infant and ending with acceptance of the actual infant. These stages are:
   a. Shock

b. Denial
c. Sadness and anger
d. Reorganization and acceptance

2. **Supportive actions** that help the parents through this tragic period include the following:
   a. The parents should be encouraged to spend as much time as possible with the infant.
   b. The infant should be shown to the parents as soon as possible, because a mental image of the anomaly is often worse than the actual malformation.
   c. Good lines of communication should be maintained, and information should be conveyed in a truthful manner.
   d. The parents need support through each stage of adjustment and should not be rushed through the various stages.
   e. Plans for adequate support of the infant and parents should be made before discharge.

C Support of the parents of a dying infant during the illness and after the death

1. **Parental reactions**
   a. **Grief** experienced after the loss of a newborn is unique in that the attachment one has for a parent, sibling, spouse, or older child has not been formed. Rather, the newborn is perceived as a part of the parent, especially the mother. As such, the grieving behavior of the parents includes both the classic grieving behaviors plus behaviors reflecting detachment, similar to the feelings experienced when a limb has been amputated. The feelings include anger, guilt, fury, helplessness, and horror.
   b. Loss of a newborn often results in a **breakdown in communication** between the parents due to their difficulty in expressing emotions and their feelings of guilt, blame, or both.
2. **Supportive actions.** The parents can best be supported through the following actions.
   a. The parents should be prepared if death is anticipated.
   b. The parents should be together when they are told of the death.
   c. Every effort should be made to allow the parents to hold the infant before and after death if they desire to.
   d. Time for the immediate grieving should be allowed to pass before discussion of autopsy and burial arrangements.
   e. Support should be offered to the parents 3 to 4 months after the death. This may be in the form of an office visit or contact with a parents' group.
   f. Autopsy reports should be made available and discussed with the parents in a timely fashion.

BIBLIOGRAPHY

Avery GB, Fletcher MA, MacDonald MG: *Neonatology: Pathophysiology and Management of the Newborn,* 5th ed. Philadelphia, JB Lippincott, 1999.

Creasy RK, Resnik R, Iams J: *Maternal-Fetal Medicine,* 5th ed. Philadelphia, WB Saunders, 2003.

Klaus MH, Fanaroff AA: *Care of the High-Risk Neonate,* 5th ed. Philadelphia, WB Saunders, 2001.

Polin RA, Fox WW: *Fetal and Neonatal Physiology,* 3rd ed. Philadelphia, WB Saunders, 2003.

Volpe JJ: *Neurology of the Newborn.* 4th ed. Philadelphia, WB Saunders, 2001.

Taeusch HW, Ballard RA, Gleason CA: *Avery's Diseases of the Newborn,* 8th ed. Philadelphia, WB Saunders, 2004.

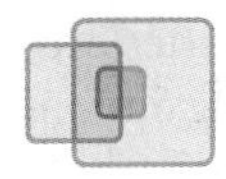

Study Questions

Directions: *Each of the numbered items or incomplete statements in this section is followed by answers or completions of the statement. Select the ONE lettered answer or completion that is BEST in each case.*

1. You are evaluating a 2-day-old term infant for discharge. You note 15 to 20 fine yellow-white tiny papules over the nose and cheeks, a nonblanching erythematous patch over the nape of the neck, and a localized area of bluish-gray discoloration over the left buttock. On further inspection you find numerous, widely scattered erythematous macules with central white pustules in a distribution that has changed during the past 24 hours according to personnel in the nursery. Finally, there is also a yellow color to the skin extending from the head to the groin region. You review each of the dermatologic findings in the infant to decide whether any of these require further consideration. Which of the following dermatologic diagnoses noted on this infant's discharge examination merits further evaluation and could potentially delay discharge?

A Salmon patch
B Jaundice
C Milia
D Mongolian spot
E Erythema toxicum

2. A 1-week-old girl presents to your office for a routine postnatal follow-up visit. The pregnancy, labor, and delivery were unremarkable except for the need for cesarean section due to breech presentation. Which of the following orthopedic conditions is this infant at highest risk for?

A Clavicle fracture
B Developmental dysplasia of the hip
C Flexion contracture of the elbow
D Lower extremity malformation
E Metatarsus adductus

3. A well-appearing full-term newborn has just been admitted to the normal newborn nursery. Upon reviewing his chart you note that his delivery was forceps assisted and that his Apgar scores were 2 at 1 minute, 8 at 5 minutes, and 9 at 10 minutes. Which of the following is a true statement regarding the Apgar score(s) in this infant?

A The 1-minute Apgar score reflects inadequate resuscitation up to that point
B The 1-minute Apgar score reflects perinatal asphyxia
C The 5-minute Apgar score reflects good ventilation
D The 5-minute Apgar score reflects the likelihood of a stable postnatal course
E The 10-minute Apgar score reflects successful prevention of neurologic damage

4. You are seeing a 12-day-old newborn in your office for bilateral eye discharge. Because the infant is currently in foster care, there is no information known about prenatal history. Postnatal history is unremarkable. She appears to have been born at term, in a tertiary care hospital, and was discharged to a foster family at 3 days of life. She has been healthy and thriving with the exception of significantly reddened eyes bilaterally and worsening greenish discharge over the last 24 hours. Which of the following is the most likely diagnosis in this infant?

A Chemical conjunctivitis
B Blocked lacrimal duct
C Chlamydial conjunctivitis
D Gonococcal conjunctivitis
E Group B streptococcus (GBS) bacteremia

5. You are looking after a 28-hour-old, intubated boy born at 24 weeks weighing 560 grams. He is currently receiving a parenteral solution of 10% dextrose plus calcium without electrolytes. At the present time, the infant weighs 490 grams. He is intubated but appears comfortable; breath sounds are clear and equal bilaterally. There is a newly audible systolic murmur consistent with a patent ductus arteriosus (PDA). Serum electrolytes are normal and urine output is appropriate. Which of the following options for fluid-care management is most appropriate for the infant at this point in time?

- A Introduce enteral nutrition consisting of fortified breast milk via gastric bolus
- B Replace 10% dextrose solution with total parenteral nutrition
- C Significant decrease in IV fluid rate of current solution given potential PDA
- D Introduce special "premie" formula for increased vitamin and mineral needs via continuous feeding
- E Significant increase in IV fluid rate of current solution plus electrolytes given dramatic weight loss

6. A 2-hour-old newborn boy was born at 28 weeks and weighs 800 grams. His respiratory status has slowly deteriorated since birth and a decision is made to intubate him in order to assist his labored respirations. Which of the following conditions has likely led to this deterioration in respiratory status?

- A Transient tachypnea of the newborn
- B Hyaline membrane disease
- C Persistent pulmonary hypertension of the newborn
- D Pneumonia
- E Sepsis

7. A 4-kg girl was born at 41 weeks' gestation. The vaginal delivery was complicated by late heart rate decelerations and amniotic fluid that contained thick, particulate meconium. The infant is intubated secondary to significant respiratory distress; in addition, 100% oxygen is administered. Despite this treatment oxygen saturations do not exceed 85%. Which of the following conditions has likely led to this deterioration in respiratory status?

- A Transient tachypnea of the newborn
- B Hyaline membrane disease
- C Persistent pulmonary hypertension of the newborn
- D Pneumonia
- E Sepsis

8. You are examining an 18-hour-old full-term infant. Of note is the fact that he appears significantly jaundiced. He is otherwise vigorous and has good urine output. He has been breastfeeding every 2 to 3 hours. Which of the following is the most likely cause of this baby's jaundice?

- A Physiologic and of little significance
- B Intolerance to his mother's breast milk
- C Improper lighting in the nursery
- D Incompatibility between blood types of mother and baby
- E A red blood cell defect such as sickle cell

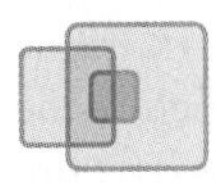

Answers and Explanations

1. The answer is B (*III C 2*). Jaundice in the neonate is first visible on the face and, as the serum bilirubin level rises, the jaundice progresses caudally to include the rest of the body and the sclerae. If not adequately evaluated and treated, jaundice can easily lead to significant and irreversible brain injury (kernicterus). Common birthmarks that are visible at birth include flat vascular nevi (i.e., salmon patch nevus and port wine stains) and mongolian spots (*see III C 8*). Benign rashes are common and include erythema toxicum neonatorum, which has a "flea-bite" appearance with scattered erythematous macules that may contain papulopustular centers filled with eosinophils and rash typically changes distribution from day to day; milia, which are fine, pinpoint, yellow-white papules caused by retained sebum that typically cover the bridge of the nose, chin, and cheeks and are transient; and neonatal pustular melanosis, which consists of small vesiculopustules that are present at birth and rupture within a few days, leaving transient pigmented macules with scaly borders.

2. The answer is B (*III C 7*). Developmental dysplasia of the hip occurs in 1 in 1000 live births and is much more common in girls and breech deliveries. Asymmetries in lower limb length, placement of medial thigh and gluteal folds, or degree of hip flexion should raise suspicion for unilateral hip dislocation. When the hips are flexed to 90 degrees, the legs normally can be abducted fully or almost fully (approximately 80 degrees) to touch the examining table. "Telescoping" of the femoral head with the subluxation (Barlow) maneuver or a palpable "thump" with the Ortolani maneuver suggests dislocation.

3. The answer is C (*II C,* Table 6-3). The 5-minute Apgar score reflects good ventilation. The Apgar score was devised as a means of assessing oxygenation, ventilation, and degree of asphyxia in a uniform manner that quickly communicates information to all persons involved in resuscitation of a newborn. The Apgar evaluation is routinely performed at 1 and 5 minutes after birth, with continuation at 10 and 20 minutes in the case of a score of < 7. Five signs—heart rate, respiratory effort, muscle tone, reflex irritability, and skin color—are examined and assigned a score of 0, 1, or 2. The Apgar score is obtained by adding all individual scores. A score of 8 to 10 reflects good oxygenation and ventilation and indicates no need for vigorous resuscitation. A score of 5 to 7 indicates a need for stimulation and supplemental oxygen. A score of < 5 indicates a need for assisted ventilation and possible cardiac support. The Apgar score at 5 minutes reflects the adequacy of resuscitation and the potential degree of perinatal asphyxia.

4. The answer is C (*III E 2*). *Chlamydia trachomatis* is the most prevalent identifiable infectious cause of neonatal conjunctivitis. The incubation period is 5 to 14 days. Conjunctivitis affects between 2% and 8% of all infants during the first month of life. Chemical conjunctivitis secondary to administration of silver nitrate drops usually appears within the first day of life and disappears within 3 to 4 days. Gonococcal ophthalmia has decreased in frequency as a result of neonatal prophylaxis. The mean incubation period is approximately 6 days, with a range of 1 to 21 days.

5. The answer is B (*IV A 1, IV B 2 b*). Preterm and other sick infants frequently require total parenteral nutrition (TPN) because of gastrointestinal disorders (e.g., neonatal necrotizing enterocolitis), other nongastrointestinal disorders (e.g., respiratory disease, sepsis, serious congenital heart disease), or immaturity of the gastrointestinal tract (e.g., impaired motility, enzyme deficiencies) as they are unable to take sufficient volume and/or adequately absorb sufficient nutrients with enteral feeds necessary to adequately meet fluid and caloric requirements for basal metabolic needs and growth needs in sick infants. Fluid balance is monitored by ongoing, frequent measurements of urine output, change in body weight, serum sodium concentration, and urine specific gravity. IV fluid infusion rates (including TPN) are fine-tuned by balancing current fluid status of the infant with established requirements for basal needs and growth. A TPN solution of dextrose, amino acids, fat, vitamins, and minerals is administered by either peripheral or central venous access and, if appropriately used, will provide adequate calories and protein to support basal needs and growth of the sick infant.

6, 7. The answers are 6-B and 7-C (*V A 2*). Hyaline membrane disease (respiratory distress syndrome of the newborn) is a respiratory disorder that primarily affects preterm infants who are born before the biochemical maturation of their lungs. The lungs are poorly compliant due to a deficiency of surfactant, resulting in the classic complex of progressive atelectasis, intrapulmonary shunting, hypoxemia, and cyanosis. Affected infants characteristically have tachypnea, grunting, nasal flaring, chest retraction, and cyanosis in the first 3 hours of life. There is decreased air entry on auscultation. Persistence of the fetal circulation, or persistent pulmonary hypertension of the newborn, is usually a disease of term infants who have experienced acute or chronic in utero hypoxia. It is seen frequently in infants who have meconium aspiration syndrome. The primary abnormality is a failure of the pulmonary vascular resistance to fall with postnatal lung expansion and oxygenation. Transient tachypnea of the newborn is thought to result from decreased lymphatic absorption of fetal lung fluid. It most commonly occurs in infants born near term by cesarean section, without preceding labor. The tachypnea is quiet or mild and usually not associated with retractions. The infant appears comfortable and is rarely cyanotic. Pneumonia is often associated with chorioamnionitis and may be caused by aspiration of infected amniotic fluid. The infectious agent may also cross the placenta, enter the fetal circulation, and spread to the lungs. Sepsis is often present. The infant has signs of respiratory distress, including tachypnea, cyanosis, and retractions. Auscultation may reveal rales, rhonchi, or diminished breath sounds. Other signs of systemic infection may be noted, including poor perfusion, hypotension, acidosis, and leukopenia or leukocytosis. Sepsis and bacterial infections most frequently are acquired via the birth canal or nosocomially. Neonatal sepsis occurs in 1% to 4% of premature infants and in $< 1\%$ of term infants. The infection is almost always bacteremic (often with seeding of the meninges by way of the blood) and associated with systemic symptoms—a condition referred to as neonatal sepsis. Signs and symptoms of bacterial infection include unexplained respiratory distress, unexplained feeding intolerance, temperature instability, hypoglycemia or hyperglycemia, and apnea.

8. The answer is D (*V C 2*). Nonphysiologic jaundice refers to hyperbilirubinemia that is secondary to a pathologic process. Nonphysiologic jaundice should always be suspected when the umbilical cord serum bilirubin concentration is elevated, the clinical appearance of jaundice is within the first 24 hours of life, or the conjugated fraction of the serum bilirubin concentration exceeds 2 mg/dL. Specific causes of nonphysiologic indirect hyperbilirubinemia include hemolytic diseases of immune cause (e.g., fetomaternal blood group incompatibilities) as well as nonimmune cause (e.g., spherocytosis, hemoglobinopathy, enzyme deficiency), extravascular blood loss and accumulation (e.g., due to cephalhematoma), increased enterohepatic circulation (e.g., due to intestinal obstruction), breastfeeding associated with poor intake, disorders of bilirubin metabolism (e.g., Lucey-Driscoll syndrome, Crigler-Najjar syndrome, Gilbert syndrome), and metabolic disorders (e.g., hypothyroidism, panhypopituitarism, galactosemia). The most common cause of nonphysiologic indirect hyperbilirubinemia is fetomaternal blood incompatibility. Physiologic jaundice refers to the increased serum concentration of unconjugated bilirubin that is observed during the first few days of life but usually does not become visible until at least the second day of life.

chapter 7

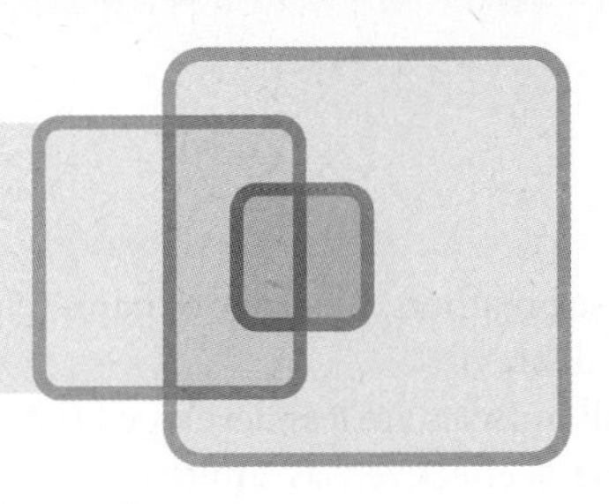

Critical Care

CHRISTOPHER L. CARROLL

I GOAL AND SCOPE OF PEDIATRIC CRITICAL CARE MEDICINE

Pediatric critical care is a specialty concerned with the management of children with failing homeostatic mechanisms. Pediatric critical care physicians frequently interact with pediatric medical and surgical subspecialists, nurses, social workers, respiratory therapists, and others to coordinate the care of patients who have complicated conditions. These health care personnel have special expertise in ventilatory support, promotion of cardiac output, treatment of acute electrolyte disorders and coma, and the nutritional interventions needed for critically ill youngsters. They are called upon to help parents make difficult decisions about therapeutic options and end-of-life care for their children.

II PEDIATRIC RESUSCITATION

A Primary concerns

1. **Basic life-support (BLS) measures** form the foundation of pediatric critical care and must precede any advanced life-support interventions. Thereafter, advanced life-support techniques should be promptly initiated.
2. "ABC" (**airway, breathing, circulation**) is the appropriate sequence of interventions in both basic and advanced life-support scenarios.
3. **Reassessment** of the patient is required after any intervention.
4. Basic and advanced life-support techniques must be supplemented with hands-on training if one is to become proficient.

III RESPIRATORY INTENSIVE CARE

A Respiratory assessment

1. Primary concerns
   a. The large majority of pediatric arrests are respiratory in origin (80%) and most of these occur in children under 1 year of age.
   b. There are key **anatomic and physiologic differences from adults** that impact the resuscitation of children.
   c. The goal of respiratory support is to maintain oxygenation and ventilation at levels that can support physiologic needs while minimizing adverse effects of therapies.
   d. **Foreign body aspiration** and **airway obstruction** should be suspected in children who have sudden onset of respiratory distress associated with gagging, coughing, or stridor.
2. Anatomic differences
   a. Prominent occiput can induce flexion of neck and airway obstruction.
   b. The tongue is proportionately larger and obstructs the airway more easily.
   c. Smaller airway diameters are more likely to be affected by obstruction/edema.
   d. The larynx is more anterior, more caudad, funnel shaped, and narrowest at the cricoid cartilage, making it more prone to subglottic stenosis.
   e. The epiglottis is larger and floppier and can lead to significant obstruction if infected.

3. Physiologic differences
   a. Infants are obligate nose breathers. Blockage of nares (e.g., sputum, choanal atresia) can cause significant respiratory distress.
   b. Cartilage and chest wall muscles are less developed (i.e., less compliant), so infants are unable to increase tidal volume as effectively as adults.
4. Clinical features of respiratory distress
   a. Respiratory rate
      (1) Tachypnea is the first sign of respiratory distress.
      (2) Patients attempt to increase ventilation, decrease PCO_2, and normalize pH by increasing minute ventilation.
      (3) However, slow or irregular breathing in an acutely ill child can reflect impending respiratory failure.
   b. Oxygen saturation
      (1) Oxygen saturation is the measure of the amount of oxygen bound to hemoglobin.
      (2) Along with PaO_2, it reflects the degree of oxygenation.
      (3) The **oxyhemoglobin dissociation curve** relates the oxygen saturation to PaO_2.
   c. Respiratory mechanics
      (1) Increased respiratory effort results from either **increased resistance** to airflow or **decreased lung compliance.**
      (2) Accessory muscle use
         (a) This occurs when the child is attempting to increase tidal volume and minute ventilation.
         (b) Examples include suprasternal ("tracheal tugging"), supraclavicular, and subcostal retractions.
         (c) Nasal flaring and "head bobbing" are particularly concerning signs.
      (3) Grunting
         (a) Grunting is produced by premature glottic closure accompanied by late expiratory contraction of the diaphragm in attempt to maintain positive airway pressure during exhalation.
         (b) It is a sign of small airway collapse, alveolar collapse, or both.
      (4) Stridor
         (a) Stridor is a high-pitched sound during inspiration that is a sign of extrathoracic airway obstruction.
         (b) Causes include tracheomalacia, infections (e.g., croup), upper airway edema, and foreign body aspiration.
      (5) Wheezing
         (a) Wheezing is a high-pitched whistling sound during exhalation that is a sign of intrathoracic airway obstruction.
         (b) When accompanied by prolonged exhalation phase, it is a further sign of small airway obstruction.
         (c) Causes include asthma, bronchiolitis, and, more rarely, foreign body aspiration.
   d. Level of consciousness/muscle tone
      (1) **Both** can be difficult to assess.
      (2) Children with impending respiratory failure may have an altered level of consciousness and hypotonia that is distinct from that of sleeping children.
5. **Respiratory failure**
   a. **Definition.** Respiratory failure occurs when dysfunction of the respiratory system results in abnormal gas exchange, resulting in hypoxemia (i.e., arterial $PO_2 < 50$ mm Hg) and/or hypercapnia (i.e., arterial $PCO_2 > 50$ mm Hg). A discussion of underlying pathophysiology can be found below.
   b. **Etiologies.** Acute respiratory failure can be caused by a variety of disorders (see Chapter 13).

B Derangements of oxygenation and ventilation

1. **Oxygenation defects**
   a. **Alveolar partial pressure of oxygen (PO_2)** depends on **barometric pressure** (PB), **water vapor pressure** (PH_2O), **the fraction of inspired oxygen** (FIO_2), **alveolar partial pressure of carbon dioxide (PCO_2),** and **respiratory quotient** (R):

   Alveolar $PO_2 = FIO_2 \times (PB - PH_2O) - PCO_2/R$

TABLE 7-1 The A-a Gradient and Arterial Hypoxemia

Cause of Hypoxemia	Gradient	Mechanism
Shunt	Increased	Unsaturated hemoglobin does not come into contact with alveolar O_2
Low $\dot{V}/\dot{Q}$ ratio	Increased	Insufficient alveolar O_2 to completely saturate hemoglobin present in pulmonary capillary
Hypoventilation	Normal	PCO_2 rises, decreasing alveolar PO_2
Diffusion defect	Increased	Oxygen diffusion is mechanically obstructed (e.g., fibrosis) or is limited by time available before exhalation
Altitude	Normal	Lower atmospheric pressure causes decreased alveolar PO_2

A, alveolar; a, arterial.

b. **Arterial PO_2** depends on the **alveolar PO_2**, the **distribution of inspired gas among the alveoli and their relationships with pulmonary capillary blood flows** ("$\dot{V}/\dot{Q}$ matching"), **diffusion** of oxygen across the alveolar-capillary membrane (which depends on time available for diffusion and is rarely clinically important), and the nature of the membrane itself.

Alveolar-arterial (A-a) oxygen gradient = alveolar PO_2 (calculated) − arterial PO_2 (measured)

c. **Several distinct pathophysiologic mechanisms may cause arterial hypoxemia. Hypoxemia may occur with or without an increase in A-a gradient** (Table 7-1). Conditions that do not increase the gradient lower arterial PO_2 by lowering alveolar PO_2; that is, they cause **hypoventilation.** Conditions that result in an increased A-a gradient **impair gas distribution or diffusion.**

d. **Arterial oxygen content** depends on hemoglobin concentration and hemoglobin saturation (the latter is a result of the arterial PO_2).

O_2 Content = [1.34 × Hemoglobin (g/dL) × % Saturation] + [0.003 × PaO_2 (mm Hg)]

where: 1.34 = milliliters of O_2 per gram of fully saturated hemoglobin, and 0.003 = milliliters of O_2 per mm Hg

e. **Overall oxygen delivery** to the tissues, in turn, is quantified by the product of the cardiac output (Q) and arterial oxygen content:

Oxygen Delivery = O_2 Content (mL/dL) × Q (L/min) × 10

f. **Utilization of oxygen** by the tissues depends on the overall oxygen delivery, subsequent distribution of nutrient capillary flow, and mitochondrial activity.

2. **Ventilation defects**
   a. PCO_2 may be elevated because of **increased CO_2 production** or **decreased alveolar ventilation.**
   b. **Alveolar ventilation** depends on **tidal volume** (Vt, the volume of gas inspired in each breath), **dead space volume** (Vd, the volume of gas inspired in each breath that does not reach functional alveoli), and **respiratory rate.**

   Alveolar ventilation = (Vt − Vd) × RR

   In the physiologic range, PCO_2 is inversely proportional to alveolar ventilation.

C Respiratory support techniques

1. **Airway positioning.** Establishing and maintaining a patent airway is the foundation of basic life support. Proper positioning of the airway can relieve obstruction and dramatically improve the condition of the child.
   a. **Children younger than 2 years.** Position the infant with the neck in a neutral position so that the tragus of the ear is level to the top of the shoulder (towel under shoulders).
   b. **Children older than 2 years**
      (1) Head tilt-chin lift procedure
         (a) This should only be used when head and neck injury are not expected.
         (b) Place one hand on the forehead and gently tilt the head back.

(c) At the same time, place fingertips under the bony part of the jaw and lift the mandible upward and outward.

(2) Jaw thrust

(a) This can be used in head/neck injury and is useful for opening the airway during bag and mask ventilation.

(b) While standing at head of the bed, place two to three fingers under each side of the lower jaw at its angle and life upward and outward.

2. **Supplemental oxygen** may be provided by nasal cannula, face mask, or tent, or in association with other techniques of assisted ventilation.

a. **Purpose.** Oxygen is used to provide sufficiently high PO_2 to maintain the body's physiologic activities. It cannot alone correct hypoventilation or hypercarbia.

b. **Limitations**

(1) **Toxicity.** Prolonged administration of high concentrations of oxygen damages the alveolar membrane. Because the time and concentration thresholds for toxicity are inexact, it is prudent to use the lowest oxygen concentration compatible with acceptable physiologic status in individual patients.

(2) **Effectiveness.** Simple supplemental oxygen is useful for treating diseases that cause moderate $\dot{V}/\dot{Q}$ mismatch. However, when severe $\dot{V}/\dot{Q}$ mismatch or intrapulmonary shunting occur, little response will be obtained. In general, if adequate oxygenation ($PO_2 > 60$ mm Hg) is not attained by administration of 60% O_2, an additional pressure-based modality is needed to recruit alveoli for gas exchange.

3. **Alveolar recruitment techniques and pharmacologic adjuncts**

a. **Continuous positive airway pressure (CPAP)** or **positive end-expiratory pressure (PEEP)**

(1) CPAP and PEEP improve end-expiratory lung volumes in patients with poor lung compliance, thereby decreasing shunt and improving $\dot{V}/\dot{Q}$ ratios and lung compliance (Figure 7-1).

(2) They decrease work of breathing and improve oxygenation.

(3) It is called CPAP during spontaneous respiration and PEEP during mechanical ventilation.

b. **Bilevel positive airway pressure (BiPAP)**

(1) BiPAP augments a patient's respirations with pressure assistance through a tightly fitting face mask in both inspiratory and expiratory phases (i.e., "bilevel").

(2) When the patient begins to inhale, the BiPAP machine senses the pressure drop in the circuit and gas flow is supplemented to a preset pressure level.

(3) BiPAP can sometimes support the patient's respirations enough to avoid intubation and mechanical ventilation.

(4) It is not effective if the face mask cannot be tolerated or in **apneic patients.**

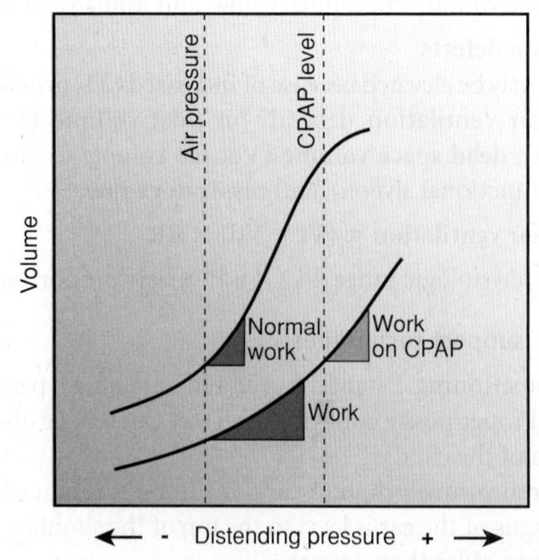

FIGURE 7-1 Effect of the use of continuous positive airway pressure (CPAP) on end-expiratory lung volumes in respiratory failure.

c. **Helium-oxygen mixtures (Heliox)**
   (1) Less viscous than nitrogen-oxygen in room air, these mixtures promote laminar gas flow and reduce airway resistance at points of obstruction.
   (2) They may be used during spontaneous or mechanical ventilation.
   (3) These mixtures are used in conditions where airflow is critically reduced by obstruction of large airways (e.g., **croup**) or small airways (e.g., **asthma**).
   (4) To derive benefits, 60% to 80% helium must be used, so they may not be practical in patients requiring high concentrations of supplemental oxygen.

d. **Bronchodilating agents**
   (1) These agents can reduce airway resistance by increasing the diameter of the smaller airways (see Chapter 13).
   (2) They can be administered orally, intravenously, or as aerosols (either intermittently or continuously).

e. **Artificial airways**
   (1) Nasopharyngeal tubes, endotracheal tubes, and tracheostomy tubes can improve airway mechanics by bypassing proximal obstructions.
   (2) Tracheostomy tubes can also improve alveolar ventilation by decreasing anatomic dead space and airway resistance.

3. **Mechanical ventilation**
   a. **Positive-pressure ventilation** supplies gas directly to the trachea through an endotracheal tube or tracheostomy. The delivery of gas is controlled by manipulating flow rate, inspiratory time, volume, and pressure. All modes use PEEP to improve end-expiratory lung volumes.
      (1) **Volume-limited ventilation**
         (a) Volume-limited ventilation delivers gas with a predetermined tidal volume over a predetermined inspiratory time at a preset rate.
         (b) Peak inspiratory pressure is determined by the patient's lung compliance and the set tidal volume.
         (c) **Flow pattern** may be constant or decelerating. Constant gas flow patterns have a constant rate of gas delivery during the inspiratory cycle. A decelerating flow pattern provides most of the gas early in inspiration decelerating over time. Decelerating flow patterns may improve gas distribution in some patients in a fashion similar to pressure-limited ventilation (see below).
         (d) Peak inspiratory pressure must be followed for elevated pressures ($\geq$ 35 cm H_2O).
         (e) Ventilating with low tidal volumes (6 mL/kg vs. 12 mL/kg) has been shown to improve outcomes, including survival in patients with severe lung disease.
      (2) **Pressure-limited ventilation**
         (a) Pressure-limited ventilation delivers gas with a predetermined inspiratory pressure over a predetermined inspiratory time at a preset rate.
         (b) Tidal volume depends on the patient's lung compliance and the present inspiratory pressure.
         (c) Inspiratory pressure levels are maintained throughout inspiration.
         (d) Gas flow rates are very high initially and decrease over the remainder of the inspiratory period. Decelerating flow patterns are generally the most effective way to distribute gas in a patient with parenchymal lung disease.
         (e) Tidal volume must be followed for hypo- or hyperventilation.
      (3) **Pressure-support ventilation**
         (a) Pressure-support ventilation is used to augment spontaneous ventilation in intubated patients (above rate set in pressure- or volume-limited ventilation).
         (b) It provides some support for spontaneous breaths to help overcome airway resistance (from the endotracheal tube).
         (c) It can also be used without a back-up rate, effectively the equivalent of BiPAP.
      (4) **Oscillating ventilators**
         (a) Oscillating ventilators are thought to minimize ventilator-induced lung injury in patients with severely impaired oxygenation and lung compliance.

(b) They deliver gas with predetermined levels of mean airway pressure, frequency of oscillation (cycles per second, or Hz), and amplitude of oscillation. **A high constant mean airway pressure** is used to maintain small airway patency.

(c) Superimposed oscillations with minimal tidal volume and pressure amplitudes provide a wave of fresh gas that propagates into the alveoli.

IV CARDIOVASCULAR INTENSIVE CARE

A **Shock** is a complex metabolic state characterized by impaired delivery and utilization of oxygen and other substrates by the tissues.

1. **General principles**
   a. **Causes**
      (1) **Noncardiovascular causes** of shock include hypoxemia, hypoglycemia, and toxins (e.g., cyanide) that impair delivery and/or utilization of oxygen.
      (2) **Cardiovascular causes** include derangements of the three components of cardiac output: Preload (e.g., hemorrhage), contractility (e.g., myocarditis), and afterload (e.g., sepsis).
   b. **Phases.** All forms of untreated shock may progress through three phases:
      (1) **Compensated shock**—signs of shock with maintained blood pressure
      (2) **Decompensated shock**—signs of shock associated with frank hypotension
      (3) **Irreversible shock**—prolonged ischemia causing permanent organ failures
2. **Types of shock**
   a. **Hypovolemic shock** is caused by decreased circulating volume (preload; see also Chapter 14).
      (1) **Clinical features**
         (a) Tachycardia
         (b) Cool, pale extremities
         (c) Prolonged capillary refill time (> 2 seconds)
         (d) Decreased level of consciousness (late)
         (e) **Hypotension** (**very late,** signifying a > 25% decrease in blood volume)
      (2) **Physiologic responses**
         (a) Tachycardia
         (b) Decreased urine output
         (c) Vasoconstriction
         (d) Increased contractility
      (3) **Compensatory mechanisms**
         (a) Secretion of antidiuretic hormone
         (b) Secretion of aldosterone-renin-angiotensin
         (c) Increased sympathetic nervous system discharge, with secretion of endogenous catecholamines
      (4) **Therapeutic approaches**
         (a) **Primary therapy** is restoration of circulating volume with crystalloid or colloid solutions, or blood products if shock is due to hemorrhage. Rapid resuscitation (≥ 60 mL/kg in first hour) is key.
         (b) **Secondary therapy** is inotropic support, typically used as a supplemental therapy during initial resuscitation with intravenous fluids.
         (c) Fluid balance and physical examination must be frequently reassessed. If there is a poor response to fluid therapy, central venous pressure monitoring may be helpful.
   b. **Cardiogenic shock** is caused by decreased contractility.
      (1) **Clinical features**
         (a) Tachycardia
         (b) Cool, pale extremities
         (c) Delayed capillary refill
         (d) Impaired mental status
         (e) Pulmonary edema formation
         (f) Hypotension (*early,* in contrast with hypovolemic shock). **Note that clinical features are similar to hypovolemic shock.**

(2) **Physiologic responses**
   (a) Tachycardia
   (b) Decreased urine output leading to hypervolemia
   (c) Vasoconstriction causing increased afterload
   (d) Further decrease in contractility and cardiac output due to increased demands resulting from these responses
(3) **Compensatory mechanisms**
   (a) Secretion of antidiuretic hormone
   (b) Secretion of aldosterone-renin-angiotensin
   (c) Increased sympathetic nervous system discharge, with secretion of endogenous catecholamines
(4) **Therapeutic approaches**
   (a) **Inotropic support** (i.e., dopamine, dobutamine, epinephrine, or milrinone). When pharmacologic vasodilation to reduce afterload is desired in addition to inotropic support, dobutamine or milrinone are the preferred agents.
   (b) **Diuresis**
   (c) **Continuous monitoring** of cardiac rhythm, arterial blood pressure, and urine output is indicated. Central venous pressure monitoring is often helpful.

c. **Distributive shock** is caused by disordered perfusion of tissue beds, often caused by **sepsis** or **toxins.**
(1) **Clinical features**
   (a) **Early signs** include tachycardia, fever, low diastolic pressure, normal or slightly increased systolic pressure, bounding pulses, initially brisk capillary refill, low urine output, and impaired level of consciousness.
   (b) **Late signs** are similar to those seen in cardiogenic shock.
(2) **Physiologic responses**
   (a) **Tachycardia**
   (b) **Increased contractility** may occur early, with subsequent deterioration if treatment is unsuccessful.
(3) **Therapeutic approaches**
   (a) Monitor cardiac rhythm, arterial and central venous pressure, and urinary output; pulmonary arterial catheterization may be helpful.
   (b) Attempt to correct triggering derangement.
   (c) Maintain circulating blood volume.
   (d) Provide inotropic support.
   (e) In refractory cases with persistent hypotension, promote vasoconstriction with α-adrenergic agents (i.e., norepinephrine or vasopressin).

B Postoperative cardiovascular management

1. **Acute management.** Patients who have undergone cardiopulmonary bypass for open heart procedures frequently exhibit decreased myocardial contractility for the first 24 to 48 postoperative hours. Patients who have undergone ventriculotomy are at risk for further decrements of cardiac output.
   a. Preload, afterload, and rhythm are closely monitored and kept in a narrow physiologic range to promote adequate cardiac output. In most patients, electrocardiogram (ECG) and arterial and central venous pressures are continuously monitored. When indicated, left atrial or pulmonary artery pressures may also be measured.
   b. Cardiac output may be supported by infusion of **inotropic agents** such as dopamine, dobutamine, epinephrine, or milrinone.
   c. In addition to inotropic support, perfusion may be enhanced by afterload reduction with **vasodilators** such as nitroprusside.
   d. Electrolytes (particularly potassium and calcium) and acid-base balance are also closely monitored and maintained in a narrow physiologic range to promote cardiac output.
2. **Complications**
   a. **Pleural** or **pericardial effusions** may appear as early as the first postoperative week as part of the **postpericardiotomy syndrome.** These fluid collections usually disappear without treatment, but should be monitored until they do so, and may require drainage if cardiac output

or ventilation is significantly impaired. Alternatively, aspirin or steroids may be effective in subacute cases.

b. Patients who have intracardiac repairs may acquire **conduction defects** that predispose them to dysrhythmias and necessitate suppressant medication. On rare occasions, they may require **implantable pacemakers** or **defibrillators.**

c. Patients who receive indwelling grafts or valve devices are at increased risk for **thrombogenesis** and **bacterial colonization.** Such complications may lead to **stroke** or **endocarditis.** Chronic anticoagulant therapy is used to prevent thrombus formation in recipients of heart valves.

C Dysrhythmias Only unstable dysrhythmias require emergent treatment. Dysrhythmias that are not associated with circulatory instability may usually await definitive evaluation by a pediatric cardiologist before treatment (see Chapter 12).

1. **Bradydysrhythmias.** Most episodes of bradycardia in children are caused by hypoxemia; therefore:
   a. **Oxygenate and ventilate,** and then reassess.
   b. If bradycardia persists despite adequate oxygenation and ventilation, drug therapy with epinephrine should be initiated. If the bradycardia still does not respond, **atropine** should be administered.
   c. If these modalities are ineffective and bradycardia persists, **ventricular pacing** should be considered.

2. **Tachydysrhythmias.** Cardiovascular compromise is a result of reduced diastolic cardiac filling time, which causes inadequate stroke volume.
   a. Determine whether the rhythm is **narrow complex** or **wide complex.** If the rhythm is a narrow-complex tachycardia, distinguish **sinus tachycardia** from **supraventricular tachycardia** (SVT) (Table 7-2).
   b. **Sinus tachycardia** in a stable patient may be the result of fever, anxiety, dehydration, or pain. Treat the source of the tachycardia, not the rapid heart rate per se.
   c. **Supraventricular tachycardia** is diagnosed in patients who have regular rhythms, heart rates between 180 and 240 beats per minute, and no visible P waves on the ECG. Patients who have **stable SVT** are treated with intravenous **adenosine** (rapid bolus of 0.1 mg/kg). If a patient with SVT becomes **unstable, synchronized cardioversion,** starting at 0.5 to 1 joules per kilogram (J/kg) of discharge, is used. If cardioversion is to be attempted and the patient is conscious, sedation should be given before the procedure and the physician must be prepared to assist ventilation.
   d. **Unstable, wide-complex tachycardia** is assumed to be **ventricular tachycardia.** If a patient with such a condition has **palpable pulses,** he or she is treated with **synchronized cardioversion** as described above. If the patient becomes **pulseless, defibrillation** with 2 J/kg is recommended.

TABLE 7-2 Distinguishing Sinus Tachycardia from Supraventricular Tachycardia

Measurement	Sinus Tachycardia	Supraventricular Tachycardia
Heart rate	Usually < 200, but may exceed 200	Usually > 230
Electrocardiogram	P waves seen Variability	No P waves seen Very regular
History	Identifiable cause for increased rate (e.g., fever, dehydration, respiratory distress, agitation)	Nonspecific symptoms
Physical examination	Consistent with history	Instability greater than suggested by history Congestive heart failure may be present in infants

e. A pediatric cardiologist should be contacted as soon as possible to coordinate further therapy. However, **treatment of unstable patients should not be delayed.**

V NEUROLOGIC INTENSIVE CARE

A Intracranial pressure

1. **Normal physiology**
   a. **Intracranial pressure (ICP)** is determined by the relationship of the **volume of the intracranial contents** with the **capacity of the skull.** Normal ICP is ≤ 10 mm Hg.
   b. The intracranial contents usually consist of brain tissue (80%), cerebrospinal fluid (CSF; 12%), blood (8%), and extracellular (interstitial) fluid (< 1%).
   c. Cerebral blood flow normally remains stable over a wide range of systemic blood pressures. This phenomenon is called **autoregulation.**
2. **Pathophysiology**
   a. Causes of increased ICP include:
      (1) Increased cerebral mass (e.g., brain tumor, traumatic hemorrhage)
      (2) Increased CSF volume (e.g., hydrocephalus)
      (3) Increased intravascular blood volume (e.g., arteriovenous malformation)
      (4) Increased interstitial fluid (cerebral edema)
      (5) Presence of extravascular fluid collections (e.g., epidural, subdural, subarachnoid, or intracerebral hemorrhages)
   b. Compensatory mechanisms
      (1) Shunting of blood out of the venous sinuses to the central veins of the chest
      (2) Shunting of CSF out of the ventricles into the spinal cord
      (3) Expansion of cranial sutures and fontanelles in infants
   c. When intracranial volume overwhelms these compensation mechanisms, intracranial pressure rises rapidly and cerebral blood flow is impeded. If the situation is not reversed, uncal **herniation** and **brain death** will occur due to cerebral ischemia.
3. **Treatment** for increased ICP
   a. **Intubation.** Although initially children with increased ICP often have hyperventilation, subsequent loss of airway control and hypoventilation are common with worsening intracranial hypertension. Whenever possible, intubation of these patients should be undertaken by people who have both the necessary technical skills and knowledge about the risks and benefits of medications used in this scenario.
   b. **Monitoring**
      (1) **Pulse oximetry** and **cardiac rate and rhythm** should be monitored continuously.
      (2) Arterial pressure should be continuously assessed in patients at risk for increased ICP.
      (3) **Central venous pressure monitoring** helps to guide intravenous fluid administration. It is important to maintain a euvolemic state in patients who have increased ICP.
      (4) ICP may be measured directly by a number of devices. Obtained values may be used to calculate the **cerebral perfusion pressure (CPP),** defined as:

      CPP = (Mean arterial blood pressure) − ICP

      Improved patient outcomes have been associated with maintenance of CPP above approximately 50 mm Hg in infants and 70 mm Hg in older children.
   c. **Reduction of volume of intracranial contents.** When CPP is unacceptably low because ICP is elevated (> 20 mm Hg), reduction of ICP may be accomplished by:
      (1) Resection of tumor or other space-occupying lesions
      (2) Removal of CSF directly from the cerebral ventricles via a ventriculostomy device
      (3) Reduction of interstitial fluid/edema
         (a) **Cerebral edema** of the **vasogenic type** (e.g., associated with trauma or tumors) may be amenable to osmotic therapy and other modalities described in the following sections. In contrast, **ischemia** causes cell death and **cytotoxic edema,** which rarely responds significantly to therapy.
         (b) **Osmotic agents** such as mannitol (0.25–1.0 g/kg/dose) reduce ICP within minutes and are a mainstay of therapy. Within an hour of administration, **osmotic diuresis**

occurs. It is important to anticipate this fluid loss and prevent intravascular volume depletion. Although it is true that overhydration can be harmful by promoting cerebral edema formation, systemic dehydration is also injurious because it causes secondary ischemia to brain cells.

(4) Reduction of cerebral blood volume

(a) When autoregulation is intact, **hyperventilation** (PCO_2 between 30 and 35 mm Hg) reduces ICP because cerebral blood flow is directly proportional to PCO_2 in the physiologic range (20–60 mm Hg). However, overzealous hyperventilation (< 25 mm Hg) may worsen pre-existing cerebral ischemia, so this modality has become a second-line therapy, except when **immediate** reduction in ICP is necessary to stave off incipient herniation.

(b) **Short-acting barbiturates** (e.g., pentobarbital) constrict cerebral blood vessels and also decrease cerebral metabolic demand. Both of these effects reduce cerebral blood volume and may, therefore, reduce ICP.

(c) Modest (30%) elevation of the head in a midline position may promote drainage of venous blood into the internal jugular veins without jeopardizing cerebral perfusion.

B Brain death

1. **General principles**

a. All states now recognize the concept of brain death as well as somatic death. Brain death is characterized by **complete and irreversible brain and brainstem failure.** The criteria for determining brain death are medical and not legal. Brain death is invariably followed by somatic death (usually within several days).

b. **Assessment.** Brain death is difficult to evaluate in young children due to developmental issues. On rare occasions, states of apparent clinical brain death have been followed by prolonged survival and some degree of recovery in very young infants and, more frequently, in premature babies. Therefore, suggested guidelines for the determination of brain death in infants differ from those for older children or adults. One set of such guidelines is summarized in Table 7-3.

2. **Physical examination** must be performed when the body temperature is > 35°C (96°F), blood pressure is within normal limits for age, and no medications or toxins are present in concentrations that may cause reversible coma resembling brain death. Brain-dead patients often poorly control body temperature or vasomotor tone, so they may require artificial warming or use of pressor drugs to attain an acceptable status for the examination. An examination revealing any level of brain function in the following ways is *incompatible* with the diagnosis of brain death:

a. **Demonstrable cortical functions**

(1) Any pain response other than simple stereotypical withdrawal (which may reflect only spinal cord integrity)

(2) Preservation of muscle tone (nonflaccid limbs)

(3) Voluntary movement, localization, or decorticate or decerebrate posturing

TABLE 7-3 Guidelines for Pediatric Brain Death Determination

Age Range[a]	Observation Period	EEG Testing
7 d to 2 m	Two examinations separated by 48 h	Two examinations separated by 48 h
2 mo to 1 y	Two examinations separated by 24 h	Two examinations separated by 24 h
Older than 1 y	Two examinations separated by 12–24 h	None required; observation period may be reduced if isoelectric EEG is obtained

EEG, electroencephalogram.
[a] No guidelines exist for premature infants or full-term infants during the first week of life.
Reprinted with permission from Report of special task force: guidelines for the determination of brain death in children. *Pediatrics* 80:298–300, 1987.

b. **Demonstrable midbrain functions**
   (1) **Oculocephalic reflexes** ("doll's eyes")
   (2) **Oculovestibular reflexes** ("cold-caloric" responses)
c. **Demonstrable cranial nerve functions**
   (1) Pupillary reflex
   (2) Corneal reflex
   (3) Gag reflex
   (4) Sucking movements
d. **Respiratory drive** is assessed with an **apnea test.**
   (1) The patient is **preoxygenated** with 100% O_2 for 5 minutes, and minute ventilation is adjusted so that the patient is eucapnic (i.e., PCO_2 is 35–45 mm Hg) at the beginning of the test.
   (2) **The ventilator rate** is turned to zero, and apneic oxygenation is continued. Heart rate and pulse oximeter values are monitored while the patient is continuously observed for any respiratory efforts for up to 10 minutes, or until heart rate or saturation levels fall to unacceptable levels.
   (3) **An arterial blood gas sample** is drawn at the end of the testing period, before reinstituting mechanical ventilation. The PCO_2 level must rise by 20 mm Hg and be associated with respiratory acidosis without spontaneous ventilation for the test to be consistent with a diagnosis of brain death.

3. **Neurophysiologic testing** may be used to corroborate the diagnosis of brain death.
   a. **Electroencephalography** (EEG) is mandated in some published guidelines for determination of brain death in children younger than 1 year of age (see Table 7-3).
   b. **Brain-evoked potentials** (auditory- or somatosensory-evoked responses) may be used to assess transmission of external stimuli.
   c. **Four-vessel cerebral angiography** may be used to evaluate cerebral blood flow. Brain death is associated with absence of cerebral blood flow. This test is very invasive, is technically demanding, and may not be possible in a child who is too unstable to tolerate movement to an angiography suite.
   d. **Isotope brain scanning** may also be used to assess cerebral blood flow. Absence of intracranial blood flow supports a diagnosis of brain death.

VI TRAUMA

A General principles

1. **Epidemiology**
   a. **Injuries** are the leading cause of death in children older than 1 year (see Chapter 2).
   b. **Inflicted trauma (child abuse)** is a frequent cause of death in children between 1 month and 1 year of age. Between 1300 and 4000 children each year die as a result of child abuse (see Chapter 3).

2. **Management.** Pediatric trauma victims are best treated in a hospital by pediatric surgeons, neurosurgeons, and critical care specialists who work collaboratively in a pediatric intensive care unit. They should be rapidly transferred to such a facility after initial stabilization.

B Initial assessment of the critically injured pediatric patient

1. Immediate assessment is made of **airway stability** (while maintaining cervical spine protection), **respirations,** and **circulation.** Large-bore intravenous access is established at this time.

2. A rapid **physical examination** is done to assess external evidence of trauma, bleeding, and neurologic status.

3. Initial **emergent interventions** (*see VI C*) are performed.

4. **Radiographs,** including cervical spine radiographs, are done rapidly, preferably in an appropriately equipped trauma room rather than in a radiology unit.

5. **Blood tests** are performed, including arterial blood gas, hematocrit, coagulation studies, electrolytes, hepatic enzymes, amylase, and lipase.

6. The **bladder is catheterized,** and urine is then evaluated for flow and presence of blood.
7. **Further radiologic tests,** such as head or abdominal computed tomography (CT) scans, are done if indicated.

C Therapy Patients who have major injuries should be observed and treated in a pediatric intensive care unit.

1. **Airway instability** is treated by endotracheal intubation, tracheotomy, or cricoidotomy.
2. **Respiratory failure** is treated with mechanical ventilation and, when necessary, by placement of thoracostomy tubes to drain pneumothorax and/or hemothorax.
3. **Hypoperfusion** is treated by administration of isotonic crystalloid, colloid, or blood. In the appropriate setting, pericardiocentesis may be indicated to treat cardiac tamponade resulting from hemopericardium. Inotropic support may be required.
4. **Surgical intervention** is guided by the patient's status and the results of the diagnostic evaluation.

D Specific injuries

1. **Head trauma.** A minority (< 20%) of pediatric patients with severe head injuries have **intracranial lesions** amenable to surgery. More often, they have **acute axonal injuries** with concurrent **cerebral edema** and increased ICP. Intracranial pressure monitoring devices are commonly placed to guide therapies in these patients.
2. **Child abuse.** Infants who have intracranial injuries suggestive of child abuse must be completely evaluated for other **occult injuries,** especially fractures (see Chapter 3).
3. **Hepatic and splenic lacerations** are best diagnosed by abdominal CT examination. Surgical repair or resection is rarely required; usually such lesions undergo spontaneous tamponade and heal.
4. **Spinal cord trauma**
   a. **Evaluation** of spinal cord structural integrity and neurologic function should be done immediately in all cases of multiple or severe trauma. Cervical support should be continued until the entire cervical spine, including the odontoid, has been adequately evaluated. The comatose *drowning* victim must also be evaluated for cervical trauma, which may have occurred during an unwitnessed diving accident.
   b. **Complications.** Unrecognized fractures or dislocations of the spinal column may lead to paraplegia, quadriplegia, or death.
   c. **Therapy**
      (1) **Stabilization of the vertebral column** with a cervical collar is indicated in the acute setting. Thereafter, halo traction or operative spinal fusion is used to treat chronic instability.
      (2) **Glucocorticoid administration** in the initial posttrauma period may limit the ultimate magnitude of neurologic deficits.
      (3) Patients who have spinal cord injury may suffer acute secondary ischemia from *spinal shock.* Therapy for spinal shock includes intravenous fluids and pressor medications.

VII NUTRITIONAL SUPPORT DURING CRITICAL ILLNESS

A Nutrition in high-stress states (sepsis and multiple trauma)

1. **Metabolic pathophysiology**
   a. Secretion of counterregulatory hormones (e.g., endogenous catecholamines, glucocorticoids, glucagon) leads to relative insulin resistance and **hyperglycemia.**
   b. Hyperpyrexia, increased cardiac demands, and wound healing cause a **marked increase in metabolic activity, oxygen and energy consumption,** and **carbon dioxide generation.**
   c. These increased metabolic demands lead to a requirement for **increased alveolar ventilation** and may predispose to **respiratory failure.**
   d. In the absence of adequate caloric and protein sources, muscle proteins are broken down to supply amino acids for gluconeogenesis and protein synthesis.

e. These processes may lead to **severe malnutrition,** anergy, and infectious complications unless intervention is provided.
f. **Hyperglycemia** has been linked to increased multiorgan system failure in critically ill adults. Tight control of hyperglycemia with insulin infusion protocols can improve outcomes in critically ill adults and may also be useful in children.

2. **Nutritional support**
a. In general, **enteral feedings** are preferable. Even small volumes ("trickle feedings") promote gut endothelial integrity and thereby reduce bacterial translocation from gut lumen to the bloodstream.
b. Multiple organ system failures or abdominal trauma may prevent early enteral feeding. In this case, parenteral alimentation should be established.
c. The goal is to eventually attain a **positive nitrogen balance.** This requires higher protein-to-calorie ratios than a normal diet because carbohydrates are processed inefficiently by the body during stress states.
d. **Providing fat** in the early period prevents essential fatty acid deficiency and may decrease carbon dioxide production by lowering the respiratory quotient.
e. Current recommendations are to administer 1.2 to 1.4 times a patient's estimated basal caloric needs during critical illness. Overfeeding has also been associated with increased morbidity and mortality and should be avoided.

VIII ETHICAL ISSUES IN PEDIATRIC INTENSIVE CARE

A Do not resuscitate (DNR) orders

1. **Areas of potential conflict.** By definition, minors are not legally competent, and therefore are unable to create a **"living will"** or **durable power of attorney** before catastrophic, life-threatening illness or injury occurs. Therefore, decisions about resuscitation must be based on the **substituted judgment** of others, usually parents. Disagreements with the medical care team about the most appropriate course of action may arise.
2. **Ethical resolution.** In the absence of parental mental incompetency or evidence of child abuse or neglect, the parents are usually accepted as the advocates for the child's best interests.
a. When parents and caregivers disagree about the appropriate aggressiveness of future therapies, it is often helpful to convene a multidisciplinary meeting with the family to discuss pertinent issues. When consensus cannot be reached, medical interventions are continued as further discussions proceed.
b. Occasionally, families and caregivers cannot resolve their differences, which results in consultation with the hospital ethics committee. Extremely rarely, persistent unresolvable disagreements about DNR status are taken to the state legal system.

B

Removal of supportive therapy may be requested by families or recommended by physicians in situations in which a child has minimal likelihood of survival or attainment of an acceptable level of function. The substituted judgment of the family is required in these instances (*see VIII C*).

1. **Areas of potential conflict**
a. Although current mainstream opinion holds that there is no ethical difference between not starting a therapy and withdrawing it at a later time, disagreements may still occur. Recent court cases have supported the "no difference" position.
2. **Ethical resolution**
a. Where legally permissible, discontinuation of life-supporting therapy for a pediatric patient who is not brain dead is predicated on consensus of parents and physicians.
b. Occasionally, irreconcilable disagreements between families and caregivers may be brought to the hospital ethics committee, the court system, or both.

C Religious objections to therapy

1. **Areas of potential conflict**
a. Free exercise of religion by a family may conflict with both the state's interest in the welfare of a child and the child's right to adequate care.

b. Examples of such conflicts may be seen in children of Jehovah's Witnesses who require blood transfusion or the children of faith healers who need antibiotics for life-threatening infections or treatment of other severe illness or injury.

2. **Ethical resolution**

a. The legal and ethical consensus is that an adult may refuse treatment for him- or herself, but that the child's right to treatment is safeguarded by the state when lack of treatment will make death or injury likely or certain.

b. Because such an act by the state does represent infringement of the parents' right to free exercise of religion, court orders for such treatment are given only when evidence for clear danger of injury without therapy is provided.

BIBLIOGRAPHY

Behrman RE, Kliegman RM, Jenson HB (eds): *Nelson Textbook of Pediatrics.* Philadelphia, WB Saunders, 2003.

Fuhrman BP, Zimmerman JZ (eds): *Pediatric Critical Care.* St. Louis, Mosby, 2005.

Ralston M, Hazinski MF, Zaritsky AL, et al. (eds): *PALS Provider Manual.* Dallas, American Heart Association, 2006.

Report of special task force: guidelines for the determination of brain death in children. *Pediatrics* 80:298–300, 1987.

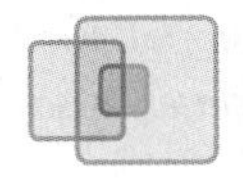

Study Questions

***Directions:** Each of the numbered items or incomplete statements in this section is followed by answers or completions of the statement. Select the ONE lettered answer or completion that is BEST in each case.*

1. A young infant is rushed to the emergency department. The child is cyanotic, is breathing with gasping respirations, and has a heart rate of 40 beats per minute. Which of the following is the most appropriate intervention that should be performed first in this child?

A Intraosseous cannulation
B Synchronized cardioversion
C Chest compressions
D 100% oxygen by face mask or hood
E Bag-and-mask ventilation with 100% oxygen

2. A 2-year-old previously healthy boy with no prior history of wheezing is noted to be wheezing when his mother picks him up from day care. On arrival to your office, the infant is awake and alert with good oxygen saturations, mild to moderate accessory muscle use, and focal wheezing in the right chest. Which of the following is the most appropriate next step in the management of this child?

A Reassurance and follow-up in your office again tomorrow
B Prescription of an oral β-agonist medication for wheezing
C Prescription of an inhaled β-agonist medication for wheezing
D Chest radiography
E Referral to a pulmonologist

QUESTIONS 3–4

A 6-month-old infant girl is seen in the emergency department with a 3-day history of vomiting and profuse watery diarrhea. On initial physical examination, she has unlabored respirations at a rate of 40/minute, heart rate of 180/minute, and poor responsiveness to noxious stimulation. Her central pulses are bounding, but distal pulses are thready with a capillary refill time of 7 seconds. Blood pressure is 80/40 mm Hg.

3. Which of the following is TRUE regarding this child's condition relative to definitions of shock?

A By definition, she is in hypovolemic shock
B By definition, she is in cardiogenic shock
C By definition, she is in distributive shock
D By definition, she is not in shock as she has normal blood pressure for age
E By definition, she is unlikely to be in shock as she has gastroenteritis

4. Which of the following is the most appropriate therapy in the early management of this child?

A Fluid bolus to restore circulating blood volume
B β-Blocking agent to decrease heart rate and thereby decrease oxygen consumption
C Inotropic support with an α-adrenergic medication to increase both contractility and vasoconstriction
D Afterload reduction with nitroprusside to reduce the resistance to cardiac output
E Antibiotic administration to treat the presumed infection

Directions: *Each set of matching questions in this section consists of a list of 4 to 6 lettered options followed by several numbered items. For each numbered item, select the ONE lettered option that is most closely associated with it. Each lettered option may be selected once, more than once, or not at all.*

QUESTIONS 5–8

For each case patient described below, select the principal cause of tissue hypoxia.

A Decreased alveolar PO_2
B Decreased arterial PO_2
C Decreased arterial oxygen content
D Decreased cardiac output

5. A child with newly diagnosed leukemia is hospitalized with a hemoglobin concentration of 3 g/dL.

6. A child experiences respiratory distress and decreased activity tolerance while vacationing in the Grand Teton Mountains.

7. A child is seen at the emergency department with weak respirations and severe hypovolemic shock from diarrhea and dehydration.

8. A newborn is extremely cyanotic in room air. Evaluation reveals pulmonary atresia and a large ventricular septal defect.

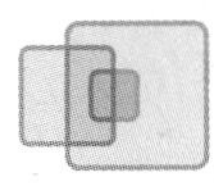

Answers and Explanations

1. The answer is E (*II A 2*). The first intervention in the patient who has cardiopulmonary failure is provision of adequate ventilation. If vital signs improve with bag-and-mask ventilation or subsequent intubation, respiratory failure was the source of the condition. Transition to a shock state after ventilation is ensured implies that circulatory compromise is the etiology, and further interventions are guided by the remainder of the assessment. (Remember the ABCs of resuscitation.)

2. The answer is D (*III A 1 d; III A 4 c* [5]). In young children with acute onset of wheezing, foreign body aspiration must be considered. This is especially true in this child, with no infectious symptoms, acute onset, and focality of wheezing. Evaluation with chest radiography is the appropriate next step as reassurance without treatment or workup could have dangerous consequences; this stage of investigation typically does not require referral to a pulmonologist. Inhaled β-agonist therapy may be instituted as therapy if there is no foreign body; however, oral β-agonist therapy has no role in the acute management of wheezing.

3. The answer is A (*IV A 2*). This child exhibits many of the features of hypovolemic shock. There are poor distal pulses, markedly prolonged capillary refill time, and evidence of impaired vital organ function (decreased mental status). In addition, the clinical history is consistent with dehydration. Gastroenteritis is a common cause of hypovolemic shock in this age group and a leading cause of mortality in developing countries. Hypotension is a late finding in hypovolemic shock.

4. The answer is A (*IV A 2 a*). The goal in treatment of hypovolemic shock is to restore circulating blood volume and prevent deterioration into irreversible, multiple organ system failure. First-line therapy is fluid resuscitation; inotropic support is secondary. In this case, a β-blocking agent to decrease heart rate and thereby decrease oxygen consumption would be harmful to the patient. Afterload reduction would also be harmful to the patient during the acute phase by dropping the arterial blood pressure. Although antibiotic coverage may be important, fluid resuscitation is paramount.

5–8. The answers are 5-C, 6-A (*III B 1, Table 7-1*), **7-D,** and **8-B** (*Table 7-1*). Severe anemia causes a marked decrease in arterial oxygen content by decreasing the amount of oxygen bound to hemoglobin. This is independent of arterial PO_2, which remains normal. Breathing at high altitudes is associated with lower barometric pressure, which lowers alveolar PO_2. A child who has low cardiac output from hypovolemic shock breathes ineffectively due to diminished oxygen delivery to the respiratory muscles. A child who has cyanotic congenital heart disease has right-to-left intracardiac shunting. Arterial PO_2 is diminished despite normal alveolar PO_2 and lung structures because the blood does not contact alveolar gas.

chapter **8**

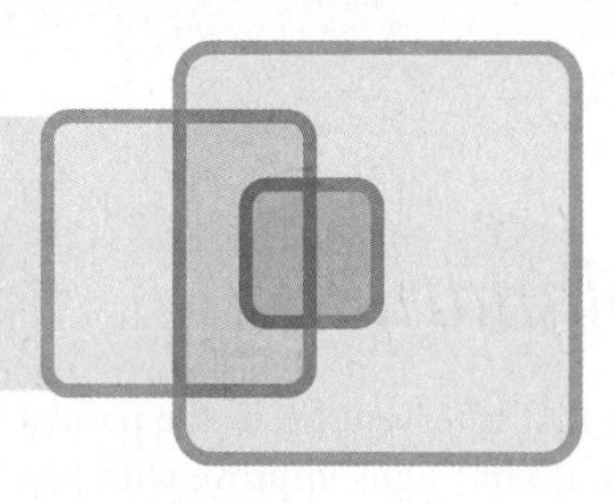

Genetic Disorders and Dysmorphology

MARY-ALICE ABBOTT

I MEDICAL GENETICS: OVERVIEW

A **Definition** Genetic differences manifest themselves throughout the lifespan and significantly influence medical practice, contributing to congenital malformations (birth defects), metabolic diseases, abnormal growth patterns, dysmorphic syndromes, neurologic conditions (e.g., hearing loss), and the development of common adult-onset disorders and cancer. The entire spectrum of human development is guided by the interaction of genetic makeup and the environment. Most birth defects are caused by environmental factors, genetic alterations, or a combination of both. As knowledge and technology in the field of **medical genetics** continue to advance rapidly, physicians and society are continually faced with challenging ethical questions.

B The **categories** of conditions with a genetic cause or component include **single gene disorders**, **chromosomal abnormalities**, and **multifactorial or complex disorders**.

C **Incidence** Single gene disorders appear to affect 2% of the overall population throughout the lifespan. In the pediatric population, there is a high rate of single gene disorders in hospitalized children (6%–8%). Seven in 1000 liveborn infants have chromosomal disorders and perhaps 5% of children have a multifactorial condition. Adults are also affected by genetic differences; it is estimated that > 60% of adults are affected with a multifactorial condition.

D **Genetic counseling** is the process whereby trained professionals communicate complex medical and genetic information to patients and their families in a **nondirective**, but supportive, fashion. This counseling is of value to individuals who have a positive history of genetic disorders and to those who are at increased risk for having a child with a genetic condition or birth defect. **Genetic counseling** should provide information regarding the specific diagnosis, mode of inheritance, and recurrence risk, both for the parents and the affected individual. Likewise, genetic counselors provide direct support to families and help families make contact with other affected families or support groups.

1. **Establishing an accurate diagnosis** allows better medical management of affected individuals, because the natural history of etiologically separate disorders with similar manifestations may be very different.
2. **Evaluating recurrence risk.** Once a diagnosis has been made, the pattern of inheritance, if any, is known and it becomes possible to discuss recurrence risks and **prenatal diagnostic options** for future pregnancies.
   a. If a couple has a child who has a specific genetic condition, that couple's risk (with each pregnancy) includes their risk of having a child with the specific condition in addition to the population risk of 3% for other birth defects.
   b. If a birth defect is caused by a known environmental agent (e.g., radiation, alcohol), the risk for recurrence of the specific birth defect in future pregnancies can sometimes be eliminated.
3. **Pedigree analysis** is the first step in most genetic counseling. A four-generation pedigree is constructed for each family, including all medical information.

TABLE 8-1 Populations at Increased Risk for Specific Genetic Disorders

Population	Disease
Northern European Caucasian	Cystic fibrosis
African descent	Sickle cell disease
Ashkenazi Jews, French Canadians	Tay-Sachs disease
Mediterranean descent	α-Thalassemia
Southeast Asians	β-Thalassemia

a. **Ethnic background** is ascertained for all family members because some conditions (especially autosomal recessive disorders) occur with increased frequency in specific populations. Certain ethnic subgroups are at increased risk for having children with specific autosomal recessive disorders due to the increased likelihood of common ancestors and a small genetic pool (Table 8-1).
b. **Family history of congenital anomalies** and **pregnancy loss** is noted because this information may give clues to genetic disorders.
c. **Parental consanguinity** is noted because this leads to an increased risk for having a child with a birth defect, particularly an autosomal recessive disorder or multifactorial disorder since people who are related are more likely to carry the same rare mutations than are those who are not related.

E **Prenatal diagnosis** A variety of procedures and tests are available for detection of birth defects and genetic disorders before delivery, beginning with the first trimester. Early detection affects how the physician manages the remainder of the pregnancy, delivery, and neonatal period. There may be therapeutic options available to prevent development of abnormalities (e.g., in utero treatment of congenital adrenal hyperplasia). Detection of congenital anomalies in pregnancy also allows parents the option of pregnancy termination or additional time for emotional adjustment. Indications for prenatal testing are listed in Table 8-2. Available prenatal diagnostic procedures include the following:

1. **Screening tests**
   a. **Maternal serum screening** measures levels of maternal blood for up to four fetoplacental products: **α-fetoprotein (AFP),** unconjugated estriol, human chorionic gonadotrophin, and inhibin-A.
      (1) An elevated AFP level indicates increased risk for neural tube defects, other open defects (e.g., omphalocele), and fetal bleeding.
      (2) A low AFP, with characteristic patterns of elevation or decrease in unconjugated estriol and human chorionic gonadotropin (hCG) levels, may be found in pregnancies at risk for trisomies 18 and 21, as well as for Turner syndrome (45,X).
      (3) Other characteristic patterns of elevation or depression of these markers may suggest certain rarer disorders.
      (4) There is no risk to the pregnancy associated with maternal serum screening; therefore, it is offered to every pregnant woman at 15 to 17 weeks' gestation.

TABLE 8-2 Some Indications for Prenatal Testing

Indication	Risk
Women 35 y of age or older	Down syndrome, other aneuploidies
Elevated maternal serum AFP concentration	Open defect (e.g., neural tube defect)
Low maternal serum AFP concentration	Down syndrome
Prior history of autosomal trisomy	Trisomy
Parent with balanced chromosome translocation	Unbalanced karyotype
Family history of genetic disorder or carrier parent	Specific disorder in family
Family history of isolated structural defect	Same structural defect

AFP, α-fetoprotein.

b. **First-trimester screening** is available at 11 to 13 weeks' gestation and uses a combination of an ultrasound (nuchal translucency) measurement with maternal serum markers (free β-hCG and pregnancy-associated plasma protein A [PAPP-A]) to identify pregnancies at risk for chromosomal abnormalities (e.g., trisomy 21 and 18) and other fetal problems (e.g., genetic syndromes, congenital heart defects).

c. **Fetal ultrasound** is a safe test that can be offered in pregnancies for which there is a risk of structural fetal anomalies or growth abnormalities.

(1) **Level I** ultrasound is performed in most obstetric office settings to evaluate fetal size, growth, number of fetuses, and viability. If abnormalities are suspected, most patients are referred for level II ultrasound.

(2) **Level II** ultrasound is offered at centers that specialize in the care of high-risk pregnancies and management of fetal abnormalities. Major structural abnormalities of most organ systems can be diagnosed and evaluated. Level II ultrasound may be performed in conjunction with amniocentesis (*see I E 2*) or chorionic villus sampling (*see I E 2*).

(3) **Fetal echocardiography,** typically performed at 22 weeks' gestation, can accurately diagnose most significant structural heart defects.

2. **Diagnostic Testing**

a. **Amniocentesis**

(1) **Technique**

(a) **Timing.** Amniocentesis is usually performed at approximately 15 to 20 weeks' gestation.

(b) **Procedure.** In routine amniocentesis, a needle is inserted into the amniotic cavity and approximately 20 mL of amniotic fluid is removed. The fluid and living fetal cells it contains are evaluated for fetal chromosome anomalies, specific DNA analysis, biochemical abnormalities, and/or AFP level.

(2) **Complications** occur in 1 in 200 to 1 in 400 cases and include:

(a) **Spontaneous labor,** leading to spontaneous abortion

(b) **Amniotic fluid leakage,** leading to spontaneous labor or oligohydramnios

(c) **Needle puncture of the fetus** (rare), because the procedure is done under ultrasound guidance

(d) **Infection** (rare, because the procedure is done aseptically)

(3) **Indications.** Amniocentesis is primarily offered to women whose risk for having an affected fetus is greater than the risk for complications from the procedure. This high-risk group includes those listed in Table 8-2.

b. **Chorionic villus sampling (CVS)**

(1) **Technique**

(a) **Timing.** CVS is usually performed between 10 and 12 weeks' gestation.

(b) A catheter is placed through the cervix via the transvaginal route under ultrasound guidance, or a needle is inserted transabdominally into the developing placenta. Chorionic villus cells of the placenta are aspirated for chromosomal, DNA, or biochemical studies.

(2) **Complications.** Compared to amniocentesis, CVS poses a greater risk (~1%) for fetal loss and maternal infection (chorioamnionitis).

(3) **Advantages.** A major advantage of CVS is the early gestational age at which the test is offered. If an abnormality is detected and the parents opt to terminate the pregnancy, the procedure may be less psychologically traumatic and of lower risk at or before 12 weeks (when CVS results are available) than at 18 to 20 weeks (when amniocentesis results are available).

(4) **Disadvantages**

(a) The CVS process only collects fetal cells and does not allow withdrawal of amniotic fluid for AFP or other biochemical testing.

(b) Due to the possibility of chromosomally differing cell lines in the chorionic villi (**mosaicism;** *see V A*), CVS results are occasionally ambiguous, which necessitates further evaluation with amniocentesis.

c. **Percutaneous umbilical blood sampling** is a procedure in which fetal blood is obtained from the umbilical cord under ultrasound guidance but without direct visualization. The test is used for chromosome analysis and biochemical study of fetal blood. The complication risk of the procedure is 2% to 3%.

d. Fetoscopy

(1) **Technique.** Fetoscopy is an infrequently used procedure whereby a small fiberoptic instrument is inserted transabdominally, under ultrasound guidance, into the uterine cavity where the fetus is visualized and can be examined. The technique can also be used to obtain **fetal skin biopsy specimens** for prenatal diagnosis of genetic skin disorders such as ichthyosis.

(2) **Complications.** The risk of this procedure is approximately 3% to 5%, with complications involving bleeding, pregnancy loss, infection, and amniotic fluid leakage.

e. Preimplantation diagnosis is possible for some disorders, including carriers of some chromosomal translocations, using in vitro fertilization techniques.

(1) **Gametes** are harvested from the parents, and fertilization is allowed to take place in vitro.

(2) After several cell divisions in culture, one to a few cells are dissected from the **blastocyst** for genetic analysis. If normal, the embryo is implanted into the woman's uterus using standard techniques.

II DYSMORPHOLOGY: OVERVIEW

A **Dysmorphism** is an abnormality in form or structural development. The presence of abnormal physical features often suggests an underlying (usually genetic) disorder and sometimes portends the presence of other (internal) abnormalities of form or function.

1. Dysmorphic features are those that fall outside the range of normal.

a. Dysmorphic features fall into three major categories: **Malformations, deformations,** and **disruptions** (Table 8-3).

b. Objectively measurable features. For many features there are objectively measurable norms. For example, individuals in whom the distance between the pupils (interpupillary distance) is measurably smaller than normal have **hypotelorism,** and patients whose distance is greater than normal have **hypertelorism.**

c. Subjectively observable features require careful observation. Some features must be judged subjectively by contrast with the normal population.

(1) Examples of subjectively observable dysmorphic features include a flat facial profile, a small chin, a down-turned mouth, an abnormally folded ear, and abnormal palmar creases.

(2) The features of a dysmorphic-appearing child should be compared to familial characteristics. One or more dysmorphic features may be present in otherwise normal individuals.

2. Minor anomalies are unusual morphologic features, present in $< 4\%$ of the population, that themselves are of no serious medical or cosmetic consequence to the patient. Examples include ear pits, toe syndactyly, curved fifth fingers, and unusual ear shape.

a. The significance of minor anomalies is that they serve as valuable clues to a possible underlying pattern of malformation or isolated major internal malformations.

b. The presence of **two or more minor anomalies** should lead to a more extensive evaluation of the patient.

TABLE 8-3 Categories of Birth Defects and Dysmorphism

Category	Pathogenesis	Causes
Malformations	Poor tissue formation	Genetic Teratogenic
Deformations	Abnormal mechanical forces	Crowding Oligohydramnios Abnormal position
Disruptions	Destruction of normal tissue	Amniotic bands Thrombosis

B Congenital anomalies/birth defects

1. **Definition.** Medically significant birth defects are congenital anomalies that require some form of medical intervention. Birth defects range in severity from relatively minor anomalies (e.g., polydactyly) to severe or systemic conditions (e.g., hydrocephalus, trisomy 18).
2. **Incidence.** The population risk for medically significant birth defects is approximately 3% of all liveborn infants. However, not all birth defects are detected at birth; for example, some forms of kidney disorders, congenital heart disease, and mental retardation are diagnosed later in life. Congenital anomalies cause more than 20% of all infant deaths, and 9% of deaths in children ages 1 to 9 years.
3. **Etiologic classification.** The entire spectrum of human development is guided by the interaction of genetic makeup and the environment. Most birth defects are caused by environmental factors, genetic alterations, or a combination of both.

C **Syndromes** are recognizable patterns of abnormalities that are known or presumed to be the result of a single cause. This may include internal and/or external abnormalities that may be structural and/or functional. Recognizable patterns of dysmorphic features, with or without other abnormalities, often constitute syndromes; Down syndrome is a classic example of dysmorphic features in a recognizable pattern (Figure 8-1, *IV B 1*). Some syndromes, however, have no associated dysmorphic features.

1. All of the findings of a specific syndrome need not be present in a given individual who has the syndrome. Persons who have the same syndrome share a number of findings, but not necessarily any one feature or any specific combination of them. In most cases, no one feature is pathognomonic for a syndrome.
2. It is not uncommon for the findings characteristic of a syndrome to develop over time, so that it is not always possible to make a diagnosis in a very young child.
3. Syndromes can be sporadic and of unknown cause, or caused by single gene abnormalities, chromosomal anomalies, teratogens, or deformations.

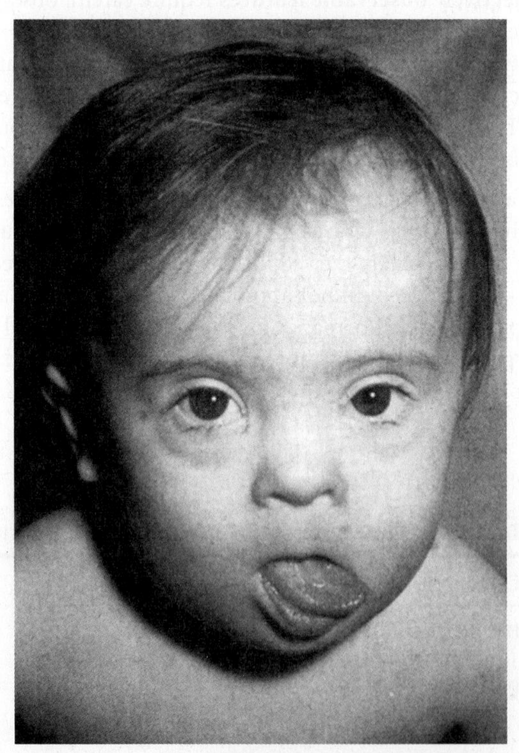

FIGURE 8-1 Characteristic dysmorphic features in an infant with Down syndrome. Note small palpebral fissures with epicanthal folds, flat nasal bridge, small nose and mouth, protruding tongue, and small chin. Brushfield spots can be seen on the iris. (Photograph courtesy of K. Jones, M.D.)

TABLE 8-4 Evaluation for Patterns of Malformation

Evaluation	Examples of Areas of Focus
Family history	Consanguinity Similar problems Other birth defects Abnormal mental development Pregnancy loss
Prenatal history	Mechanical forces Teratogen exposure
Physical examination	Dysmorphic features Growth Development
Neurologic examination	Asymmetry Vision, hearing problems Altered tone
Laboratory studies	Chromosome analysis Prenatal infection titers Metabolic studies
Imaging studies	Computed tomography or magnetic resonance imaging scan of the brain Ultrasound of heart or kidneys Skeletal radiographs

D Patient evaluation The presence of dysmorphic features in a patient should lead to the search for other abnormalities and an underlying disorder. A careful evaluation of the dysmorphic child is important so that a diagnosis can be reached (Table 8-4). With current knowledge and technology, a diagnosis can be made in approximately 50% of dysmorphic children.

1. **Prenatal history** should pay particular attention to potential causes of abnormal features such as oligohydramnios, abnormal uterine structure, abnormal fetal position, abnormal fetal activity, twinning, fibroids, medications, and use of alcohol or illicit drugs.
2. **Developmental** and **behavioral histories** often give clues to specific disorders.
3. **Physical examination** should focus on seeking a pattern of features that has been previously described.
4. **Testing** should be directed by the clinical findings and may be broad (e.g., metabolic screening tests), focused (e.g., chromosome analysis or microarray), or specific (e.g., molecular testing for a specific disease or mutation).

III SINGLE GENE DISORDERS

A General characteristics Each human normally has approximately 30,000 **genes** that are packaged in the 46 chromosomes (22 pairs of **autosomes** and 1 pair of **sex chromosomes**). All genes come in pairs except for some genes on the Y chromosome. More than 5000 different single gene disorders have been described, which are classified by their mode of inheritance (i.e., autosomal dominant, autosomal recessive, X-linked, or maternal).

B Detection The completion of the Human Genome Project and the recent availability of high throughput sequencing techniques have made DNA-based molecular testing for many genetic disorders, including analyses of large and complex genes, feasible in a clinical setting. In addition to direct DNA sequencing, other molecular techniques such as Southern blot analysis to detect large gene deletions and allele-specific oligonucleotide (ASO) testing to detect common point mutations remain important methods as well. Genetic testing is particularly useful to confirm a suspected diagnosis in an affected individual and/or to make prenatal testing of at-risk individuals possible.

C **Autosomal dominant conditions** occur when one gene of a gene pair is altered or mutated.

1. **General characteristics**
   a. **Defect.** Autosomal dominant conditions are often caused by a **mutation in a gene coding for a structural protein** or in a protein involved in a signaling or other developmental pathway.
   b. **Recurrence risk.** Any individual with an autosomal dominant condition has a 50% chance of passing on the mutant gene to each offspring. Thus, each child of an affected individual has a 50% chance of being affected.
   c. **Inheritance.** A mutant gene is usually inherited from one parent who is affected with the same condition. Sometimes, an individual will be the first person in a family to display an autosomal dominant trait. This is caused by a **new (de novo) mutation** of that gene in the ovum or spermatocyte that produces the affected individual. The recurrence risk for the parents of a child who has a new mutation is very low (i.e., equivalent to the chance that another spontaneous mutation will occur). However, the risk for the offspring of the affected individual is 50%. Rarely, unaffected parents may have more than one child affected by an autosomal dominant disorder. In some cases this is caused by gonadal (germline) mosaicism in one of the parents, wherein a mutation arose in some of his or her developing germ cells. Thus, these individuals are not affected, but they can pass on the mutation to their offspring (*see V A*).
   d. **Clinical features**
      (1) It is common for autosomal dominant genes to cause conditions that manifest differently and vary in degree of severity among affected individuals. This is called **variable expressivity.** For example, in polycystic kidney disease, some people have early renal failure, whereas others exhibit only hypertension with normal renal function at the same age. The severity or type of expression of an autosomal dominant disorder in an offspring is usually independent of the way the parent is affected.
      (2) Likewise, carriers of some autosomal dominant mutations may have no identifiable abnormality, whereas others in the family with the mutation have a recognizable disorder. This is called **decreased penetrance.** An example of this phenomenon is seen in some instances of familial **polydactyly** where some obligate carriers of the mutation do not have polydactyly.
      (3) A mutant dominant gene often has an effect on more than one tissue or organ system, a phenomenon known as **pleiotropy.**
2. **Marfan syndrome** is an autosomal dominant disorder with a prevalence of about 1 to 5 in 10,000. Marfan syndrome demonstrates variable expressivity, pleiotropy, and a high rate of new mutation.
   a. **Defect**
      (1) Marfan syndrome is caused by a mutation in the fibrillin-1 gene (*FBN1*), located on the long arm of chromosome 15. The abnormal protein product contributes to defective connective tissue.
         (a) A large number of different mutations in the gene have been identified in people who have clinically diagnosed Marfan syndrome.
         (b) Clinical diagnosis is the mainstay of diagnosis (see below). Direct molecular testing can be used to confirm a diagnosis. However, the detection rate is $< 100\%$; that is, a mutation may not be detectable in a clinically affected individual.
   b. **Clinical features** are listed in Table 8-5 and illustrated in Figure 8-2.
      (1) **Diagnostic criteria** have been formulated by consensus among experts in the field.
         (a) Once the diagnosis is considered, the various manifestations should be specifically investigated by skeletal measurements, ophthalmologic evaluation, and echocardiography. Other evaluations may be needed in equivocal cases.
         (b) Homocystinuria, a metabolic disorder that has significant clinical overlap with Marfan syndrome, should be ruled out by quantitative measurement of total homocysteine (*see III D 3*).
      (2) **Diagnostic challenges.** Only approximately 75% of affected people have an affected parent, due to the high incidence of new dominant mutations in Marfan syndrome. Variability in both severity and manifestations can also make it difficult to prove a positive family history. It is often necessary for the parents and siblings of a possibly affected individual to be evaluated.

TABLE 8-5 Clinical Features of Marfan Syndrome

Skeletal	Long, thin face, limbs, and digits Disproportionate tall stature High arched palate Sternum deformity (asymmetric pectus excavatum/carinatum) Hypermobile joints Scoliosis
Cardiac	Aortic root dilatation Mitral valve prolapse Risk for aortic aneurysm rupture
Ophthalmologic	Lens subluxation Flat corneas Severe myopia
Pulmonary	Spontaneous pneumothorax Emphysema

3. **Predisposition to cancer** can be inherited, usually in an autosomal dominant manner.
   a. A variety of genetic syndromes have an increased risk of both cancer and the developmental abnormalities that characterize the particular disorder. Examples include:
      (1) **Beckwith-Wiedemann syndrome,** characterized by generalized overgrowth; macroglossia (large tongue); neonatal hypoglycemia; omphalocele or other umbilical abnormalities; and predisposition to cancers, including Wilms tumor, hepatoblastoma, and nephroblastoma. Beckwith-Wiedemann syndrome is usually caused by a new mutation but can be inherited from a parent.
      (2) **Neurofibromatosis type I** is characterized by the presence of fibromatous tumors of the skin and multiple café au lait spots. Patients with this genetic disorder have an increased risk of pheochromocytoma, fibrosarcoma, neurofibrosarcoma, and some other malignancies, as well as nonmalignant central nervous system (CNS) tumors such as optic glioma.
   b. In other individuals, the genetic abnormality exhibits itself exclusively as a predisposition to cancer. Typically in these conditions, although children carry the mutated gene, the cancers develop during the adult years (see also Chapter 16). Familial adenomatous polyposis (FAP), however, is a cancer predisposition syndrome that can have serious medical and oncologic consequences for adolescents.

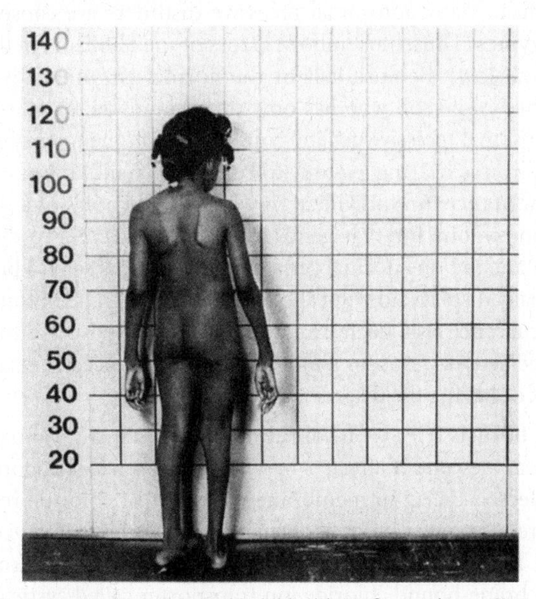

FIGURE 8-2 Characteristic body habitus in a 3-year-old child with Marfan syndrome. Note tall stature; thin body habitus with long limbs, long hands, and long flat feet; and scoliosis. (Photograph courtesy of R. Pyeritz, M.D.)

TABLE 8-6 Selected Cancer Predisposition Syndromes

Mechanism	Syndrome	Gene	Inheritance	Types of Cancer
Oncogene	Multiple endocrine neoplasia 2A, 2B, and 3	RET	AD	Pheochromocytoma, medullary thyroid carcinoma
Tumor suppressor	Multiple endocrine neoplasia 1	MEN1	AD	Various endocrine tumors, ovarian, bronchial carcinoma, other
	Breast/ovarian cancer	BRCA1 and 2	AD	Breast, ovarian, prostate, other
	Li-Fraumeni	p53	AD	Osteosarcoma, breast, many others
	Familial adenomatous polyposis	APC	AD	Colon (polyposis)
	Von Hippel-Lindau disease	VHL	AD	Cerebellar hemangioblastoma, renal cell carcinoma pheochromocytoma, other
DNA repair	Hereditary nonpolyposis colon cancer (HNPCC)	MLH1, MSH1 MSH6, others	AD	Colon (nonpolyposis)
Chromosome breakage	Ataxia-telangiectasia	ATM	AR[a]	Leukemia, breast

AD, autosomal dominant; AR, autosomal recessive.
[a] Heterozygotes for the mutation may also have an increased risk of cancer, including breast.

(1) Cancer can develop when **oncogenes,** whose expression are normally tightly regulated, are overexpressed.
(2) **Tumor suppressor genes** cause cancer when their normal function, usually involved in cell cycle regulation, is lost.
(3) Cancer may also develop in patients with mutations in genes involved in DNA repair, or with mutations that predispose to chromosomal rearrangements.
(4) Table 8-6 lists several of the more well-defined inherited cancer predisposition syndromes.

D **Autosomal recessive disorders** occur when both alleles carry mutations.

1. **General characteristics**
   a. **Defect.** Many autosomal recessive disorders are caused by mutations in genes coding for **enzymes.** Thus, most inborn errors of metabolism are the result of autosomal recessive genes (see below). Because half of the normal enzyme activity is adequate under most circumstances, a person who has only one mutant gene will not be affected. There are many other autosomal recessive genetic conditions not due to enzymatic defects, such as congenital non-syndromic hearing loss due to connexin 26 mutations.
   b. **Inheritance.** An individual in whom both copies of a gene pair have mutations is said to be **homozygous** for that gene. In autosomal recessive disorders, an individual who has one mutant and one normal gene for a gene pair is said to be **heterozygous** for that gene pair and usually displays no clinical effects from the single mutant gene.
   c. **Recurrence risk.** Each parent of a child who has an autosomal recessive disorder is presumed to be heterozygous for a mutation in the involved gene; each child of such a couple has a 25% risk of having the disorder.
2. **Cystic fibrosis** (CF) is one of the most common autosomal recessive disorders in Caucasians of European descent. It affects *1 in 3000* newborns in this population (see Chapters 11 and 13).
   a. **Defect.** A defect in membrane transport of chloride results in an inability to clear mucous secretions in the lungs and causes decreased pancreatic exocrine function.
   (1) The protein product of this gene, located on the long arm of chromosome 7, is a membrane-bound chloride ion transporter called cystic fibrosis transmembrane conductance regulator (CFTR).

(2) Close to 1000 different mutations and polymorphisms of this gene have been identified, with significant ethnic variation in the frequency of different mutations. Some correlations between specific mutations and clinical severity (genotype-phenotype) have been made.

(3) The Δ-F508 mutation—a deletion of three base pairs, leading to loss of a phenylalanine (F) residue at amino acid position 508 of the CFTR protein—is found in 70% of U.S. CF patients.

b. **Clinical features and course** (see Chapters 11 and 13). Some individuals identified as having two CF mutations have mild or no manifestations (e.g., nonclassic CF and isolated congenital bilateral absence of the vas deferens).

c. **Diagnosis**

(1) Although **sweat chloride testing** remains the mainstay of clinical diagnosis, direct DNA analysis can identify 90% of chromosomes carrying a specific CF mutation. Individuals of non-European descent are more likely to have a rare or unique mutation; therefore, molecular diagnosis in this population is less efficient.

(2) **Prenatal diagnosis** can be accomplished if mutations have been identified in the parents. **Carrier testing** is available to women of reproductive age (and their partners if necessary).

(3) Identification of a mutation allows accurate screening for carrier status in unaffected relatives.

(4) **Cystic fibrosis screening** has been added to the panel of conditions screened for in many states' newborn screening programs. Typically, newborn screening for CF is via a tiered approach: Blood spots are first tested for immunoreactive trypsinogen level (IRT), followed by DNA testing for the most common CF mutations on the subset of samples with the highest IRT levels. This screening method identifies not only the majority of neonates with CF, but also many carriers.

3. **Inborn errors of metabolism.** Genetic defects involving many of the more than 10,000 metabolic processes of the body are single gene disorders, usually inherited as autosomal recessive traits, although a few are X-linked (e.g., ornithine transcarbamylase deficiency [see *III D 3 g (2)*]), autosomal dominant (e.g., porphyria), or due to mutations in mitochondrial DNA (*see III D j*).

a. **Incidence and epidemiology**

(1) Although individual metabolic disorders are rare, as a group they are relatively common and are responsible for a significant amount of neonatal disease, mental retardation, and mental illness.

(2) Symptoms of a metabolic disorder may be seen at birth or may occur at any age, depending on the specific defect.

(3) Many inborn errors of metabolism are being identified in the immediate neonatal period due to the increased use of tandem mass spectroscopy in state newborn screening (NBS) programs.

b. **Defect**

(1) Metabolic disorders are usually caused by specific **defects in enzyme structure or function** or abnormalities of proteins that transport **metabolites to cells or across cell membranes.** The consequent metabolic alterations manifest as physiologic disturbances, mental deficiencies, or both.

(2) These diseases may cause symptoms by several mechanisms:

(a) Some conditions are due to an inability to synthesize chemicals needed for important biologic processes.

(b) Conversely, some metabolic defects are due to the inability to break down and excrete by-products of normal metabolism. Symptoms may be due to a generalized buildup of toxic by-products (e.g., isovaleric academia) or excessive tissue-specific storage of metabolic by-products (e.g., the mucopolysaccharidoses [*see III D i*]).

(c) Other metabolic diseases are due to defects in energy metabolism. Medium-chain acyl CoA dehydrogenase deficiency (MCADD) leads to a block in the catabolism of stored fats during fasting, which clinically manifests as recurrent hypoketotic hypoglycemia with fasting or catabolism or even sudden death.

TABLE 8-7 **Categories of Common Metabolic Disorders**

Category	Common Examples
Disorders of amino acid and organic acid metabolism	Phenylketonuria, homocystinuria, isovaleric acidemia
Disorders of ammonia metabolism	Ornithine transcarbamylase deficiency
Disorders of carbohydrate metabolism	Galactosemia, glycogen storage diseases
Disorders of lysosomal storage	Hunter syndrome (mucopolysaccharidosis)

(3) The **symptoms** of metabolic disorders are determined both by the nature of the abnormal compounds and the pattern of tissues and biologic processes involved.

c. Categories of common metabolic disorders are listed in Table 8-7.

d. Some **clinical features** are especially suggestive of inborn errors of metabolism.

(1) **Vomiting** and metabolic **acidosis** after initiation of feeding with breast milk or formula may herald a disorder of **amino acid or carbohydrate metabolism.**

(2) **Unusual odor of urine** or **sweat** may be seen in several conditions. For example, **maple syrup urine disease** is named for the odor of burnt sugar given off by the urine of affected children.

(3) **Hepatosplenomegaly** can be caused by metabolic disorders in which there is an accumulation (storage) of metabolites within the cells of the liver and spleen.

(4) **Mental retardation** may be caused by inborn metabolic errors. Metabolic defects are especially likely when there is evidence of neurologic deterioration. **Brain atrophy** or other toxic effects can be caused by harmful effects of circulating metabolites, such in phenylketonuria (PKU). Hydrocephalus with mental retardation can result from the inability to metabolize intracellular substances, such as in the **mucopolysaccharidoses.**

(5) Severe metabolic **acidosis** with a high **anion gap** can be caused by the presence of abnormal metabolites, most commonly relating to defects of **amino** and **organic acid metabolism.**

(6) **Hyperammonemia** is usually associated with urea cycle disorders and organic acid disorders.

(7) A family history of **early infant death** should suggest the possibility of an inborn error in metabolism.

(8) **Growth retardation** is frequently seen in infants who have inborn errors of metabolism.

(9) **Seizures** are a common manifestation of a metabolic disturbance.

e. Diagnosis. In most recognizable metabolic disorders, enzyme activity or a specific metabolite can be directly measured as abnormal. In some errors of metabolism, it is possible to detect heterozygous carriers of the condition and/or make a prenatal diagnosis by performing biochemical testing of amniocytes or chorionic villus tissue. An increasing number of inborn errors may be diagnosed by identification of the specific gene mutation. When a specific gene mutation has been identified in a family, testing to determine carrier status, prenatal diagnosis, and/or preimplantation genetic diagnosis are available.

f. Disorders of amino acid and **organic acid metabolism**

(1) **General features**

(a) **Defect.** These disorders usually involve a block in a synthetic or degradative pathway, causing buildup of either the precursor or catabolites of the precursor.

(b) **Clinical features**

(i) Symptoms, which usually begin in early infancy, are the result of inadequate synthesis of necessary metabolic compounds. Excess precursors or their metabolites may interfere with normal metabolic function and regulation (e.g., by causing severe acidosis or alkalosis).

(ii) Symptoms may become evident after the initiation of protein-containing feedings, which increase the substrate for the deficient enzyme.

(c) **Diagnosis.** Specific diagnosis requires evaluation of urine and plasma for the concentration of amino acids, organic acids, and their metabolites.

(d) **Therapy.** Some of these disorders are untreatable and associated with early death or mental retardation. Others are treatable with dietary manipulation or replacement of deficient cofactors. Most organic acid disorders lead to decreased level of consciousness, mental and neurologic deficiency, and death in infancy or childhood.

(2) **PKU,** the best studied and most common of the amino acid disorders, occurs in 1 in 12,000 liveborn infants.

(a) **Defect.** The majority of cases result from a deficiency of the enzyme phenylalanine hydroxylase, which prevents conversion of phenylalanine to tyrosine, with subsequent buildup of toxic metabolites.

(b) **Clinical features.** Unlike most amino acid disorders, PKU is not symptomatic early in infancy. Symptoms are seen later in infancy and during childhood, if the disorder is untreated.

(i) The most significant manifestation is moderate to severe **mental retardation.**

(ii) **Neurologic manifestations,** including hypertonicity and tremors and behavior disorders, are common.

(iii) Because there is a block in the conversion of phenylalanine to tyrosine, **hypopigmentation** is a common sign (tyrosine is a necessary intermediate in production of the pigment melanin).

(c) **Prevention of mental retardation** in PKU can be achieved by early identification of the defect and restriction of dietary intake of phenylalanine.

(i) All 50 states in the United States and most developed countries have mandatory newborn screening programs to identify infants who have PKU, so that the diet can be initiated sufficiently early to prevent mental retardation. PKU was the first disorder for which population-based screening was initiated. Since then, states have expanded their newborn screening panels to include a number of other conditions, most of which have a genetic etiology or component (e.g., fatty acid oxidation disorders, CF, hemoglobinopathies, hearing loss).

(ii) Dietary restriction should start very early in infancy (by age 1 month) to be optimally effective, and lifelong restriction is recommended to prevent loss of intellectual capability.

(iii) **Maternal PKU.** Individuals with PKU who maintain careful dietary management are able to live normal lives. However, females with PKU who have discontinued dietary restriction are at substantially increased risk for having children who have birth defects, especially microcephaly, congenital heart disease, and mental retardation (see environmental agents) (*see VI E 2*).

g. **Disorders of ammonia metabolism** occur in at least 1 in 50,000 newborns.

(1) **General features**

(a) **Defect.** Disorders of the urea cycle are associated with hyperammonemia, because they disrupt the conversion of ammonia to urea for excretion from the body.

(b) **Clinical features**

(i) Ammonia levels usually rise after initiation of protein-containing feedings or breastfeeding.

(ii) Affected children are well at birth but become progressively more lethargic, and seizures or decreased level of consciousness may develop.

(2) **Ornithine transcarbamylase deficiency (OTCD)**

(a) **Defect.** OTCD is a prototypic disorder of ammonia metabolism. Unlike most inborn errors of metabolism, it is an X-linked condition.

(i) Although primarily males are severely affected, female carriers may manifest symptoms because of skewed X-inactivation (*see III E 1 a*).

(ii) Allelic heterogeneity (different mutations in the same gene) exists, so that some affected males (or females) have a more or less severe mutation and clinical course.

(b) **Clinical features**

(i) Typically, overwhelming illness develops in affected males within 24 to 48 hours after initiation of protein-containing feedings. The newborn becomes progressively lethargic and may manifest seizures and a decreased level of consciousness as serum ammonia levels rise to > 500 μM and, frequently, to > 1000 μM.

(ii) Female carriers may have headache and vomiting after high-protein meals and, later, learning disabilities or an altered response to a protein load.

(c) Therapy and prognosis

(i) Treatment may be attempted with intravenous fluids, glucose, and agents that exploit alternative pathways for nitrogen excretion (e.g., benzoic acid, phenylacetate).

(ii) Early aggressive treatment can improve the prognosis for survival and function, but the outlook often remains poor unless the infant is managed prospectively from birth (prenatal diagnosis or suspicion based on positive family history). Even then, the management is complex and demanding of the parents.

(iii) Other urea cycle disorders (e.g., citrullinemia, argininosuccinic aciduria, carbamyl phosphate synthetase deficiency) have similar clinical courses to OTCD. Arginase deficiency tends to occur with less severe hyperammonemia and with progressive spastic quadriplegia and mental retardation.

h. Disorders of carbohydrate metabolism

(1) Galactosemia is a severe example of an inborn error of carbohydrate metabolism.

(a) Defect. It is an autosomal recessive disorder of lactose metabolism most commonly caused by deficiency of the enzyme **galactose 1-phosphate uridyltransferase,** resulting in impaired conversion of galactose 1-phosphate to glucose 1-phosphate.

(b) Clinical features are noted within a few days to weeks after initiation of formula or breast milk feedings. Initial symptoms include hepatomegaly, vomiting, anorexia, aminoaciduria, and growth failure.

(c) Diagnosis is suspected by detection of non–glucose-reducing substances in the urine (galactose and galactose 1-phosphate) and is confirmed by demonstrating absence of galactose 1-uridyltransferase activity in erythrocytes. Galactosemia is a component of most states' newborn screening panels because it is largely treatable when diagnosed early.

(d) Therapy for galactosemia is the elimination of all infant formulas and foods containing galactose (soy based infant formulas and other foods).

(i) Treated individuals often have normal intelligence if the diagnosis is made and treatment is initiated early. However, even in treated individuals, there is an increase in the incidence of learning disorders. Affected females have a high incidence of ovarian hypofunction and premature ovarian failure.

(ii) Untreated infants often die, either from failure to thrive or *Escherichia coli* sepsis. Untreated survivors suffer from growth retardation, mental retardation, and cataracts.

i. Mucopolysaccharidoses (MPSs) are a group of disorders characterized by deficiency of lysosomal enzymes responsible for intracellular catabolism of mucopolysaccharides. All are autosomal recessive conditions except for **Hunter syndrome** (MPS type II; iduronate 2-sulfatase deficiency), which is an X-linked disorder (*see III E*). The incidence of this group of disorders is 1 in 25,000 newborns.

(1) Clinical features are caused by intracellular accumulation (storage) of mucopolysaccharides and are generally not apparent at birth.

(a) All tissues can be affected, but effects are most commonly seen in the liver and spleen (hepatosplenomegaly); skeleton (skeletal dysplasia, joint contracture); brain (megalencephaly, mental retardation); heart (aortic and mitral valve incompetence); and respiratory system (tracheal stenosis).

(b) Mucopolysaccharidoses are usually associated with deterioration of neurologic function and progressive mental retardation. In some MPSs (e.g., Morquio syndrome), the CNS is unaffected and intelligence is normal.

(2) Diagnosis of a mucopolysaccharidoses is suggested by the presence of specific mucopolysaccharides in the urine. The diagnosis is confirmed by performing specific enzyme assays on leukocytes or fibroblasts.

(3) **Treatment options** have become available for some of the MPS disorders. These aim to replace the missing/nonfunctional enzyme. Approaches to this include bone marrow or umbilical cord stem cell transplant and enzyme replacement therapy (ERT). ERT is achieved by performing intravenous infusions of exogenous recombinant enzyme, specific to the underlying disorder, at regular intervals. ERT has been shown to decrease some of the somatic manifestations, such as cardiac and airway problems, but has not impacted the progressive CNS dysfunction. There is some evidence to suggest that there may be positive effects on the CNS with stem cell transplants.

j. Disorders of mitochondrial energy metabolism are a highly variable group of diseases due mainly to defects in the function of the electron transport chain or associated enzymes (e.g., those involved with β-oxidation of fats [OXPHOS]).

(1) The mitochondrion is a membrane-bound intracellular structure containing many of the enzymes involved in cellular energy metabolism.

(a) It carries some of its own genetic information in the form of a small circular genome (mitochondrial DNA [mtDNA]), although most mitochondrial enzymes are encoded by nuclear DNA and transported into the mitochondria by a targeted active process. The mitochondrial genome is exclusively inherited from the mother through the several hundred mitochondria in the cytoplasm of the ovum.

(b) The resulting phenotypes are considered to be energy-deficient states.

(c) Organs and physiologic processes that are highly energy dependent are preferentially affected, causing:

(i) CNS dysfunction, such as developmental delay or seizures, or abnormalities of hearing or vision

(ii) Myopathies, both peripheral and cardiac

(iii) Intestinal dysfunction, such as transport dysfunction and chronic diarrhea

(2) Disorders of mitochondrial energy metabolism can occur due to mutations in nuclear DNA (typically autosomal recessive) or in mtDNA.

(a) Because mitochondria are inherited only through the mother, disorders due to mutations in the mitochondrial DNA can produce a unique pedigree pattern or **maternal inheritance.**

(b) **Heteroplasmy** refers to the observation that the relative population of mutant mitochondria can vary within different tissues in an individual and between individuals in the same family.

(i) There can be variation in the affected organ, with the defects being functional, not structural.

(ii) There can be variation over time, usually increased severity.

(3) **Diagnosis**

(a) **Lactate, pyruvate,** and the ratio of lactate to pyruvate may be elevated in either blood or cerebrospinal fluid, or both.

(b) **Measurement** of other substances, such as ammonia, carnitine, and urine organic acids, may also be useful in diagnosing these disorders.

(c) **Definitive diagnosis** rests in demonstration of a specific enzymatic defect in lymphocytes, fibroblasts, hepatocytes, or muscle cells, or in identification of a pathologic DNA mutation (nuclear or mtDNA).

E **X-linked disorders** occur when a male inherits a mutant gene on the X chromosome, which is always maternal in origin. Common X-linked disorders include hemophilia A, color blindness, Duchenne muscular dystrophy, and fragile X syndrome.

1. General characteristics

a. Inheritance

(1) The affected male is termed **hemizygous** for the abnormal allele because he has only a single X chromosome and a single copy of X-linked genes. Males are more severely affected because they do not have a second X chromosome to compensate for the effects of the abnormal allele.

(2) The mother of the affected individual is usually **heterozygous** for the abnormal allele because she has two X chromosomes, one normal and one abnormal allele. Because one

of the X chromosomes in each cell is inactivated (with the majority of the genes on that chromosome not transcribed) in a random fashion (**Lyon hypothesis**), female heterozygotes may demonstrate partial manifestations of the disorder. It is estimated that up to one third of lethal X-linked disorders are due to new mutations.

b. **Recurrence risks** for X-linked disorders depend on whether the mother or the father has the abnormal gene.

(1) **If the mother carries one abnormal allele,** with each pregnancy there is a 50% chance that the abnormal allele will passed on. If the offspring inheriting the abnormal allele is a daughter, she, too, will be a carrier (heterozygote). If the offspring inheriting the abnormal allele is a son, he will be affected (hemizygote). Thus, each daughter has a 50% chance of being a carrier, and each son has a 50% chance of being affected.

(2) **If the father carries the abnormal allele** and thus is **affected,** he can pass that abnormal gene only to his daughters, and all his daughters will be carriers. Because the Y chromosome is normal, all his sons will be unaffected. **There is no direct male-to-male transmission in linked conditions.**

2. The **dystrophinopathies** (including Duchenne and Becker muscular dystrophy) are X-linked conditions caused by mutations in the very large DMD gene encoding the protein dystrophin, a component of the complex of proteins that provides structural support to the sarcolemma. Women who carry a DMD mutation may have milder manifestations of the condition, particularly cardiac problems. Full expression of the condition is seen in affected boys. Mothers of affected boys have a one-third chance of NOT carrying a mutation (denovomutations). Mutation analysis is available, but detection of a mutation, particularly in carrier females, is not always possible.

F **Y-linked genes.** The Y chromosome contains a number of unique genes without specific counterparts on the X chromosome. Although no abnormalities of these genes have yet been associated with congenital anomalies, genes associated with male infertility have been identified.

IV CHROMOSOME DISORDERS

A **General characteristics** An alteration in the amount or nature of chromosome material is usually associated with birth defects or other abnormalities. Chromosome disorders are seen in approximately 5 in 1000 liveborn infants (0.5%). Most chromosome defects arise **de novo** (i.e., no other family member has a defect).

1. **Defect.** The defects are usually classified as abnormalities of **number** or **structure** and **content.** They may involve either the **autosomes** or the **sex chromosomes;** conditions due to autosomal abnormalities are usually more severe than those due to sex chromosome abnormalities.

a. **Numeric defects** are deviations from **euploidy** (normal number of chromosomes, 46). Examples of numeric chromosome abnormalities **(aneuploidy)** include trisomy 21 (Down syndrome), trisomy 18, trisomy 13, Klinefelter syndrome (47,XXY), and Turner syndrome (usually 45,X).

b. **Structural defects** result from chromosome breakage and rearrangement. Possibilities include unbalanced translocation, (micro)deletion, duplication, inversion, and isochromosome. Examples of disorders due to structural chromosome abnormalities include microdeletion of 22q11 (*see IV D 1 c [1]*), cri du chat syndrome (5p deletion) (*see IV D 1 c [2]*), and Wilms tumor with aniridia (11p deletion). Prader-Willi syndrome (*see V B 2*) is commonly associated with a (micro)deletion within the maternally derived chromosome 15q.

2. **Indications for chromosome analysis**

a. Chromosomal abnormalities often result in poor growth and short stature. They may rarely be associated with overgrowth.

b. Children who have **recognizable phenotypes** (clinical features) consistent with known chromosomal disorders should have confirmatory chromosome studies.

c. Children who have **multiple congenital abnormalities** or **dysmorphic features** with no clinically identifiable cause require chromosome studies.

d. Chromosome studies should be part of the genetic evaluation of children who have **mental retardation** or speech or other developmental delays, with no identifiable cause.

e. Parents who have had **recurrent (two or more) pregnancy losses** should undergo chromosome studies. Of couples with two or more miscarriages, 5% will have one member with a balanced reciprocal chromosome translocation.

(1) Miscarriage can result when an embryo or fetus has inherited an unbalanced variant of such a chromosome translocation that is incompatible with life.

(2) Such couples are at risk for having a liveborn child who has multiple congenital anomalies and developmental disabilities due to an unbalanced variant of the translocation; thus, these couples should be offered prenatal diagnosis.

f. Chromosome studies are valuable for aiding in the diagnosis and management of patients who have **ambiguous genitalia.**

g. Sex chromosome abnormalities may be found in males and females who have **infertility.**

h. Chromosome studies from bone marrow samples of patients who have **leukemia** often demonstrate abnormalities.

i. Solid tumors often contain cytogenetic alterations, which may give clues to their genetic origin.

3. Methods of chromosome analysis. Chromosome studies can be performed on any tissue in which cells are actively undergoing mitosis.

a. A **karyotype** is an ordered arrangement of the chromosomes that is made from micrographs. Chromosome banding patterns (visible through staining techniques) are used to analyze chromosome structure. The **high-resolution,** or prometaphase, **chromosome analysis** captures cells in an early stage of the mitotic cycle, so the chromosomes are longer and have more regions (bands) visible for analysis.

b. Peripheral blood lymphocytes are the most commonly studied tissue because blood is easily obtained.

(1) The T cells are stimulated with phytohemagglutinin, which causes the cells to undergo mitosis.

(2) Results from peripheral blood chromosome studies usually take a minimum of 3 days to obtain, because that is the time required for the cells to enter metaphase (when the chromosomes are compacted and most easily stained and visualized).

c. Fluorescence in situ hybridization (FISH) is a technique that uses fluorescently labeled DNA probes specific to a given chromosome segment to rapidly identify the origin of extra or missing genetic material—for example, trisomy or components of a translocation, deletion, or duplication. **FISH-based techniques** are particularly useful for detecting specific, very small deletions, especially those that are not visible by standard prometaphase analysis (*see IV A 3 b*). The gene-rich material in the chromosomal telomeres is difficult to analyze on routine chromosome analysis. FISH-based techniques are available to examine the subtelomeric regions of all chromosomes (subtelomeric FISH).

d. Bone marrow studies. Bone marrow cells are constantly undergoing mitosis, making it possible to obtain results within 6 hours of obtaining a sample.

(1) The most common use of bone marrow chromosome studies is for evaluation of leukemia. The exact type of chromosomal anomaly in leukemic cells aids in diagnosis, management, and determination of prognosis (see Chapter 16).

(2) Bone marrow chromosomes may be studied when management decisions regarding newborn infants who have multiple birth defects may be altered by knowing whether there is a chromosome abnormality associated with a very poor prognosis (e.g., trisomy 18 [*see IV B 3*]).

e. Organ tissue studies. Chromosome studies can also be performed on solid tissues and organs. Usually, it takes at least 3 to 4 weeks for solid tissue cells to grow in culture before chromosome analysis can be performed.

(1) Occasionally it is not possible to obtain peripheral blood, as in the case of a stillborn fetus. Another source of cells is then used for chromosome analysis, usually fibroblasts from a skin biopsy. Fibroblasts may be viable and culturable for many hours after the fetal demise.

(2) In the case of chromosome mosaicism, tissue biopsy specimens (usually taken from the skin) are grown in culture to diagnose or confirm the defect.

f. Chromosome microarray (CMA) analysis is a new molecular testing technique used to analyze genomic/genetic material. It can detect small duplications and/or deletions (copy number variations). It does not provide structural information about the chromosomes.

B Numeric autosomal abnormalities (aneuploidy) Characteristic phenotypes are associated with specific autosomal trisomies. **Trisomy** refers to the fact that three—rather than the normal two—copies of a specific chromosome are present in the cells of an individual. Such trisomies almost always occur because of a meiotic division error called **nondisjunction** in either the oocyte or the spermatocyte. Only a few trisomies are found in liveborn infants; others are seen only in spontaneously aborted fetuses.

1. **Down syndrome (DS)** is the most common autosomal trisomy compatible with life.
   a. **Types of defects.** The most common karyotype associated with DS is trisomy 21, although some cases result from translocations or, more rarely, mosaicism.
      (1) **Trisomy.** Ninety-five percent of children with DS have 47 chromosomes, with three number 21 chromosomes. Trisomy 21 occurs in 1 in 700 liveborn infants.
         (a) The risk for having a child with an extra chromosome 21 increases with **advancing maternal age.** This risk rises dramatically after 35 years of age. Most children who have trisomy 21 are born to women younger than 35 years of age, however, because most females give birth before 35 years of age. The reason for the increased incidence of trisomy 21 in fetuses of older mothers is not well understood. The extra chromosome comes from the father in only a small percentage of cases.
         (b) The empirically observed **recurrence risk** for parents of children who have trisomy 21 is ~1% (unless the age-related risk is greater).
      (2) **Translocation.** Four percent of children with DS have 46 chromosomes, with a translocation of the third number 21 chromosome to another chromosome—usually chromosome number 13, 14, 15, 21, or 22.
         (a) Of all cases of translocation DS, three fourths are **de novo** (i.e., not familial).
         (b) One fourth of translocation cases are **familial,** meaning that one of the parents has a balanced translocation involving one number 21 chromosome and another chromosome. In these cases, the empirically observed **recurrence risk** may be as high as 15% in future pregnancies (depending on which other chromosome is involved and on the sex of the partner carrying the balanced translocation). In the rare situation of a familial 21;21 translocation, the recurrence risk is 100%.
      (3) **Mosaicism.** One percent of children with DS have chromosome mosaicism, with some cells having 46 chromosomes (two number 21 chromosomes), and some cells having 47 chromosomes with three number 21 chromosomes. The mosaicism results from either a mitotic division error that occurred during early embryonic development or loss of the third chromosome 21 in an early cell line. Children with mosaic DS may have a milder clinical presentation than those with trisomy 21 in all of their cells.
   b. **Clinical features.** Children with DS have a characteristic appearance that can be defined in terms of their dysmorphic features. A number of other characteristic functional and structural abnormalities are part of the recognizable syndrome. **Clinical findings** and **complications** of trisomy 21 are listed in Table 8-8. Figure 8-1 demonstrates the characteristic facial findings. **Cardiac defects,** especially endocardial cushion defects and septal defects, are seen in close to 50% of persons who have DS.
   c. **Prognosis.** With improved medical, educational, and vocational management, life expectancy for many individuals with DS is well into adulthood. Therefore, issues relating to employment, financial security, health care, and living situation must be addressed. Semi-independent living is achievable for many adults with DS.
2. **Trisomy 13.** From 1 in 4000 to 1 in 10,000 newborns are affected by trisomy 13.
   a. **Types of defects**
      (1) **Trisomy.** Seventy-five percent of cases of trisomy 13 are caused by an extra chromosome 13 as a result of parental meiotic nondisjunction. There is a relationship between the occurrence of trisomy 13 and advanced maternal age, although it is not as strong as that for trisomy 21.
      (2) **Translocation.** Twenty percent of cases of trisomy 13 are the result of translocation involving chromosome 13.
         (a) Three fourths of these cases are **de novo.**
         (b) One fourth of these cases are caused by a familial translocation involving the number 13 chromosome, and in these cases the empirically observed **recurrence risk** can be as high as 14% in future pregnancies.

TABLE 8-8 Clinical Findings and Complications of Trisomies 21, 13, and 18

System	Trisomy 21	Trisomy 13	Trisomy 18
Growth	Short stature	Intrauterine growth retardation	Intrauterine growth retardation
Head	Microcephaly Brachycephaly (flat occiput)	Microcephaly Open scalp lesion (cutis aplasia)	Microcephaly Prominent occiput
Face	Flat facial profile Short, up-slanting palpebral fissures Brushfield spots of the iris Flat nasal bridge Epicanthal folds Small mouth with protruding tongue Small, retroplaced mandible Small ears with abnormal shape	Cleft lip (may be bilateral) Cleft palate (may be bilateral) Microphthalmos Colobomata of the eye	Small-appearing face Micrognathia (small mandible)
Neck	Excess posterior skin	Usually normal	Usually normal
Thorax	Short sternum	Usually normal	Short sternum
Cardiac	Endocardial cushion defects Ventriculoseptal defect	Variety of cardiac defects	Variety of cardiac defects
Gastrointestinal	Duodenal atresia Hirschsprung disease	Omphalocele	Usually normal
Extremities	Short hands and fingers Incurved fifth fingers (clinodactyly) Single palmar crease Wide gap between first and second toes	Polydactyly of hands and feet	Overlap of second finger on third, fourth finger on fifth Fixed finger contractures Lack of interphalangeal flexion creases Rocker bottom feet
Genitalia	Small external genitalia	Genital malformations (may be ambiguous in males)	Usually normal
Neurologic	Mental retardation (mean IQ, 50) Developmental delay Hypotonia Alzheimer-like dementia (third and fourth decades)	Severe mental retardation Holoprosencephaly Other CNS malformations	Severe mental retardation CNS malformations Hypertonia (after initial hypotonia) Occasional neural tube defects
Skeletal	Hypoplastic middle phalanx of fifth finger Cervical spine subluxation (risk for spinal cord injury)		Hip dislocation
Other	Hypothyroidism Leukemia		

IQ, intelligence quotient; CNS, central nervous system.

(3) **Mosaicism.** Five percent of the cases of trisomy 13 are mosaic for normal 46-chromosome cell lines and cell lines with 47 chromosomes with an extra number 13 chromosome.

b. **Clinical features** of trisomy 13 are listed in Table 8-8.

c. **Prognosis** for patients with trisomy 13 is extremely poor: 50% of patients die before 1 month of age, 70% die before age 6 months, and 90% die before age 1 year.

3. **Trisomy 18** occurs in 1 in 8000 liveborn infants. There is a relationship between advanced maternal age and the occurrence of trisomy 18, but this is less marked than that seen in trisomy 21 and trisomy 13.
   a. **Types of defects.** Trisomy 18 is rarely caused by a chromosomal translocation.
      (1) Ninety percent of the cases of trisomy 18 are a result of **meiotic nondisjunction.**
      (2) Ten percent of the cases of trisomy 18 are mosaic—either caused by a postzygotic (postfertilization) mitotic nondisjunction or by loss of the third chromosome 18 in an embryonic cell line.
   b. **Clinical features** of trisomy 18 are listed in Table 8-8. The variability and subtlety of the dysmorphic features can sometimes make this condition difficult to recognize.
   c. **Prognosis** for patients who have trisomy 18 is poor: 30% of patients die within 1 month of birth, and 90% die before 1 year of age.

C **Sex chromosome disorders** involve abnormalities in the number or structure of the X or Y chromosome.

1. **Turner syndrome** affects 1 in 3000 newborn girls.
   a. **Types of defects.** In Turner syndrome, the second X chromosome is either missing or abnormal. Several different chromosomal anomalies can result in the Turner phenotype.
      (1) In 55% of girls who have Turner syndrome, there is a 45,X karyotype.
      (2) In 25% of patients, the structure of one of the X chromosomes is altered. The structural anomaly is usually a **deletion** of a segment of the chromosome or a duplication of the long or short arm of the chromosome, with a subsequent loss of the other arm (called an **isochromosome**).
      (3) In 15% of patients, there is **mosaicism** for two or more cell lines, one of which is usually 45,X, and the other is 46,XX or 46,XY. A third cell line may be present, most commonly leading to a karyotype of 45,X/46,XX/47,XXX.
   b. **Recurrence risk** for parents of a girl who has Turner syndrome is the same as the general population risk (i.e., 1 in 2500 liveborn girls, or, more accurately, 1 in 5000 liveborn infants).
   c. **Clinical features** of Turner syndrome may be noted at birth, although many girls are not diagnosed until puberty.
      (1) **Dysmorphic features** include **lymphedema** of hands and feet at birth, a shield-shaped chest, **webbing of the neck,** cubitus valgus (increased carrying angle), short stature (average adult height is 135 cm [53 inches]), and multiple pigmented nevi.
      (2) **Functional** and **structural abnormalities**
         (a) **Gonadal dysgenesis** is present in 100% of individuals and is associated with primary amenorrhea and lack of typical pubertal development due to absence of ovarian hormones. It is important to replace ovarian hormones at puberty as part of the management of girls with Turner syndrome. With rare exceptions, women are unable to become pregnant.
         (b) **Gonadoblastoma** (a tumor of abdominally located gonads with Y-containing cells) may develop in patients who have a cell line with a Y chromosome. It is essential to perform bilateral gonadectomy in girls who have such a cell line.
         (c) **Renal anomalies,** present in 40% of patients, include duplication of the collecting system and horseshoe kidney.
         (d) **Congenital heart disease** occurs in 20% of patients. Defects include aortic stenosis, bicuspid aortic valve, and coarctation of the aorta. Dissecting aortic aneurysm in young adulthood may be a life threatening complication.
         (e) **Autoimmune thyroiditis** is common.
         (f) Intelligence usually falls within the normal range. However, **specific learning disabilities** are common, particularly in visuospatial organization.
   d. **Diagnosis.** The diagnosis of Turner syndrome is made by chromosome analysis. Evaluation of 30 cells is standard, so that low level mosaicism can be detected.
      (1) Some of these girls have mosaic Turner syndrome, and a skin biopsy is necessary to find the mosaicism in fibroblasts.

(2) A phenotypically similar but genetically unrelated condition is **Noonan syndrome,** which, unlike Turner syndrome, is an autosomal dominant condition, affects males and females equally, and has a number of additional clinical findings.

e. **Prognosis** depends on the type and severity of malformations. Lifespan probably is normal in most cases. The availability of recombinant growth hormone has allowed women with Turner syndrome to achieve a more typical adult height.

2. **Klinefelter syndrome** affects 1 in 800 newborn boys and is caused by an extra X chromosome.

a. **Types of defects**

(1) In 80% of boys who have Klinefelter syndrome, there is a **47,XXY karyotype.**

(2) In 20% of patients, there is mosaicism with one cell line having a **47,XXY karyotype.**

b. **Recurrence risk** for Klinefelter syndrome is the same as the general population risk (i.e., 1 in 1600 liveborn infants).

c. **Clinical features** are variable and nonspecific.

(1) Boys are usually **taller than expected** for their family, with an arm span generally greater than their height.

(2) The **testes remain small,** and there is hyperplasia of Leydig cells and greatly diminished spermatozoa production, with infertility. This represents **seminiferous tubule dysgenesis.**

(a) Serum testosterone concentration is usually low.

(b) At puberty, boys are **incompletely masculinized** and usually have more female body habitus, female escutcheon, and decreased body hair. Treatment with testosterone leads to more complete masculinization.

(c) **Gynecomastia** is a common feature, which may account for the increased rate of male breast cancer observed in males with 47,XXY.

(3) The mean IQ is 90, and there is a slight increase in the incidence of mild mental retardation.

(4) **Behavioral problems** and **immaturity** are common. Some of the behavioral and social adjustment difficulties may improve with testosterone replacement therapy.

D Structural chromosome abnormalities Most structural chromosome abnormalities are associated with well-characterized phenotypes; however, some are not. In some cases, parental chromosome analysis is important in determining the clinical relevance of a subtle chromosomal (e.g., subtelomere) abnormality. Some chromosomal differences are familial in nature and of no clinical significance.

1. **Partial deletions/duplications**

a. **Types of defects**

(1) Some syndromes can be caused by the loss of chromosome material from the ends of a chromosome (terminal deletions), the most distal gene-rich telomeres **(subtelomeric chromosome deletions),** or loss of material from the middle or inner portion of a chromosome **(interstitial deletion).** Some deletions occur frequently and have a recognizable pattern, such as deletion of chromosomal region 22q11 (*see IV D 1 c [1]*). Duplications may also cause recognizable syndromes (duplication 22q11 causes cateye syndrome).

(2) Although most chromosome deletions arise **de novo,** terminal deletions (and very rarely interstitial deletions) may result from the child inheriting a chromosome translocation in an **unbalanced form** (unequal exchange of material between two chromosomes) from a parent who has a balanced reciprocal translocation (equal exchange of material between two chromosomes). In cases of deletions, it is necessary to perform karyotypes of both parents to rule out a parental balanced rearrangement (see Figure 8-3).

(3) A family history of recurrent pregnancy loss may be found when parents have balanced chromosome translocations because other family members may also carry the translocation.

(4) **Contiguous gene deletion syndromes** refer to phenotypes resulting from the absence of several neighboring genes.

(a) These defects cause recognizable but variable conditions, often with several diverse manifestations.

(b) In some cases, microdeletions are visible by high-resolution chromosome analysis; in others, they are not. In these cases, FISH-based technology is necessary to detect the deletion.

(c) An example of a contiguous gene syndrome is **Williams syndrome,** which is due to a small deletion on the long arm of chromosome 7, including the elastin gene.

(i) Patients missing only the elastin gene have isolated congenital cardiovascular findings, typically supravalvular aortic stenosis.

(ii) Patients missing additional genetic material in the region have Williams syndrome, with mild mental retardation, characteristic facial appearance, characteristic behavioral profile ("cocktail party personality"), hypercalcemia, and hyperextensible joints, as well as supravalvular aortic stenosis.

(iii) These additional findings are presumed to be due to the loss of other genes in the region.

b. Terminal deletions. Children with terminal deletions typically have growth deficiency, mental retardation, dysmorphic features, and multiple malformations, although there is a wide range of phenotypes.

c. Examples of disorders caused by partial deletions

(1) **22q11** deletion syndrome has an estimated prevalence of 1 in 4000 in the population. In some cases, the deletion is detected on routine chromosome analysis, but many cases can be detected only with FISH for the 22q11 region.

(a) The same microdeletion has been shown to cause **DiGeorge syndrome, velocardiofacial syndrome, conotruncal heart anomaly-face syndrome,** and **some apparently isolated conotruncal heart defects.**

(b) There are a wide variety of manifestations in patients who have this deletion.

(i) **Clinical findings** are described in Table 8-9.

(ii) Some infants have severe congenital heart disease, cleft palate, and/or immunodeficiency.

(iii) Other patients may have no readily observable abnormalities.

(iv) A variety of congenital heart defects have been found in these patients, most of **conotruncal origin.**

(v) More than half of patients who have type B interrupted aortic arch are found to have deletion 22q11.

(c) Parents of affected children should also be tested because studies have shown a 10% incidence of familial deletion, occasionally in a normal-appearing parent.

(2) **Cri du chat syndrome** occurs in 1 in 50,000 newborns.

(a) **Defect.** The syndrome is caused by a deletion of material from the terminal end of the short arm of chromosome 5 (**5p-**).

TABLE 8-9 Clinical Findings in Deletion 22q11 Syndrome

Growth	Mild short stature
Craniofacial	Cleft palate (without cleft lip)
	Velopharyngeal insufficiency (hypernasal speech)
	Small ears, unusual ears; Tubular nose
	"Squared-off" nasal tip
	Mild malar hypoplasia
Cardiac	Most commonly conotruncal defects
Immunologic	Thymic aplasia (T-cell deficiency)
Extremities	Long-appearing tapered fingers
Endocrine	Hypocalcemia (may be transient)
Neurologic	Low IQ to mild mental retardation
	Learning disabilities
Behavior	Attention deficit disorder
	Difficulty with social interaction
Psychiatric	Bipolar disorder
	Other affective disorders
	Psychotic symptoms

IQ, intelligence quotient.

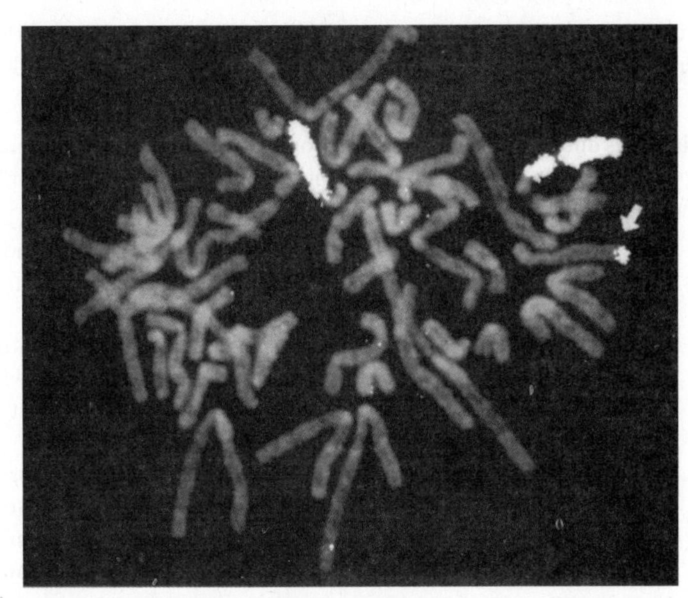

FIGURE 8-3 Chromosome painting using fluorescence-tagged DNA library for chromosome 14. There is a translocation involving the long arms for chromosomes 13 and 14. The proband has two normal chromosomes 14 and a derivative 13 with a small piece of 14 translocated to it. (Photograph courtesy of S. Schwartz, Ph.D.)

(b) **Clinical features**

(i) Affected children have a characteristic cat-like cry.

(ii) Profound mental retardation and CNS abnormalities are consistent findings.

(iii) Congenital heart disease is common, as are ocular malformations (e.g., cataracts, optic atrophy).

(c) **Prognosis.** Patients can survive into adulthood.

2. **Partial trisomy**

a. **Defect.** Partial trisomy results when extra chromosome material is found in the karyotype, but there is less than an entire extra chromosome present.

(1) The extra chromosome material can occur at the end of the long or short arm of the chromosome, or it may be inserted within the normal chromosome.

(2) Occasionally a small piece of extra chromosomal material, with or without a centromere, is found in the karyotype. This is referred to as a **marker** chromosome. Some small marker chromosomes do not cause any phenotypic effect. When a marker is diagnosed prenatally, demonstration that one of the clinically normal parents also has the marker is reassuring that the prognosis is good for the fetus.

b. **Clinical features.** The origin of the extra chromosome material determines the phenotypic effect. When the extra material is autosomal in origin, dysmorphic features, growth insufficiency, malformations, and developmental abnormalities are commonly seen.

c. **Diagnosis**

(1) **High-resolution banding** or **FISH** can sometimes identify the origin of the extra chromosome material, especially if it is large.

(2) **Parental karyotypes** should be obtained because the partial trisomy sometimes results from a balanced parental translocation (Figure 8-3).

V NONTRADITIONAL INHERITANCE

A number of conditions have been identified where the inheritance pattern does not follow the standard patterns originally described by **Mendel** (e.g., autosomal dominant, autosomal recessive, or X-linked).

A **Mosaicism** refers to the presence of two or more cell lines with different chromosome compositions in an individual. Mosaicism occurs as a result of mitotic nondisjunction after fertilization. The genetic change is not carried by a parent, so the risk for recurrence of a child with mosaicism is usually negligible. The phenotype is affected by the number and tissue distribution of abnormal versus normal cells. Mosaicism can be a feature in single gene disorders (neurofibromatosis type 1) or chromosomal disorders (Turner syndrome, Down syndrome).

B **Disorders due to genetic imprinting.** Some genes are expressed differently, depending on the parent from whom the gene was inherited. This differential modification, or marking, of genes is a normal phenomenon known as genetic imprinting.

1. Some genes are inactivated when inherited from the father, and others are inactivated when inherited from the mother. These **inactivated genes** are not transcribed into gene products to the same extent as the gene from the other-sex parent.
   a. In **genetic imprinting,** the gene is intact and normal, but has somehow been modified so that its expression is modulated, depending on the parent from whom it was inherited. **Hypermethylation** of the gene, preventing transcription, is the most commonly recognized mechanism of imprinting.
   b. Imprinting is a **reversible process.** When the gene is processed during gametogenesis, the imprint is erased and reset, determined by the sex of the transmitting parent.
   c. Only a relatively small proportion (< 5%) of the genes in the human genome are known to be affected by imprinting. The pattern of imprinting is complex and can vary from tissue to tissue.
2. **Prader-Willi syndrome (PWS)** was the first disorder recognized as involving imprinted genes. PWS occurs in 1 in 15,000 newborns.
   a. **Defect.** This syndrome is associated with absence of paternally contributed genes on the long arm of chromosome 15(q11-q13).
      (1) In the normal individual, the maternal contribution to the relevant region of chromosome 15 is not expressed; there is gene expression from only the paternal copy. In PWS, the paternal copy of these genes has either been deleted or is missing due to maternal uniparental disomy (*see V B 2 a [3] and V C*) or is abnormally imprinted, so that no active copies of these genes are present.
      (2) Approximately 70% of patients who have PWS have a chromosome deletion detected by high-resolution chromosome analysis, FISH, or molecular genetic analysis. The deleted chromosome is always of paternal origin. Methylation analysis detects all cases of PWS.
      (3) Approximately 25% of patients with PWS who have a normal-appearing chromosome complement are missing the paternal contribution to 15q due to absence of the entire paternal chromosome 15 and presence of two number 15 chromosomes of maternal origin. This is called maternal **uniparental disomy** (UPD).
         (a) Two copies of chromosome 15 are required for survival. For most of the genes on this chromosome, it does not matter whether the genes are maternal or paternal in origin, because most of the genes on chromosome 15 are not imprinted.
         (b) UPD probably occurs because of nondisjunction, which leads to a trisomy followed by loss of the chromosome from the parent who contributes only one copy to the trisomy. In PWS, the trisomy would contain one paternal 15 and two maternal 15s, and would be followed by loss of the paternal 15.
      (4) A small proportion of patients (approximately 5%) have a chromosome translocation or other structural rearrangement involving 15q. This is associated with either UPD or a small deletion.
      (5) A few patients have PWS because of a defect in switching the imprint when the father passes on his maternally inherited (imprinted) chromosome 15.
   b. **Recurrence risk.** The empiric recurrence risk is < 1 in 100, unless the chromosome 15 deletion is the result of an imprinting defect, parental translocation, or, rarely, some other rearrangement.
   c. **Clinical features**
      (1) Children with PWS have severe **infantile hypotonia** associated with feeding difficulties and **failure to thrive** in infancy. Later (between 1 and 4 years of age), **central obesity** develops in these children due to an appetite disorder. An abnormal satiety mechanism leads these individuals to eat large amounts of food unless strict dietary control is enforced.
      (2) **Developmental delay** is a major feature. Most patients are mildly mentally retarded, although there is a range of IQs observed. Behavior problems are common. A charac-

teristic personality type is seen, typically with temper tantrums, difficulty with change in routine, and obsessive-compulsive features.

(3) **Dysmorphic features** include narrow bifrontal diameter, almond-shaped palpebral fissures, a downturned mouth, and small hands and feet.

(4) **Hypogonadotrophic hypogonadism** is present, which manifests as small genitalia and incomplete puberty.

(5) There is mild **short stature** in adulthood.

d. **Prognosis.** Lifespan is shortened only by the complications of obesity (e.g., diabetes mellitus, hypoventilation).

e. **Treatment.** Recombinant **growth hormone** is now used to treat individuals with Prader-Willi syndrome from infancy to adulthood with improvement in growth and early motor development and weight control with increased lean muscle mass. Behavioral interventions with strict supervised adherence to diet and exercise allow individuals to maintain a healthy weight.

3. Much is yet to be learned about the impact of genetic imprinting in causing human genetic disorders. It is known that many imprinted genes are growth related, and abnormalities relating to the "dose" (i.e., zero, one, or two active copies) of imprinted genes often cause undergrowth or overgrowth.

C Uniparental disomy When UPD for a chromosome occurs, it can have three different consequences.

1. If there are no imprinted genes and no abnormal genes on the chromosome, no consequences are expected. This has been reported for several chromosomes, including 1, 3, 4, 13, 21, and 22.
2. If there are one or more imprinted genes, an abnormality may ensue, as is the case in PWS and several other recognized conditions, including **Angelman syndrome** (associated with absence of maternally inherited 15[q11q13]) and **Beckwith-Wiedemann syndrome** (associated with imprinted genes on 11p). Effects of UPD have also been described for chromosomes 6, 7, and 14.
3. In UPD, the two chromosomes from the same parent can be the two different chromosomes in that parent **(heterodisomy)** or duplicate copies of only one of the parent's chromosomes **(isodisomy).** In the latter case, a recessive mutation present in a single nonimprinted gene on that duplicated chromosome could result in an autosomal recessive disorder, even though only one parent was a carrier. This has been identified in a number of instances, after being first recognized in a case of **cystic fibrosis.**

D Trinucleotide (or triplet) repeat expansion Some genetic diseases have been recognized to become more severe, or to occur at an earlier age, in successive generations. A molecular basis for this phenomenon, called **anticipation,** has been shown for disorders due to elongation of repeated stretches of three nucleotides.

1. **Defect.** Normally these genes have a small number of copies of the repeated sequence (e.g., < 37 CAG trinucleotide repeats in Huntington disease).

   a. During meiosis the number of repeats may increase. The mechanism for this expansion is not well understood.

   b. For some disorders there may be an intermediate stage, called a **premutation,** where there is expansion beyond the normal range, but not enough to cause the disorder. Premutations are more likely to expand in future meioses.

   c. There is frequently a predilection for expansion during meiosis in parents of one sex. This is condition-specific, and may involve the mother (e.g., fragile X syndrome and myotonic dystrophy) or the father (e.g., Huntington disease and spinocerebellar ataxia type I).

   d. The expanded trinucleotide repeat may involve:

   (1) A coding region of the gene (exon)—for example, Huntington disease (coding for a polyglutamine tract)

   (2) A noncoding region of the gene (intron)—for example, Friedreich ataxia

   (3) A genetic sequence outside of the gene in the 5′ or 3′ untranslated region—for example, the fragile X gene (*FMR1*) and the myotonic dystrophy gene (*DMPK*), respectively

2. **Clinical features.** There is wide variety in the age of onset and clinical course in these disorders. However, all of the disorders described to date that are due to trinucleotide repeat expansion primarily involve neurologic phenotypes (Table 8-10).

TABLE 8-10 Examples of Disorders Caused by Trinucleotide Repeat Expansions

Disorder	Inheritance	Trinucleotide Sequence	Number of Repeats: Normal	Number of Repeats: Affected	Clinical Findings
Myotonic dystrophy	AD	CTG	5–27	> 50 May be > 1000	Myotonia Muscle wasting Cataract Cardiac conduction defect Smooth muscle abnormalities Testicular atrophy Frontal baldness Hypotonia and respiratory distress in congenital form Mental retardation in congenital form
Huntington disease	AD	CAG	9–37	> 37	Chorea Dementia Psychiatric symptoms (especially depression) Onset third to fourth decade
Spinocerebellar ataxia type I	AD	CAG	19–38	40–80	Cerebellar ataxia Chorea Hyperreflexia Onset third to fourth decade
Friedreich ataxia	AR	GAA	7–20	> 100	Cerebellar ataxia Absent deep tendon reflexes Dysarthria Cardiomyopathy Onset second to third decade May also be due to other mutations in the gene
Fragile X syndrome	XLR	CGG	6–52	> 200	Mental retardation Macrocephaly Post pubertal Macroorchidism Dysmorphic features
X-linked spinal and bulbar muscular atrophy	XLR	CAG	19–25	> 40	Facial fasciculation Bulbar signs Muscle weakness Androgen deficiency Onset in third decade

AD, autosomal dominant; AR, autosomal recessive; XLR, X-linked recessive.

3. **Inheritance.** Most of these disorders are inherited in an autosomal dominant manner. Table 8-10 shows some examples of the known triplet repeat disorders, including three that do not have autosomal dominant inheritance. Fragile X is a notable exception (X linked).

VI ENVIRONMENTAL FACTORS

A General principles An individual's environment (pre- and postnatal) can have modifying effects not only on development, but also on the continued expression of many genes. **Environmental factors** are known to cause at least 10% of all birth defects. Individuals with different genetic backgrounds may exhibit variable responses to the same environmental exposures.

B **Teratogens** are environmental agents that increase the risk for a **specific** congenital malformation or a specific pattern of anomalies by interfering with embryonic or fetal organogenesis, growth, or cellular physiology, or by disrupting previously normal tissue. A general increase in all malformations is usually due to increased reporting in cases where there is an undesired outcome or side effect (i.e., bias of ascertainment). Usually, not every exposed fetus shows the effect of a teratogen. Genetic factors in the mother or fetus may affect the impact of teratogens.

1. **Proving** the relationship between a substance to which a fetus is exposed and a birth defect involves the consideration of several important factors.
2. **Timing of exposure.** Exposure to a teratogen before implantation (days 7–10 postconception) will either result in loss of the embryo or no effect. Morphogenesis occurs for only the first 8 to 12 weeks, so that any structural abnormality in tissue development must occur before 12 weeks' gestation. Thereafter, growth and CNS development are primarily affected.
3. **Dosage is important.** For many teratogens there is a threshold below which no effect is demonstrable.
4. **Genetic background** of the mother and, especially, the fetus determines whether a specific fetus will be affected (e.g., only 11% of fetuses whose mothers take hydantoins during pregnancy will exhibit fetal hydantoin syndrome).

C **Infectious agents,** especially **"TORCH" organisms** (including *Toxoplasma gondii,* rubella virus, cytomegalovirus, and herpes simplex virus), are known to be responsible for a significant proportion of birth defects (see Chapter 6).

D **Medication, drugs,** and **chemicals** can interfere with embryonic and fetal development.

1. **Anticonvulsant drug (ACD)** exposure during pregnancy can cause fetal damage. A specific pattern of anomalies including fetal growth disturbance and skeletal and CNS abnormalities is seen in some infants exposed to **hydantoins.** Valproic acid is associated with increased risk of neural tube defects. Fetal effects have also been described with other ACDs. However, because prolonged seizures during pregnancy may also cause fetal damage, current management goals for pregnant women with seizure disorders are monotherapy with the lowest effective dose of ACD, along with careful monitoring, during pregnancy.
2. **Thalidomide** exposure during pregnancy has been associated with limb malformations and cleft palate.
3. **Retinoic acid** exposure during pregnancy, especially exposure to isotretinoin, results in brain, ear, and heart malformations.
4. **Tetracycline** exposure causes dark staining of teeth.
5. **Other teratogenic chemicals** have been described, including anticoagulants, antithyroid medications, cancer chemotherapeutic agents, angiotensin-converting enzyme inhibitors, iodine-containing agents, lead, lithium, and mercury.

E **Maternal metabolic disorders** can also adversely influence fetal development.

1. **Diabetes.** Infants of diabetic mothers have a 10% to 15% risk for birth defects, particularly those involving the heart, skeleton, brain, and spinal cord. The causative factor is believed to be hyperglycemia. Careful control of diabetes before conception and throughout pregnancy decreases the risk for birth defects.
2. **Phenylketonuria.** Infants of mothers who have PKU are exposed during pregnancy to excess metabolites of the amino acid phenylalanine. Brain and congenital heart defects occur in nearly every fetus exposed to uncontrolled maternal PKU. Dietary control in the mother significantly decreases this risk and should begin before conception (*see III D 3 f [2][c][iii]*).

F **Mechanical forces**

1. **Intrauterine mechanical forces** can result in **deformations.**
   a. Intrauterine tumors or fibroids or abnormal uterine anatomy may result in a fetus that is constrained, thereby causing breech presentation, facial distortions, developmental dysplasia of the hip, or club feet.
   b. Inadequate amniotic fluid (oligohydramnios) results in severe fetal constraint and may also be associated with hypoplasia of the lungs.

2. **External mechanical forces** can result in **disruptions of fetal blood supply.** These forces can include the formation of bands of tissue from the amniotic sac that can cause limb hypoplasia or transverse amputations.
   a. Similar patterns of abnormality due to vascular disruption can be seen in fetuses exposed to cocaine in utero.
   b. A deceased co-twin can also cause vascular disruption.

G Maternal alcohol use Alcohol is the most common teratogen to which the fetus may be exposed. The amount of alcohol consumed appears to correlate with the degree of adverse effect on the fetus. A genetic predisposition may play a significant role in determining which fetuses will be severely or mildly affected by maternal alcohol use and which will be unaffected, although specific genetic factors have not yet been identified. The timing of the alcohol use also plays a role in determining alcohol's effect on the developing fetus.

1. **Fetal alcohol syndrome** (FAS) represents a frequent and striking example of a teratogenic disorder.
   a. **Incidence**
      (1) In most populations, fetal alcohol syndrome occurs in 1 to 2 per 1000 newborns, and it is estimated that an additional 7 in 1000 may exhibit milder effects often with neurodevelopmental abnormalities. The syndrome affects 30% to 45% of the offspring of females who consume more than four to six alcoholic drinks per day while pregnant.
      (2) An estimated 10% to 20% of cases of mild to moderate mental retardation are the result of the effects of alcohol in utero.
   b. **Clinical features** of fetal alcohol syndrome include evidence of maternal alcohol use, pre- and postnatal growth deficiencies, physical features characteristic of FAS (facial dysmorphisms—small eyes, hypoplastic midface, long smooth philtrum), and anomalies such as joint contractures, cardiac and kidney malformations, and CNS dysfunction (mean intelligence quotient [IQ] of 63, infantile tremulousness, childhood hyperactivity) (Figure 8-4).
2. **Fetal alcohol *spectrum* disorders.** In those offspring of alcoholic females who do not manifest the complete fetal alcohol syndrome, one or more of the anomalies seen in that syndrome can sometimes be found (e.g., a pattern of alcohol-related neurodevelopmental defects has been

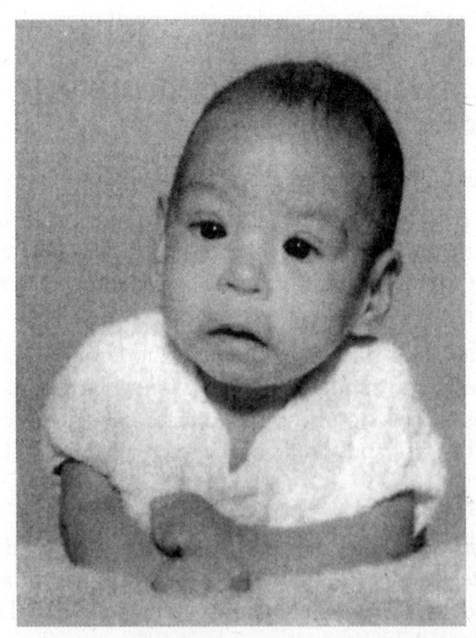

FIGURE 8-4 Characteristic dysmorphic facial features in an infant with fetal alcohol syndrome. Note mild ptosis; epicanthal folds; flat nasal bridge, short nose; long, smooth philtrum; and thin upper vermilion border. (Photograph courtesy of T. Kellerman.)

described in exposed children). It is important to rule out other causes for the abnormalities before ascribing the effects to alcohol exposure, as alternative diagnoses may have different associated findings and recurrence risk.

3. **Miscarriage.** There is an increased risk of miscarriage, which is proportional to the amount of alcohol consumed.
4. **Other effects.** Lesser amounts of alcohol have been shown to produce milder symptoms in a proportion of exposed offspring, particularly with regard to size and behavior. There are no data supporting a "safe" amount of alcohol use during pregnancy. Thus, alcohol is to be avoided entirely during pregnancy.

H **Environmental pollutants** of various types have been suggested as possible teratogens, although it has been very difficult to study such agents. Birth defects registries, which exist in many states, may be helpful in implicating or absolving specific environmental pollutants as causes of birth defects.

VII MULTIFACTORIAL DISORDERS

A General characteristics

1. **Multifactorial or complex disorders** are conditions that are believed to be caused by a combination of genetic and environmental (nongenetic) factors. Many birth defects and common disorders of midlife are ascribed to multifactorial inheritance.
2. **Incidence** is variable for the different multifactorial disorders, but is frequently as high as 1 in 1000, or even more common for some conditions, such as congenital heart disease.
3. **Recurrence risk.** Individuals who have a multifactorial disorder or who have a child with a multifactorial disorder have approximately a 2% to 5% empiric risk for recurrence of the disorder with each subsequent pregnancy.
   a. Unlike single gene disorders, the recurrence risk for multifactorial disorders increases with an increasing number of affected relatives and increasing severity of the disorder.
   b. The male (M)-to-female (F) ratio differs for several multifactorial disorders (e.g., developmental dysplasia of the hip [F > M] and cleft lip [M > F]). When this is the case, the recurrence risk for first-degree relatives is greater when the affected individual is of the less-often-affected sex.
   c. The recurrence risk is greater when the affected individual is more severely affected. For example, the recurrence risk is greater when a child has bilateral cleft lip and palate compared to isolated cleft lip.
4. **Examples.** Common multifactorial disorders include:
   a. **Common birth defects** (e.g., club foot, cleft lip with or without cleft palate, neural tube defects [meningomyelocele, anencephaly], congenital heart defects, developmental dysplasia of the hip, and pyloric stenosis)
   b. **Mental retardation** (when a specific cause is not identified)
   c. **Affective disorders** (e.g., bipolar disorder)
   d. **Common disorders of midlife** (e.g., hypertension, hyperlipidemia, diabetes mellitus, coronary artery disease, cancer)

B **Neural tube defects,** including meningomyelocele and anencephaly (see Chapter 18), occur in 1 to 2 in 1000 newborns in the United States.

1. **Risk factors.** Anencephaly and meningomyelocele represent variable expression of the same disorder. A person at risk for this disorder may have a child with either manifestation. Neural tube defects show classic multifactorial inheritance, but the incidence varies due to a number of factors.
   a. **Geographic location** is important, with the incidence being highest in Ireland and Wales.
   b. **Economic class** is another important variable, with higher incidence in poorer groups.
   c. **Maternal age** is a factor. There is a bimodel distribution, with both teenage mothers and older mothers are at increased risk.
   d. **Prenatal exposure** to known contributory environmental factors, such as valproic acid and maternal diabetes, results in an increased risk.
2. **Recurrence risk** increases with each additional first-degree relative who is affected.

a. For a couple with one child who has a NTD, the recurrence risk for each subsequent child to be affected is 3% to 5%, increasing to 7% to 10% after a second affected child is born.
b. A person who has a meningomyelocele has a 2% to 4% risk of having an affected child with each pregnancy.

3. **Preventive therapy**
   a. Current studies demonstrate that the recurrence risk for neural tube defects may be lowered significantly by taking 4 mg of **folic acid** daily from the time of conception through the time of formation of the neural tube (end of first trimester). As a result, many physicians recommend starting a prenatal vitamin preparation that contains adequate folate before conception.
   b. Studies also suggest that taking 0.4 mg of folic acid daily beginning **before conception** and continuing through the second month of gestation (after neural tube closure is complete) may significantly lower the incidence of neural tube defects in the general population.

C **Orofacial clefts** are common birth defects with multifactorial inheritance.

1. **Cleft lip with or without cleft palate** is seen in 1 to 2 per 1000 liveborn infants.
   a. **Risk factors**
      (1) Twice as many boys are born with cleft lip, with or without cleft palate, as girls.
      (2) The incidence of cleft lip is highest in Asian and some Native American populations, and lowest in African Americans.
   b. **Differential diagnosis.** There are more than 50 syndromes that include cleft lip with or without cleft palate, and these must be excluded before making the diagnosis of isolated (i.e., multifactorial) cleft lip with or without cleft palate. These syndromes may be autosomal dominant, autosomal recessive, X-linked, chromosomal, or sporadic. Cleft lip may be associated with exposure to **teratogenic agents.**
   c. **Recurrence risk**
      (1) Recurrence risk if one child or one parent is affected is 3% to 5%.
      (2) Recurrence risk if two children or one child and one parent are affected is 10%.
      (3) Recurrence risk is higher if affected individuals have bilateral cleft lip and palate or if females are affected.
2. **Cleft palate** is a multifactorial condition distinct from cleft lip with or without cleft palate that is seen in 1 in 2000 liveborn infants.
   a. **Risk factors**
      (1) Girls are affected more frequently than boys.
      (2) The recurrence risks for cleft palate without cleft lip are similar to those for cleft lip with or without cleft palate; however, there is no increased risk for having a child with cleft lip.
   b. **Differential diagnosis.** There are more than 150 syndromes that involve cleft palate; therefore, other abnormalities must be excluded before making a diagnosis of isolated cleft palate.
   c. Another form of cleft palate is caused by **micrognathia (hypoplastic mandible)** and projection of the tongue posteriorly during development, preventing closure of the palate. This phenomenon is called **Pierre Robin sequence.**
      (1) The cleft is usually U-shaped.
      (2) The **recurrence risk** is generally low because the Pierre Robin sequence is usually sporadic; however, the Pierre Robin sequence can be associated with syndromes such as **Stickler syndrome, 22q11 deletion syndrome,** and **Treacher Collins syndrome.** When a syndrome is present, the recurrence risk depends on the inheritance of the syndrome. There are more than 50 syndromes in which the Pierre Robin sequence is a feature.

BIBLIOGRAPHY

Buyse ML (ed): *The Birth Defects Encyclopedia.* Cambridge, MA, Blackwell Scientific, 1990.
Cassidy SB, Allanson JE: *Management of Genetic Syndromes,* 2nd ed., Hoboken, Wiley Liss, 2005.
Gelehrter TD, Collins FS, Ginsberg D: *Principles of Medical Genetics,* 2nd ed. Baltimore, Williams and Wilkins, 1998.
Gorlin RJ, Cohen MM, Levin JS: *Syndromes of the Head and Neck,* 3rd ed. New York, Oxford University Press, 1990.
Jones KL: *Smith's Recognizable Patterns of Human Malformation,* 6th ed. Philadelphia, WB Saunders, 2006.
McKusick VA: *Mendelian Inheritance in Man,* 12th ed. Baltimore, Johns Hopkins University Press, 1998. (Online: www.ncbi.nlm.nih.gov/Omim/)

Nussbaum RL, McInnes RR, Willard HF (eds): *Thomson and Thompson Genetics in Medicine*, 6th ed. Philadelphia, WB Saunders, 2001.

Rimoin DL, Connor JM, Pyeritz RE (eds): *Emory and Rimoin's Principles and Practice of Medical Genetics,* 3rd ed. New York, Churchill-Livingstone, 1996.

Scriver CR, Beaudet AL, Sly WS, et al. (eds): *The Metabolic and Molecular Bases of Inherited Disease,* 7th ed. New York, McGraw-Hill, 1995.

Stevenson RE, Hall JG, Goodman RM (eds): *Human Malformations and Related Disorders.* New York, Oxford University Press, 1993.

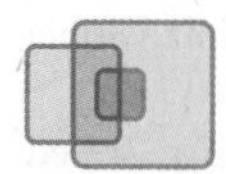

Study Questions

Directions: *Each of the numbered items or incomplete statements in this section is followed by answers or completions of the statements. Select the ONE lettered answer or completion that is BEST in each case.*

1. A newborn girl has been diagnosed as having phenylketonuria (PKU), the most common disorder of amino acid metabolism, through state newborn screening. Which of the following consequences will early initiation of dietary treatment protect this child from?

A Seizure disorder
B Hypoglycemia
C Mental retardation
D Hearing loss
E Failure to thrive

2. A young woman with PKU should be counseled preconceptually about the risk of birth defects in her offspring. Which of the following is the most important thing that she can do preconceptionally to decrease the risk of birth defects in her offspring?

A Monitor her urine for ketones
B Dietary restriction of phenylalanine
C Daily folic acid supplementation
D Initiate a low-protein diet
E Monitor her blood sugar

3. You learn that the father of your 12-year-old pediatric patient has recently received a clinical diagnosis of Marfan syndrome. Which of the following evaluations is most important for your patient?

A Echocardiography
B Arm span-to-height ratio
C Homocystinuria level
D Spine and chest radiographs
E Ophthalmologic exam

4. You are asked to counsel a couple whose first child was born with a neural tube defect. The pregnancy history, the infant's physical examination, and the family history are unrevealing. The parents want to know what caused the child's birth defect. Which of the following is the most likely cause of their child's birth defect?

A It is the result of a teratogen
B It is the result of low maternal serum α-fetoprotein level
C It is the result of a spontaneous mutation
D It is the result of a multifactorial phenomenon
E It is the result of a chromosomal imbalance

5. A 5-year-old child has coarse facial features, hand contractures, hepatosplenomegaly, and progressive loss of developmental milestones. Which of the following disorders is the most likely diagnosis in this child?

A Mucopolysaccharidosis
B Congenital disorder of glycosylation
C Aminoaciduria
D Urea cycle enzyme deficiency
E Hereditary fructose intolerance

6. A pregnant woman is referred for genetic counseling. She has ingested significant amounts of alcohol throughout pregnancy. During the session, the genetic counselor describes the clinical problems that may occur in children secondary to maternal alcohol ingestion during pregnancy. Which of the following constellation of findings is most consistent with a diagnosis of fetal alcohol syndrome?

A A large for gestational age child with omphalocele
B A dysmorphic child with tetralogy of Fallot and hypocalcemia
C A hypotonic child with up-slanting palpebral fissures and a single palmar crease
D A small for gestational age child with narrow palpebral fissures and smooth philtrum
E A child with a neural tube defect

7. A 26-year-old woman gives birth to a child with trisomy 21 Down syndrome. Which of the following should you counsel about the chance that a subsequent pregnancy will be affected with a trisomy?

A The risk is $< 1\%$, given her age
B The risk can be increased by prenatal exposure to teratogens
C The risk can be decreased by prenatal supplementation with folic acid
D The risk is as high as 25%
E The risk is approximately 1%

8. An otherwise healthy, normally grown 5-year-old boy without striking dysmorphic features has significant developmental delay. He has a 3-year-old brother who is not yet talking. Which of the following evaluations is indicated for this patient?

A Myotonic dystrophy testing
B Fragile X molecular studies
C Methylation for Prader Willi syndrome
D Serum α-fetoprotein testing
E Uric acid level

Directions: *Each set of matching questions in this section consists of a list of 4 to 6 lettered options followed by several numbered items. For each numbered item, select the ONE lettered option that is most closely associated with it. Each lettered option may be selected once, more than once, or not at all.*

QUESTIONS 9–12

For each of the following pregnant patients, select the optimal first test that should be offered to the woman for prenatal diagnosis.

A Level II (specialized) fetal ultrasound
B Amniocentesis or chorionic villus sampling
C Maternal serum (triple/quad) screening
D Periumbilical blood sampling
E Fetoscopy

9. A 27-year-old woman in her 18th week of pregnancy; both the patient and her husband are heterozygous for the sickle cell mutation.

10. A 30-year-old woman with a negative family history for birth defects and genetic disorders who is 16 weeks pregnant.

11. A 29-year-old woman who previously had a child with microcephaly.

12. A 22-year-old woman in her 10th week of pregnancy whose husband is a carrier of a familial balanced translocation.

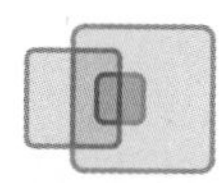

Answers and Explanations

1 and 2. The answers are 1-C and 2-B (*III D 3 f 2*). Phenylketonuria is an autosomal recessive disorder of amino acid metabolism that is characterized by a lack of conversion of phenylalanine to tyrosine. Dietary restriction of phenylalanine should start early in infancy (by age 1 month) and be maintained throughout life, because this measure will prevent the mental retardation and neurologic and behavior problems characteristic of the untreated disorder. Lifelong therapy is especially important for females with PKU who are at a high risk for giving birth to children with microcephaly and congenital heart disease when they are off dietary restriction during pregnancy. Also, adolescents and adults who stop dietary restriction have been shown to have decreased cognitive function. Because tyrosine is essential to the production of the pigment melanin, hypopigmentation is a common sign of untreated PKU. Although prenatal use of folic acid has been shown to decrease the incidence of neural tube defects, in this individual, the overall risk of neural tube defects (1 in 500 in the United States) is lower than the risk of the teratogenic effects of maternal hyperphenylalaninemia.

3. The answer is A (*III C 2, Table 8-5*). Marfan syndrome is an autosomal dominant disorder of connective tissue caused by mutations in the fibrillin gene. Each offspring of an affected individual is at 50% risk of inheriting the condition. Major manifestations include a characteristic body habitus (i.e., long, thin digits and limbs with increased arm span-to-height ratio; loose joints; scoliosis; and chest deformity), aortic dilatation, mitral valve prolapse, lens dislocation, and myopia. The most serious medical consequence of this condition is aortic root dilation, which in some cases can lead to sudden death due to rupture.

4. The answer is D (*VII B*). Neural tube defects are due to a defect of closure of the neural groove. Failure of cranial closure results in anencephaly, and distal failure to close results in meningomyelocele (spina bifida); both conditions occur on the basis of a multifactorial disorder with two possible manifestations. The recurrence risk for neural tube defects increases with each additional first-degree relative who is affected. A couple with one affected child and no other family history has a 3% to 5% risk of having another child with a neural tube defect; the risk is higher after a second affected child is born. High maternal serum α-fetoprotein levels, which reflect an abnormal opening between the fetus and amniotic fluid, occur in 85% of pregnancies in which a neural tube defect is present. Neural tube defects rarely are part of a syndrome. Neural tube defects can be due to teratogens (e.g., valproic acid), but in this case there is no history of prenatal exposures.

5. The answer is A (*III D 3 i*). The mucopolysaccharidoses are caused by an inability to catabolize one of several glycosaminoglycans that make up the intracellular substance and are lysosomal storage disorders. Therefore, mucopolysaccharides accumulate in skin (causing coarse features), internal organs (causing hepatosplenomegaly), and the brain (causing progressive intellectual impairment). Disorders of glycosylation, amino acid metabolism, urea cycle enzyme deficiency, and hereditary fructose intolerance are not associated with storage of metabolites.

6. The answer is D (*VI G 1, 2*). Alcohol exposure during gestation can produce a child who has some or all of the features of the fetal alcohol syndrome, or the exposure can have no recognizable effect. Clinical features of fetal alcohol syndrome include central nervous system abnormalities (e.g., intellectual defects, microcephaly); growth deficiencies; facial dysmorphisms including narrow palpebral fissures, smooth philtrum and thin upper lip, and flat midface; and other structural anomalies (e.g., congenital heart disease). Neither Beckwith/Wiedemann syndrome, Down syndrome, nor chromosome microdeletions occur at increased frequency as a result of maternal alcohol use. Neural tube defects may be due to teratogens such as valproate, but are rarely associated with prenatal alcohol use.

7. The answer is E (*IV B 1*). Down syndrome, the most common chromosome abnormality seen in liveborn infants (population incidence of ~1 in 700), is caused by trisomy of chromosome 21. The trisomy usually results from maternal nondisjunction during meiosis; however, no preventable mechanism has ever been identified. The extra chromosomal material results in a characteristic pattern of dysmorphic features and mental disability, with an increased risk for internal malformations, especially congenital heart defects and duodenal atresia. Mental retardation generally is moderate, with the average intelligence quotient being 50. For each of this couple's subsequent pregnancies, there is an increased risk of aneuploidy, including trisomy 21, of ~1%. When maternal age-related risk for aneuploidy is > 1%, this risk estimate prevails.

8. The answer is B (*III E 1, Table 8-10*). Mental retardation has many causes, including fragile X syndrome, chromosome abnormalities, metabolic disorders, and heritable syndromes. Fragile X syndrome is an important consideration particularly in boys with mental retardation, and undoubtedly in brothers with mental retardation. With an unremarkable past medical history and normal growth, metabolic causes are less likely. Serum α-fetoprotein testing is used for prenatal screening or screening for cancer. Although myotonic dystrophy can affect intelligence, neurologic features such as ptosis and hypotonia are prominent. Similarly, Prader/Willi affects cognitive function, but infantile hypotonia and failure to thrive followed by hyperphagia are characteristic. Uric acid is a screen for Lesch-Nyhan syndrome, which is characterized by mental retardation and self-destructive biting of fingers and lips.

9–12. The answers are 9-B (*I E 2*), **10-C** (*I E 1*), **11-A** (*I E 1* [*C*]), and **12-B** (*I E 2*). Amniocentesis is a procedure performed as early as 12 weeks' gestation for various analyses of amniotic fluid, including the study of specific biochemical or DNA markers in the cells or fluid. Chorionic villus sampling is performed at 8 to 11 weeks' gestation and can provide fetal cells for biochemical or DNA analysis; amniotic fluid is not available by this technique. Sickle cell disease is an autosomal recessive disorder for which DNA-based testing is available. When both parents are heterozygotes, their child has a 25% chance of being affected. Amniocentesis and chorionic villus sampling provide material containing fetal DNA that can be analyzed for the sickle cell mutation.

Maternal serum screening, using maternal biomarkers including AFP, can be considered in every pregnancy, because it carries no risk and can raise suspicion of either an open defect (e.g., neural tube defect) or chromosomal aneuploidy.

Microcephaly can be genetic and may be diagnosed in utero through accurate head measurements by ultrasound, because norms exist for head size at each gestational age.

A familial balanced translocation predisposes the couple to having chromosomally unbalanced offspring with abnormal phenotype. Amniocentesis or chorionic villus sampling allows determination of fetal chromosome constitution. Percutaneous umbilical blood sampling will also detect a chromosomal alteration, but this procedure carries a higher risk.

chapter **9**

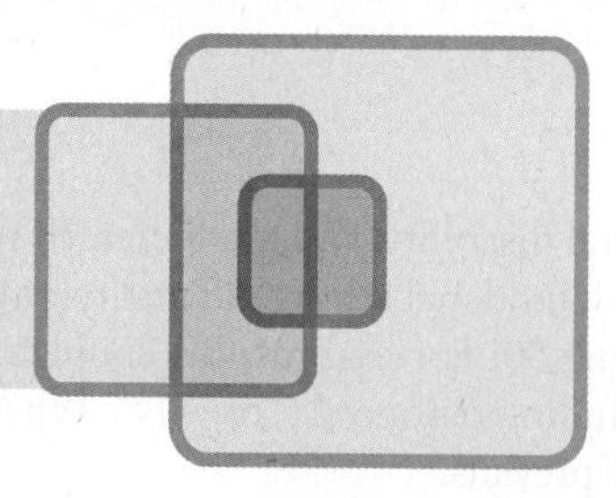

Immunologic, Allergic, and Rheumatologic Diseases

HILLARY HERNANDEZ-TRUJILLO • MARSHALL GRODOFSKY • BARBARA EDELHEIT

I INTRODUCTION

The human immune system is an essential defense mechanism that allows us to live in harmony with the outside world. When certain components are missing or overly abundant, the balance of our immune system can be shifted so that we are unable to fight particular infections (**immunologic disorders**), we overreact to our environment (**allergic disorders**), or we even mistake ourselves for the enemy (**autoimmune disorders**). The next four sections describe this delicate balance and what happens when disruptions occur.

II HOST DEFENSE SYSTEMS AND IMMUNOLOGIC DEFICIENCIES

The host defense system is a dynamic network of cellular and humoral elements working in concert to allow the host to **distinguish between self and nonself** in order to recognize foreign substances and eliminate, neutralize, or metabolize those substances. Functions of the immune system include resistance to microbial invasion, maintenance of homeostasis, and surveillance against transformed or malignant cells.

A Evaluation for immunodeficiency disorders

Any patient who has a history of frequent infections, trouble clearing infections, or susceptibility to opportunistic infections should be evaluated for an immunodeficiency.

1. **History of infections.** Severe, recurrent, or persistent infections strongly suggest an immunodeficiency disorder. It is important to discover the **age of onset** as the younger the age at onset, the more serious the immunodeficiency, unless the immune deficiency is acquired. Also, the **site of infection** can be an important clue as serious sites of infection (as in meningitis, organ abscess, pneumonia, sepsis, or generalized dermatitis) suggest an underlying immunodeficiency. Often, these patients will present with infections in multiple organ systems, chronic skin infections, or even failure to thrive. Typically, the **causative agents** are important to know as well, as they can provide clues as to which type of immunodeficiency is present.
2. **Family history.** A pedigree chart is helpful because many immunodeficiency disorders are autosomal recessive or X-linked.
3. **Social history.** It is important to know if the person is an IV drug user, their sexual orientation, if they were exposed to blood products before testing began, or if they have recently moved from an endemic region.
4. **Adverse reactions to drugs and vaccines.** For example, polio and blood product transfusion reactions occur more commonly in patients who have immunodeficiency disorders.
5. **Physical findings** that relate to immune deficiency are presented in Table 9-1.
6. **Laboratory testing.** Information about immune function can be obtained from a number of tests (Table 9-2).

B Nonspecific (innate, nonadaptive) host defenses

1. **Barriers** act as a front line of defense. There are two types: **Anatomic** barriers such as skin, cilia, and mucus, and **biochemical** barriers such as lysozyme, lactoferrin, and gastric acid. Any barrier

TABLE 9-1 Physical Findings Related to Immune Deficiency

Organ System	Finding	Immune Deficiency
Growth/development	Failure to thrive	SCID
Facial features	Micrognathia, low-set ears, hypertelorism, short philtrum of upper lip	DiGeorge anomaly
Skin/oral mucosa	Candidiasis, eczema, pyoderma, desquamative erythroderma	SCID, DiGeorge anomaly Wiskott-Aldrich syndrome, phagocytic defects, antibody deficiency, Omenn disease
Eyes	Conjunctival telangiectasia	Ataxia-telangiectasia
Lymphoid system	Hepatosplenomegaly	Phagocytic defects, CVID, Bruton disease (XLA)
	Absent tonsils	
Cardiovascular	Congenital heart disease, conotruncal defects	DiGeorge anomaly
Neuromuscular	Ataxia, cerebellar tetany (newborn)	Ataxia-telangiectasia, DiGeorge anomaly
Skeletal	Arthritis, dwarfism, flaring and cupping deformity of the ribs	Bruton disease (XLA), short-limb dwarfism, ADA deficiency

SCID, severe combined immunodeficiency disease; CVID, common variable immunodeficiency disease; XLA, X-linked agammaglobulinemia; ADA, adenosine deaminase deficiency.

TABLE 9–2 Tests of Immune Competence

Screening Tests

Nonspecific tests
- Absolute granulocyte count
- Total hemolytic complement (CH_{50}; for primary complement deficiency)
- Nitroblue tetrazolium test of neutrophil function (for chronic granulomatous disease)
- Flow cytometry (for leukocyte adhesion molecules on surface of monocytes)

Tests of humoral (B-cell) immunity
- Quantitation of serum immunoglobulins
  - Isotypes—IgG, IgM, IgA, IgE
  - IgG subclasses
- Tests for specific IgM antibodies to ABO blood groups (serum isohemagglutinin levels)
- Patient's antibody response after immunization for diphtheria and tetanus toxoids or pneumococcal polysaccharide antigens, if older than 2 y
- Antibody response after infection to respiratory viruses
- Enumeration and phenotyping of B cells in blood

Tests of cellular (T-cell) immunity
- Absolute lymphocyte count
- Chest radiograph for thymus shadow (only in first few days of life)
- Delayed hypersensitivity skin tests to recall antigens
- Enumeration and phenotyping of T cells and T-cell subsets

Special Immunologic Tests

B-cell tests
- Polyclonal B-cell–induced immunoglobulin production in vitro
- Tests of immunoregulation by T cells of immunoglobulin synthesis

T-cell tests
- Lymphocyte blast transformation response to mitogens, antigens
- Mixed lymphocyte culture assays
- Tests of lymphocyte-mediated cytotoxicity

Ig, immunoglobulin.

TABLE 9-3 Phagocyte Disorders

Disorder	Inheritance	Clinical Features	Therapy
Chronic granulomatous disease	X-linked (67%); autosomal recessive (33%)	Infections with catalase-positive bacteria and fungi affecting skin, lungs, liver; granuloma formation; NBT test diagnostic	Antibiotics; γ-interferon
Myeloperoxidase deficiency	Autosomal recessive	Fungal infections (candidiasis) in deep tissues, especially in presence of diabetes	Antibiotics
Leukocyte adhesion deficiency	Autosomal recessive	Delayed separation of the umbilical cord; skin infections; otitis media; pneumonia; gingivitis; periodontitis	Antibiotics
Abnormal chemotaxis	Variable	Recurrent skin infections with staphylococci, enteric bacteria	Antibiotics

NBT, nitroblue tetrazolium dye.

defect leaves the host susceptible to acquiring infections more frequently and more easily than humans with intact barrier protection.

2. **Cells** involved in nonspecific defense include leukocytes, mast cells, macrophages, cells of the reticuloendothelial system, dendritic cells, endothelial cells, platelets, and natural killer cells.
   a. **Phagocyte disorders** (Table 9-3) may include dysfunction in adherence to vascular endothelium, lack of recognition and migration toward a chemical stimulus (chemotaxis), or deficiency in phagocytosis and intracellular killing.
      (1) **Clinical features** include being prone to infections with bacteria of low virulence (i.e., *Staphylococcus aureus* and Gram-negative enteric bacteria), frequent/recurrent infections due to the inability to accumulate neutrophils at the sites of infection, or a history of delayed separation of the umbilical cord (> 6 weeks after birth) and poor wound healing.
3. **Plasma or soluble factors** include proteins of the complement and coagulation pathways, proteins of the kinin-kallikrein system, acute-phase proteins, and fibronectin.
   a. **Complement disorders** include a dysfunction in the activation of the complement (C) system via either the classic or alternative pathway. Faulty complement activation or regulation can lead to immune-mediated damage of host tissues and various disorders.
      (1) **Genetics.** Most genetically determined complement deficiencies are inherited as autosomal recessive disorders. C1 inhibitor deficiency is inherited as an autosomal dominant trait.
      (2) **Clinical features** are summarized in Table 9-4.
4. **Factors released from cells** include lysosomal enzymes, mediators of anaphylaxis, α- and β-interferons, interleukins (ILs), and chemokines.

C. **Specific (adaptive) host defenses** involve an **immunogenic** response to foreign materials, followed by specific recognition and long-term memory of the **antigen** that caused the initial **immune response.**

1. **Humoral immunity** defends primarily against the extracellular phases of bacterial and viral infections and includes components such as **B lymphocytes** (B cells), **plasma cells, immunoglobulins** (IgG, IgM, IgA, IgD, and IgE), and the **cell-derived soluble factors** (e.g., cytokines).
   a. **B-cell deficiency disorders** (Table 9-5) are defects or deficiencies of B cells that can lead to various antibody deficiencies, or **hypogammaglobulinemias.** These patients will suffer from recurrent infections.

TABLE 9-4 Clinical Features of Congenital Complement Deficiencies

Deficiency	Features
Deficiency of early complement components (C1, C2, C4)	Collagen vascular disorders (e.g., systemic lupus erythematosus [SLE]) and increased susceptibility to pyogenic infections
C3 deficiency	Severe pyogenic infections; SLE and glomerulonephritis
Deficiency of late complement components (C5, C6, C7, C8)	Systemic *Neisseria* species infections, such as meningococcal sepsis and meningitis, and disseminated gonococcal infections
Abnormalities of the control proteins of the alternative pathway (factors H and I, properdin)	Recurrent infections
Deficiency of complement inhibitors (C1 esterase inhibitor)	Recurrent angioedema

TABLE 9-5 B-Cell Deficiency Disorders

Disorder	Inheritance	Clinical Features	Therapy
X-linked agammaglobulinemia (Bruton disease)	X-linked	Recurrent pyogenic infections; infections of lungs, sinuses, middle ear, skin, central nervous system	Immune serum globulin; antibiotics
Transient hypogammaglobulinemia of infancy	Unknown	Recurrent pyogenic infections; frequent in families with other immunodeficiencies	Antibiotics; immune serum globulin (selected patients)
Selective immunoglobulin deficiency (IgA, IgM, IgG subclasses)	Various(IgA deficiency only); autosomal recessive; unknown	Recurrent infections of lungs, sinuses; gastrointestinal disease; allergy; frequent in families with common variable immunodeficiencies	Antibiotics; immune serum globulin (IgG subclass deficiencies with specific antibody deficiency)
Immunoglobulin deficiency with increased IgM (and IgD)	X-linked; autosomal recessive; unknown	Infections of lungs, sinuses, middle ear; increased frequency of autoimmune disease	Immune serum globulin; antibiotics
Common variable immunodeficiency	Autosomal recessive; unknown	Infections of lungs, sinuses, middle ear; giardiasis; malabsorption; autoimmune disease	Immune serum globulin; antibiotics
Transcobalamin II deficiency	Autosomal recessive	Recurrent infections; megaloblastic anemia; intestinal villous atrophy; defective granulocyte bactericidal activity	Immune serum globulin; high dose of vitamin B_{12}
X-linked hypogammaglobulinemia with growth hormone deficiency	X-linked	Recurrent pyogenic infections; short stature	Immune serum globulin; growth hormone
Functional or specific antibody deficiency with normal total immunoglobulins and normal IgG subclasses	Unknown	Recurrent sinopulmonary infections	Antibiotics; immune serum globulin

Ig, immunoglobulin.

(1) **Most common infections are extracellular** and include pyogenic and enteric bacteria, because patients are deficient in serum opsonins necessary for phagocytosis; enteric viruses that may lead to a dermatomyositis-like disease (i.e., poliovirus, echovirus, coxsackievirus); or diseases such as *Giardia lamblia* (IgA deficiency).

(2) **Sites of infection** include the skin; middle ear; conjunctiva; sinuses; meninges; and the respiratory, urinary, and gastrointestinal tracts.

2. **Cellular immunity** defends against intracellular organisms and provides immune surveillance against malignant cells and foreign tissue. Components of cellular immunity include **T lymphocytes** and their subsets and **immune-modifying, cell-derived factors** (e.g., ILs, chemokines, and γ-interferon).

a. **T-cell deficiency disorders** (Table 9-6) result from abnormalities in T-cell functions. Antibody production is also likely to be affected in patients who have severe T-cell abnormalities because T cells are important immunoregulators of B-cell differentiation and function, resulting in combined T- and B-cell immune deficiencies.

(1) **Recurrent infections** are also common in patients who have cellular immunodeficiencies and the most common causative agents are **intracellular pathogens** such as herpesviruses, mycobacteria, *Candida, Pneumocystis carinii,* and *Toxoplasma.*

(2) **Sites of infection** can be either local or systemic.

(3) **Congenital T-cell immunodeficiencies** represent a complex spectrum that includes defects in lymphoid stem-cell differentiation, which result in severe combined immunodeficiency disorders, as well as isolated defects that affect only cell-mediated immunity to one particular pathogen.

b. **Acquired immune deficiency syndrome (AIDS)** is a disorder associated with a profound deficiency in T-cell immunity and, in children, T-cell and B-cell abnormalities.

(1) **Causative agent. Human immunodeficiency virus type 1 (HIV-1),** a retrovirus, is the cause of AIDS.

(2) **Transmission** of HIV occurs via sexual contact, IV drug use with needle/syringe sharing, blood or blood product transfusion, and organ transplantation, and from mother to baby during childbirth or breastfeeding. The risk of transmission via blood, blood products, or organ transplantation has diminished greatly as a result of efficient screening of blood and organ donors and pretreatment of plasma products. The average risk of perinatal transmission is 15% to 35% for babies born to untreated infected mothers and is reduced by two third if zidovudine is given to the infected mother during the last two trimesters of pregnancy and to the infant during the first 6 weeks of life. Breastfeeding can also transmit HIV infection to an infant.

(3) **Immunologic abnormalities associated with HIV infection** include a progressive depletion of CD4 T cells, resulting in a decrease in the ratio of CD4 T cells to CD8 T cells; impaired T-cell immunity even when CD4 T cells are present in normal numbers; impaired mononuclear macrophage function; and impaired production of specific antibody despite a polyclonal increase in serum immunoglobulins.

(4) **Diagnosis of HIV infection** is done by serologic testing via enzyme-linked immunosorbent assay (ELISA), Western blot, polymerase chain reaction (PCR) for HIV p24 antigen, or HIV RNA, or HIV culture of blood lymphocytes. Maternal antibodies may persist for up to 18 months in exposed infants; hence, with few exceptions, positive HIV serologic findings in such infants are not diagnostic until after 18 months.

(5) **Prognosis.** The majority of children who have HIV infection will eventually die from complications of AIDS. Infants who have significant clinical disease in the first year of life tend to progress most rapidly. Those infants remaining asymptomatic into the second year are likely to remain relatively disease free for several years. Some may even reach adolescence.

(6) **Clinical features** can range from mild to severe. Recurrent upper respiratory infections and otitis media can be markers for mild disease, whereas chronic oral candidiasis, diarrhea, failure to thrive, anemia, and a variety of infectious diseases that reflect some degree of immunodeficiency can indicate moderate disease. Severe disease is marked by AIDS-defining conditions that are opportunistic infections such as *P. carinii* pneumonia,

TABLE 9-6 T-Cell and Combined T-Cell and B-Cell Deficiency Disorders in Children

Disorder	Inheritance	Clinical Features	Therapy
Severe combined immunodeficiency disorders—gene defects in:		Recurrent infections; wasting; chronic diarrhea; failure to thrive; graft versus host disease; opportunistic infections (e.g., *Pneumocystis carinii*)	Bone marrow transplantation
IL-2 receptor γ chain	X-linked		
	Autosomal recessive		
ZAP-70 tyrosine kinase			
Jak 3 kinase			
CD3γ, CD3ϵ subunits			
Defects of the purine salvage pathway Adenosine deaminase deficiency Purine nucleoside phosphorylase deficiency	Autosomal recessive	Recurrent infections; dysostosis (in some adenosine deaminase deficiency); anemia and mental retardation (purine nucleoside phosphorylase deficiency)	Bone marrow transplantation; enzyme replacement therapy
DiGeorge anomaly (third and fourth pharyngeal pouch syndrome) CATCH 22 syndrome	Embryologic defects	Hypoparathyroidism (hypocalcemia); facial abnormalities; congenital heart disease; infections; chromosome 22 microdeletions (22q11)	Thymus graft with or without bone marrow transplantation
Autoimmune lymphoproliferative syndrome (Fas gene mutations)	Autosomal recessive	Massive nonmalignant lymphoid organ and lymph node enlargement; autoimmune disease; double negative (CD4–, CD8–) T cells	Supportive, steroids
Major histocompatibility complex deficiency	Autosomal recessive	Intestinal malabsorption; recurrent infections; failure to thrive	Bone marrow transplantation
Type I deficiency[a]			
Type II deficiency[b]			
Chronic mucocutaneous candidiasis	Autosomal recessive	Chronic candidal infection of the skin, nails, scalp, and mucous membranes; autoimmune endocrine disorders	Topical and systemic antifungal agents; transfer factor; thymus transplantation
Ataxia-telangiectasia	Autosomal recessive	Oculocutaneous telangiectasia; progressive cerebellar ataxia; bronchiectasis; malignancy; defective chromosomal repair; raised α-fetoprotein level	Bone marrow transplantation
Wiskott-Aldrich syndrome	X-linked	Eczema; thrombocytopenia; susceptibility to infections; malignancy; small, defective platelets	Bone marrow transplantation; antibiotics; splenectomy

CATCH 22, cardiac defects, abnormal facies, thymic hypoplasia, cleft palate, hypocalcemia.
[a] TAP transporter defect.
[b] Gene defects of CIITA or RFX-5 (regulators of class II major histocompatibility complex gene transcription).

Mycobacterium avium complex, candidal esophagitis, disseminated cryptococcosis, toxoplasmic encephalitis, cryptosporidiosis, disseminated tuberculosis, and wasting syndrome.

(7) **Progressive neurologic disease** can be manifested by developmental delay, encephalopathy, paresis, dystonia, and peripheral neuropathy. Cerebral atrophy and intracranial calcifications may be seen on computed tomography scan.

(8) **Therapy.** General management includes antiretroviral therapy, treatment of secondary infections, prophylaxis against *P. carinii* pneumonia, and nutritional support.

(a) **Antiretroviral therapy.** A combination of two reverse transcriptase inhibitors and one protease inhibitor is recommended. A change in all three retroviral drugs is recommended if drug resistance develops. Patients are monitored by viral load and CD4 counts.

(b) **Prophylaxis for *P. carinii* pneumonia** is indicated if the CD4 T-cell number is $< 500/\mu L$. The **drug of choice is trimethoprim-sulfamethoxazole (TMP-SMX),** which is given three times a week.

D **Programmed cell death (PCD)** is a critical balance of cell growth, cell differentiation, and cell elimination.

1. Cells undergoing PCD (**apoptosis**) exhibit morphologic changes very different from cell necrosis and characteristically do not elicit an inflammatory response as necrosis does. The process of PCD occurs in all tissues of the body through a complex pathway of intracytoplasmic enzymes that eventually leads to nuclear fragmentation and specific cleavage of cellular DNA.

2. **Disorders of programmed cell death (apoptosis)** are divided into two categories: **Congenital defects** and **acquired defects.** A congenital defect in the expression of the Fas membrane receptor leads to an autoimmune lymphoproliferative syndrome. An acquired defect in the *bcl-2* gene leads to overexpression, which results in B-cell lymphoma.

III HYPERSENSITIVITY REACTIONS

The same immunologic mechanisms that protect the host can cause tissue damage if they occur in exaggerated or inappropriate form.

A **Types of hypersensitivity** The widely accepted classification divides these mechanisms into four types of hypersensitivity reactions. Many immunopathologic processes are mediated by more than one type of hypersensitivity reaction.

1. **Type I (immediate-type, atopic, or reaginic) hypersensitivity reactions.** An allergen reacts and cross-links IgE antibodies, which triggers the IgE receptors on mast cells and basophils to release pharmacologic mediators (e.g., histamine). Examples of type I reactions include allergic rhinitis, asthma, and anaphylactic shock (e.g., insect sting and drug reactions).

2. **Type II (antibody-dependent cytotoxic) hypersensitivity reactions.** Antibody (usually IgG or IgM) binds to cell-associated antigens, which leads to either complement-mediated tissue injury or cytotoxicity by antibody-dependent cell-mediated lysis via the Fc receptors on effector cells. An example of a type II reaction is autoimmune hemolytic anemia.

3. **Type III (immune complex-mediated) hypersensitivity reactions.** Complexes composed of antigen and antibody activate complement and mediate an inflammatory reaction. An example of a type III reaction is acute glomerulonephritis.

4. **Type IV (cell-mediated or delayed) hypersensitivity reactions.** These reactions are caused by antibody-independent mechanisms involving sensitized T cells and cytokines. Examples of type IV reactions include contact dermatitis and graft rejection.

B **Role in autoimmune disease** For unknown reasons, the body's self-recognition system sometimes goes awry, so that substances in the body's own tissues become **autoantigens,** and the stage is set for the development of an **autoimmune disease.** Autoimmune disorders usually are type II or type III hypersensitivity reactions, but also may include type IV processes.

IV ALLERGIC DISORDERS

A **Principles of IgE-mediated allergic disorders** IgE was originally called the **reaginic** or **atopic antibody,** because it was known to react with the antigens that cause symptoms in atopic individuals.

1. **Pathogenesis of IgE-mediated allergies.** IgE binds to surface receptors on **mast cells** and **basophils,** thereby sensitizing these cells. When these sensitized cells come in contact with a **specific antigen,** they release **mediators** of inflammation and **triggers** of the immediate allergic reaction. The mediators act rapidly on local tissues, causing the patient's symptoms. In many allergic disorders, the immediate, short-lived inflammatory episode is followed 4 to 8 hours later by a second event that persists for 24 to 48 hours. These **late-phase allergic reactions,** which are mediated by CD4 + T cells, contribute to the clinical manifestations and prolonged inflammation in asthma (see Chapter 13), allergic rhinitis, and other atopic diseases.
2. **Evaluation for allergic disorders**
   a. **History.** LISTEN TO YOUR PATIENT! Many times, patients will present with complaints of symptoms when exposed to certain things or report things they try to avoid. Often, parents will already have an idea when something makes their child's asthma or eczema worse. In most cases, a diagnosis can be made through history alone. Patients generally go to an allergist for confirmation of their suspicions via testing and for aid with management of symptoms.
      (1) **Variations in symptoms** can provide clues to the allergen. Symptoms may vary with **time** by being seasonal, perennial, monthly, diurnal, or nocturnal. The can also vary by **location** as they may occur indoors, outdoors, at school, at work, at home, or even within certain rooms.
      (2) **Environment.** Symptoms may be induced by exposure to specific allergens or made worse by irritants such as tobacco smoke, perfumes, and wood-burning stoves.
      (3) **Family history** regarding atopic disorders such as asthma, rhinitis, and eczema should be explored. If one parent is atopic, there is a 25% to 30% chance of atopy in the child; if both parents are atopic, then the incidence increases to more than 50%.
   b. **Physical examination.** Refer to Table 9-7 for signs and symptoms commonly associated with allergic disorders.
   c. **Testing and evaluation**
      (1) **Pulmonary function testing** may be helpful (see Chapter 13).
      (2) **Skin testing** is based on the antigen-IgE reaction that occurs on the surface of mast cells in the skin. A small amount of presumed antigen is administered as a solution into the superficial layers of the skin by a surface scratch, a needle-prick through a drop of the antigen solution, or intracutaneous injection. Controls used for skin testing include histamine (positive) and solvent or vehicle (negative). A positive reaction will produce a wheal-and-flare reaction at the skin test site.

TABLE 9-7 Common Signs and Symptoms of Allergic Disease

Target Tissue	Sign or Symptom
Skin	Dermatitis, eczema, urticaria, angioedema
Eyes	Pruritus, tearing, burning, photophobia, chemosis, allergic shiners, conjunctival injection, palpebral and bulbar conjunctiva papillae
Ears	Fullness, popping, serous otitis media, hearing loss
Nose	Congestion, sneezing, pruritus, rhinorrhea, snoring, anosmia, epistaxis, clear secretions, pale and boggy turbinates, polyps, adenoidal hypertrophy
Throat	Pruritus, scratchiness or soreness, postnasal mucous discharge, hoarseness, halitosis, cobblestoning of posterior pharyngeal wall, high-arched palate, malocclusion of teeth
Chest	Cough, tightness, dyspnea, wheezing
Gastrointestinal	Dysphagia, abdominal cramps, bloating, diarrhea

TABLE 9-8 Drug Therapy for Allergic Disorders

Drug	Target Tissue	Actions
β_2-adrenergic agonists	Bronchial smooth muscle, respiratory epithelium	Relax smooth muscles, increase mucus flow, increase ciliary action
Theophylline	Bronchial smooth muscle, diaphragm muscles	Blocks adenosine receptors, increases contractility, relaxes smooth muscles
Cromolyn	Mast cells	Inhibits mediator release
Nedocromil	Mast cells, eosinophils	Inhibits mediator release
Anticholinergics	Smooth muscle	Antagonize muscarinic receptor action of acetylcholine
Antihistamines	H_1-receptors	Block effects of histamine
Leukotriene modifiers	Inflammatory cells, endothelial cells	Inhibit 5-lipoxygenase, inhibit LTD receptor
Glucocorticosteroids	Inflammatory cells	Inhibit arachidonic acid metabolism Stabilize cell membrane Inhibit cytokine production
	Vasculature	Decrease capillary permeability

LTD, leukotriene D.

(3) **Quantitation of total and specific IgE**

(a) **Total serum IgE levels** are determined by a paper radioimmunosorbent test. At birth, cord serum contains virtually no detectable IgE. Serum concentrations in children increase slowly, reaching adult levels at 5 to 7 years of age. Not all atopic subjects have high IgE levels and vice versa.

(b) **Antigen-specific IgE levels** in serum can be determined by a radioallergosorbent test (RAST). However, this in vitro analog of testing is ten times less sensitive than intracutaneous skin testing.

(4) **Challenge testing.** A presumed allergen can be administered directly to the mucosa of the target organ to identify the relationship between direct contact with the allergen and development of symptoms.

3. **Drug therapy for allergic disorders** is presented in Table 9-8.

B **Anaphylaxis** is an acute, life-threatening systemic reaction caused by an IgE-mediated hypersensitivity reaction and characterized by urticaria-angioedema, acute airway obstruction, and circulatory collapse. **Anaphylactoid reactions** are clinically identical to anaphylaxis but are caused by the nonimmunologic release of mediators from mast cells and basophils, such as by complement-derived anaphylatoxins.

1. **Pathogenesis**
   a. The most common causes are **drugs** (e.g., antibiotics, intravenous contrast), Hymenoptera (bee) **stings, foods,** and **latex** products, particularly in high-risk groups who are repeatedly exposed to latex products such as health care professionals and patients who have spina bifida.
   b. The **route of allergen administration** most commonly is parenteral or via ingestion. Inhalation is less common.
   c. The **onset of anaphylaxis** occurs within a few minutes to hours after antigen exposure. Systemic manifestations are caused by the release of inflammatory mediators from mast cells and basophils.
2. **Clinical features of anaphylaxis** are delineated in Table 9-9.
3. **Therapy MUST BE IMMEDIATE** and should focus on the ABCs of critical care. Therapies may include:
   a. **Epinephrine** is the first-line approach to the treatment of anaphylaxis.
   b. **Antihistamines** are only helpful for symptomatic relief of urticaria but ***will not stop the progression of anaphylaxis***!

TABLE 9-9 Clinical Manifestation of Anaphylaxis

Target Tissue	Signs or Symptoms
Skin	Urticaria, angioedema, flushing, itching
Respiratory	Nasal congestion, sneezing, rhinorrhea, hoarseness, stridor, dyspnea, bronchospasm, hypoxia
Cardiovascular	Dizziness, syncope, hypotension, arrhythmia, palpitations, substernal pain
Gastrointestinal	Nausea, vomiting, diarrhea, dysphagia, abdominal cramps
Neurologic	Headache, seizure
Genitourinary	Urgency

c. **Fluid therapy and vasopressors** are given for treating circulatory collapse and maintaining blood pressure.

d. **Airway maintenance and bronchodilating drugs** may be necessary.

e. **Corticosteroids** can be administered in severe anaphylaxis.

f. **Oxygen** should be given if the patient is cyanotic or has a low PO_2.

g. **Glucagon,** in addition to epinephrine, can be given for those patients who take a β-blocker medication, as they may be resistant to the effects of epinephrine alone due to the β-blockade.

h. The patient should be **observed** for at least 4 to 6 hours after stabilization to watch for late-phase rebound, which can be just as severe as the initial event.

4. **Prevention** involves avoidance of known antigens, use of emergency epinephrine self-administration kits, and use of allergy identification bracelets.

C **Allergic rhinitis** is a disorder of the nasal mucosa characterized by nasal blockage, rhinorrhea, sneezing, and pruritus.

1. **Pathophysiology.** Mast cells in the nasal mucosa regulate the local blood flow in the mucosa by a controlled release of vasoactive mediators. Release of histamine causes itching, sneezing, and hypersecretion. Parasympathetic nerve pathways also play a major role in hypersecretion and congestion. Both early- and late-phase inflammatory processes occur.

2. **Classification and clinical features**

a. **Seasonal allergic rhinitis** (hay fever)

(1) **Symptoms** include congestion; pruritus; increased thin, watery, clear mucous secretions (rhinorrhea); loss of the senses of smell and taste; chronic cough and clearing of the throat due to postnasal discharge; and chronic malaise and fatigue. Epistaxis, nasal or sinus polyps, and persistent serous otitis media and sinusitis may also be significant problems.

(2) **Physical findings that are characteristic** include transverse nasal crease, dark shadows under the eyes ("allergic shiners"), and dental malocclusion. The **nasal turbinates** are edematous and pale, with a bluish tinge; they are covered with a thin, clear secretion. **Postnasal drainage** of secretions may result in cobblestoning of the posterior pharyngeal wall. **Other findings** can include conjunctivitis, nasal polyps, and sinusitis.

(3) **Nasal mucosal scrapings** show large numbers of eosinophils.

b. **Chronic or perennial rhinitis** may have an allergic or nonallergic basis.

c. **Vasomotor rhinitis** results from local autonomic imbalance.

3. **Inhalant or airborne allergens**

a. **Pollens** constitute one of the most important groups of allergens. Ragweed, other weeds, grasses, and trees are the most common offenders. To cause clinically significant sensitization, a pollen must be produced in large quantities by a common plant and must be dispersed by wind rather than insects. There is often a **seasonal occurrence** that varies with geographic location and the time of year of pollination. For example, grass pollen is present in the spring and early summer, whereas ragweed is present in the late summer and early fall.

b. **Molds or fungi.** Spores are ubiquitous in the environment; molds are especially present in places of high humidity and warmth. Mold allergies are most common in the fall and early spring.

c. **Household dust** allergen is the feces of the dust mite. Dust mite-sensitive patients have perennial symptoms but usually are worse in the late fall and winter.

d. **Cockroach antigens** are important allergens in the inner city home environment and cause significant allergy especially related to asthma.

e. **Animal allergens.** Dander, dried saliva, urine, and feathers are the major allergens. **Cats are the most highly allergenic of the common household pets.**

4. **Other contributing factors** include **irritants** (smoke, perfumes, etc.), weather conditions, temperature changes, infections, air pollution, endocrine hormone imbalance, and stress.

5. **Therapy**

a. **Avoidance** is the single most direct and safe mode of treatment. Often this will require actions such as removal of a pet from the home. After removal of a pet, animal allergens may persist for a year or longer.

b. **Drug therapy** is directed at preventing mast cell degranulation and blocking the effects of the released mediators.

(1) **Antihistamines** are useful for controlling rhinorrhea and pruritus. They are classified as first and second generation. First-generation antihistamines are overall more sedating than the second-generation variety.

(2) **Decongestants** are useful for reducing congestion.

(3) **Cromolyn sodium** blocks mediator release from mast cells and is effective in treating both early- and late-phase allergic reactions.

(4) **Corticosteroids** mainly affect late-phase allergic reactions.

(5) **Atropine-like drugs** are useful for treating vasomotor rhinitis.

c. **Desensitization (immunotherapy)** can be useful in patients who have clear-cut seasonal allergic rhinitis caused by the inhalant pollen allergens.

D Allergic diseases of the eyes and ears

1. **Allergic conjunctivitis** is usually caused by inhalant allergens.

a. **Clinical features** include tearing, itching, edema (chemosis), and redness of the conjunctiva. The **cornea is not involved;** thus, no scarring occurs.

b. **Therapy** is **primarily drug therapy** with combination ocular decongestant-antihistamine preparations, oral antihistamines, topical mast cell stabilizers, or topical nonsteroidal anti-inflammatory drugs.

2. **Vernal conjunctivitis** is a severe, bilateral inflammatory disorder that occurs mainly in the spring and summer in preadolescent boys (male-to-female ratio is 3:1). The disease tends to resolve after puberty and is often seen concomitantly with eczema, asthma, or atopic dermatitis.

a. **Clinical features** include intense itching, tearing, photophobia, and a stringy ocular mucous discharge that contains numerous eosinophils. Physical findings include giant papillae or cobblestoning of the upper tarsal conjunctiva. Vernal conjunctivitis **can result in corneal damage,** with ulceration and scarring.

b. **Therapy** is with mast cell stabilizers, a topical antihistamine, and, if necessary, topical or systemic corticosteroids or even topical cyclosporine.

3. **Eyelid allergic disease** can occur in patients who have **atopic dermatitis** or **eczema.** Clinical features can range from a scaly, edematous, crusty exudate to keratoconjunctivitis, cataracts, or keratoconus.

4. **Serous otitis media** and **middle ear effusions** may be allergy related. In allergic children, adenoidal hypertrophy contributes to obstruction of the eustachian tube.

E Atopic dermatitis (eczema)

This common pruritic skin disorder usually begins in infancy and has a chronic fluctuating course with seasonal variations. In 50% of patients, the skin problem starts in the first year of life; in up to 80%, onset is before 5 years of age.

1. **Immunologic aspects** of atopic dermatitis are elevated serum IgE levels in 85% of patients, with most patients having immediate skin reactivity to a variety of environmental allergens. Other

atopic diseases are often present such as asthma or allergic rhinitis. A family history is a strong indicator for developing atopy.

2. **Clinical features** are characterized by a chronic or relapsing course.
   a. **Pruritic dermatitis** has a typical morphology and distribution. In infants and young children, the facial and extensor surfaces are affected. Lesions tend to be erythematous, papulovesicular, and exudative. In older children, the distribution is more on the flexural surfaces, and lesions are more dry and lichenified.
   c. **Other clinical features** include cheilitis, infraorbital folds, anterior neck folds, white dermatographism and a delayed blanch response, and facial pallor associated with infraorbital darkening.
3. **Complications** include repeated cutaneous infections and possible keratoconus. Anterior or posterior subcapsular cataracts are rare before puberty.
4. **Therapy** is directed toward suppressing the itch-scratch cycle by using oral **antihistamines**. Skin **moisturizers** are used to maintain skin hydration and prevent drying. **Antibiotics** may be necessary for patients who have weepy lesions and pyoderma. **Topical corticosteroids** are used only in patients who have severe atopic dermatitis.

F **Urticaria and angioedema** **Urticaria** (hives) are evanescent wheals of varying size that affect the superficial layers of the epidermis and mucous membranes. **Angioedema** is similar but involves the deeper layers of the dermis and submucosal or subcutaneous tissues.

1. **Pathogenesis**
   a. **Type I hypersensitivity reactions** are a common cause of urticaria and angioedema. Hymenoptera stings, drugs, and certain foods are common causes of IgE-mediated urticaria and angioedema. Other immunologic processes associated with urticaria include viral, parasitic, fungal, and certain bacterial infections.
   b. **Immune complex disease and cutaneous vasculitis** are associated with activation of the complement system and generation of anaphylatoxins. Radiocontrast dyes and blood transfusions can induce complement-mediated urticaria or angioedema. Hereditary angioedema is caused by the deficiency or dysfunction of the C1 esterase inhibitor.
   c. **Nonimmunologic mechanisms** also cause urticaria and angioedema such as nonspecific release of histamine from mast cells or basophils that can be caused by morphine, codeine, curare derivatives, bacterial toxins, crustacean secretions, and snake venom. Some substances (i.e., aspirin and preservatives) activate the arachidonic acid pathway, with production of leukotrienes.
   d. **Physical agents** also can induce urticaria by this mechanism, as in dermatographism (from pressure), solar urticaria, aquagenic urticaria, cold urticaria, heat-induced urticaria, and cholinergic urticaria.
2. **Clinical features and diagnosis**
   a. **Urticarial lesions** usually appear at multiple sites, and last < 24 hours. Lesions do not result in discoloration of the skin. If a *bruise-like* discoloration remains after the urticarial lesion disappears, vasculitis should be considered. **Acute urticaria** can last for a few days, most often due to food, drug, or viral illness. **Chronic urticaria** lasts longer than 6 weeks and often the cause is not identified.
   b. **Evaluation** should be directed at a **good history** to determine a causative agent. Skin testing or RAST for specific IgE antibodies can be helpful to confirm the allergen, although in 70% of cases an etiology is never identified. Physical urticaria can be diagnosed by using the stimulating agent, such as an ice cube, to evaluate for cold urticaria. A subgroup of patients with urticaria have autoantibodies to thyroid antigens and thus can be treated with low-dose thyroid replacement hormone.
3. **Therapy**
   a. **Antihistamines** (H_1-receptor antagonists) are the principal drug for the management of urticaria and angioedema. Some patients who have chronic urticaria unresponsive to H_1-receptor antihistamines may respond to therapy with both H_1- and H_2-receptor antihistamines. Tricyclic antidepressants may also be helpful in treating chronic urticaria.

b. **Cyproheptadine** is recommended for cold urticaria.
c. **Systemic corticosteroids** should be used only in patients who have severe, acute urticaria and angioedema and patients who have an underlying disorder (e.g., vasculitis) that calls for the use of these drugs.

G Food allergy

1. **Pathogenesis**
   a. An inappropriate response to an ingested food is referred to as an **adverse food reaction.** Both **immunologic** and **nonimmunologic** (food intolerance) **mechanisms** cause adverse food reactions.
   b. **Immune-mediated reactions** include reactions to milk, soy, eggs, fish, peanuts, and wheat. Preservatives are a minor cause of food reactions.
   c. **Nonimmunologic reactions to foods** include the toxic or pharmacologic effects of bacterial toxins or chemical additives, a nonimmunologically mediated histamine release, an inborn enzyme deficiency, psychological reactions, and intrinsic gastrointestinal disease.
2. **Clinical features.** Food allergy can be expressed through a variety of clinical symptoms. Some patients have **abdominal symptoms**, such as nausea, vomiting, abdominal pain, bloating, or diarrhea. There may be an associated **swelling of the lips** and tingling of the mouth or throat. Other patients may have **anaphylaxis**, asthma, rhinorrhea and congestion, **urticaria**, **angioedema**, **eczema**, and joint pain.
3. **Diagnosis.** The classic diagnostic tests used in allergy will not reliably identify a food allergy. The diagnosis of food allergy is best made by **oral challenge testing** in which the food is given and effects on the target organ are evaluated.
4. **Therapy.** Elimination or **avoidance** of the offending food substance from the diet is the major approach to the treatment of patients who have food allergy. Other precautions include the availability of **epinephrine** (EpiPen) for treating anaphylaxis and a medical alert bracelet.

H Allergic reactions to stinging insects are type I hypersensitivity reactions. Between 0.5% and 5% of the population experience a systemic reaction after a sting, but death from insect allergy in children is very rare.

1. **Clinical features** can range from mild symptoms, such as **urticaria** and pruritus, to **angioedema** or life-threatening **anaphylactic shock. Large local reactions** that exceed 5 cm and occur within 24 to 72 hours after the sting are probably delayed hypersensitivity reactions. Subsequent reactions to insect stings are not worse, so someone with urticaria will not have anaphylaxis with the next sting.
2. **Diagnosis** is generally identified from the **history** and by skin testing with purified venoms or by in vitro testing with RAST.
3. **Therapy** is mainly preventive and patients should avoid using perfumes and wearing brightly colored clothes and should not walk barefoot outdoors. They should also carry **epinephrine** in case anaphylaxis follows an insect sting. **Immunotherapy** is indicated for those individuals who are at risk for severe cardiovascular systemic reactions and fatal anaphylaxis.

I Adverse drug reactions have many causes and up to 70% to 80% of adverse drug reactions are **predictable adverse reactions** that result from the pharmacologic actions of a drug. **Unpredictable adverse reactions** can result from immunologic hypersensitivity, an underlying genetic susceptibility, or idiosyncrasy. Immunologic reactions require prior exposure or at least 7 days of continuous therapy with the drug in question.

1. **Development of a drug allergy**
   a. Few drugs are large enough molecules to serve as complete antigens. Drugs (or their metabolites) that can serve as **haptens** are most likely to cause sensitization.
   b. **Topical application** causes sensitization more often than other routes of drug administration, probably because the carrier proteins for the drug haptens are readily available in the skin.
   c. **Intermittent courses of moderate doses of a drug** are more likely to predispose to sensitization than prolonged treatment courses.

d. **Atopy.** Although the incidence of adverse drug reactions is the same for atopic and nonatopic patients, an atopic person is more prone to the development of severe reactions.

2. **Clinical features**
   a. **Drug eruptions** can take many forms as the **skin** is the most common site of drug hypersensitivity reactions. Exanthematous eruptions, urticaria, angioedema, and photosensitivity are most common and relatively mild, whereas **epidermal necrolysis** and **Stevens-Johnson syndrome** can be fatal.
   b. **Anaphylaxis** occurs most commonly with **parenteral** administration.
   c. **Serum sickness (type III hypersensitivity)** can be induced by various drugs, notably the penicillins, as well as the foreign protein in serum.
      (1) **Symptoms** usually develop in 7 to 12 days but may be accelerated in patients previously exposed to the drug. Symptoms include urticaria, angioedema, erythema multiforme, fever, and arthritis.
      (2) **Therapy.** Reactions can be controlled by antihistamines or, in severe cases, corticosteroids. There are no sequelae.
   d. **Other manifestations of drug allergy** include drug fever, a reaction resembling systemic lupus erythematosus (SLE) (*see VIII A*), hemolytic anemia, thrombocytopenia, purpura, asthma, hypersensitivity pneumonitis, hepatocellular damage, cholestasis, peripheral neuritis, and, rarely, seizures.

3. **Examples of drug allergies**
   a. **Penicillin and its derivatives** cause many cases of allergic drug reactions.
      (1) **Mechanism.** Metabolites of penicillin are haptens and bind with proteins to form antigenic groups known as **the major determinant** and **several minor determinants.**
      (2) Although the **cephalosporins** have a similar structure to penicillin, a person who is sensitive to penicillin has only an 8% cross-reactivity with the second- and third-generation cephalosporins.
   b. **Aspirin** can cause reactions that appear to be allergic in nature, such as urticaria, angioedema, or asthma. Reactions to aspirin are probably not IgE mediated, but instead may be related to perturbations of the arachidonic pathways associated with increased production of **leukotrienes**, because the structurally unrelated nonsteroidal anti-inflammatory drugs can produce similar reactions.
   c. Other significant hypersensitivity reactions to drugs include those to **insulin** and **anticonvulsants.**
   d. Adverse reactions to radiocontrast media, various opioids, vancomycin, angiotensin-converting enzyme inhibitors, and local anesthetics may be mediated by nonimmunologic release of mediators from mast cells.

V POSTINFECTIOUS ARTHRITIS

A Reactive arthritis During the recovery period from an infectious illness (e.g., gastroenteritis, upper respiratory illness), the body's immune response may cause arthritis.

1. A common example is **transient synovitis** (previously called toxic synovitis), in which a child, commonly age 3 to 10, has sudden pain in the hip, often referred to the thigh or groin. There is a history of a prodromal upper respiratory infection. There is pain with range of motion of the hip and hip ultrasound may demonstrate fluid in the synovial space.
2. The patient does not require antibiotics, as this is a response to a prior viral infection, not an active infectious agent in the joint. The course is self-limited and should resolve in 1 to 2 weeks.

B Lyme arthritis is the second most common manifestation of Lyme disease in children. It is a late complication of the disease and most typically is a monoarthritis that presents as a diffusely swollen joint without extreme pain (see Chapter 10).

C Acute rheumatic fever and poststreptococcal reactive arthritis

1. **Rheumatic fever** is a multisystem, nonsuppurative, inflammatory disease triggered by a group A β-hemolytic streptococcal (GABHS) infection of the upper respiratory tract. The disease occurs

after a latent period of 1 to 3 weeks following streptococcal pharyngitis. Patients who develop rheumatic fever have a marked tendency to suffer recurrent attacks after subsequent GABHS infections of the upper respiratory tract. Rheumatic fever is a potentially serious disease because it may cause permanent damage to heart muscle and valves (**rheumatic heart disease**).

a. **Incidence.** The peak incidence of initial and recurrent attacks of rheumatic fever is between 5 and 15 years of age.

b. **Clinical features**

(1) **Polyarthritis**—usually with fever—is the presenting finding in approximately 75% of patients. The arthritis chiefly affects large joints, is characteristically migratory, and is painful out of proportion to objective findings of redness and swelling. There are no sequelae.

(2) **Carditis** is the most serious of the clinical manifestations because it is the only one that may lead to chronic sequelae. It occurs in approximately 50% of patients and may be asymptomatic, unless pericarditis or heart failure is present. A pansystolic, blowing mitral murmur is the hallmark. Less common is a diastolic aortic murmur heard along the left sternal border. Murmurs may remain but often disappear if recurrences of rheumatic fever are prevented.

(3) **Chorea** occurs in from 10% to 30% of the patients. Often insidious in onset, initially there is emotional lability followed by characteristic, random, jerky movements and muscle weakness. Chorea runs a self-limited course of 6 to 13 weeks' duration, and recovery is complete.

(4) **Less common** but very **characteristic findings** include **subcutaneous nodules** (small, painless swellings found overlying bony prominences) and **erythema marginatum** (a pink, evanescent rash over the trunk).

c. **Diagnosis**

(1) There is no specific diagnostic laboratory test for rheumatic fever. The diagnosis is based on the widely accepted **Jones criteria,** which classify the manifestations as **major** and **minor** according to their diagnostic importance.

(2) Table 9-10 shows how Jones criteria can be used to help diagnose rheumatic fever.

(a) The presence of two major criteria or of one major and two minor criteria indicates a high probability of rheumatic fever if supported by evidence of a preceding streptococcal infection. This evidence includes an elevated or rising streptococcal antibody titer or a positive throat culture result for group A streptococcus.

(b) The absence of a preceding streptococcal infection should make the diagnosis suspect, except in situations in which rheumatic fever is first discovered after a long latent period from the antecedent infection (e.g., chorea, indolent carditis).

(3) **Laboratory tests**

(a) **Streptococcal antibody tests** (e.g., antistreptolysin O) are useful for documenting a recent streptococcal infection and the erythrocyte sedimentation rate and C-reactive protein tests can provide evidence of an inflammatory process.

TABLE 9-10 Jones Criteria for Guidance in the Diagnosis of an Initial Attack of Rheumatic Fever

Major Manifestations	Minor Manifestations
Carditis	Clinical
Polyarthritis	Fever
Chorea	Arthralgia
Erythema marginatum	Laboratory
Subcutaneous nodules	Elevated acute-phase reactants
	ESR
	C-reactive protein
	Prolonged PR interval on ECG

ESR, erythrocyte sedimentation rate; ECG, electrocardiogram.
Based on Special Writing Group of the Committee on Rheumatic Fever, Endocarditis, and Kawasaki Disease of the Council on Cardiovascular Disease in the Young of the American Heart Association: Guidelines for the diagnosis of rheumatic fever. Jones criteria, 1992 update. *JAMA* 268:2069–2073, 1992.

TABLE 9-11 Clinical and Laboratory Characteristics of Poststreptococcal Reactive Arthritis (PSRA) and Acute Rheumatic Fever (ARF)

Characteristics	PSRA	ARF
Antecedent group A streptococcal infection	Yes	Yes
Onset of arthritis after infection	< 2 wk	2–3 wk
Migratory arthritis	No	Yes
Axial arthritis	Yes	No
Heart involvement	6%	50%
Response to ASA	Not dramatic	Dramatic
Association with HLA-B27	No	No
Association with HLA-DRb	DRB1*01	DRB1*16

ASA, acetylsalicylic acid.
Cassidy and Petty Textbook of Pediatric Rheumatology, Table 31-8. Adapted from Ahmed S., Ayoub, EM, Scornik JC, et al: Poststreptococcal reactive arthritis: clinical characteristics and associations with HLA-DR alleles. *Arthritis Rheum* 41:1096–1102, 1998. Copyright ©1998 John Wiley and Sons, Inc. Reprinted with Permission of Wiley-Liss, Inc., a subsidiary of John Wiley & Sons, Inc.

(b) **Throat culture is not very helpful,** because it is usually negative by the time signs of rheumatic fever appear.

d. **Therapy** includes the following:
  (1) **Salicylates** to control fever and joint manifestations
  (2) A short course (2–4 weeks) of **corticosteroid therapy** for treating severe carditis. If there is evidence of heart failure, anticongestive measures are required.

e. **Prevention of recurrences.** Once the diagnosis is established, the patient should be given either 600,000 to 1.2 million U of **benzathine penicillin G** as one injection or therapeutic doses of oral penicillin for 10 days. Penicillin-allergic patients can be treated with erythromycin. Long-term prophylaxis with an injection of benzathine penicillin every 3 or 4 weeks will prevent streptococcal infections and recurrences of rheumatic fever. Prophylaxis should be continued for a minimum of 5 years and at least until the patient is 21 years of age if there is residual heart disease.

2. **Poststreptococcal reactive arthritis** is the name given to a condition of polyarthritis seen in a patient following a streptococcal infection who does not fulfill the Jones criteria. This entity is believed to fall on a continuum of conditions related to the immune response to GABHS. This type of arthritis is distinguished from the arthritis in acute rheumatic fever (ARF) as shown in Table 9-11.

VI CHRONIC ARTHRITIS OF CHILDHOOD

The criteria for the diagnosis of **chronic inflammatory arthritis** in childhood include age younger than 16 and objective arthritis of more than one joint lasting 6 weeks or longer. The nomenclature for the different types of chronic arthritis is confusing and debate continues as to the ideal classification system. The American College of Rheumatology described the term ***JRA*** **(*juvenile rheumatoid arthritis*)** in the 1970s. The term ***juvenile chronic arthritis*** was developed by the European League Against Rheumatism, and most recently, in 1997, a group of experts proposed the term ***juvenile idiopathic arthritis*** **(*JIA*).** Each group describes the distinctions slightly differently.

A **Pauciarticular (oligoarticular) JIA** refers to a chronic type of childhood arthritis affecting four or fewer joints. It is generally a disease of toddlers, with the most common age group 1 to 3 years. It affects girls more commonly at a ratio of 5:1 and accounts for about **60%** of patients with juvenile arthritis. This is the group of children at highest risk for associated asymptomatic **uveitis,** which occurs in 15% to 20% of these patients.

1. These children commonly have positive **antinuclear antibody (ANA)** results; other tests including rheumatoid factor (RF), complete blood count (CBC), and erythrocyte sedimentation rate (ESR) are typically normal, without evidence of systemic inflammation.
2. These children are usually well managed with nonsteroidal anti-inflammatory drugs (NSAIDs) and intra-articular steroid injections.
3. Typically, there is a favorable outcome with respect to the joints, though the eye disease may result in long-term complications. **Children with a positive ANA must be screened three to four times yearly for evidence of iritis;** children who are ANA negative need twice yearly screening.

B **Polyarticular JIA** accounts for about **30%** of children with chronic juvenile arthritis.

1. The International League of Associations for Rheumatology (ILAR) criteria divide patients into two distinct groups based on the presence or absence of the **rheumatoid factor.**
   a. In general, **RF-negative** patients are younger children with large joint, symmetric involvement.
   b. The **RF-positive** patients are preteens to teens, more commonly girls, with symmetric, small joint involvement of their hands.
2. These children often have laboratory results consistent with a **systemic inflammatory process** such as elevated white blood cell counts and platelet counts, anemia, and elevated erythrocyte sedimentation rates.
3. Screening for inflammatory eye disease is important; the frequency is based on the presence or absence of the ANA.
4. **Treatment** is often with NSAIDs, but often requires other classes of disease-modifying antirheumatic drugs (DMARDS) such as weekly, low-dose methotrexate; tumor necrosis factor inhibitors such as etanercept, infliximab, and adalimumab; systemic corticosteroids; and other medications.

C **Systemic onset JIA (SOJIA)** accounts for about **10%** of patients with JIA. This type of arthritis may occur at any age, though it is rare in infants. It occurs equally in boys and girls. Systemic onset juvenile arthritis is a diagnosis of exclusion. Children often present with high fevers of unknown origin. If in doubt, it is appropriate to evaluate for infectious or malignant conditions as well.

1. The **fever pattern** is typically quotidian, with a daily or twice-daily fever spike with a return to normal or below normal during the day.
2. An evanescent **salmon-colored rash** comes with the fever spikes.
3. Many patients have **Koebner phenomenon,** in which a lesion may be elicited by scratching the skin.
4. Children often have associated hepatosplenomegaly, lymphadenopathy, pericarditis, or pleuritis.
5. Laboratory parameters show marked systemic inflammation and usually ANA and RF tests are negative.
6. **Treatment** for these patients usually includes systemic corticosteroids, NSAIDs, and often other DMARDs.
7. A potentially devastating complication of SOJIA is **macrophage activating syndrome,** a disseminated intravascular coagulopathy-type disorder with significant morbidity and mortality.

VII SPONDYLOARTHROPATHIES

Refer to a group of forms of arthritis that affect the joints of the axial skeleton, as well as involve peripheral large joints. There is also an association of these diseases in patients with the **antigen HLA-B27.**

A **Juvenile ankylosing spondylitis (JAS)** usually occurs in older children and teens, with a higher prevalence in boys by 7:1. This generally presents as arthritis in the joints of the lower extremities, lower back pain, and **enthesitis**—inflammation of the areas of insertion of tendons, ligaments, or fascia into bone. These patients may have an acute iritis, which presents as a red painful eye, rarely with long-term damage. Cardiovascular disease is uncommon, but patients with JAS are at risk of aortic insufficiency. Treatment of JAS includes NSAIDs as well as other DMARDS.

TABLE 9-12 Criteria for Diagnosis and Classification of Juvenile Psoriatic Arthritis

ILAR Criteria
Arthritis and psoriasis
OR
Arthritis and at least two of the following:
Dactylitis
Nail pitting or onycholysis
Family history of psoriasis in a first-degree relative
Exclusions
Presence of rheumatoid factor
Presence of systemic onset juvenile arthritis
Presence of a family history of B27-associated disease
Onset of arthritis in a male with HLA-B27 after the age of 6 y

ILAR, International League of Associations for Rheumatology.
From Petty RE, Southwood TR, Manners P, et al.: International League of Associations for Rheumatology classification of juvenile idiopathic arthritis: second revision, Edmonton 2001. *J Rheum* 31:390–392, 2001.

B Psoriatic arthritis A child may meet criteria for psoriatic arthritis without having the presence of psoriasis (or they may later develop psoriasis) (Table 9-12). One should suspect psoriatic arthritis in a child presenting with a **dactylitis** (sausage digit). These children also need screening for asymptomatic inflammatory eye disease at least every 6 months. Treatment is similar to that for other forms of JIA.

C Inflammatory bowel disease (IBD)-associated arthritis Approximately 7% to 21% of children with IBD have associated arthritis (see Chapter 11). The arthritis tends to involve the large joints of the lower extremities with associated enthesitis. More commonly, the arthritis is active during periods of flare of the gut inflammation. Inflammation of the sacroiliac joints, commonly seen in JAS, is not seen as often in patients with IBD-associated arthritis. Treatment for the bowel disease is often effective in controlling the arthritis and the use of NSAIDs is discouraged due to the risk to the gastrointestinal system.

VIII SYSTEMIC CONNECTIVE TISSUE DISEASES

A Systemic lupus erythematosus

1. SLE is a multisystem, autoimmune inflammatory disorder of unknown etiology. It is characterized by the presence of autoantibodies, the **ANA** being the most sensitive and positive in 98% of patients. There are other autoantibodies such as ds-DNA ab, anti-Ro, Anti-La, anti-Sm, and anti-RNP antibodies that have greater specificity but lower sensitivity.
2. SLE is rare under age 5 and uncommon between 5 and 10 years of age, and in adolescence the incidence becomes similar to that in adults. It is more common in girls than boys by 5 to 10:1.
3. SLE should be suspected in a teenage girl with unexplained fevers, weight loss, and fatigue, as well as more specific findings described in Table 9-13. It can also present more acutely with severe compromise such as acute psychosis, seizures, pulmonary hemorrhage, renal failure, and other life-threatening, emergent situations.
4. **Laboratory findings**, in addition to the presence of autoantibodies, may include neutropenia, anemia, and thrombocytopenia. Elevations in acute-phase reactants such as ESR are seen. It is critical to send urinalysis to evaluate for renal involvement.
5. **Treatments** are varied, depending on the organ system involved. Most patients are given hydroxychloroquine as an immunomodulatory agent. Patients require systemic corticosteroids, tapered to the lowest possible dose. Other medications include immunosuppressive drugs such as azathioprine, cyclophosphamide, and mycophenolate mofetil. If anticardiolipin antibodies are

TABLE 9-13 American College of Rheumatology 1997 Criteria (Four of the 11 Criteria Are Needed)

Malar (butterfly) rash
Discoid—lupus rash
Photosensitivity
Oral or nasal mucosal ulcerations
Nonerosive arthritis
Nephritis: Proteinuria > 0.5 g/day or cellular casts
Encephalopathy: Seizures or psychosis
Pleuritis or pericarditis
Cytopenia
Positive immune serology: ds-DNA, anti-Sm, positive anticardiolipin antibodies based on (a) positive IgG or IgM anticardiolipin antibodies or (b) lupus anticoagulant or (c) false-positive VDRL
Positive ANA

Ig, immunoglobulin.
Adapted from Ferraz MB, Goldenberg J, Hilario MO, et al.: Evaluation of the 1982 ARA lupus criteria data set in pediatric patients. *Clin Exper Rheumatol* 12:83–87, 1994.

present, one may need anticoagulant therapy. Other important features of care include sun protection, good nutrition, and calcium and vitamin D supplementation.

B **Juvenile dermatomyositis (JDM)** is an uncommon, idiopathic, inflammatory disease affecting striated muscle and skin. Children present with complaints suggesting proximal muscle weakness, such as difficulty with stairs or combing their hair. The rash is usually quite suggestive of the diagnosis with purple discoloration of the eyelids (heliotrope suffusion) and red, raised, scaly lesions on the knuckles, elbows, and knees (Gottron papules). Elevations in the muscle enzymes help confirm the diagnosis. A T2-weighted magnetic resonance image of the thigh can demonstrate muscle edema and inflammatory changes. Biopsy can be done if the diagnosis is uncertain. Treatment generally consists of systemic corticosteroids and methotrexate, and, more recently, intravenous immunoglobulin (IVIG) has been advocated by many experts. The efficacy of hydroxychloroquine is controversial. While there is a high rate of associated malignancy in adults with dermatomyositis, this association does not occur in children with JDM.

C **Scleroderma** may be **localized** or **systemic.**

1. **Localized scleroderma** is more frequent than systemic sclerosis, though still uncommon. Often the term ***morphea*** is used to describe the lesions. There are different types of morphea, with linear morphea being the most common in childhood. Typically, there is initially a localized area of erythema or waxy induration that evolves into an area of indurated, tight, shiny, bound-down skin with eventual softening and improvement. The prognosis is generally benign, with a mean length of symptoms of 3 to 5 years.
2. **Systemic sclerosis** is very uncommon in childhood. It is a systemic disease of unknown etiology causing tight thickened skin and internal organs.

IX VASCULITIS

Refers to inflammation of blood vessels. There are many types of vasculitis and classification remains challenging. Most commonly, the vasculitides are categorized by the size of the involved vessels. The most common types of vasculitis seen in the pediatric population are **Henoch-Schönlein purpura (HSP)** and **Kawasaki disease (KD)**.

A **HSP** is a small-vessel, immune complex vasculitis that presents in children ages 3 to 15. It appears as a characteristic, nonthrombocytopenic purpura generally involving the lower extremities and buttocks. One may see associated edema of the lower extremities. Gastrointestinal involvement,

TABLE 9-14 Criteria for the Diagnosis of Kawasaki Disease

Fever for more than 5 d (4 d if treatment with IVIG eradicates fever) plus at least four of the following clinical signs not explained by another disease process:
- Bilateral conjunctival injection
- Changes in the oropharyngeal mucous membranes, including one or more of injected and or fissured lips, strawberry tongue, and injected pharynx
- Changes in the peripheral extremities, including erythema and/or edema of the hands and feet (acute phase) or periungual desquamation (convalescent phase)
- Polymorphous rash, primarily truncal, nonvesicular
- Cervical lymphadenopathy with at least one node > 1.5 cm

Modified from Centers for Disease Control: Revised diagnostic criteria for Kawasaki Disease. *MMWR Morb Mortal Wkly Rep* 39:27–28, 1990.

demonstrated by colicky pain, occurs in approximately two thirds of children. There is a risk of intussusception. Renal involvement occurs in one third of children and includes a range of findings from microscopic hematuria and proteinuria to nephrotic syndrome or acute renal failure. A small percentage has long-term renal disease. Treatment is generally supportive with fluids and pain control. Glucocorticoids are generally not required. In two thirds of children, the illness resolves within 4 weeks; some children continue to have flares of rash and belly pain for several months. Prognosis is usually excellent.

B. **KD** is a medium-size vessel vasculitis that occurs commonly in childhood, most often in children younger than age 5. Diagnosis requires fever for > 5 days with four of five of the other criteria (Table 9-14). The main complication and risk of KD is **cardiovascular disease** (see also Chapter 12). The risk of coronary damage is 25% in untreated patients.

1. **Laboratory markers** demonstrate systemic inflammation including elevated white blood cell count, ESR, and platelets (which often reach > 1 million during the second week of illness). Urinalysis reveals a sterile pyuria. Liver function tests demonstrate elevations of transaminases.
2. **Treatment** of KD includes admission to the hospital, cardiology evaluation, IVIG, high-dose acetylsalicylic acid (ASA) until the fever resolves, and then low-dose ASA for the antiplatelet effect.

BIBLIOGRAPHY

Cassidy JT, Petty RE, Laxer RM, et al. (eds): The Textbook of Pediatric Rheumatology, 5th ed. Philadelphia, Elsevier Saunders, 2005.

Kay AB: Allergy and allergic diseases—first of two parts. *N Engl J Med* 344:30–37, 2001.

Kay AB: Allergy and allergic diseases—second of two parts. Allergic diseases and their treatment. *N Engl J Med* 344:109–114, 2001.

Rosen FS, Cooper MD, Wedgwood RJP: The primary immunodeficiencies. *N Engl J Med* 333:431–438, 1995.

Supplement to the Journal of Allergy and Clinical Immunology. Mini-primer on allergic and immunologic diseases. *J Allergy Clin Immunol* 117:S429–493, 2006.

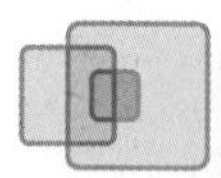

Study Questions

Directions: *Each of the numbered items or incomplete statements in this section is followed by answers or completions of the statement. Select the ONE lettered answer or completion that is BEST in each case.*

1. A 12-month-old boy was born to a 22-year-old HIV-infected mother who died only 2 months after delivery. At 12 months, the child appears healthy and is growing and developing well, but his blood test results are positive for HIV antibodies. Which of the following does this blood test indicate?

- A The child is definitely infected with HIV
- B Maternal antibodies are still present in the boy's blood
- C The positive HIV antibody test result could be the result of paternal antibodies
- D The test is not diagnostic, and the child remains in the category E, or indeterminate, classification
- E Maternal antibodies to HIV are more likely to cause positive HIV serologic test results than antibodies produced in children

2. A 6-year-old girl experiences her second episode of meningococcal meningitis. Which of the following is the most likely immunodeficiency disorder in this child?

- A Neutrophil dysfunction
- B Deficiency of complement component C3
- C Deficiency of C1 esterase inhibitor
- D Deficiency of complement component C6
- E Deficiency of T cells

3. A 6-year-old boy complains of itchy eyes, watery nose, and sneezing starting mid-May and lasting through June. Which of the following is the first drug of choice or modality in your treatment of this child?

- A Antihistamines and topical nasal corticosteroids
- B Avoidance of the offending allergen
- C Desensitization
- D Oral steroids
- E Antibiotics

4. A teenager who gets stung by a bee develops urticaria within 30 minutes of the sting. Which of the following is this reaction is most likely mediated by?

- A Complement component C3
- B IgE antibodies
- C Neutrophils
- D T cells
- E IgA antibodies

5. A teenage African American girl presents to your office with complaint of unexplained fevers, 10-lb weight loss, and swelling of her knees and ankles. On physical exam you see a thin, ill-appearing teen who has swelling and pain with range of motion of her wrists, knees, and ankles. Lab results demonstrate anemia, elevated ESR, positive ANA, positive ds-DNA antibody, and urinalysis with moderate blood and protein. Which of the following is the most likely diagnosis?

- A Pauciarticular juvenile idiopathic arthritis
- B Acute rheumatic fever
- C Systemic lupus erythematosus
- D Juvenile dermatomyositis
- E Henoch-Schönlein purpura

Directions: *Each set of matching questions in this section consists of a list of 4 to 6 lettered options followed by several numbered items. For each numbered item, select the ONE lettered option that is most closely associated with it. Each lettered option may be selected once, more than once, or not at all.*

QUESTIONS 6–9

For each of the following patients, select the most likely immune deficiency disorder.

A Chronic granulomatous disease
B X-linked agammaglobulinemia
C Complement C2 deficiency
D DiGeorge anomaly

6. A patient is initially seen with a malar facial rash, arthritis, and a cutaneous vasculitis

7. A patient has recurrent bilateral lobar pneumonia

8. A patient is initially seen with oral candidiasis, a history of tetany in the newborn period, and tetralogy of Fallot

9. A patient is initially seen with cervical lymphadenitis from which *Klebsiella pneumoniae* is cultured

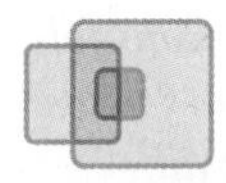

Answers and Explanations

1. The answer is D (*II C 2 b [4]*). In this case, detection of HIV antibody could be the result either of maternal antibody or antibody produced by an infected child. Hence, we can say only that the child was perinatally exposed and remains in the indeterminate classification as maternal antibodies may persist in the infant for up to 18 months.

2. The answer is D (*II B 3 a, Table 9-4*). A deficiency of one of the late-acting complement components results in recurrent *Neisseria* infections. Deficiency of the complement component C3 results in bacterial infections, particularly with enteric Gram-negative bacteria. Neutrophil dysfunction usually results in infection with Gram-positive organisms. T-cell immunodeficiencies result in viral, parasitic, and fungal infections. C1 esterase inhibitor deficiency is associated with recurrent angioedema.

3. The answer is A (*IV C 5 b [1]*). Although desensitization therapy may be useful in the treatment of allergic rhinitis, the most direct and safest approach to therapy for allergies to pollens is a combination of antihistamines and topical nasal steroids. Avoiding allergens can also be very helpful, if feasible. Oral steroids should only be used for severe symptoms, and in these cases drug use should be limited to 3 to 5 days.

4. The answer is B (*III A*). Type I hypersensitivity reactions are mediated by IgE antibodies. Type III hypersensitivity reactions are mediated by IgG antibodies, complement, and neutrophils. Type IV hypersensitivity reactions are mediated by T cells.

5. The correct answer is C (*VIII A*). SLE occurs in teens as often as in the adult population. The incidence is increased in African Americans. SLE often presents with general symptoms such as fevers and weight loss. More specific features would include arthritis and proteinuria and hematuria. The anemia and elevated ESR are also common but not specific. The ANA is present in about 98% of patients with SLE but it is nonspecific. The ds-DNA is a specific test suggesting SLE. Children with pauciarticular JIA are not systemically ill and should have four or fewer swollen joints. They commonly have a positive ANA (75% of the time), but they never have positive ds-DNA antibodies. They should not have proteinuria and hematuria. A patient with ARF should have a history of a preceding streptoccocal infection and should not have anti-ds DNA or renal involvement. Children with JDM should have a history of weakness as well as information about abnormal muscle enzymes. HSP may have renal involvement and arthritis but should have a history of purpuric lesions.

6. The answer is C (*Table 9-4*). Patients who have congenital complement deficiencies are initially identified with a connective tissue disease such as systemic lupus erythematosus.

7. The answer is B (*Table 9-5*). Recurrent pneumonia caused by virulent bacteria such as *Pneumococcus, Haemophilus,* or *Streptococcus* species is seen in patients who have antibody deficiency such as X-linked agammaglobulinemia.

8. The answer is D (*Table 9-6*). Candidiasis should be a "red flag" for a T-cell deficiency as seen in patients who have DiGeorge anomaly, born without a thymus or with only the remnants of the thymus gland.

9. The answer is A (*Table 9-3*). Patients who have chronic granulomatous disease (CGD) have an increased frequency of skin infections and pyogenic adenitis. Although *Staphylococcus* is a common organism in their infections, patients with CGD also have infections caused by certain Gram-negative (low virulence) organisms, such as *Escherichia coli, Klebsiella* species, *Proteus* species, and other organisms that are catalase positive.

chapter **10**

Infectious Diseases

MELISSA R. HELD • PETER KRAUSE

I INTRODUCTION

A Significance of infectious diseases Infectious diseases are the leading cause of morbidity in infants and children. Since the introduction of effective vaccines, the incidence of certain infections (e.g., smallpox, polio, diphtheria, measles, mumps, rubella, pertussis, tetanus, *Haemophilus influenzae* type b) has been reduced dramatically; however, only smallpox has been eradicated worldwide. Antimicrobial compounds have markedly improved the prognosis associated with many infections, but the emergence of resistant strains has required the continued development of new antimicrobial agents.

II FEVER OF UNKNOWN ORIGIN AND FEVER WITHOUT LOCALIZING SIGNS

A Definitions

1. **Fever** has no universally recognized definition. A practical definition of fever in children is a rectal temperature above 100.4°F (38°C). Oral temperatures usually are approximately 1°F lower than rectal temperatures. The higher the temperature is, the greater the risk of having a bacterial infection.
2. **Fever of unknown origin** suggests that a child has been febrile for more then 10 days without an identifiable cause. Fever of fewer then 10 days without an identifiable cause is referred to as **fever without localizing signs.**

B Diagnosis Fever must be documented (rectal temperatures for infants and young children) and a careful history and physical examination must be performed.

1. The age of the child and other risk factors for a serious bacterial illness must be assessed.
   a. **Workup** of infants younger then 28 days of age and all toxic-appearing infants regardless of age should include a complete blood count (CBC), blood culture, urinalysis and urine culture, and spinal fluid analysis. A chest radiograph may be clinically indicated. These infants should be hospitalized and started on parenteral antibiotic therapy.
   b. The management of non–toxic-appearing infants and children 1 month to 3 years of age who have fever and no localizing signs is more variable. Generally, antibiotics are withheld until a definitive diagnosis is made.
2. **Observation** is an important part of the examination and may include elements of how the child interacts with his or her environment using descriptive terms such as "irritable," "consolable," "lethargic," or "playful."

III BACTEREMIA AND SEPSIS

A Definitions

1. **Bacteremia:** Bacteria in the blood
2. **Systemic inflammatory response syndrome (SIRS): Systemic responses to a variety of processes, including:**
   a. Pulse rate over 90 beats per minute
   b. Respiratory rate over 20 per minute

c. Temperature > 100.4°F (38°C) or < 95°F (35°C)
d. PCO_2 < 37 mm Hg
e. White blood cell (WBC) count > 10,000/mm^3 or < 4000/mm^3
f. Band count > 20

3. **Sepsis:** Infection plus variety of processes including two or more SIRS criteria
4. **Septicemia:** Infection in the *blood* plus two SIRS criteria
5. **Severe sepsis:** Sepsis plus organ dysfunction
6. **Septic shock:** Sepsis plus hypotension (systolic blood pressure < 90) despite fluid resuscitation
7. **Multiple organ dysfunction syndrome (MODS):** Altered organ function in an acutely ill patient. Intervention to maintain homeostasis is usually required.

B **Occult bacteremia** is defined as bacteremia in febrile children up to age 3 years who initially have no focal sign of infections but who subsequently have a blood culture that grows a bacterial pathogen.

1. **Incidence and etiology.** *Streptococcus pneumoniae* was the most common etiologic agent prior to the introduction of the conjugated pneumococcal vaccine given to infants. Prior to vaccination, the incidence of occult bacteremia ranged from 1.5% to 2%.
2. **Clinical features. Signs and symptoms usually consist of a temperature of at least 102°F (38.9°C) without an obvious focus of infection.**
3. **Diagnosis.** Laboratory workup consists of a WBC count and blood culture.
4. **Therapy.** Empiric antibiotic therapy may be used while awaiting culture results, depending on the likelihood of soft tissue complications.

C Sepsis in infants under 2 months of age

1. **Incidence and etiology.** The most common causative agents are group B streptococcus and *Escherichia coli.*
2. **Clinical features.** Fever is typically present without an obvious focus of infection.
3. **Diagnosis.** Workup includes CBC, blood culture, urinalysis and urine culture, and spinal fluid analysis. A chest radiograph may be clinically indicated.
4. **Therapy** consists of parenterally administered ampicillin and an aminoglycoside, or ampicillin and cefotaxime.

D Sepsis in infants over 2 months of age

1. **Incidence and etiology.** Causative agents include *S. pneumoniae* and *Neisseria meningitides.*
2. **Clinical features** include fever without an obvious focus of infection.
3. **Diagnosis.** Workup includes CBC, blood culture, urinalysis and urine culture, and spinal fluid examination if indicated by clinical or laboratory results.
4. **Therapy** is a parenterally administered third-generation cephalosporin such as ceftriaxone. Vancomycin should also be added if bacterial meningitis is suspected.

E Sepsis in the immunocompromised patient Defects in immune function may be congenital or acquired (see Chapter 9) and include disorders of humoral immunity (antibody and complement defects), cellular immunity (neutrophil, monocyte, and lymphocyte defects), and structural immune mechanisms (e.g., compromised skin integrity, splenic dysfunction). Patients with cancer may have a low neutrophil count (below 500/mm^3) due to chemotherapy.

1. **Etiology** includes *Pseudomonas aeruginosa,* Gram-negative enteric rods, and *Staphylococcus aureus. Staphylococcus epidermidis* is a common cause of sepsis in children who have central venous or intra-arterial catheters.
2. **Clinical features.** Fever may be the only manifestation of life-threatening sepsis in immunocompromised children. These patients must be examined carefully for a focus of infection, including the oral and rectal areas.

3. **Diagnosis.** Laboratory evaluation includes WBC count, chest radiograph (if clinically indicated), and cultures of the blood and urine.
4. **Therapy.** Empiric therapy usually consists of vancomycin (if the patient has a central catheter) and ceftazidime.

IV CENTRAL NERVOUS SYSTEM INFECTIONS

A **Meningitis** refers to any inflammation of the meninges.

1. **Classification and etiology.** There are two major classifications of meningitis: **Bacterial and aseptic.** These usually can be distinguished on the basis of cerebrospinal fluid (CSF) characteristics.
   a. In **bacterial meningitis,** CSF may show an increased WBC count with a predominance of neutrophils, an increased protein level, a lowered glucose level, and, frequently, the presence of bacteria on Gram stain.
      (1) In **neonates,** the most common causes are group B streptococci, *E. coli,* other coliform bacteria, and *Listeria monocytogenes.*
      (2) In **infants and children,** the most common causes are *S. pneumoniae* and *N. meningitidis.* Rare causes include *Borrelia burgdorferi* (the cause of Lyme disease) and *Mycobacterium tuberculosis.*
   b. In **aseptic meningitis,** the CSF does not contain bacteria. It is characterized by a mildly elevated WBC count with a predominance of mononuclear cells, a normal or mildly elevated protein level, and a normal glucose level. **The cause of aseptic meningitis usually is viral.** The most common viral causes of meningitis in infants and children are enteroviruses (e.g., coxsackieviruses, echoviruses) and herpes simplex virus.
2. **Clinical features.** The early signs and symptoms of meningitis are less specific in young infants than in older children. Generally, the clinical manifestations are more severe with bacterial meningitis than with viral meningitis.
   a. **Central nervous system involvement** manifests as severe headache, lethargy, confusion, irritability, seizures, vomiting, and a bulging fontanelle.
   b. **Meningeal involvement** manifests as neck or back pain and **Brudzinski sign** (i.e., neck flexion causes flexion of the legs) and **Kernig sign** (i.e., inability to extend the leg after the thigh is flexed to a right angle with the axis of the trunk). **Nuchal rigidity** is a sensitive sign in children older than 12 months.
   c. **Nonspecific features** include fever, irritability, poor feeding, and petechial lesions (most commonly seen with meningitis due to *N. meningitidis*).
3. **Diagnosis. Bacterial meningitis is a medical emergency. A lumbar puncture should be performed immediately.** In cases of viral meningitis, viral culture results of CSF are positive in less than half of patients. Cultures of tissue or fluid other than CSF may help establish the specific cause of meningitis (e.g., a blood culture for bacteria or throat and rectal cultures for virus).
   a. **Normal CSF values** are presented in Table 10-1.
   b. **CSF findings in bacterial and viral meningitis** are shown in Table 10-2.
   c. **Contraindications to lumbar puncture.** The decision to perform a lumbar puncture is based on clinical suspicion of bacterial meningitis. Contraindications may include increased intracranial pressure due to a space-occupying lesion, shock, respiratory failure, or a bleeding diathesis.

TABLE 10-1 Normal Cerebrospinal Fluid Values

	Opening Pressure (mm Hg)	WBC Count	PMNs (%)	Protein (mg/dL)	Glucose (% of Serum)
Neonate	< 60	< 30	< 40	< 180	> 50
Infant/child	< 90	< 10	< 10	< 50	> 50

PMNs, polymorphonuclear cells; WBC, white blood cell.

TABLE 10-2 CSF Findings in Bacterial and Viral Meningitis

Parameter	Bacterial Meningitis	Viral Meningitis
CSF pressure	Increased	Increased
WBC count	100–10,000	10–500
WBC type	Predominantly PMN	Predominantly mononuclear
Protein content (mg/dL)	> 40	> 40
Glucose content (mg/dL)	< 40 (< 50% blood glucose)	Normal
Gram stain/culture	Positive for bacteria	Negative
Latex agglutination	Positive for bacteria	Negative

CSF, cerebrospinal fluid; PMN, polymorphonuclear cell; WBC, white blood cell.

4. **Therapy for bacterial meningitis**
   a. **Antimicrobial therapy. Initial therapy** (before identification of the causative organism) **is based on patient age.**
      (1) **Neonates and infants younger than 2 months** are usually given ampicillin and an aminoglycoside, or ampicillin and cefotaxime. Ampicillin is active against group B streptococci and *L. monocytogenes.* Cefotaxime is active against group B streptococci and coliform bacteria, and aminoglycosides are active against coliform bacteria.
      (2) **Infants and children older than 2 months** are usually given ceftriaxone or cefotaxime, plus vancomycin. Ceftriaxone and cefotaxime are active against *S. pneumoniae* and *N. meningitidis,* whereas vancomycin is active against cephalosporin-resistant *S. pneumoniae.*
   b. The **duration of therapy** varies by age and causative organism.
   c. **Supportive care** consists of fluid restriction to minimize cerebral edema, maintenance of intravascular volume with fluid replacement therapy, anticonvulsants (if seizures are present), and assisted ventilation (for respiratory failure).
   d. **Corticosteroid therapy** for children who have pneumococcal or meningococcal meningitis has not been definitively shown to be beneficial.
   e. **Follow-up care.** Neurologic evaluation at the time of discharge from the hospital might include a vision test, hearing test, and formal developmental assessment. Periodic monitoring of neurologic and developmental status should be carried out for at least 2 years.

B **Encephalitis** is an inflammation of the brain parenchyma leading to cerebral dysfunction.

1. **Etiology.** A specific pathogen is not identified in approximately 75% of the annual cases of acute encephalitis that occur in the United States. Viral causes are the most common.
   a. **Herpes simplex virus** is the most common cause of sporadic acute encephalitis in the United States.
      (1) Herpes simplex virus type 2 usually is the cause of encephalitis in neonates.
      (2) Herpes simplex virus type 1 causes most cases of encephalitis in older children.
   b. **Arboviruses** occasionally cause encephalitis outbreaks during the summer because these viruses are transmitted by insects (usually mosquitoes). Important arboviral causes of encephalitis in the United States include:
      (1) California encephalitis virus
      (2) St. Louis encephalitis virus
      (3) Eastern equine encephalitis virus
      (4) Western equine encephalitis virus
      (5) West Nile virus
   c. **Enteroviruses** (i.e., coxsackieviruses and echoviruses) cause encephalitis outbreaks during the summer and early fall.
   d. **Infections occasionally associated with encephalitis** include *Bartonella henselae* (cat-scratch disease), *M. tuberculosis, B. burgdorferi* (Lyme disease), varicella-zoster virus, *Mycoplasma pneumoniae,* Epstein-Barr virus (infectious mononucleosis), human herpesvirus 6, Rocky Mountain spotted fever, measles, mumps, and rubella.

2. **Clinical features** may vary but usually include the following symptoms.
   a. **Early signs and symptoms are nonspecific** and typical of acute systemic illness (e.g., fever, headache, vomiting, upper respiratory tract symptoms).
   b. **Neurologic signs and symptoms** develop abruptly. Most commonly, there is a decreased level of consciousness, which may range from confusion to deep coma. Seizures, paralysis, and abnormal reflexes are also common. Increased intracranial pressure can result in papilledema.
3. **Diagnosis.** A complete history includes an evaluation of all possible exposures to infected people, insects, or animals. Laboratory tests can be used to confirm the diagnosis of encephalitis and sometime identify an etiology.
   a. **Lumbar puncture and CSF examination** are essential. **Typical CSF findings** include increased intracranial pressure, variable pleocytosis (generally 10–500 cells/mm^3) with a predominance of mononuclear cells, increased protein level ($>$ 40 mg/dL), and a normal glucose level.
   b. CSF should be examined directly and cultured for bacteria, mycobacteria, fungi, and viruses.
   c. **Polymerase chain reaction** (PCR) may be performed for detection of herpes simplex in CSF.
   d. **Brain biopsy** may be performed to obtain tissue specimens for culture and rapid viral antigen tests.
   e. **Serologic tests** (e.g., hemagglutination inhibition, complement fixation, enzyme-linked immunosorbent assay [ELISA]) may be used to detect viral antibodies. The diagnosis of arboviral encephalitis is best confirmed by serologic tests.
   f. **Electroencephalograms, computed tomography (CT), magnetic resonance imaging (MRI), and brain scans** may reveal focal or generalized abnormalities in patients who have encephalitis.
4. **Therapy**
   a. **Antimicrobial therapy. Acyclovir is the drug of choice for treatment of herpes simplex encephalitis.** There is no specific therapy for other types of viral encephalitis.
   b. **Supportive care**
      (1) Patients who have encephalitis should be placed in an **intensive care** unit, with close **cardiac monitoring** and placement of an **intracranial pressure transducer** if intracranial pressure is moderately to severely increased.
      (2) **Phenobarbital** may be given to prevent convulsions.
      (3) Severe cerebral edema can be decreased by using corticosteroids, mannitol, and diuretics.

V UPPER AIRWAY INFECTIONS

A **Otitis media,** or inflammation of the middle ear, is one of the most common infections of childhood. Otitis media is classified as **acute** or **chronic.**

1. **Etiology**
   a. **Bacteria** are the primary agents of otitis media.
      (1) The most **common causes** in all age groups are *S. pneumoniae* (25%–40% of cases), unencapsulated strains of *H. influenzae* (15%–25% of cases), and *Moraxella catarrhalis* (12%–20% of cases).
      (2) **Less common causes** include group A β-hemolytic *Streptococcus*, also known as *Streptococcus pyogenes* (acute form), *S. aureus*, and *P. aeruginosa* or *Mycobacterium* (chronic form).
   b. **Viruses** are not important direct causes of otitis media. However, viral upper respiratory tract infections commonly result in obstruction of the eustachian tube, which allows bacteria to multiply in the middle ear space.
2. **Predisposing factors** associated with increased incidence include otitis media occurring in the first 6 months of life, immunodeficiency, structural defects that impair eustachian tube function (e.g., cleft palate), day care attendance, and siblings who have recurrent otitis media.
3. **Clinical features of otitis media** are often variable and nonspecific.
   a. **Classic signs and symptoms of acute otitis media** (AOM) include pain in one or both ears (otalgia), irritability in an infant or toddler, and a bulging and erythematous tympanic membrane. A discharge may be present (otorrhea).

TABLE 10-3 Characteristics of Three Upper Airway Infections

Characteristic	Viral Croup and Spasmodic Croup	Tracheitis	Epiglottitis
Etiology	Respiratory viruses, including parainfluenza viruses and influenza viruses	Respiratory viruses and bacteria, including *Staphylococcus aureus, Streptococcus pyogenes,* and *Streptococcus pneumoniae*	*Haemophilus influenzae* type b
Common age of occurrence	3 mo–3 y	3 mo–5 y	2–7 y
Clinical features			
Onset	Variable (12–48 h)	Gradually progressive (12 h–7 d)	Rapid (4–12 h)
Fever	Variable (100°F–105°F)	Variable (100°F–105°F)	High (≥ 103°F)
Hoarseness and barking cough	Yes	Yes	No
Dysphagia	No	No	Yes
Course of obstruction	Variable progression	Variable progression, usually severe	Rapid progression
Lab findings			
Leukocyte count	Mildly elevated band form count	Variable, possibly increased	Usually markedly elevated with increased band forms
Roentgenogram	Subglottic narrowing on PA radiograph	Subglottic narrowing on PA radiograph; irregular soft tissue density within trachea on lateral radiograph	Swollen epiglottis on lateral radiograph
Treatment	Humidification, epinephrine, corticosteroid	Humidification, antibiotic, intubation	Antibiotic, intubation

PA, posteroanterior.

b. **Common signs and symptoms of chronic otitis media** include hearing impairment, perforation of the tympanic membrane, and otorrhea.

c. **Nonspecific signs and symptoms** include fever, irritability, mild upper respiratory tract symptoms, vomiting, and diarrhea.

4. **Diagnosis.** A certain diagnosis of AOM meets all three of the criteria: Rapid onset, presence of middle ear effusion, and signs and symptoms of middle-ear inflammation.
   a. **Otoscopy and tympanometry** are used to provide the basis for a diagnosis of otitis media.
      (1) **Bulging of the tympanic membrane**—as evidenced by partial or total loss of the light reflex or bony landmarks—and diffuse erythema generally are accepted as reliable indications of otitis media. Erythema can result from crying or fever and, by itself, does not establish the diagnosis.
      (2) **Fullness or bulging of the tympanic membrane** has the highest predictive value. Reduced or impaired mobility of the membrane can be assessed with a pneumatic otoscope.
      (3) **Tympanic membrane compliance** can be determined more objectively using a tympanometer.
   b. **Needle aspiration and culture of the middle ear** contents is the most reliable method for confirming the presence of infection and can be used to identify the causative agent. Only rarely is this procedure necessary.

5. **Therapy**
   a. **Acute otitis media**
      (1) **Initial treatment** is directed against the most commonly encountered bacteria, *S. pneumoniae* and *H. influenzae.* The drug of choice is amoxicillin, which usually is effective against both of these organisms. However, observation without use of antibacterial agents in a child with uncomplicated AOM is an option for selected children based on diagnostic certainty, age, illness severity, and assurance of follow-up.

(2) If there is a poor response to initial therapy, **alternative antibiotic regimens** are used including amoxicillin-clavulanate, cefuroxime, cefpodoxime, or cefdinir. Azithromycin or clarithromycin, erythromycin-sulfisoxazole, or sulfamethoxazole-trimethoprim can be used in children with penicillin or cephalosporin allergies. A single intramuscular injection of ceftriaxone is also adequate in treating AOM.

(3) Standard duration of therapy is 10 days but in children over 6 years with mild to moderate disease, a 5- to 7-day course is usually adequate.

(4) A **tube** may be inserted through the tympanic membrane to promote drainage of the middle ear space.

b. **Chronic otitis media**

(1) **Chronic suppurative otitis media.** The classic symptoms are otorrhea and hearing loss. The pathogens are usually mixed and commonly include *S. aureus, P. aeruginosa,* or both.

(2) **Otitis media with effusion (OME).** Chronic OME may be related to infection but also to such conditions as allergy and immunologic disorders. OME is common following acute otitis media. It may persist for several months, and then usually resolves spontaneously. Treatment is controversial. Placement of tympanostomy tubes is recommended in children who have had persistent middle ear effusion for more than 3 months that is unresponsive to antibiotic therapy.

B **Otitis externa** (swimmer's ear) is inflammation of the outer ear canal, usually caused by *S. aureus.* Other causative organisms include *P. aeruginosa* and *E. coli.* Purulent drainage from the canal and slight pain often occur. Therapy consists of local antibiotic ear drops.

C **Sinusitis** is an inflammation of the mucous membrane lining the paranasal sinuses, which may be **acute** or **chronic.**

1. **Acute and chronic forms**

a. **Acute sinusitis** may involve one or more sinuses. Inflammation of the ethmoid sinuses (**ethmoiditis**) is most common in children, because these are the only sinuses that are fully developed at birth. The maxillary sinuses may also be involved but are not clinically important until after 18 months of age. **Frontal sinusitis and sphenoidal sinusitis** are rare before 10 years of age, because these sinuses begin to develop after 6 years of age.

b. **Chronic sinusitis** occurs after prolonged episodes of untreated or inadequately treated acute sinusitis that result in permanent changes in the mucosal lining of the sinus.

2. **Predisposing factors** include viral upper respiratory tract infection, allergy (allergic rhinitis), and asthma. Other contributing factors include periodontal disease, rapid changes in altitude, swimming, trauma, exposure to tobacco smoke, and immunologic defects.

3. **Etiology.** Acute sinusitis is caused by several bacterial pathogens.

a. The **predominant microorganisms** include *S. pneumoniae,* unencapsulated strains of *H. influenzae,* and *M. catarrhalis.*

b. **Viral infections** or **allergies** are usually predisposing factors for bacterial infection in the sinuses.

4. **Clinical features**

a. **Common symptoms** in children older than 5 years are fever, facial pain, headache, and sore throat. Younger children may have nasal discharge, cough that persists longer than 10 days, eye swelling, and fever.

b. **Suggestive signs** include periorbital swelling, localized tenderness to pressure, and malodorous breath.

5. **Diagnosis** is best made by suggestive clinical findings.

a. **Radiographs** should be used in select circumstances and interpreted with caution, as even the common cold can cause radiologic evidence of sinusitis. **Sinus CT scanning** gives the best views of the sinuses.

b. **Transillumination** of the frontal and maxillary sinuses may provide valuable information for the diagnosis of sinusitis in older children.

c. **Sinus aspiration and culture** can identify the specific microbial cause of sinusitis. Rarely is it needed to confirm the diagnosis in children.

6. **Therapy**
   a. **Antimicrobial therapy**
      (1) **Initial treatment** of acute sinusitis should be with a narrow-spectrum antibiotic such as high-dose amoxicillin for most children.
   b. **Sinus irrigation** or **surgical drainage** of the sinuses is indicated in patients who do not respond to antimicrobial therapy or those with intraorbital or intracranial complications, such as orbital cellulitis, cavernous sinus thrombosis, meningitis, or brain abscess.

D **Infections of the oral cavity** **Gingivitis** and **stomatitis** refer to inflammatory disease of the gingivae (gums) and oral mucosa, respectively. Combined inflammation of the gingivae and oral mucosa is termed gingivostomatitis.

1. **Herpetic gingivostomatitis**
   a. **Incidence.** Herpetic gingivostomatitis is the most common type of gingivostomatitis in children. Primary infection usually occurs before age 5.
   b. **Etiology.** Herpetic gingivostomatitis is caused by herpes simplex virus (herpes simplex virus type 1 more than type 2).
   c. **Pathogenesis.** Primary infection affects the mouth and gums, whereas recurrent disease usually affects the junction of the lip and skin (**herpes labialis**) and is less severe than the primary infection. Recurrent herpes labialis may be precipitated by stress, sun exposure, or illness.
   d. **Clinical features.** Primary herpetic gingivostomatitis causes painful, erythematous, edematous, and ulcerative lesions on the buccal mucosa, gums, and, sometimes, hard palate and tongue. Fever is usually present, often to a temperature of 105°F (40.6°C). The infection occurs after a 3- to 9-day incubation period, improves after 3 to 5 days, and usually resolves within 2 weeks.
   e. **Therapy.** Young children often will refuse to eat or drink and may require rehydration. Orally administered acyclovir may decrease the severity of illness if started within 24 to 48 hours after onset.
2. **Herpangina.** Characteristic oropharyngeal lesions are one of the protean manifestations of enteroviral infections.
   a. **Etiology and incidence.** Coxsackieviruses (types A and B) and echoviruses are the causative agents. Infection is most common in summer and fall, when enteroviruses are prevalent.
   b. **Clinical features** include **fever, sore throat, and pain on swallowing.** Fever may be sudden and high, up to 106°F (41.1°C). Headache, myalgia, and vomiting may also occur. The **characteristic lesions** are 1- to 2-mm vesicles and ulcers surrounded by an erythematous ring measuring up to 10 mm in diameter. The lesions occur in the posterior pharynx, including the anterior tonsillar pillars, soft palate, uvula, tonsils, and pharyngeal wall. The fever subsides in 2 to 4 days, but the ulcers may persist for a period of up to 1 week.
   c. **Therapy** is supportive. Hydration may be needed.
   d. **Hand-foot-and-mouth disease** is another infectious disease caused by enteroviruses, which is characterized by vesicular lesions of the mouth, hands, and feet.
4. **Candidal gingivostomatitis. "Thrush"** is the term used to describe gingivostomatitis due to infection by *Candida* sp., usually *Candida albicans.*
   a. **Incidence.** Candidal gingivostomatitis is common in newborns. The condition usually clears by 3 months of age, except in severely debilitated infants. Oral antibiotic therapy may predispose an individual to thrush. When candidal gingivostomatitis occurs after the first year of life, a defect of cell-mediated immunity should be considered.
   b. **Clinical features** include grayish-white lesions on the buccal mucosa and dorsum of the tongue. Both yeast forms and pseudohyphae are seen on Gram stain. Culture on blood agar will yield *Candida* sp. organisms.
   c. **Therapy** consists of administering a solution of **nystatin** orally four times daily for 1 week. Retreatment sometimes is necessary. **Clotrimazole troches,** fluconazole, or ketoconazole are effective alternatives.

E **Pharyngitis** "Acute pharyngitis" refers to any of the numerous inflammatory conditions involving the pharynx. Most often caused by a virus, the most clinically significant cause of acute pharyngitis is group A β-hemolytic *Streptococcus.* Because penicillin is effective against streptococcal but not viral pharyngitis, it is important to recognize streptococcal pharyngitis so that its symptoms can be alleviated and its complications (*see V E 5*) can be prevented.

1. **Epidemiology.** Streptococcal pharyngitis is one of the most common respiratory tract infections of childhood. All age groups may be affected but the peak incidence occurs in children between the ages of 5 and 15 years. Incidence is highest in winter and spring.
2. **Clinical features**
   a. **Symptoms** may vary widely from very mild to severe. In **older children,** there is an abrupt onset of fever and sore throat accompanied by headache and malaise. **Younger children** may initially be seen with nausea, vomiting, and abdominal pain.
   b. **Physical signs** may include fever, tonsillar enlargement with exudates, edema, erythema, and lymphoid hyperplasia of the pharynx, tender anterior cervical lymph nodes, and petechiae on the soft palate.
3. **Diagnosis**
   a. **Differential diagnosis**
      (1) Viruses include Epstein-Barr virus (*see VIII C*), adenovirus, herpes simplex virus, enterovirus, influenza virus, and parainfluenza virus.
      (2) **Bacterial causes** include *M. pneumoniae, Neisseria gonorrhoeae, Arcanobacterium haemolyticum,* and hemolytic streptococcal groups other than A (e.g., groups C and G).
   b. **Throat culture** is the traditional method for diagnosis of streptococcal pharyngitis.
   c. **Rapid diagnostic test kits** have been developed for office use. These involve the extraction of streptococcal antigens from throat swabs, so that the antigens can be identified using immunologic methods such as enzyme immunoassay.
4. **Therapy**
   a. The **treatment of choice** for streptococcal pharyngitis in children is oral **penicillin V** given two to three times daily for 10 days. Intramuscular benzathine penicillin G is appropriate alternative therapy.
   b. **Penicillin-allergic patients** may be given any one of several **alternative antibiotics.**
      (1) Oral **erythromycin** is the favored alternative, given in the form of erythromycin estolate or erythromycin ethylsuccinate in two to four divided doses.
      (2) Narrow-spectrum (first-generation) cephalosporins are an acceptable alternative; however, as many as 5% of penicillin-allergic people with also be allergic to cephalosporins.
5. **Complications**
   a. **Suppurative complications** include peritonsillar cellulitis or abscess, retropharyngeal abscess, suppurative cervical lymphadenitis, acute otitis media, and acute sinusitis.
   b. The delayed, **nonsuppurative complications** of streptococcal pharyngitis are more significant: Acute rheumatic fever (see Chapter 9) and acute glomerulonephritis (see Chapter 14).

F **Cervical adenitis** refers to inflammation and enlargement of the lymph nodes of the neck. Swollen and tender cervical lymph nodes are common in children. In many cases, the illness is self-limited (as in cervical adenitis associated with a viral infection); however, in other cases the illness requires prompt and specific treatment, such as cervical adenitis due to *S. aureus* or group A *Streptococcus.*

1. **Etiology** is quite variable but usually related either to bacterial infection of the oral cavity or other areas of the head and neck (e.g., streptococcal pharyngitis) or to viral upper respiratory tract infection.
   a. **Common agents.** *S. aureus* and group A *Streptococcus* are the most frequently identified; in addition, group B *Streptococcus* are common causes in neonates. Studies have also implicated anaerobic bacteria, either alone or as a polymicrobial infection.
   b. **Less common agents**
      (1) **Cat-scratch disease** primarily affects children and is an important cause of cervical adenitis. The causative organism is *B. henselae.* Transmission is usually by a cat scratch but occasionally from another animal or plant thorn.
      (2) Several species of **atypical mycobacteria** cause cervical adenitis in infants and young children. The most common of these are *Mycobacterium scrofulaceum* and *Mycobacterium avium-intracellulare.*

(3) **Other agents** of childhood cervical adenitis include Ebstein-Barr virus, cytomegalovirus, *M. tuberculosis, Francisella tularemia, Yersinia pestis* (plague), *Histoplasmosis,* and *Toxoplasma gondii.*

2. **Clinical features**
   a. **General description.** Swollen, tender nodes are typically found in a single location of the neck. **Bilateral involvement** suggests a nonspecific or viral infection, which usually resolves spontaneously. **Unilateral involvement** with nodes that are more severely swollen (3–6 cm in diameter), tender, and warm suggests a pyogenic infection. Fever may or may not be present.
   b. In **cat-scratch disease,** which is unilateral, the involved nodes may be quite large and, in 10% to 25% of cases, these nodes are suppurative. Low-grade fever and a transient maculopapular rash may also be noted.
   c. In **atypical mycobacterial infection,** the cervical adenitis usually involves the submandibular or submaxillary nodes, is unilateral, and runs an indolent course. Fever and other systemic signs are usually absent.

3. **Diagnosis**
   a. **Medical history and physical examination** should include information concerning the duration of the lymphadenopathy, recent upper respiratory tract infections, contact with pets (especially cats), and exposure to individuals who have tuberculosis. All node sites should be examined, with dimensions noted. Liver and spleen size should also be noted.
   b. Specific determination of the cause of cervical adenitis usually is not attempted if the child has only slightly enlarged and minimally tender lymph nodes. A **diagnostic workup** is performed if the child has a moderate fever and systemic symptoms when first examined, a large (> 3 cm) or fluctuant node is found, findings suggest an unusual cause, or empiric antibiotic therapy has failed (*see V F 4*).
      (1) **Needle aspiration, incision and drainage, or excision and biopsy** are the most direct methods for identifying the cause of cervical adenitis.
      (2) A **tuberculin skin test** should be considered in all children with cervical adenitis.
      (3) **Serologic tests** may help to identify viruses (e.g., Ebstein-Barr virus), certain bacteria (e.g., *B. henselae, Francisella tularensis*), and protozoa (*T. gondii*).
      (4) Other diagnostic tests include Gram stain and culture of any focus of infection, blood culture, complete blood count, chest radiograph, and ultrasound of the node to identify pus or loculation.

4. **Therapy**
   a. Cervical adenitis that is characterized by only **slight enlargement** (< 3 cm) and **minimal tenderness** of the lymph nodes should be closely observed but otherwise is untreated.
   b. Cervical adenitis that is characterized by more severe enlargement and tenderness is usually treated first with empiric antibiotic therapy for 10 to 14 days.
      (1) Choices for empiric therapy include **cephalexin, cefadroxil,** and **clindamycin.** If periodontal disease is suspected, clindamycin or **amoxicillin-clavulanate** is preferred based on their activity against oral anaerobes.
   c. For moderate to severe infections, a needle aspiration or incision and drainage may be necessary.
      (1) Intravenous therapy with **cefazolin, nafcillin, oxacillin,** or **clindamycin** may be empirically started, until culture results are known. Clindamycin therapy provides good anaerobic coverage if there is evidence or suspicion of periodontal disease. After discharge from the hospital, therapy can be changed to an oral antibiotic.
      (2) **Cervical adenitis associated with cat-scratch disease** is usually self-limited and requires only analgesics. Antibiotic therapy may be considered in patients who have more severe cases and might include oral trimethoprim-sulfamethoxazole, or parenteral rifampin, azithromycin, or gentamicin, although efficacy of antibiotic therapy has not been demonstrated. Suppuration may occur and can be managed with needle aspiration.
      (3) **Cervical adenitis due to atypical mycobacteria** is treated with excision of infected nodes. Antituberculous drug therapy alone is usually unsuccessful, although it may be used in addition to surgical excision.

G **Acute infectious laryngitis** is common and usually occurs in association with the common cold and influenza. Infectious laryngitis is often included as part of the croup syndrome.

H Infections of the larynx and trachea (Table 10-3)

1. **Croup** is a general term used to describe several acute conditions (both infectious and noninfectious) involving the larynx and, to a lesser extent, the trachea and bronchi. Croup syndromes are characterized by a distinctively brassy cough combined with one or more of the following: Hoarseness, inspiratory stridor, and signs of respiratory distress due to laryngeal obstruction. In clinical practice, the term *croup* is usually used to describe acute laryngotracheitis (viral croup) and acute spasmodic laryngitis (spasmodic croup). **Acute laryngotracheitis** is the most common of the clinical entities termed *croup.*
   a. **Etiology.** Acute laryngotracheitis is caused primarily by respiratory viruses, most commonly **parainfluenza virus.**
   b. **Clinical features.** Symptoms are often worse at night and persist for several days. Onset may be gradual.
      (1) Patients are initially seen with symptoms of **upper respiratory tract infection,** followed after several days by the characteristic **barking cough, inspiratory stridor,** and **respiratory distress.**
      (2) **Fever** is variable, but can be high.
      (3) **Hoarseness and aphonia** are common.
   c. **Diagnosis** is made clinically but can be aided by radiography of the larynx, which reveals subglottic narrowing. An anteroposterior view of the neck shows the classic narrowing of the trachea ("church steeple" sign).
   d. **Therapy** for viral croup is mainly directed at improving air exchange and is mainly supportive.
      (1) **Home care.** Patients who have mild illness may be treated at home with humidified air from a hot shower or bath, hot steam from a vaporizer, or "cold steam" from a nebulizer.
      (2) **Hospitalization.** Patients with cyanosis, decreased level of consciousness, progressive stridor, or a toxic appearance should be hospitalized. Cold, humidified oxygen should be provided, and the patient should be observed closely in case emergency intubation is needed. But otherwise, the patient should be disturbed as little as possible.
      (3) **Racemic epinephrine** (2.5% solution delivered by nebulizer) has been shown to improve air exchange in these patients. This drug should be used in moderately ill, hospitalized patients and it may eliminate the need for intubation during the 24 to 48 hours when the illness is most severe. Racemic epinephrine's effects are transient; thus, it is not recommended for outpatient use.
      (4) **Corticosteroids** have been the subject of much debate, but they may be helpful for patients who are severely ill. Parenteral and oral **dexamethasone** and nebulized corticosteroids have been shown to lessen the severity and duration of symptoms.
2. **Laryngotracheobronchitis,** or bacterial tracheitis, is far less common than laryngotracheitis or acute spasmodic laryngitis, but is more severe. It is often caused by a combination of bacterial and respiratory viral pathogens. Severe tracheal obstruction with copious, thick secretions is common.
   a. **Etiology.** Laryngotracheobronchitis is caused by **parainfluenza** or **influenza viruses** and often a bacterial **coinfection,** including *S. aureus, S. pneumoniae,* or *H. influenzae* type b.
   b. **Clinical features.** Laryngotracheobronchitis is usually similar in onset to laryngotracheitis but results in more serious illness.
   c. **Therapy.** Treatment is similar to that of acute laryngotracheitis, with the exclusion of steroids and racemic epinephrine and the inclusion of antibiotics. Intubation with vigorous suctioning of the airway to remove secretions is usually necessary.

I **Acute epiglottitis** is a rapidly progressive infection of the epiglottis and contiguous structures that may cause life-threatening airway obstruction (Table 10-3).

1. **Etiology and incidence.** Almost all cases of acute epiglottitis in children are caused by ***H. influenzae* type b**. The incidence of acute epiglottitis has markedly decreased due to the use of the *H. influenzae* type b vaccine.

2. **Clinical features.** The abrupt onset of high fever, moderate to severe respiratory distress, and stridor in a child who is sitting forward with his or her mouth open and drooling are symptoms highly suggestive of acute epiglottitis.

3. **Diagnosis**

   a. **Physical examination** should be done quickly and with care to minimize anxiety and keep the child calm. The diagnosis is based on finding a swollen, cherry-red epiglottis. It is essential to **visualize the epiglottis with a laryngoscope or bronchoscope in an operating room,** with complete cardiorespiratory support. Visualization of the epiglottis in other settings by depressing the tongue is contraindicated because of the possibility of inducing airway obstruction.

   b. **Radiography.** Lateral neck radiographs of the nasopharynx and upper airway are useful in mild cases in determining whether epiglottitis is present. The presence of the "thumbprinting" sign is a common radiographic marker for epiglottitis.

   c. **Culture** of the epiglottis and blood should be obtained for identification of the causative organism and its antimicrobial susceptibility pattern.

   d. **Differential diagnosis.** The major differential considerations are acute laryngotracheitis (viral croup) and bacterial tracheitis. Epiglottitis has a more abrupt onset and more severe symptoms.

4. **Therapy**

   a. **Ventilatory support.** After visual confirmation of epiglottitis, the patient should be intubated and given ventilatory support until edema subsides, usually after several days.

   b. **Intravenous antibiotic therapy** is given for 7 to 10 days and is directed against *H. influenzae* type b. The initial agent of choice is a third-generation cephalosporin. Therapy can be directed after sensitivity patterns are identified.

   c. **Contraindications.** Racemic epinephrine and corticosteroids should not be given to these patients.

J **Mumps** is a highly contagious, acute viral disease. The most characteristic feature is painful enlargement of the salivary glands, primarily the parotid glands. The disease is almost always benign and resolves spontaneously. Active immunization with live attenuated mumps virus vaccine is effective for prevention of mumps and has few side effects (see Chapter 1).

VI LOWER RESPIRATORY TRACT INFECTIONS

A **Bronchiolitis** is an acute viral infection of the bronchioles.

1. **Epidemiology.** Bronchiolitis is a common lower respiratory tract illness of children younger than 2 years (due to their small airways), with a peak incidence at 6 months of age. Most cases occur in the winter and early spring months.

2. **Etiology.** More than 50% of cases are caused by respiratory syncytial virus (RSV). Other causes include human metapneumovirus, parainfluenza virus, and adenovirus.

3. **Pathophysiology.** Bronchiolitis causes inflammation of bronchioles, with narrowing of bronchial diameter that leads to hyperinflation and atelectasis. Young infants with bronchiolar obstruction are more likely to have extensive atelectasis with increased hypoxia and respiratory distress than are older children.

4. **Clinical features**

   a. **Symptoms**

      (1) The onset of bronchiolitis is characterized by mild upper respiratory tract symptoms, which last several days and may be accompanied by a mild fever (temperature of 101°F–102°F [38.4°C–38.9°C]).

      (2) Lower respiratory tract involvement follows, with gradual development of respiratory distress (i.e., paroxysmal cough, wheezing, tachypnea, dyspnea) accompanied by irritability and decreased appetite.

   b. **Physical signs** of bronchiolitis include tachypnea, flaring of the alae nasi, and, occasionally, cyanosis. Rales and expiratory wheezes are characteristic. Neonates may present with apnea.

5. **Diagnosis** of bronchiolitis is usually made on the basis of the history, physical examination, and classic, confirmatory radiographic findings, including hyperinflation and occasional scattered areas of consolidation due to atelectasis. The WBC count and differential are usually within normal range.
   a. **Diagnosis of the specific agent** of bronchiolitis can be made by rapid tests for viral antigen in the nasopharynx (especially immunofluorescence for respiratory syncytial virus), viral cultures, or observation of a rise in serum antibody titers.
   b. **Differential** diagnosis should include asthma as well as congestive heart failure, foreign body in the lung or trachea, pertussis, chlamydial infection, cystic fibrosis, and bacterial pneumonia.
6. **Therapy**
   a. **Hospitalization.** In some children—especially infants who have congenital heart disease, cystic fibrosis, bronchopulmonary dysplasia, or other underlying pulmonary disease—respiratory distress progresses rapidly and is severe enough to require that the patient be hospitalized with **assisted ventilation.** The mortality rate among these patients is much higher than in those who have mild to moderate bronchiolitis.
      (1) Supportive therapy is the mainstay of therapy, with some patients requiring oxygen saturation monitoring and support. Nasal suctioning of secretions can be helpful.
      (2) Very young infants may require temporary cardiopulmonary monitoring for apnea.
   c. Ribavirin has in vitro activity against RSV but is not routinely recommended.
7. **Prevention**
   a. **Palivizumab** (Synagis) is a humanized mouse monoclonal antibody administered intramuscularly on a monthly basis during the RSV season to reduce the risk of hospitalization in high-risk children. It is not used to treat RSV infection.
   b. Respiratory syncytial virus immune globulin intravenous (RSV-IGIV) is no longer routinely available.

B **Pneumonia** refers to inflammation of the lung parenchyma (i.e., the portion of the lower respiratory tract consisting of the respiratory bronchioles, alveolar ducts, alveolar sacs, and alveoli). There are numerous infectious causes of pneumonia, including viruses, bacteria, fungi, parasites, and rickettsiae. Although most cases of childhood pneumonia are caused by viruses, antibiotics are prescribed because the precise cause is usually not determined.

1. **Bacterial pneumonia**
   a. **Etiology**
      (1) **Common bacterial causes. Pneumococcal pneumonia** is the most common typical bacterial pneumonia in children of all ages. Group A *Streptococcus* and *S. aureus* are other causes. Group B *Streptococcus* is a cause of pneumonia in infants under 3 months.
      (2) **Other bacterial causes** of pneumonia in children include Gram-negative enteric organisms, *M. pneumoniae, Chlamydia species,* anaerobes (especially in patients at risk for aspiration), *H. influenzae* type b, and *M. tuberculosis.*
   b. **Clinical features**
      (1) **Older children** who have bacterial pneumonia are typically first seen with mild upper respiratory tract symptoms (e.g., cough, rhinitis), followed by the abrupt onset of fever, tachypnea, chest pain, and shaking chills. Physical examination often reveals lateralizing chest signs, such as decreased breath sounds and rales on the affected side.
      (2) **Younger children** (i.e., < 6 years) who have bacterial pneumonia may initially be seen with nonspecific manifestations of infection, including fever, malaise, gastrointestinal complaints, restlessness, apprehension, and chills. **Respiratory signs** may be minimal and include tachypnea, cough, grunting respirations, and flaring of the alae nasi. Signs of pneumonia may also be subtle in the young infant, with absence of rales and rhonchi.
   c. **Diagnosis**
      (1) **Laboratory findings** include peripheral blood leukocytosis with a preponderance of neutrophils and dense, focal infiltration visible on chest radiograph.
      (2) **Specific diagnosis** can be made from culture or rapid antigen testing of the blood, alveolar fluid, pleural fluid, or urine. Fluid may be obtained by lung biopsy, lung puncture, thoracentesis, or bronchoscopy. Although Gram stain and culture of the sputum is often helpful in identifying the pathogen, sputum usually is difficult to obtain from children.

d. Therapy. There is no universally accepted antibiotic regimen for treatment of presumed bacterial pneumonia. In addition to the following general guidelines, such factors as age, severity of illness, presence of illnesses in the child's family, and results of laboratory studies must be considered when an antibiotic is chosen.

(1) **Neonates** who have pneumonia should be hospitalized and treated empirically intravenously either with ampicillin and an aminoglycoside (e.g., gentamicin) or with ampicillin and cefotaxime or ceftazidime. If there is reason to suspect staphylococcal infection, a penicillinase-resistant penicillin should be used in addition to these antibiotics. Supportive care also plays an important role with intravenous fluids, supplemental oxygen, ventilatory support, and chest physical therapy.

(2) **Children younger than 6 years** who have mild to moderate illness can be observed closely at home and given high-dose amoxicillin (80–100 mg/kg/day). Children who have more severe illness require hospitalization and an intravenous antibiotic such as cefuroxime or ceftriaxone. For the most severely ill patients, initial therapy should consist of very broad-spectrum coverage such as oxacillin or vancomycin plus ceftazidime or an aminoglycoside.

(3) **Children older than 6 years** who have mild to moderate illness are given an oral penicillin or second-generation cephalosporin, or if *M. pneumoniae* is the likely cause, erythromycin or azithromycin (*see VI B 3*). Children who have severe illness are hospitalized and treated with the same antibiotics as for children younger than 6 years of age.

2. Viral pneumonia

a. Etiology. A virus is the most common cause of pneumonia in children. **RSV is the most common viral cause;** other common causes include parainfluenza virus, adenovirus, and enterovirus. Less common causes of pneumonia in children include rhinovirus, influenza virus, cytomegalovirus, varicella-zoster virus, and herpes simplex virus.

b. Clinical features. The clinical presentation of viral pneumonia, like that of bacterial pneumonia, begins with several days of rhinitis and cough, followed by fever and more pronounced respiratory tract symptoms, such as dyspnea and intercostal retractions. In general, the symptoms of viral pneumonia are less fulminant than those of bacterial pneumonia.

c. Diagnosis

(1) **Laboratory findings** include a preponderance of lymphocytes observed on CBC and diffuse, bilateral infiltrates visible on chest radiograph.

(2) **Specific diagnosis** can be made by rapid tests for viral antigen (e.g., immunofluorescence) and culturing nasopharyngeal and rectal specimens for viruses.

d. Therapy for viral pneumonia at one time was limited to supportive care; however, the introduction of antiviral chemotherapy has allowed for specific therapy.

(1) **Antiviral therapy**

(a) **Acyclovir** has been used to treat pneumonia caused by herpes simplex virus or varicella-zoster virus. This drug is given by intravenous infusion over a period of 7 to 10 days.

(b) Influenza can be treated with amantadine, rimantadine, zanamivir, or oseltamivir depending on the age of the patient, whether the agent is influenza A or B, and the resistance patterns common that year.

(2) **Supportive care** includes administration of intravenous fluids and supplemental oxygen as well as ventilatory support and chest physical therapy.

3. Other causes of pneumonia

a. *M. pneumoniae* is the most common nonviral cause of pneumonia in children older than 6 years. The peak incidence of *M. pneumoniae* pneumonia is between the ages of 5 and 15 years.

(1) **Clinical features.** In general, *M. pneumoniae* pneumonia is less severe than traditional bacterial pneumonia and often is referred to as "walking pneumonia." Hospitalization rarely is necessary.

(a) The **onset of illness** is gradual; fever, headache, and malaise are experienced for 2 to 4 days before respiratory tract symptoms develop.

(b) **Symptoms.** A nonproductive cough is the characteristic respiratory tract symptom. Pharyngitis is also common.

(2) **Diagnosis**

(a) **Laboratory findings.** The CBC often is within normal limits, but leukocytosis with a shift to the left may be noted. The infiltrate on chest radiograph is usually interstitial in appearance, but it may be focal. Cold agglutinin levels are usually elevated (> 1:64) during the first week of illness, but these levels may not be elevated in young children.

(b) **Specific diagnosis** is made by demonstration of an elevation in antibody titer in convalescent-phase serum or isolation of *M. pneumoniae* from sputum or throat culture.

(3) **Therapy. Erythromycin** or azithromycin is used for treatment of *M. pneumoniae* pneumonia.

VII FEVER AND RASH (TABLE 10-4)

A **Meningococcemia** is caused by *N. meningitides,* a Gram-negative diplococcus.

1. **Epidemiology.** Most disease is caused by five serotypes (A, B, C, Y, and W-135). The disease is spread from asymptomatic carriers of the organism in the nasopharynx. Peaks of disease occur in children under 5 years of age and in adolescents. The incubation period ranges from 1 to 10 days but is usually < 4 days.
2. **Clinical features.** Invasive infection with the organism can result in meningococcemia, meningitis, or both. Fever, chills, and a progressive rash (macular, papular, petechial, or combination) can be of sudden onset but patients may not initially appear toxic. **Waterhouse-Friderichsen syndrome** includes acute adrenal insufficiency, purpura, disseminated intravascular coagulation, shock, coma, and sometimes death. Mortality can be high.
3. **Diagnosis.** Cultures of blood and CSF are indicated. Cultures of the rash or other body fluids may also reveal the organism.
4. **Treatment.** Penicillin G should be given for patients with invasive disease. Alternative agents include ceftriaxone, cefotaxime, and ampicillin. Five to seven days of treatment is usually adequate.

B **Measles (rubeola)** is an acute, highly contagious viral disease that occurs chiefly in young children living in densely populated areas. Measles is caused by a **paramyxovirus** (the measles virus).

1. **Epidemiology.** Although measles is uncommon in developed countries where vaccine is used, it continues to be a major health problem worldwide.

TABLE 10-4 Exanthems: Etiology and Clinical Features

Exanthem	Etiology	Incubation Period	Prodrome	Most Common Rash	Complications
Measles (rubeola)	Measles virus	8–12 d	2–4 d	Maculopapular, beginning on head	Pneumonia, otitis media, encephalitis
Rubella	Rubella virus	12–23 d	Children: None Adults: 1–5 d	Maculopapular	Arthritis, congenital rubella syndrome
Roseola	Human herpes virus 6	~9 d	3–7 d	Maculopapular 3–4 d after fever	Convulsions, encephalitis
Erythema infectiosum (Fifth disease)	Parvovirus B19	4–20 d	2–3 d	"Slapped cheeks" reticular	Arthritis, aplastic crisis, fetal hydrops, death
Varicella	Varicella-zoster virus	10–21 d	Children: None Adults: 1–2 d	Vesicles in "crops" beginning on trunk	Bacterial skin infection, meningitis, encephalitis
Scarlet fever	*Streptococcus pyogenes*	1–7 d	1–2 d	Generalized, finely punctate	Rheumatic fever, glomerulonephritis
Rocky Mountain spotted fever	*Rickettsia rickettsii*	1–14 d	1–5 d	Papular, petechial, purpuric	DIC, shock, pneumonia, cardiac failure

DIC, disseminated intravascular coagulation.

2. **Clinical features.** The clinical course of measles has three stages.
   a. An **incubation period** extends from 8 to 12 days after initial exposure to the virus; signs and symptoms are absent during this stage.
   b. A **prodrome** follows, consisting of malaise, fever (temperatures up to 105°F [40.6°C]), cough, coryza, conjunctivitis, and **an erythematous maculopapular rash.** Within 2 or 3 days after the onset of symptoms, **Koplik spots** (small, irregular, red spots with central gray or bluish-white specks) appear on the buccal mucosa.
3. **Diagnosis** can usually be made on the basis of observed characteristic clinical findings. A fourfold or greater rise in hemagglutination inhibition antibodies over 2 or 3 weeks confirms the diagnosis.
4. **Therapy** is mainly supportive. Vitamin A administration should be given to children 6 months to 2 years when hospitalized with measles or in children older than 6 months who have certain risk factors (immunodeficiency, moderate to severe malnutrition, impaired intestinal absorption).
5. **Prevention**
   a. A live attenuated vaccine given alone or as part of the measles, mumps, and rubella (MMR) vaccine is highly effective in preventing measles (see Chapter 1). The vaccine may provide protection if given within 72 hours of measles exposure.
   b. Immunoglobulin (IG) can be given to modify or prevent measles if given within 6 days of exposure.
6. **Complications** are rare but may occur, especially in malnourished, vitamin A–deficient, or immunocompromised children. Measles complications include pneumonia, encephalitis, subacute sclerosing panencephalitis (SSPE), pericarditis, and hepatitis. The mortality rate is low in healthy children.

C **Rubella (German measles)** is a viral disease that usually is innocuous when acquired postnatally; however, it can have devastating effects when a fetus is infected transplacentally during maternal infection. **Prevention** of rubella is effected by a live attenuated vaccine, which is usually given at age 12 to 15 months and again at school entry (4–6 years old) as part of the MMR vaccine (see Chapter 1).

D **Roseola infantum (exanthem subitum)** is a common, acute disease of infants and young children, which is caused by human herpesvirus 6.

1. **Clinical features**
   a. **Onset.** The illness usually begins with an **abrupt fever** characterized by temperatures of 103°F to 106°F (39.5°C–41.1°C). The fever persists for 1 to 5 days, although the child appears well and has no physical findings to explain the fever.
   b. The temperature usually returns to normal by the third or fourth day of illness, and a **macular** or **maculopapular rash** appears on the trunk and spreads peripherally. The rash often resolves within 24 hours.
   c. **Leukocyte count** may initially be as high as 20,000/mm^3, with a shift to the left. By the second day of illness, leukopenia and neutropenia are noted.
2. **Therapy.** Most cases are benign and self-limited.

E **Erythema infectiosum (fifth disease)** is a mild, self-limited systemic illness accompanied by a distinctive rash. It occurs primarily in epidemics involving children, although adults infrequently are affected. It is caused by **parvovirus B19.**

1. **Clinical features**
   a. Usually there is no prodrome and fever may be absent or only low grade. Systemic symptoms, especially recurrent arthralgias, occur more frequently in adults.
   b. The **rash progresses through three stages.**
      (1) The rash begins as a marked **erythema of the cheeks,** which gives a "slapped cheek" appearance.
      (2) An **erythematous, maculopapular rash** then involves the arms and spreads to the trunk and legs, producing a reticular pattern.
      (3) The third stage is characterized by fluctuations in the severity of the rash upon exposure to hot and cold. The rash lasts 2 to 3 weeks but may persist for several months, with low-grade fever.

2. **Therapy** consists of supportive measures. Intravenous immunoglobulin should be considered for chronic infection that may develop in immunocompromised patients.
3. **Complications** (e.g., arthritis, hemolytic anemia, encephalopathy) are rare. Parvovirus B19 infection during pregnancy can cause fetal hydrops and death. Transient arrest of erythrocyte production (aplastic crisis) may occur in patients who have hemoglobinopathies such as sickle cell anemia.

F Varicella-zoster infections

1. **Definitions**
   a. **Primary infection results in varicella (chickenpox),** a highly contagious disease, occurring primarily in children younger than 10 years of age. It usually is a mild, self-limited disease in otherwise healthy children, but it may be a severe or even fatal illness in immunocompromised children.
   b. **Zoster (shingles)** represents a reactivation of varicella infection, occurring predominantly in adults who previously had varicella and who have circulating antibodies. Zoster can occur in children but is uncommon under 10 years of age. Zoster is an acute infection characterized by crops of vesicles confined to a dermatome and often accompanied by pain in the affected dermatome.
2. **Clinical features**
   a. **Varicella**
      (1) After an **incubation period** ranging from 10 to 21 days (usually 14–16 days), a prodrome begins that consists of mild fever, malaise, anorexia, and, occasionally, a scarlatiniform or morbilliform rash.
      (2) The **characteristic pruritic rash** begins the day following the start of the prodrome, appearing first on the trunk and spreading peripherally.
         (a) The rash begins as red papules and develops rapidly into clear "teardrop" vesicles that are approximately 1 to 2 mm in diameter on an erythematous base. The vesicles become cloudy, breaking down into thin ulcerative lesions that crust before healing.
         (b) The lesions occur in widely scattered "crops," so that several stages of the lesions are usually present at the same time. Vesicles may occur on mucous membranes.
      (3) The **severity of the illness** ranges from a few lesions associated with a low-grade fever, to hundreds of lesions associated with temperatures up to 105°F (40.6°C), to fatal disseminated disease in immunocompromised children. In most children, varicella manifests as a generalized rash with mild fever and mild systemic symptoms.
      (4) **Infectious period.** Patients are infectious beginning approximately 24 hours before the appearance of the rash until all lesions are crusted, which usually occurs 5 to 7 days after the onset of the rash.
   b. **Zoster**
      (1) **Onset.** Attacks of zoster may begin with pain along the affected sensory nerve that is accompanied by fever and malaise.
      (2) A **vesicular eruption** similar to the vesicular form of varicella then appears in a dermatome area and usually clears in 7 to 14 days, but can last as long as 4 weeks.
      (3) The lesions are infectious if there is either direct contact or a susceptible individual inhales aerosolized infected epithelial cells.
3. **Diagnosis of both varicella and zoster** is usually made clinically.
   a. Vesicular fluid or a scab can be tested by PCR. PCR or direct fluorescent antibody tests are the diagnostic methods of choice.
   b. A rise in immunoglobulin G (IgG) antibody from acute and convalescent titers can confirm a diagnosis.
4. **Therapy**
   a. **Uncomplicated cases of varicella or zoster** require only supportive therapy.
   b. Administration of **varicella vaccine** to susceptible people 12 months of age or older should be given as soon as possible (ideally within 72 hours).
   c. For susceptible individuals who have not had varicella, **prophylaxis with IGIV** (one dose) within 96 hours of exposure should be given. Immunocompromised patients who develop varicella or disseminated zoster should be **treated with intravenous acyclovir.**
   d. **Oral acyclovir** is generally not recommended for immunocompetent children and adolescents.

5. **Prevention** is effectively achieved through the use of varicella vaccine (see Chapter 1).
6. **Complications**
   a. The **most common** complications of a varicella-zoster infection include encephalopathy, cerebellitis, Guillain-Barré syndrome, aseptic meningitis, pneumonia, hepatitis, thrombocytopenic purpura, purpura fulminans, cellulitis, abscess formation, and arthritis. Varicella is an important risk factor for severe, invasive β-hemolytic *Streptococcus* disease.
   b. **Progressive varicella** (with meningoencephalitis, pneumonia, and hepatitis) occurs in immunocompromised children and is associated with a mortality rate of approximately 20%.

G **Scarlet fever** is an acute illness characterized by fever, pharyngitis, and an erythematous rash caused by group A *Streptococcus* strains that produce erythrogenic toxin. The disease usually is associated with pharyngeal infections but, in rare cases, follows streptococcal infections at other sites (e.g., wound infections, impetigo). Scarlet fever is rare in infancy.

1. **Clinical features.** The **characteristic rash** is erythematous and finely punctate, and blanches with pressure. It appears initially on the trunk and becomes generalized within a few hours to several days. The face is flushed with circumoral pallor and there is increased erythema in the skin folds (Pastia lines). The skin may feel rough (**"sandpaper-like"**). The rash fades over 1 week and is followed by desquamation, which may last for several weeks. A **strawberry tongue** (rough, erythematous, swollen) and pharyngeal erythema with exudate may be present.
2. **Diagnosis** is made on the basis of the clinical presentation and the isolation of *Streptococcus* on throat culture or wound site.
3. **Therapy** for scarlet fever is the same as that for streptococcal pharyngitis, consisting of 10 days of orally administered penicillin.
4. **Complications.** Both suppurative (e.g., cellulitis) and nonsuppurative (e.g., glomerulonephritis, rheumatic fever) complications can occur with scarlet fever, just as with streptococcal pharyngitis (*see V E*).

H **Rocky Mountain spotted fever** is an acute febrile illness characterized by the sudden onset of fever, headache, myalgia, mental confusion, and rash. The disease may be severe, leading to shock and death in 5% to 7% of patients, even with appropriate antimicrobial therapy. Most cases are in children under 15 years of age.

1. **Etiology and epidemiology**
   a. Rocky Mountain spotted fever is a **tick-borne illness** caused by *Rickettsia rickettsii,* which is widespread in the United States but most predominant in the southeastern states. Incubation period is approximately 1 week.
   b. The principal **vectors** of Rocky Mountain spotted fever are *Dermacentor andersoni,* the **wood tick,** which is found in the West and is most active during the spring, and *Dermacentor variabilis,* the **dog tick** that is found in the East and is most active during the summer.
2. **Clinical features**
   a. The clinical onset of Rocky Mountain spotted fever is abrupt and follows an incubation period that averages approximately 7 days (usually 2–8 days after an infected tick bite). Typical initial presentations include fever, chills, headache (can be generalized and severe), signs of meningoencephalitis (irritability, confusion, delirium), myalgias, conjunctivitis with photophobia, nonpitting edema, and a rash.
   b. A **characteristic rash** develops on the third to fifth day of illness. The lesions begin as rose-colored, blanching macules on the hands, wrists, feet, and ankles, which spread to involve the entire body. The rash then becomes more **papular, petechial, and eventually purpuric** if treatment is delayed.
3. **Diagnosis** is made primarily on the basis of clinical appearance and history (a history of tick bite exists in 60%–85% of cases). Isolation of the organism is difficult and dangerous; serologic confirmation generally takes 7 to 10 days and may be delayed for 5 or more weeks if antibiotics are begun early. If a specialized laboratory is available, rapid diagnosis can be made using immunofluorescence.

4. **Therapy**
   a. **Antibiotic therapy.** Doxycycline is the drug of choice; chloramphenicol or a fluoroquinolone is an alternative choice.
   b. **Supportive therapy** is essential for patients who have serious illness, such as those in shock.
5. **Prevention** includes wearing protective clothing, using tick and insect repellent, and removing ticks promptly and properly.
6. **Complications** of Rocky Mountain spotted fever include focal neurologic deficits, coma, renal failure, disseminated intravascular coagulation, gangrene of the distal extremities and scrotum, pneumonia, and shock that can possibly lead to death.

VIII OTHER SYSTEMIC INFECTIONS

A **Lyme disease** is a multisystem inflammatory disease that primarily affects the skin, joints, and nervous system.

1. **Epidemiology.** Lyme disease is the most common vector-borne disease in the United States. It has been reported in 47 states, but the major foci are in the Northeast; upper Midwest; and, to a lesser extent, the northwest United States. Lyme disease is transmitted to humans through the bite of an Ixodid tick. The incubation period from the tick bite to appearance of a single or multiple erythema migrans lesion ranges from 1 to 55 days (median 11 days). Late manifestations can occur months to years later.
2. **Etiology.** Lyme disease is caused by the spirochete *B. burgdorferi.* The white-footed mouse is the major reservoir for *B. burgdorferi* in the northeastern and midwestern United States. The white-tailed deer is an important host for the tick.
3. **Clinical features** are divided into three stages.
   a. **Early, localized infection** is characterized by an expanding erythematous, annular skin lesion (erythema migrans); fever; headache; fatigue; arthralgias; myalgias; neck pain; and back pain.
   b. **Early, disseminated infection** is characterized by multiple erythema migrans, aseptic meningitis, cranial neuropathies (especially of the facial nerve), radiculoneuritis, and carditis/heart block (rare in children).
   c. **Late infection** is characterized by asymmetric, pauciarticular arthritis (especially of the knee); polyneuropathy; and encephalopathy. Arthritis is much more common than neurologic disease.
4. **Diagnosis** is made by the presence of erythema migrans in a patient who lives in an endemic area. In the absence of erythema migrans, the diagnosis is based on the presence of clinical findings consistent with Lyme disease and laboratory evidence (usually based on serologic tests) of an infection with *B. burgdorferi.*
5. **Therapy.** For early localized disease, oral doxycycline (8 years or older) or amoxicillin or cefuroxime (all ages) is used for a 14- to 21-day course. For early disseminated and late disease, the same oral regimens are used for multiple erythema migrans or isolated facial palsy (21–28 days) and arthritis (28 days). For persistent or recurrent arthritis, carditis, or meningitis, ceftriaxone or penicillin (intravenous) can be used for a 14- to 28-day course.
6. **Complications.** With appropriate antibiotic therapy, the long-term outcome is excellent regardless of the stage of disease at which therapy is initiated. In a very small proportion of patients, chronic arthritis or chronic neurologic disease may develop despite appropriate antibiotic therapy.

B **Kawasaki disease** is a generalized vasculitis of unknown cause that is a leading cause of acquired heart disease in children who live in the United States. Clinical and epidemiologic characteristics suggest an infectious agent. Infection may lead to an immune-mediated disease in certain genetically predisposed children (see Chapter 9).

C **Infectious mononucleosis** is an acute infection characterized by fever, sore throat, lymphadenopathy, splenomegaly, atypical lymphocytosis, and the presence of heterophil antibody. Infectious mononucleosis most often affects adolescents and young adults.

1. **Etiology.** Infectious mononucleosis is caused by Epstein-Barr virus, a herpesvirus. Cytomegalovirus and *T. gondii* cause illnesses that are virtually indistinguishable from Epstein-Barr virus–induced mononucleosis.
2. **Clinical features** of infectious mononucleosis are highly variable. Symptoms are usually less severe in younger children than in older children, adolescents, or adults. A prodrome of malaise, fever, and headache may prevail for 3 to 7 days before the onset of more profound symptoms.
   a. **Fever** is invariably present and may last as long as 21 days. Temperature may reach as high as 104°F (40°C).
   b. **Pharyngitis** occurs in approximately 80% of patients and may be severe. Although group A *Streptococcus* may be cultured from these patients, the incidence of streptococcal pharyngitis in patients who have infectious mononucleosis is not increased compared with otherwise healthy controls.
   c. **Lymphadenopathy** is usually generalized and most often involves the cervical nodes.
   d. **Splenomegaly** is noted in most patients who have infectious mononucleosis.
   e. **Rash** occurs in approximately 5% of patients and can appear quite variable. Administration of ampicillin to patients who have infectious mononucleosis produces a rash in 90% to 100% of such patients, which is pruritic and maculopapular and may appear after cessation of antibiotic treatment.
   f. **Other clinical findings** include fatigue, eyelid edema, abdominal pain, and, rarely, jaundice.
3. **Diagnosis.** Suggestive laboratory tests include a predominance of mononuclear cells on CBC (more than 50% mononuclear cells), more than 10% atypical lymphocytes, and elevated levels of serum transaminases. Laboratory confirmation of infectious mononucleosis consists of positive serologic findings. Several serologic tests have been developed.
   a. Nonspecific tests for heterophil antibody, including the Paul Bunnell test and slide agglutination reaction, are commonly available.
   b. **Commercial heterophil antibody kits** (e.g., the Monospot test) are simple, rapid, and fairly sensitive. The test results are usually positive within the first week of infection and remain positive for several months. However, only 80% of patients with Epstein-Barr virus infection have positive test results. Also, for unknown reasons, children younger than 5 years of age with Epstein-Barr virus infection often have false-negative results on Monospot testing.
   c. **Antibodies to Epstein-Barr virus.** Patients who have infectious mononucleosis produce antibodies to various specific antigens, including Epstein-Barr viral capsid antigen (VCA), Epstein-Barr nuclear antigen (EBNA), and Epstein-Barr virus–induced early antigen (EA).
      (1) **Antibodies to VCA** (initially IgM, followed by IgG) peak in the second or third week of illness and persist for life.
      (2) **Antibodies to EA** appear early in the course of illness and disappear 2 to 6 months later.
      (3) **Antibodies to EBNA** appear 3 to 4 weeks after the onset of infection and probably persist for life.
4. **Therapy** is supportive. Convalescence may take weeks to months and is relatively shorter in younger patients compared with older patients. **Corticosteroids** generally are used in patients with:
   a. Impending airway obstruction
   b. Severe thrombocytopenia
   c. Hemolytic anemia
5. **Complications**
   a. **Splenic rupture,** due either to trauma or spontaneous occurrence, is a rare complication. Patients should be advised not to engage in any contact sports until they are fully recovered and splenomegaly has resolved.
   b. **Airway obstruction** due to tonsillar or pharyngeal hypertrophy is also rare.
   c. **Neurologic complications** are usually self-limited and reversible and include aseptic meningitis, encephalitis, myelitis, peripheral neuropathies, and Guillain-Barré syndrome.
   d. **Icteric hepatitis** occurs in approximately 5% of patients, whereas subclinical hepatitis occurs in approximately 20% to 40%. Acute liver failure is rare.

e. **Other rare complications** include autoimmune hemolytic anemia, thrombocytopenia, neutropenia, acute renal failure, complete heart block, myositis, pericarditis, pneumonia, acrocyanosis, and immunologic disorders (e.g., impaired cell-mediated immunity, agammaglobulinemia).

IX CARDIAC INFECTIONS

A. **Infective endocarditis** is an inflammatory disorder, mainly of the cardiac valves, that results from infection by any of several types of microorganisms, including bacteria, fungi, and rickettsiae.

1. **Etiology. Viridans streptococci** are the most common cause of infective endocarditis in children. However, this etiologic agent has decreased in importance since the introduction of antimicrobial therapy. ***S. aureus*** and ***S. epidermidis*** have become progressively more important causes of infective endocarditis because of the increased use of indwelling intravascular devices and cardiothoracic surgery.
2. **Epidemiology.** Pediatric patients who are at greatest risk for infective endocarditis include those who have congenital heart disease, acquired valvular heart disease (e.g., rheumatic carditis), prosthetic valves, and valves damaged from intravenous catheters. Adolescent drug abusers and children who have central venous or arterial lines demonstrate an increased risk for the disease.
3. **Pathogenesis**
   a. **Endocarditis** develops when a jet of blood, turbulence, or trauma leads to **cardiac endothelial damage.** A sterile clot or vegetation forms that serves as the nidus for bacterial infection. In most cases, **oral bacteria,** which intermittently invade the bloodstream, infect the damaged endothelium.
   b. **Vegetations** consisting primarily of fibrin, platelet aggregations, and bacterial masses form on the valve leaflet. They may be single or multiple and range in size from a few millimeters to several centimeters. Pieces of the vegetations may break off and cause embolization (e.g., splinter hemorrhages, Roth spots).
4. **Clinical features**
   a. **Early manifestations.** Infants and children who have early infective endocarditis may be nearly free of symptoms, with fatigue sometimes the only manifestation of disease. Fever, malaise, and weakness are common. The classic signs of endocarditis (e.g., splinter hemorrhages, changing heart murmurs) are not always evident. Other signs may occur include cardiomegaly, splenomegaly, petechiae, weight loss, and clubbing of the fingers.
   b. **Late manifestations** of infective endocarditis classically include such lesions as **Roth spots** (retinal hemorrhages with clear centers), **Janeway lesions** (flat, painless hemorrhagic macules on the hands or feet), and **Osler nodes** (pea-sized painful nodules, usually on the fingers). Any of these lesions infrequently occur in appropriately treated patients.
5. **Diagnosis**
   a. **Laboratory findings.** The erythrocyte sedimentation rate (ESR) is usually elevated but may be normal early in the course of the illness. The leukocyte count may be normal or elevated. Microscopic hematuria may occur.
   b. **Blood cultures** are critical for the diagnosis of infective endocarditis, because they identify the causative agent in more than 90% of cases. It rarely is necessary to obtain more than four cultures, but at least three blood cultures should be obtained during the first 24 hours of hospitalization.
   c. **Echocardiography** is helpful for establishing the presence and location of vegetations.
6. **Therapy.** When untreated, this infection is almost always fatal.
   a. **Antibiotic therapy. Intravenous antibiotics** are usually given for 4 weeks, except for patients who either have staphylococcal endocarditis or an artificial valve, for whom 6 weeks of therapy is preferred. **Initial therapy** usually consists of **ampicillin plus gentamicin,** unless staphylococci are suspected, in which case **oxacillin or vancomycin and gentamicin** are given.
   b. **Surgical intervention** (for removal of vegetations or valve replacement) may be required for patients who fail to respond to medical treatment.

7. **Complications** of infective endocarditis must be anticipated and, with early intervention, may be minimized or even prevented. Important sequelae of infective endocarditis include:
   a. **Emboli** to the brain, lungs, coronary arteries, or any peripheral artery
   b. **Mycotic aneurysms,** which are infected aneurysms of the arterial vessels in the brain
   c. **Congestive heart failure,** which usually results from valvular dysfunction
   d. **Local cardiac abscesses,** which can manifest as aneurysm or persistent fever
   e. **Drug reactions**
   f. **Autoimmune phenomena** (e.g., nephritis, arthritis)
   g. **Depression,** which can occur as a result of the prolonged hospitalization

B **Myocarditis** is an infection of the myocardium (i.e., the muscle of the heart). It occurs infrequently in children. Most cases of myocarditis are caused by enteroviruses, predominantly coxsackie B virus and echovirus.

1. **Clinical features** include fever, congestive heart failure, and arrhythmias. The electrocardiogram is abnormal, with ST-segment depression and T-wave inversion.
2. **Therapy** for patients who have viral myocarditis is supportive.

C **Pericarditis** is an inflammation of the pericardium. The most common causes of pericarditis are bacteria—especially *S. aureus, S. pneumoniae,* and *N. meningitidis*—and viruses—especially coxsackie B virus, echovirus, influenza virus, and adenovirus. Other causes include fungi and *M. tuberculosis.*

1. **Clinical features**
   a. **Left shoulder pain and back pain,** which decrease when the patient is sitting, are characteristic of pericarditis. Fever, tachypnea, tachycardia, cough, and decreased heart sounds due to pericardial fluid and pericardial friction rub are also common.
   b. **It is important to recognize significant pericardial fluid accumulation,** which can lead to cardiac tamponade. Signs of tamponade include neck vein distention on inspiration and paradoxical pulse. The essential features of paradoxical pulse are a greater than normal inspiratory decrease in arterial blood pressure and an absence of the normal inspiratory fall in venous pressure.
2. **Diagnosis**
   a. **Electrocardiographic findings** with pericarditis include a low-voltage QRS complex, ST-segment changes, and T-wave inversion. Electrical alternans may occur with large pericardial effusions. This phenomenon consists of changing electrical amplitude of the T-wave and QRS complex with the cardiac cycle.
   b. **Chest radiography** reveals a rapidly increasing cardiothoracic ratio without increasing pulmonary vascular markings.
   c. **Echocardiography** allows an estimate of the amount of pericardial fluid and is the most sensitive means of demonstrating pericardial fluid.
3. **Therapy** for severe cases of pericarditis involving cardiac tamponade consists of pericardial drainage and supportive measures, such as the administration of oxygen and isoproterenol. Prolonged antibiotic therapy is given for cases of pericarditis due to bacteria.

X SKIN, JOINT, AND BONE INFECTIONS

A Skin infections

1. **Impetigo**
   a. **Etiology.** Two variants, **nonbullous impetigo** and **bullous impetigo,** are typically caused by *S. aureus* or group A *Streptococcus.*
   b. **Clinical features** may vary but usually include a small erythematous papule or vesicle that enlarges, ruptures, and partially crusts (honey-colored crust). Lesions are usually found on the face, although other body sites can be found.
   c. **Diagnosis** is usually clinical but a bacterial culture of the lesion can be performed.
   d. **Treatment.** Penicillin should be used only when group A *Streptococcus* is identified. Otherwise, a semisynthetic penicillin, first- or second-generation cephalosporin, or amoxicillin-clavulanate should be used.

2. **Cellulitis** is a localized, acute inflammation of the skin and subcutaneous tissue characterized by erythema and warmth. Cellulitis may also arise from underlying osteomyelitis, septic arthritis, sinusitis, or deep wound infection.
   a. **Etiology.** Most cellulitis in children is caused by group A β-hemolytic *Streptococcus* or *S. aureus.*
   b. **Clinical features**
      (1) **Trauma-related cellulitis.** Cellulitis that occurs after some form of skin trauma (e.g., wound, burn, surgery, insect bites) is usually caused by group A *Streptococcus* or *S. aureus.*
         (a) **Erysipelas** refers to an acute infection of the skin and superficial subcutaneous tissues that is characterized by a sharply demarcated, firm, raised border. *Streptococcus* is the predominant cause.
         (b) Local trauma, with or without marked cellulitis, may give rise to **lymphangitis** occurring as a thin line of redness from the point of trauma to the draining regional node. Group A *Streptococcus* is the primary cause.
      (2) **Cellulitis unrelated to trauma** may be caused by *S. aureus,* group A *Streptococcus, S. pneumoniae,* or rarely, *H. influenzae* type b.
   c. **Diagnosis**
      (1) **Blood culture** results from patients who have cellulitis are sometimes positive for group A *Streptococcus, S. aureus, S. pneumoniae,* or *H. influenzae* type b.
      (2) **Aspiration** of material from the leading edge or center of the area of cellulitis and culture may yield the etiologic agent.
      (3) **Culture** of material that has drained from a wound associated with cellulitis is helpful for defining the cause.
   d. **Therapy.** Children who have cellulitis sometimes are hospitalized and given parenteral antibiotics, such as oxacillin, cefazolin, or ceftriaxone, which are effective against the likely pathogens. Hospitalization is indicated for patients who have ocular cellulitis (periorbital and orbital cellulitis). Outpatient treatment of cellulitis includes cephalexin, dicloxacillin, amoxicillin-clavulanic acid, and cefuroxime.

3. **Abscess** represents a deeper skin infection than cellulitis; in addition, it contains pus.
   a. **Etiology.** Abscesses are usually caused by *S. aureus* or group A *Streptococcus.*
   b. **Therapy.** Treatment of superficial abscesses consists of warm compresses until the abscesses become fluctuant. Surgical drainage is necessary if spontaneous drainage has not occurred. Appropriate antibiotics are indicated.

B **Septic arthritis** occurs when bacteria from the circulation enter the joint space. It may also occur from direct implantation of bacteria due to osteomyelitis or penetrating trauma. Septic arthritis may cause destruction of articular cartilage because of a lack of normal nutrients in the synovial fluid or as a result of purulent exudate and increased pressure in the joint space. The joints usually involved are the knee (40%), hip (20%), ankle (15%), elbow (15%), wrist (5%), and shoulder (5%).

1. **Etiology.** Blood culture results are positive in up to 50% of patients who have septic arthritis.
   a. **Neonates.** Group B *Streptococcus, S. aureus,* and enteric Gram-negative rods are the most common pathogens in this age group.
   b. **Older children.** *S. aureus* is the most common pathogen. Other causes include group A *Streptococcus, S. pneumoniae, N. meningitidis,* and, uncommonly, *H. influenzae* type b. *N. gonorrhoeae* causes septic arthritis in adolescents.

2. **Clinical features.** In most children, the affected joint is warm, swollen, and very painful when moved. Septic arthritis in a young infant may manifest simply as fever and poorly localized pain in the affected extremity. **Signs and symptoms** associated with a septic hip often are subtle and, in an infant, may be limited to a limp or a fixed, flexed hip.

3. **Diagnosis**
   a. **Synovial fluid analysis.** Joint aspiration is necessary for the diagnosis of septic arthritis, and it has the additional benefit of decreasing pressure in the joint space. Gram stain, culture, WBC count, and protein and glucose concentrations of the synovial fluid are obtained.
   b. **Laboratory findings.** The peripheral WBC count is usually elevated, with a shift to the left, and the ESR is usually elevated.

c. **Imaging results.** Radiographs frequently show widening of the joint space. Ultrasonography is useful for demonstrating fluid in joint infections, especially in the hip. MRI may be useful in distinguishing joint infections from cellulitis or deep abscesses. A gallium scan shows increased uptake of gallium in the involved joint.

d. **Differential diagnosis** of septic arthritis includes other causes of monoarticular arthritis, including *M. pneumoniae, M. tuberculosis, C. albicans,* Lyme disease, toxic synovitis, trauma, juvenile rheumatoid arthritis, and Reiter syndrome.

4. **Therapy**

a. Empiric antibiotic therapy should initially consist of parenteral antibiotics to treat the likely pathogens (i.e., oxacillin plus cefotaxime or an aminoglycoside for neonates, and oxacillin plus ceftriaxone for children older than 3 months of age). Antibiotics should be continued for a minimum of 3 weeks. In some cases, subsequent high-dose oral therapy can be substituted for parenteral therapy.

b. Drainage of the joint space by needle aspiration or surgical excision is important to remove inflammatory material. Septic arthritis of the hip requires immediate surgical drainage, because the blood supply of the femoral head may be compromised, which carries the risk of serious sequelae.

C **Osteomyelitis** refers to inflammation of the bone. Osteomyelitis in children occurs most frequently in the long bones of the lower extremities and, to a lesser extent, of the upper extremities.

1. **Etiology**

a. ***S. aureus*** and ***S. pyogenes*** account for more than 90% of bacterial isolates in childhood osteomyelitis.

b. ***Salmonella*** species are common pathogens in patients who have sickle cell anemia.

c. ***P. aeruginosa*** is a common pathogen in patients who have puncture wounds of the foot.

2. **Pathogenesis.** The tortuous course of the nutrient vessels in the metaphyseal region of bone cause bacteria to be trapped there. The metaphysis is located between the epiphysis (growth plate) and the diaphysis (shaft of the bone). If pus develops, it generally moves laterally to the subperiosteal space and lifts the periosteum off the shaft of the bone.

3. **Clinical features**

a. In **young infants,** fever may be the only manifestation of osteomyelitis.

b. Fever and localized bone tenderness are the most common symptoms in **older children.** Local swelling, redness, warmth, and, rarely, suppuration may subsequently occur.

c. Approximately half the patients have a **history of minor trauma.**

4. **Diagnosis**

a. **Hematologic findings.** The **WBC count** and **ESR** are usually elevated. The ESR is useful for monitoring therapy. **Blood culture** results are positive in approximately 50% of patients.

b. **Imaging results**

(1) The result of a **bone scan** using technetium 99m phosphate is usually positive 24 hours after symptoms begin; this finding provides strong evidence of osteomyelitis.

(2) **Radiographic** results do not become positive (radiolucency of bone) until 10 to 12 days after the onset of symptoms. Bone abscess should be suspected if the periosteum is separated from the shaft of the bone (periosteal elevation).

(3) **MRI** or **CT scans** are more specific than a radiograph but usually are not performed unless the diagnosis is questionable or a patient has a prolonged or difficult clinical course.

c. **Aspiration** of the affected site is desirable to recover the causative organism and determine whether an abscess is present, which would require surgical drainage. Aspiration and drainage are essential if a bone abscess or an unusual organism (e.g., *P. aeruginosa* from a puncture wound) is suspected.

5. **Therapy**

a. **Antibiotic therapy** initially should consist of a parenteral antistaphylococcal antibiotic (e.g., oxacillin or cefazolin), unless a Gram-negative organism or methicillin-resistant *S. aureus* is suspected. Appropriate antibiotic therapy is continued for a minimum of 4 weeks. In some cases, an oral antibiotic can be substituted after 1 week of parenteral antibiotics.

b. **Surgical drainage** is necessary in addition to antibiotics for successful treatment of bone abscess.

6. **Complications.** Chronic osteomyelitis may occur if treatment of acute osteomyelitis is inadequate, especially if a bone abscess is not properly drained. Joint infection may occur with osteomyelitis, especially in neonates and when the disease affects the shoulder or hip.

BIBLIOGRAPHY

American Academy of Family Physicians, American Academy of Otolaryngology-Head and Neck Surgery, and American Academy of Pediatrics Subcommittee on Otitis Media With Effusion: Clinical practice guideline. Otitis media with effusion. *Pediatrics* 113:1412–1429, 2004.

Committee on Infectious Diseases, American Academy of Pediatrics: *The Red Book. Report of the Committee on Infectious Diseases,* 27th ed. Elk Grove Village, IL, American Academy of Pediatrics, 2006.

Feigin RD, Cherry JD (eds): *Textbook of Pediatric Infectious Diseases,* 5th ed. Philadelphia, WB Saunders, 2003.

Jenson HB, Baltimore RS (eds): *Pediatric Infectious Diseases. Principles and Practice.* Norwalk, Conn, Appleton & Lange, 2002.

Mandell GL, Douglas RG, Dolin R (eds): *Principles and Practice of Infectious Diseases,* 6th ed. New York, Churchill-Livingstone, 2004.

Remington JS, Klein JO (eds): *Infectious Diseases of the Fetus and Newborn Infant,* 6th ed. Philadelphia, WB Saunders, 2005.

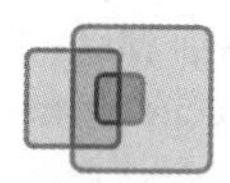

Study Questions

Directions: *Each of the numbered items or incomplete statements in this section is followed by answers or completions of the statement. Select the ONE lettered answer or completion that is BEST in each case.*

1. A 1-year-old boy is brought to the emergency room with a 10-hour history of fever and now changes in mental status. Physical examination reveals a lethargic child who has a temperature of 103°F (39.5°C), a respiratory rate of 35, blood pressure of 60/30, a full fontanelle, and a petechial rash. Which of the following is the most appropriate first step in management?

- A Blood culture, urine culture, and lumbar puncture
- B Gram stain of the petechiae
- C Immediate administration of intravenous fluids, blood culture, and antibiotics
- D Administration of corticosteroids
- E Examination of the fundi

2. A 6-year-old girl is initially seen with a nonsuppurative and moderately tender anterior cervical lymph node that measures 2 cm × 4 cm. Which of the following is the most appropriate initial therapy?

- A Amoxicillin
- B Cephalexin
- C Erythromycin
- D Penicillin
- E Incision and drainage

3. A previously healthy 13-year-old boy has a mild pneumonia characterized by a nonproductive cough. There are patchy bilateral infiltrates on chest radiograph. Which of the following antibiotics is most appropriate for treatment in this case?

- A Cephalexin
- B Amoxicillin
- C Azithromycin
- D Penicillin
- E Trimethoprim-sulfamethoxazole

4. A 3-month-old infant who has bronchopulmonary dysplasia is admitted to a hospital with fever, wheezing, and respiratory distress. A chest radiograph shows hyperinflation and extensive bilateral, interstitial infiltrates. Complete blood cell count results are normal, and the results of a rapid test for respiratory syncytial virus are positive. Blood cultures are obtained. Which of the following is the most appropriate therapy?

- A Intravenous ampicillin
- B Intravenous ceftriaxone
- C Oral amoxicillin
- D Supportive therapy
- E Palivizumab

5. A 2-year-old child is noted to have an erythematous, bulging right tympanic membrane. Which of the following are the two most likely bacterial causes of this illness?

- A *Streptococcus pyogenes* and *Staphylococcus aureus*
- B *Haemophilus influenzae* and *Staphylococcus aureus*
- C *Haemophilus influenzae* and *Streptococcus pneumoniae*
- D *Streptococcus pneumoniae* and *Staphylococcus aureus*
- E *Moraxella catarrhalis* and *Streptococcus pyogenes*

6. A 4-year-old boy is initially seen with a low-grade fever, nasal discharge, and a cough that is present both day and night but is worse at night. These clinical findings have persisted without improvement for 14 days. A sinus radiograph shows complete opacification of the maxillary sinuses bilaterally. Which of the following is the most accurate statement regarding the most appropriate treatment of acute sinusitis in this child?

A Amoxicillin is the drug of choice for antimicrobial therapy
B Sinus irrigation should be performed in addition to antimicrobial therapy
C Antihistamines should be prescribed in addition to antimicrobial therapy
D Intranasal steroids should be prescribed in addition to antimicrobial therapy
E Trimethoprim-sulfamethoxazole is the drug of choice for antimicrobial therapy

7. A 6-month-old infant has a high fever (106°F [41.1°C]) and gets a sepsis workup that includes a lumbar puncture. The CSF results are within normal limits, except for a herpes simplex virus PCR test result that is positive. The PCR test was not requested by the physician but mistakenly performed by the laboratory. It is now 48 hours later, and the infant (who was initially treated with ceftriaxone) is well. The laboratory has stored 1 mL of the CSF. Which of the following is the most appropriate next step in management?

A Complete a 10-day course of ceftriaxone
B Begin acyclovir and have the laboratory culture cerebrospinal fluid for herpes simplex virus
C Repeat the PCR test
D Begin a 21-day course of acylovir
E Perform a repeat lumbar puncture and send cerebrospinal fluid for herpes simplex culture

8. A 1-month-old infant presents with a fever of 101.8°F (38.8°C) and lethargy. You suspect that the child is septic. The white blood cell count is 18,000/mm^3. A blood culture is obtained. Which of the following are the most likely organisms to cause sepsis in this age group?

A *Streptococcus pneumoniae* and *Neisseria meningitidis*
B *Streptococcus pneumoniae* and *Staphylococcus aureus*
C Group B *Streptococcus* and *Escherichia coli*
D Group B *Streptococcus* and *Staphylococcus aureus*
E *Haemophilus influenzae*

9. A 5-year-old child comes to your office with a disseminated rash and fever. The rash is vesicular with a "teardrop" appearance to the lesions. The child has not been immunized against varicella. The child has been on high-dose steroids for over a year for another medical condition. Which of the following is the most appropriate management of this patient?

A Oral acyclovir
B Administration of varicella vaccine
C Observation only
D Hospitalization and administration of intravenous acyclovir
E Administration of intravenous varicella zoster immune globulin

10. A 12-year-old girl is hospitalized with dehydration from severe pharyngitis. On review of systems she also describes malaise and mild abdominal pain. On examination, she is febrile with otherwise normal vital signs. She has an erythematous oropharynx and shotty cervical lymph nodes. The rest of the examination is normal. You are suspicious for group A *Streptococcus* infection and start ampicillin. The next day the patient develops a generalized maculopapular rash. Which of the following is the most appropriate next step in management?

A Continue the ampicillin
B Stop the antibiotic and send a Monospot test
C Change the antibiotic to a cephalosporin
D Administer intravenous γ-globulin
E Begin treatment with oral prednisone

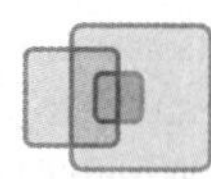

Answers and Explanations

1. The answer is C (*IV A 4*). The most appropriate initial action is blood culture and administration of intravenous fluids and antibiotics. This patient is initially seen with classic findings of meningococcal sepsis and meningitis. Although the diagnosis of meningitis and the microbiologic cause of the illness can be established by examination of CSF, a lumbar puncture should be deferred until the patient's condition is stabilized. The blood pressure indicates that the child is in shock. Initial efforts, therefore, should focus on maintaining intravascular volume by the intravenous administration of fluids. Intravenous antibiotics should also be administered promptly (preferably after a blood culture is obtained), and in this case, an appropriate choice would be a third-generation cephalosporin.

2. The answer is B (*V F 4*). The most appropriate initial therapy would be administration of cephalexin. Inflammation and enlargement of the lymph nodes of the neck, or cervical adenitis, is a common problem in children. Appropriate treatment of cervical adenitis depends on the causative microorganism and the presence or absence of pus. Initial therapy for a nonsuppurative node of moderate size and tenderness usually consists of an oral antistaphylococcal antibiotic (e.g., cephalexin or dicloxacillin; cephalexin suspension has a much better taste than dicloxacillin) for treatment of *S. aureus* and group A *Streptococcus*, which are the most likely causative organisms. Neither amoxicillin nor penicillin is usually effective against *S. aureus.* Incision and drainage are indicated only when the nodes contain pus.

3. The answer is C (*VI B 1 d* [*3*], *3 a* [*3*]). The most appropriate treatment is azithromycin. The most common nonviral causes of pneumonia in children who are older than 6 years of age are *M. pneumoniae* and *S. pneumoniae.* Pneumonia due to *M. pneumoniae* is usually milder than that due to traditional bacteria, with a gradual onset of illness that is characterized by fever, headache, malaise, and a nonproductive cough. The clinical picture described in the question, therefore, is consistent with *M. pneumoniae* pneumonia, for which the treatment of choice is azithromycin. Cephalexin, amoxicillin, penicillin, and trimethoprim-sulfamethoxazole would be effective treatment for *S. pneumoniae* pneumonia, but not for *M. pneumoniae* pneumonia.

4. The answer is D (*VI A 6 a*). Supportive therapy is the mainstay of treatment for RSV bronchiolitis. Bronchiolitis is an acute viral infection of the bronchioles, which is common in infants younger than 2 years of age. Clinical features include cough, wheezing, tachypnea, and dyspnea. Hyperinflation of the lungs typically is evident on chest radiography. Results of complete blood cell count are often normal, which reflects a viral cause. In most cases, patients recover spontaneously and do not require hospitalization or specific therapy. However, severe infection is more common among children who have underlying pulmonary disease (e.g., bronchopulmonary dysplasia). In such cases, hospitalization is necessary, and therapy includes oxygen, fluids, and possibly intubation with assisted ventilation. Palivizumab is a monoclonal antibody given to infants at high risk for infection that meet specific criteria.

5. The answer is C (*V A 1 a* [*1*]). The most likely bacterial causes of the illness described are *H. influenzae* and *S. pneumoniae.* This child is initially seen with otitis media, which is one of the most common infections of childhood. The characteristic feature of otitis media is a bulging, erythematous tympanic membrane with impaired mobility. The most common causes in all age groups are *S. pneumoniae* (25%–40% of cases) and unencapsulated *H. influenzae* (15%–25% of cases). Less common causes include *M. catarrhalis;* group A *Streptococcus*; and, for chronic otitis media, *S. aureus* and *P. aeruginosa.*

6. The answer is A (*V C 6*). The drug of choice for initial therapy of acute sinusitis is amoxicillin. Agents such as trimethoprim-sulfamethoxazole, erythromycin-sulfisoxazole, and cefuroxime should be reserved for patients who do not respond to amoxicillin or who are allergic to penicillin. Sinus irrigation or surgical drainage of the sinus is indicated only for those who do not respond to antimicrobial therapy and those who have intraorbital or intracranial complications of sinusitis. Antihistamines are not routinely prescribed in conjunction with antimicrobials, but may be helpful only in those patients who have associated allergic rhinitis. Intranasal steroids have not been proved to be of value in the treatment of acute sinusitis and should not be used to treat this infection.

7. The answer is C (*IV A 1 b, IV B 3*). When a test result is inconsistent with the clinical presentation, it should be repeated. Several findings were inconsistent with herpes simplex central nervous system infection: (a) no nuchal rigidity or decreased level of consciousness was reported in this child (although nuchal rigidity is an inconsistent finding in children under age 1 year), (b) no increase in cerebrospinal fluid leukocytes or protein was noted, and (c) the patient improved rapidly without acyclovir therapy. False-positive results from polymerase chain reaction testing may occur.

8. The answer is C (*III C 1*). Sepsis implies infection plus a variety of processes including two or more SIRS criteria, which in this case include the temperature $> 38°C$ and white blood cell count $> 10{,}000/mm^3$. Any infant under 28 days of age should have a complete workup including blood culture and complete blood count, urinalysis and urine culture, and lumbar puncture with analysis and culture. The most common causative agents in this age group are group B *Streptococcus* and *E. coli. S. pneumoniae* and *N. meningitidis* become more common in older age groups.

9. The answer is D (*VII F 4*). Uncomplicated cases of varicella or zoster require only supportive therapy. However, this child should be considered immunocompromised given the history of high-dose steroid use. Immunocompromised patients who develop varicella or disseminated zoster should be treated with intravenous acyclovir. Administration of varicella vaccine to susceptible people 12 months of age or older with whom the child has had contact should be given as soon as possible (ideally within 72 hours).

10. The answer is B (*VIII C*). Infectious mononucleosis is caused by infection with Epstein-Barr virus. Pharyngitis occurs in approximately 80% of infectious mononucleosis patients and may be severe. Although group A *Streptococcus* may be cultured from these patients, the incidence of streptococcal pharyngitis in patients who have infectious mononucleosis is not increased compared with otherwise healthy controls. Rash occurs in approximately 5% of patients with infectious mononucleosis and can appear quite variable. Administration of ampicillin to patients who have infectious mononucleosis produces a rash in 90% to 100% of such patients, which is pruritic and maculopapular and may appear after cessation of antibiotic treatment. Although it can be difficult to distinguish a rash from a drug allergy from that of other kinds of infectious-related rashes, discontinuation of the antibiotic and investigation for other etiologies is warranted. Intravenous γ-globulin is used in the treatment of Kawasaki disease. Oral steroids have occasionally been administered to patients with infectious mononucleosis for airway compromise from swelling in the back of the throat. However, corticosteroid use has not been demonstrated to alter the course of infectious mononucleosis.

chapter 11

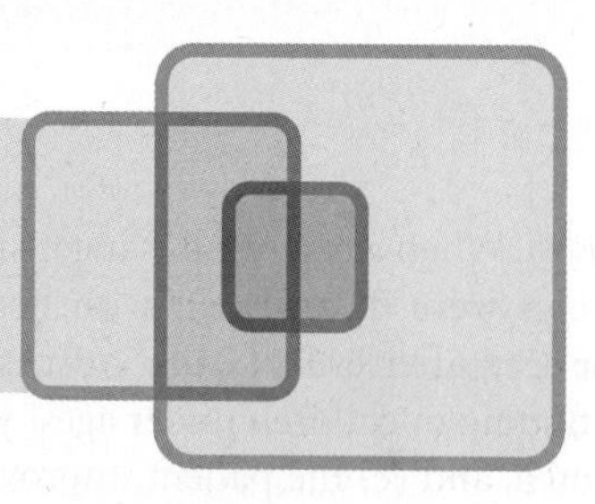

Gastrointestinal and Liver Diseases

KARAN EMERICK • FRANCISCO A. SYLVESTER

I INTRODUCTION

Gastrointestinal (GI) problems represent the second most common reason, after respiratory tract infection, for seeking medical care. The differential diagnosis and treatment of routine gastrointestinal symptoms in children (e.g., abdominal pain, vomiting, diarrhea) are often quite different from those in adults. At times, gastrointestinal symptoms may represent a nonspecific manifestation of serious infections such as pneumonia, meningitis, or pyelonephritis. The limited ability of the young child to describe his or her symptoms may make diagnosis more difficult. Subtle alterations in gastrointestinal function may adversely affect growth while causing minimal symptoms. Only careful examination of the child's growth curve may alert the physician to the possibility of underlying gastrointestinal disease.

II DISORDERS OF THE ESOPHAGUS

A Gastroesophageal reflux (GER) GER is a common disorder encountered in pediatric practice characterized by passage of stomach contents into the esophagus. Most episodes are brief, do not cause symptoms, and are promptly cleared by esophageal contractions and buffered by alkaline saliva. On occasion, gastric content can be regurgitated and spit out or reswallowed. In infants, some degree of gastroesophageal reflux is considered normal and resolves as the infant matures. When GER is unusually severe, persists beyond 18 months of age, or is associated with complications (failure to thrive, blood loss/anemia, chronic lung disease, or pain), it warrants appropriate diagnostic testing and medical or surgical management. It is important to recognize that GER is a **symptom,** not a diagnosis.

1. **Pathophysiology.** In most cases, the cause of GER is inappropriate transient relaxations of the lower esophageal sphincter, which briefly make the esophagus and the stomach a common cavity, allowing the regurgitation of gastric content into the esophagus. The pressure of the lower esophageal sphincter is normal in the majority of individuals. GER can be aggravated by esophageal inflammation (from peptic injury or eosinophilic esophagitis), esophageal dysmotility (secondary to inflammation, systemic sclerosis, cerebral palsy, myopathy, or neuropathy), obesity, chronic respiratory diseases (by augmenting negative intrathoracic pressure and cough), and diaphragmatic abnormalities.
2. **Clinical features**
   a. **Infants.** Vomiting is the most common symptom in infants and may occur immediately or hours after a feeding. The vomiting is usually effortless and painless, consisting of small amounts of curdled formula. Occasionally, vomiting may be forceful and may be confused with symptoms of pyloric stenosis. Intermittent vomiting is also common in preschool children with GER. Vomiting is nonbilious and rarely contains blood; if so, it requires additional evaluation.
   b. **School-age children** more often present with heartburn, intermittent regurgitation with reswallowing, or dysphagia. Other symptoms may include halitosis, food impaction (from esophagitis), tooth grinding, and loss of dental enamel.
3. **Diagnosis.** The diagnosis of GER is based on the history, physical examination, and exclusion of anatomic abnormalities that may predispose to the clinical features of reflux. The following tests are necessary *only* when the diagnosis is in doubt or when the presentation is dominated by one

of the complications of gastroesophageal reflux and a causal link between reflux and that complication (e.g., apnea, bronchospasm) is sought.

a. **Barium swallow** with upper gastrointestinal (UGI) radiograph is the best test for eliminating other anatomic causes of vomiting.

b. Twenty-four-hour esophageal **pH monitoring** ("**pH probe**") is still the "gold standard" for assessing and quantitating GER. A microelectrode placed in the lower esophagus measures and records intraesophageal pH. This study is most useful when trying to associate symptoms with GER (e.g., chronic cough, apnea, or seizure-like activity), but is limited because it only detects acid reflux.

c. **Esophageal impedance** consists of placing a microcatheter embedded with ring electrodes along its length in the esophagus. Upon catheter contact with liquid (irrespective of pH) or air, the electrical impedance changes. Current catheters combine impedance and pH recording. Standards to interpret its results are being developed for children.

d. **Radionuclide scans** evaluate GER by adding technetium 99m (Tc 99m) to formula or a meal and scanning the stomach to measure gastric emptying. Subsequent scanning of the lung fields can be useful in demonstrating reflux with aspiration, but the sensitivity of this method is low.

e. **Esophageal manometry** is used to measure resting lower esophageal sphincter pressure in addition to esophageal motility, which makes this modality useful to diagnose motility problems such as achalasia or scleroderma.

f. **Endoscopy** is useful to visualize the esophageal mucosa and biopsy allows histologic confirmation of esophagitis, even if the mucosa appears grossly normal.

4. **Therapy**

a. **Lifestyle changes.** Most infants who have "benign" gastroesophageal reflux can be treated conservatively with simple measures while awaiting maturation of UGI motility and resolution of symptoms. Positioning young infants with their left side down may help. Sitting in an infant car seat *increases* GER. However, elevating the head of the bed 20 degrees may help GER symptoms in older children. Thickening feedings with cereal (½ to 1 tsp cereal/ounce) improves symptoms like vomiting and irritability, and increases caloric density of the formula. In a subset of children with milk and/or soy protein allergy, a hypoallergenic formula may reduce symptoms. Smaller, more frequent feedings also help. Older children should avoid beverages with caffeine, chocolate, high-fat or spicy foods, and carbonated drinks.

b. **Medications.** Drug therapy (Table 11-1) should be reserved for patients who have complicated, symptomatic GER, including pain, feeding difficulties, respiratory complications, peptic esophagitis, and esophageal stricture.

TABLE 11-1 Pharmacologic Therapy of Gastroesophageal Reflux

Class	Drug	Mechanism	Dose
Antacid	Numerous (e.g., magnesium hydroxide, aluminum hydroxide)	Neutralizes gastric acid	0.5 mL/kg/dose 1 h postprandial every 4 h
H_2-receptor antagonist	Cimetidine	Blocks histamine receptor on parietal cell	10 mg/kg/dose qid
	Ranitidine		2 mg/kg/dose tid
	Famotidine		0.6 mg/kg/dose bid
Proton pump inhibitor	Omeprazole	Blocks H^+-K^+-ATPase pump in parietal cell membrane	1 mg/kg/dose daily 20–40 mg daily (adult dose)
Prokinetic agents	Bethanechol	Cholinergic stimulation increases LES tone	0.2 mg/kg/dose tid
	Metoclopramide	Dopamine antagonist increases LES tone, promotes gastric emptying	0.2 mg/kg/dose tid–qid
	Erythromycin	Motilin agonist	10 mg/kg/d divided tid

LES, lower esophageal sphincter; ATPase, adenosine triphosphatase; bid, twice daily; qid, four times daily; tid, three times daily.

c. **Surgery** is indicated for patients who have failed medical therapy, patients who have life-threatening or severely debilitating complications, and selected patients who have esophageal stricture or Barrett esophagus. Surgical procedures are designed to re-establish competence of the lower esophageal junction. The most commonly used procedure is the **Nissen fundoplication,** during which part of the gastric fundus is wrapped 360 degrees around the distal esophagus to create a high-pressure zone to resist gastroesophageal reflux. This can be combined with pyloroplasty and placement of gastrostomy tube as needed.

B **Eosinophilic esophagitis (EE)** is a disorder characterized by intense infiltration of the esophagus of ≥ 25 eosinophils/high power field. EE may represent a common phenotype of a heterogeneous group of disorders, including delayed hypersensitivity to food or to aeroallergens.

1. **Clinical features.** Young children with EE may present with vomiting and feeding difficulties, mimicking symptoms of GER. Older children often complain of dysphagia or have food impaction as the presenting symptom. Abdominal pain may also occur in a subset of patients.
2. **Diagnosis. Upper endoscopy** is the preferred modality, which may show multiple superficial eosinophilic microabscesses, abnormal ring-like esophageal contractions, mucosal edema, and occasionally strictures. **Biopsies** confirm the diagnosis. Special stains for mast cells may be helpful to differentiate EE from GER. Classically, pH probe studies are negative for acid GER in EE.
3. **Treatment.** Patients with EE respond to amino acid–based formulas and systemic and topical steroids (e.g., fluticasone and budesonide). An antacid is commonly used concurrently as adjuvant therapy.

C **Tracheoesophageal fistula (TEF)** The commonest form of TEF is complete esophageal atresia with a fistula connecting the distal esophagus with the trachea; this form of TEF is readily apparent at birth from the child's inability to feed or have a nasogastric tube inserted. Polyhydramnios due to inability of the fetus to swallow amniotic fluid may be a clue to this diagnosis. Rarely, a small fistula connects a patent esophagus and trachea (congenital H-type TEF) and may not cause difficulty until the child is several months of age or older. In this circumstance, the child may initially be seen with chronic coughing, especially at feedings, and with recurrent pneumonia or chronic lung disease due to aspiration. TEF requires surgical repair.

D **Esophageal damage by exogenous agents**

1. **Caustic agents** are common, accidentally ingested materials in children (See Chapter 2).
   a. Strong **alkali solutions** (e.g., lye) used as drain cleaners are most dangerous. **Acids** tend to cause more damage to the stomach than to the esophagus. The absence of oral burns or dysphagia *does not* predict the presence or degree of esophageal damage from ingestion of caustic agents. However, children may present with burns of the hands, face, and oral cavity; local pain; drooling; dysphagia, stridor, or dyspnea; abdominal and chest pain; and shock, if there is mediastinal penetration. No attempt should be made to induce vomiting or to neutralize the caustic agent. Neutralization of some chemicals releases heat, which can aggravate the injury.
   b. **Endoscopy** should be performed within 24 hours after patient stabilization under general anesthesia to document esophagitis or gastritis and the extent of the damage. Stricture formation may develop 2 to 4 weeks after ingestion and cause persistent dysphagia. A barium swallow can be performed to screen for stricture formation.
2. **Foreign bodies.** The esophagus is the most difficult portion of the gastrointestinal tract to navigate and objects that lodge in the esophagus should be expeditiously removed so that respiratory complications and esophageal ulceration and perforation do not occur. In particular, the removal of **disc batteries** should be considered an emergency. **Coins** are the most common esophageal foreign bodies found in children. American coins are not corrosive.

III DISORDERS OF THE STOMACH

A **Pyloric stenosis** is an important cause of gastric outlet obstruction and vomiting in approximately 1 in every 500 infants. It frequently affects more than one child in a family, with a male-to-female ratio of 4:1. Symptoms usually begin between 2 and 4 weeks of age, although in 5% of patients they are present shortly after birth. Projectile, nonbilious vomiting is the cardinal feature and is seen in virtually all patients. Infants often lose weight and are dehydrated. Moderate to severe **hypochloremic metabolic alkalosis** due to loss of gastric acid secondary to emesis is frequently (but not always) present. Palpation of a firm, mobile, nontender, **olive-shaped mass** in the right hypochondrium or epigastrium in the appropriate clinical setting confirms the diagnosis. If a pyloric mass cannot be palpated, ultrasonographic or radiographic evaluation (upper GI series) should be performed. Once fluid and electrolyte abnormalities are corrected, **pyloromyotomy** should be performed.

B Gastritis

1. **Pathogenesis.** ***Helicobacter pylori*** is strongly associated with gastritis in both adults and children, but most infections are asymptomatic. A small minority of patients with *H. pylori* gastritis will develop peptic ulcer disease and gastric cancer. Other causes of gastritis include food allergies, aspirin, alcohol, nonsteroidal anti-inflammatory drugs (NSAIDs), ingestion of corrosive agents, vasculitis, Crohn disease, eosinophilic gastritis, viral infection, Ménétrier disease, bile reflux, C-cell hyperplasia, and irradiation.
   a. **Clinical features** include abdominal pain and tenderness (usually epigastric), nausea, vomiting, and, occasionally, overt bleeding.
   b. **Diagnosis.** If the clinical picture warrants investigation (i.e., if there is severe pain, bleeding, or persistent vomiting), **endoscopy** can be performed. Antral gastritis with nodularity is frequently seen with *H. pylori* infection and specific histochemical stains or a rapid urease test on biopsy tissue can confirm the infection. Serologic studies may also reveal exposure to *H. pylori*, but they are not reliable indicators of active infection in children. *H. pylori* antigens can also be detected in stool. Carbon 13-labeled urea breath test is being used in some centers for the diagnosis of active *H. pylori* infection in children.
   c. **Treatment** consists of eliminating the underlying cause if known and administering an antacid for 2 to 6 weeks, depending on symptoms and histologic severity. *H. pylori* infection can be treated with combination therapy with antibiotics and a proton pump inhibitor, and several regimens are available. In the absence of ulcers, treatment for *H. pylori* in patients with abdominal pain confers a small but statistically significant benefit, so treatment should be considered on an individual basis after discussing the risk of therapy versus the risk of infection with the patient and the family.

C Peptic ulcer disease

1. **Pathogenesis.** In children, peptic ulcers are rare and usually secondary to a precipitating event (e.g., drugs, acute illness, *H. pylori* infection). They can be found in the stomach or duodenum.
2. **Clinical features.** In neonates and infants, ulcers can first present with bleeding and perforation, without preceding pain. In older children, pain becomes a more important feature and may persist for some time before the child receives medical attention. Ulcer pain may be poorly localized and may not be epigastric, as classically described in adults. Eating may or may not alleviate the pain. Nocturnal awakening may be present. Either overt or occult bleeding is seen in approximately half of school-age children with ulcer disease.
3. **Diagnosis. Endoscopic evaluation** of the upper gastrointestinal tract is the preferred method because of its superior sensitivity in detecting pathology compared with contrast radiography. Endoscopy also allows for tissue biopsy and evaluation of patterns of inflammation (e.g., allergic vs. peptic) and possible infection (e.g., *H. pylori*).
4. **Treatment** of peptic ulcer disease is similar to the treatment of gastritis (see above), except that antacid treatment is required for 6 to 8 weeks.

IV GASTROINTESTINAL HEMORRHAGE

A Pathogenesis Bleeding from the gastrointestinal tract can occur in infants and children. Usually, a careful history and physical examination, as well as consideration of the patient's age, will suggest the most likely causes. Bleeding can be secondary to coagulopathy, inflammation, ischemia, tumor, vascular lesions, or trauma, or a combination of these. It is helpful to think in terms of these broad diagnostic categories to narrow down possible etiologies in the individual patient (Table 11-2). However, attempts to make a specific diagnosis should occur only after the patient's cardiovascular status has been adequately stabilized.

B **Diagnosis** Bleeding from the gastrointestinal tract is usually a dramatic symptom that prompts immediate attention from caregivers and health providers. After a thorough hemodynamic assessment and appropriate resuscitation, the diagnostic approach to the patient with suspected gastrointestinal bleeding will involve three sequential steps:

1. **Did the patient actually bleed?** Food coloring can turn emesis and stools red, and bismuth and iron may make stools black. Amino acid–based formulas can make stool look dark green to black. Confirmation of the presence of heme protein in the stool is accomplished with a **guaiac test.**

TABLE 11-2 Differential Diagnosis of Gastrointestinal Bleeding in Children by Likely Symptom and Age at Presentation

Symptom	Infant	Child (2–12 Y)	Adolescent (> 12 Y)
Hematemesis	Swallowed maternal blood Peptic esophagitis Mallory-Weiss tear Gastritis Gastric ulcer Duodenal ulcer Gastric, duodenal duplication	Epistaxis Peptic esophagitis Caustic ingestion Mallory-Weiss tear Esophageal varices Gastritis Gastric ulcer Duodenal ulcer Hereditary hemorrhagic telangiectasia Hemobilia Henoch-Schönlein purpura	Esophageal ulcer Peptic esophagitis Mallory-Weiss tear Esophageal varices Gastric ulcer Gastritis Duodenal ulcer Hereditary hemorrhagic telangiectasia Hemobilia Leiomyoma (sarcoma) Henoch-Schönlein purpura
Painless melena	Duodenal ulcer Duodenal duplication Ileal duplication Meckel diverticulum Gastric heterotopia[a]	Duodenal ulcer Duodenal duplication Ileal duplication Meckel diverticulum Gastric heterotopia	Duodenal ulcer Leiomyoma (sarcoma)
Melena with pain, obstruction, peritonitis, perforation	Necrotizing enterocolitis Intussusception[b] Volvulus	Duodenal ulcer Hemobilia[c] Intussusception[b] Volvulus Ileal ulcer (isolated) Infectious colitis	Duodenal ulcer Hemobilia Crohn disease (ileal ulcer)
Hematochezia with crampy abdominal pain	Infectious colitis Pseudomembranous colitis Eosinophilic colitis Hirschsprung enterocolitis	Pseudomembranous colitis Ulcerative colitis Granulomatous (Crohn) colitis Hemolytic-uremic syndrome Henoch-Schönlein purpura Lymphonodular hyperplasia	Infectious colitis Pseudomembranous colitis Ulcerative colitis Granulomatous (Crohn) colitis Hemolytic-uremic syndrome Henoch-Schönlein purpura
Hematochezia without diarrhea or abdominal pain	Anal fissure Eosinophilic colitis Rectal gastric mucosa Heterotopia Colonic hemangiomas	Anal fissure Solitary rectal ulcer Juvenile polyp Lymphonodular hyperplasia	Anal fissure Hemorrhoid Solitary rectal ulcer Colonic arteriovenous malformation

[a]Ectopic gastric tissue in jejunum or ileum without a Meckel diverticulum.
[b]Classic "currant jelly" stool.
[c]Hemobilia often accompanied by vomiting and right upper quadrant abdominal pain.
Reprinted with permission from Treem WR: Gastrointestinal bleeding in children. *Gastrointest Endosc Clin N Am* 4:75, 1994.

2. **Did the bleeding originate in the upper or lower tract?**
   a. Hematemesis suggests a site proximal to the ligament of Treitz.
   b. If the clinical picture is unclear, **gastric aspiration** should be performed.
      (1) A gastric aspirate positive for blood is highly specific for upper tract bleeding. Rate of bleeding can be estimated from the nasogastric (NG) tube output.
      (2) A negative aspirate suggests lower tract bleeding, but cannot exclude an upper tract source that has stopped bleeding or a duodenal lesion with no reflux of blood back into the stomach.
3. **What is the specific source of the bleeding?** A variety of noninvasive and invasive techniques may identify the source of the bleeding.
   a. **Endoscopy** is the most sensitive and specific technique to evaluate gastrointestinal bleeding.
      (1) **Upper endoscopy** should be the first test in patients who have hematemesis or melena. Eighty percent of UGI bleeding sites can be identified. In addition to identifying the lesion and documenting the activity of bleeding, endoscopy provides potential therapy, including sclerotherapy and coagulation.
      (2) **Colonoscopy** should be the first diagnostic study in patients who have suspected colonic bleeding. Abnormal colonic mucosa will immediately alert the clinician to an infectious or inflammatory process (e.g., ulcerative colitis) or possibly identify a structural lesion (e.g., a polyp). In unstable patients who cannot be prepared for colonoscopy, a more limited sigmoidoscopy may be helpful.
      (3) **Capsule endoscopy.** This device, the size and shape of a medication capsule, is either swallowed or placed endoscopically in the duodenum. It takes multiple images as it traverses the small intestine that are transmitted to a recording device carried by the patient on a belt. It can be helpful in detecting sources of bleeding that are out of reach of conventional endoscopes. It is contraindicated in patients with suspected intestinal obstruction.
      (4) **Intraoperative enteroscopy** is reserved for those patients who continue to have significant bleeding when extensive endoscopic and radiologic test findings are negative and a small bowel source of bleeding is suspected. In this procedure, a laparotomy is performed and the bowel is telescoped over the endoscope. The cause of obscure small intestinal bleeding can be identified in approximately 80% of patients.
   b. **Radiologic evaluation**
      (1) A plain abdominal **radiograph** may exclude bowel obstruction and free intra-abdominal gas (perforated viscus).
      (2) Barium studies are contraindicated in the actively bleeding child because they are usually insensitive and will make other diagnostic testing difficult. A barium or air contrast enema may be the first diagnostic test if intussusception (*see VI A 4*) is suspected.
      (3) **Bleeding scans,** involving injection of Tc 99m pertechnetate-labeled red blood cells, may detect very slow rates of bleeding (0.1 mL/minute). Tc 99m pertechnetate injected intravenously may detect ectopic gastric mucosa in the case of Meckel diverticulum.
      (4) **Angiography** may be used to detect bleeding sites in more difficult cases and requires a higher bleeding rate (0.5 mL/minute).
      (5) **Enteroclysis** involves the intubation of the jejunum; the gradual instillation of barium, air, or methylcellulose; and evaluation of the mucosal surface of the bowel through fluoroscopy. This technique may identify the site of small bowel bleeding in 5% to 10% of patients.

C Therapy

1. **Cardiovascular resuscitation.** Immediately after ensuring the presence of an adequate airway and oxygenation, the first priority should be to restore the intravascular volume with appropriate crystalloid, colloid, or blood. The choice and volume of intravenous fluid will depend on the specific clinical circumstances. If present, coagulopathy should be rapidly corrected.

2. **Treatment of specific lesions**
   a. Different lesions discovered by endoscopy or other diagnostic tests often require specific therapeutic interventions. However, in all cases of upper gastrointestinal bleeding, an **antacid** (e.g., intravenous proton pump inhibitor) should be given. Oral sucralfate can be administered to protect and enhance the healing of mucosal lesions.
   b. **Esophageal varices** secondary to portal hypertension may be treated with a variety of techniques, including **intravenous octreotide or vasopressin** to stop the acute hemorrhage. Banding or sclerotherapy of the varices also stops bleeding and obliterates the engorged vessels. **Transjugular intrahepatic portosystemic shunt (TIPS)** is an angiographic technique in which a stent is placed within the liver through hepatic parenchyma to connect intrahepatic branches of the portal vein and hepatic veins to decompress the portal system. Finally, surgical shunts can be created between the portal and systemic venous return.
   c. Treatment of lower tract lesions depends on the cause (e.g., surgery is used for Meckel diverticulum).

V DIARRHEAL DISORDERS

A General principles Diarrheal diseases cause significant morbidity and mortality worldwide. Initial attention should be given to assessment of the degree of dehydration and electrolyte disturbances, which should be corrected. One should obtain a detailed history (e.g., age, history of travel, exposure to antibiotics, sick contacts, nocturnal awakening, nutritional status, and stool frequency, volume, and appearance). Then, to establish a differential diagnosis, a mechanism of diarrhea along with the information from the history should be considered. In general, diarrhea is caused by one of four mechanisms: **Osmotic, secretory, inflammatory,** or **functional.** However, a given disease process may cause diarrhea by more than one mechanism.

1. **Osmotic diarrhea**
   a. **Symptoms** include the passage of large, watery stools, abdominal cramping and flatulence, but no blood. Most patients do not wake up at night to pass stool. Typically there is no weight loss or other signs or symptoms of systemic involvement and physical examination is normal, except for gaseous abdominal distention in some cases. Dehydration is unusual. Laboratory evaluation is usually normal.
   b. Osmotic diarrhea is **caused** by the presence of nonabsorbable substances in the intestinal lumen that draws water from the intravascular compartment, which loosens the consistency of the stool. These substances can be either exogenous (e.g., sorbitol, high-fructose corn syrup, osmotic laxatives, excessive dietary fiber, dietary carbohydrates), or endogenous (deconjugated bile salts). Symptoms cease when the causative exogenous substance is avoided. **Carbohydrate intolerance** is a very common cause of osmotic diarrhea in school-aged children. In most cases, it is due to a primary deficiency in a brush border disaccharidase (e.g., lactase and sucrase deficiencies are the most common). However, secondary carbohydrate malabsorption may occur when there is injury to intestinal villi (e.g., from infection, celiac disease, etc.).
2. **Secretory diarrhea**
   a. Patients with secretory diarrhea have extensive losses of fluid and electrolytes due to outpouring of isotonic content into the intestinal lumen. This often leads to **dehydration,** which may be severe. Stools are liquid and clear, with no blood ("rice water" stools). In some cases, especially in diapered newborns and infants, stool can be confused with urine. Stool output continues despite fasting, and patients pass stool during sleep. Physical examination can reveal signs of dehydration and fluid-filled intestinal loops. Laboratory evaluation can reveal electrolyte abnormalities, azotemia, and acidemia.
   b. Intestinal secretion can be induced by microbial toxins (e.g., cholera), viruses (rotavirus), parasites (*Cryptosporidium, Isospora*), and neurotransmitters (e.g., vasoactive intestinal polypeptide (VIP) from ganglioneuroma or neuroblastoma), and be seen in newborns with electrolyte transport defects and microvillous inclusion disease. Diagnosis may require stool culture, intestinal biopsy, and measuring circulating levels of VIP or other mediators. Initial treatment should be aimed at restoring intravascular volume and correcting electrolyte

abnormalities. When possible, the underlying cause should be eliminated (e.g., surgical resection of a VIP-producing tumor). In selected cases, octreotide can help to reduce stool output.

3. **Inflammatory diarrhea**
   a. Children with inflammatory diarrhea can either have acute or chronic illness, depending on the causative agent or condition. **Symptoms** vary with the intestinal site that is predominantly affected. For example, colonic inflammation leads to frequent stools of small volume, with or without visible red blood, with urgency and tenesmus. Inflammation in the small bowel presents with larger, more infrequent stools, with or without dark blood, with variable urgency but no tenesmus. Dehydration may be present. Vomiting may occur. **Constitutional symptoms** are common, including weight loss, and, in some cases, fever. **Physical examination** can reveal pallor and abdominal tenderness. **Laboratory findings** may include elevated white cell and platelet counts, anemia, and elevated C-reactive protein (CRP) or erythrocyte sedimentation rate (ESR).
   b. Examples of **causes of acute inflammatory diarrhea** include bacterial infection (e.g., *Campylobacter, Escherichia coli, Salmonella, Shigella, Yersinia, Clostridium difficile, Klebsiella oxytoca*, and others) and parasites (*Entamoeba histolytica*). Specific diagnostic tests are available to detect each of these agents. **Treatment** is mostly **supportive** (rehydration, early introduction of enteral nutrition). In some cases, **antibiotic therapy** may be required due to young age, immunodeficiency, or presence of debilitating comorbidities, or to shorten disease duration.
   c. Examples of **chronic inflammatory diarrhea** are delayed hypersensitivity to protein (usually milk and/or soy), celiac disease, and inflammatory bowel disease. Each of these disorders requires specific diagnostic testing. For instance, allergy testing (prick testing, radioallergosorbent test [RAST], and patch testing) or elimination diets may be helpful to detect the offending food antigen(s) (see Chapter 9). Endoscopic biopsies may reveal eosinophilic infiltration of the gastrointestinal tract. Most patients with **celiac disease** have mild, vague symptoms. Serologic testing (antibodies to endomysium, gliadin, and tissue transglutaminase) can be used to screen for celiac disease and the diagnosis is confirmed by endoscopic biopsies of the small bowel. Treatment is the strict avoidance of dietary gluten. **Inflammatory bowel disease (IBD)** can be diagnosed with a combination of endoscopic and radiologic methods, and serologic markers are emerging as adjuvant diagnostic tools. Multiple anti-inflammatory medications are available to treat IBD.
4. **Functional diarrhea**
   a. Children can have diarrhea due to functional gastrointestinal disorders. By definition, these patients do not have any evidence of an underlying biochemical, structural, metabolic, or inflammatory cause for their symptoms. The history usually reveals a child with chronic symptoms who is otherwise well, with no growth impairment or constitutional manifestations. Stools are usually passed two to six per day, with urgency and symptom relief after defecation. Not infrequently, normal or even hard stools interrupt this pattern. Nocturnal passage of stool is very atypical. Sometimes an **exacerbating factor** such as excessive consumption of fruit juices or soda, stress, and anxiety can be identified. Physical examination and laboratory evaluation are normal.
   b. The **pathophysiology** of these disorders is incompletely understood, but it appears to involve visceral hypersensitivity, abnormalities in central gating and processing of visceral stimulation, and increased intestinal motility. **Diagnosis** is by history, physical examination, and judicious use of laboratory tests. It is important to *validate* the condition, make a *positive* diagnosis (e.g., chronic nonspecific diarrhea, irritable bowel syndrome), and offer *reassurance*. **Treatment** consists of avoiding aggravating factors, increasing dietary fiber, and occasionally using antispasmodics. More severe cases should be referred to a pediatric gastroenterologist.

VI ABDOMINAL PAIN

A Acute abdominal pain The most urgent consideration in evaluating a child who has acute abdominal pain is to determine whether there is an underlying cause requiring surgery. Most causes of abdominal pain in children do not require surgical treatment, although such causes of pain are more common in children younger than 2 years of age. Sources of pain outside the abdominal cavity (e.g., lower lobe pneumonia) must be considered in the evaluation.

1. Important **causes** of abdominal pain possibly requiring surgery (i.e., the acute abdomen) include:
   a. Intestinal obstruction due to malrotation and volvulus, intussusception, strangulated hernia, or adhesions
   b. Appendicitis
   c. Abdominal abscess
   d. Toxic megacolon
   e. Perforated intestine
   f. Cholecystitis
   g. Rupture of the spleen or other organ due to trauma
2. **Clinical features** suggesting a cause requiring surgery include:
   a. Signs of peritoneal irritation (e.g., rigidity, guarding, rebound tenderness)
   b. Bilious or feculent emesis
   c. Sudden onset of abdominal distention
   d. Absent bowel sounds or high-pitched sounds suggestive of intestinal obstruction
3. **Appendicitis** is the most common indication for acute abdominal surgery in childhood. Appendicitis occurs more frequently in children between 10 and 15 years of age. Less than 10% of patients are younger than 5 years of age.
   a. Classically, fever, vomiting, anorexia, and diffuse periumbilical pain develop. Subsequently, pain and abdominal tenderness localize to the right lower quadrant as the parietal peritoneum becomes involved.
   b. The incidence of perforation and diffuse peritonitis is high. The diagnosis is frequently delayed in a child younger than 2 years of age.
   c. Atypical presentations are common in childhood.
   d. Certain bacterial infections (e.g., *Campylobacter jejuni*, *Yersinia* species) and mesenteric adenitis may be associated with right lower quadrant pain and tenderness and may mimic appendicitis.
   e. Acute exacerbation of ileocecal Crohn disease can resemble appendicitis.
   f. The diagnosis of appendicitis should be established clinically by history and physical examination (including a rectal examination to detect tenderness or a mass). Laboratory tests may help confirm the diagnosis (elevation of white blood cells [WBCs]). An abdominal ultrasound or computed tomography (CT) scan can be used to visualize the appendix.
   g. Treatment of appendicitis is surgical.
4. **Intussusception** is the invagination (telescoping) of one part of the intestine into another. It is one of the most common causes of intestinal obstruction in infancy. As a result of impaired venous return, the affected bowel may swell, become ischemic and necrotic, and perforate, so prompt diagnosis is important to avoid this complication.
   a. Most intussusceptions are ileocolic, but ileoileal intussusception may occur in **Henoch-Schönlein purpura** (see Chapter 9). The period of peak incidence is under 2 years of age. No **lead point** for the intussusception is typically found.
   b. A specific lead point is identified in only approximately 5% of patients. Specific anatomic abnormalities leading to intussusception are more common in children older than 5 years of age. Recognizable causes of the intussusception include Meckel diverticulum, an intestinal polyp, lymphoma, or a foreign body.
   c. Bouts of irritability and colicky pain start suddenly and may subside with spontaneous reduction. Vomiting is common. Rectal bleeding may occur but only rarely in the form of the classic **"currant jelly" stools** (i.e., stools containing dark red blood and mucus).
   d. The degree of **lethargy** demonstrated by the child may be striking. At times the prominent presenting feature may be "altered consciousness."
   e. A **tubular mass** is palpable in approximately half of the patients.
   f. A plain abdominal radiograph may show a paucity of gas in the right lower quadrant or evidence of obstruction. Ultrasound shows a soft tissue mass with a laminated appearance, and a target sign on cross-sectional views. A barium enema demonstrates a coiled-spring appearance to the bowel, which is diagnostic.
   g. Treatment in uncomplicated intussusception is by **reduction** with a barium air enema. In refractory cases or with perforation, **surgery** is required.

5. Important causes of acute abdominal pain typically not requiring surgery include gastroenteritis or colitis, Henoch-Schönlein purpura, hemolytic-uremic syndrome and other types of vasculitis, fecal impaction, hepatitis, pancreatitis, vaso-occlusive crisis of sickle cell anemia, primary peritonitis, mesenteric adenitis, uncomplicated intussusception, urinary tract infection or urinary calculi, extra-abdominal causes (e.g., pneumonia, osteomyelitis, acute neurologic processes), and unusual causes (e.g., acute intermittent porphyria, familial Mediterranean fever, diabetic ketoacidosis, lead poisoning, Kawasaki disease with gallbladder hydrops, visceral larva migrans).

B **Chronic abdominal pain** is a frequent problem in children (see Chapter 4). Most often, no specific physical cause can be documented and the pain is refered to as **functional.** Two specific patterns are prominent.

1. **Infantile colic** is observed in up to 15% of otherwise healthy newborns. Symptoms and signs of colic include prolonged, inconsolable crying; crying after feedings; facial grimacing; abdominal distention; increased passage of gas; flushing; and legs held in flexion over the abdomen. In most cases, symptoms improve by 4 to 5 months of age (see Chapter 4).
2. **Functional abdominal pain syndromes** represent the most common cause of chronic abdominal pain in children. This group of disorders occurs in otherwise healthy children and includes **dyspepsia** (pain or discomfort in the upper abdomen, which may resemble peptic ulcer, bloating, early satiety, or a combination of these symptoms and are not relieved by defecation), **irritable bowel syndrome** (periumbilical abdominal pain associated with urgency to pass stool, constipation, or altered bowel pattern), and **functional abdominal pain** (abdominal pain in the periumbilical area not associated with changes in defecation). By definition, a disease process has been excluded by a careful history, physical examination, and limited diagnostic testing.
   a. **Pathogenesis.** The precise pathogenesis of functional abdominal pain syndromes is unknown, but a **biopsychosocial model** has been proposed. Visceral hypersensitivity (reaction to gut distention), disorders of pain perception and interpretation, and abnormal intestinal (primarily colonic) motility are layered upon environmental stressors and susceptible personality types.
   b. **Clinical features** include crampy or sharp abdominal pain that is centered in the midline and is diffuse, but does not radiate. It may be associated with nausea, pallor, diaphoresis, and lightheadedness. Excitement or anxiety can provoke an attack. In some cases, symptoms can affect daily activities, including school attendance.
   c. **Diagnosis.** Specific diagnostic criteria have been developed by expert consensus for each functional abdominal pain syndrome (**Rome III criteria:** www.romecriteria.org).
   d. **Therapy** consists of establishing a reassuring, therapeutic relationship with the patient and the family; validating symptoms; and making a positive diagnosis. For dyspepsia, an antacid or prokinetic may help, depending on the type of symptoms. For IBS and functional abdominal pain, dietary fiber supplementation relieves symptoms. Medications such as anticholinergic drugs, tricyclic and serotonin reuptake inhibitor antidepressants, and gabapentin are available to treat more severe pain. For some patients, cognitive behavioral therapy can help to reduce symptoms and regain function.

VII CONSTIPATION

A **General principles** Most constipated children have no underlying disorder (referred to as **functional constipation**), and treatment can be directed solely at the symptom. Formal evaluation is reserved for cases beginning at birth and those that are not responsive to standard symptomatic treatment. Specific causes include anorectal malformations, large colonic tumors, extrinsic compression of the colon, neuromuscular and primary motility disorders, medications (opiates, anticholinergics), hypothyroidism, hypercalcemia and hypokalemia, lead poisoning, infant botulism, and, rarely, celiac disease and food allergy.

1. **Pathogenesis.** Functional constipation occurs in the absence of an organic cause. In an otherwise healthy child, constipation may result simply from an episode of painful defecation, difficulties

during the period of toilet training, inattention to the urge to defecate because of involvement in other activities, or discomfort with toilet facilities in school. Frequently, a family history of constipation may be elicited. Inadequate fiber in the diet may also play a role.

2. **Clinical features**
   a. **Pattern** of defecation. A detailed history of the pattern of defecation may be difficult to obtain. Even a history of regular bowel movements does not exclude constipation, if evacuation is incomplete. In a child who has large stools, stool-withholding behavior—such as squatting, pushing, and crying—may be misinterpreted as an attempt to defecate.
   b. Accompanying **symptoms** include pain, abdominal distention, and flatulence. Occasional symptoms include rectal bleeding, poor appetite, enuresis, and a history of urinary tract infection. Rectal prolapse may rarely be seen with defecation.
   c. **Encopresis.** In cases of long-standing constipation, children may become incontinent of liquid stool and be thought to have diarrhea. This overflow incontinence is called encopresis and is present in more than 50% of children who have long-standing constipation. In some cases, encopresis may be nonretentive and secondary to psychiatric disorders (see Chapter 4).
3. **Diagnosis**
   a. **Physical examination** of the abdomen may reveal distention or palpable fecal masses. The perianal area should be examined for congenital or acquired abnormalities, including trauma. Digital rectal examination is necessary to evaluate the sphincter and estimate the amount of stool in the ampulla.
   b. When no underlying disorder is identified by history and physical examination, a favorable response to treatment supports the diagnosis of functional constipation.
   c. Treatment failure or relapse should prompt investigation of an underlying disorder with appropriate radiographic and laboratory studies.
4. **Therapy** for functional constipation. An individualized, multifaceted treatment program should be designed.
   a. **Medications** are continued until a regular pattern of defecation is established, and then they are slowly tapered. In older children, laxative therapy is commonly required for at least 6 to 12 months and occasionally longer.
      (1) In infants, stool softening may be accomplished by adding apple or pear juice. Extra fiber in the form of barley malt extracts or methylcellulose may also help. Occasionally, a natural barley malt laxative (Maltsupex) or lactulose may be used to achieve softer, more frequent stools. Because of the risk of aspiration pneumonitis, mineral oil is usually avoided in children under 12 months of age.
      (2) In older children, polyethylene glycol (without electrolytes), mineral oil, or mild laxatives such as senna derivatives are commonly used.
      (3) In cases of severe constipation, a period of aggressive treatment including enemas (otherwise to be avoided) may be required.
      (4) For **fecal impaction,** a balanced polyethylene glycol-electrolyte solution administered by the oral or nasogastric route is safe, prompt, and effective in cleansing the bowel and may avoid prolonged use of enemas or the need for manual disimpaction.
   b. Other measures include high-fiber diet, fiber supplements, and reinforcement of regular toilet use. Psychological evaluation may be necessary to address emotional factors resulting in voluntary withholding. Biofeedback training may be beneficial, especially in those children who have chronic functional constipation and rectal dyssynergia on anorectal manometry.

VIII INFLAMMATORY BOWEL DISEASE

A General principles IBD encompasses two chronic entities, **ulcerative colitis** and **Crohn disease.** In ulcerative colitis, inflammation is limited to the superficial layers of the colonic mucosa. In Crohn disease, inflammation may occur in any part of the gastrointestinal tract and affects the full thickness of the bowel wall. In some patients, the distinction between the two can be challenging, especially when inflammation is limited to the colon (**indeterminate colitis**).

TABLE 11-3 Comparative Pathologic and Clinical Features of Ulcerative Colitis and Crohn Disease

Feature	Ulcerative Colitis	Crohn Disease
Location	Colon only Proctitis Left sided Pancolitis	Mouth to anus 60% ileocolonic 30% Small bowel 10% Colonic
Histology	Mucosal inflammation Diffuse involvement Crypt abscesses Crypt distortion	Transmural inflammation Skip areas Aphthoid lesions Fissuring ulceration Granuloma Fibrosis
Clinical features		
Diarrhea	++→++++	0→++++
Rectal bleeding	++→++++	0→++++
Abdominal pain	0→++	++→++++
Abdominal mass	0	0→++++
Weight loss	0→+	+→++++
Short stature	0→+	0→++++
Perirectal disease	0	0→++++
Carcinoma risk	+→++++	0→+
	Extraintestinal manifestations (Ulcerative colitis, Crohn disease) Arthritis Ankylosing spondylitis Erythema nodosum Pyoderma gangrenosum Uveitis/episcleritis Stomatitis Sclerosing cholangitis	

1. **Pathogenesis.** IBD occurs due to a confluence of factors, including **genetic susceptibility** and **environmental triggers.** It is currently thought that susceptible individuals mount a chronic, inappropriate inflammatory response to normal commensal flora, which leads to gastrointestinal symptoms.
2. **Clinical features.** Patients can present at any age, but the peak incidence of IBD in children is in preadolescents and adolescents. Children with ulcerative colitis typically present with bloody, loose stools, with urgency and tenesmus. Systemic symptoms are usually not prominent. Children with Crohn disease may debut with symptoms ranging from isolated growth failure and perianal abscess to diarrhea, weight loss, and fever (Table 11-3).
3. **Diagnosis.** In the presence of symptoms consistent with a diagnosis of IBD, hematologic, biochemical, radiographic, and endoscopic studies may be performed. Typical laboratory findings include anemia, thrombocytopenia, elevated ESR and CRP, and decreased serum albumin. In Crohn disease, small bowel series may show narrowing and nodularity of bowel loops, especially in the terminal ileum. In ulcerative colitis, colonoscopy will reveal diffuse inflammation starting in the rectum, whereas in Crohn disease inflammation tends to be patchy.
4. **Therapy.** In children, current treatment paradigms include nutritional rehabilitation, promotion of normal growth and development, identification and treatment of psychological comorbidities, and mucosal healing with anti-inflammatory therapies. The choice of specific medications is guided by disease location and severity (Table 11-4). In cases in which complications arise (e.g., intra-abdominal abscess, intestinal obstruction, bleeding, perforation) or the disease cannot be managed medically, surgery is indicated.

TABLE 11-4 Anti-Inflammatory Medical Treatment of Inflammatory Bowel Disease

Medications	Crohn Disease	Ulcerative Colitis
5-Aminosalicylates (5-ASA)	Mild to moderate colonic disease (Pentasa also treats small bowel disease)	Mild to moderate disease Rectal preparations are available to treat distal colonic inflammation
Corticosteroids	Moderate to severe disease	Moderate to severe disease Rectal preparations are available to treat distal colonic inflammation
Antibiotics (metronidazole, ciprofloxacin)	Mild to moderate colonic disease	Not effective
Nutritional therapy	Mild to moderate small bowel disease Efficacy in colonic disease may be less	Not effective
Thiopurines	Effective in maintenance of remission Take 3–6 mo to reach peak effect	May be effective in maintenance of remission
Methotrexate	Effective in maintenance of remission	Not effective
Biologicals (infliximab, adalimumab)	Moderate to severe disease	Moderate to severe disease

IX LIVER DISEASE

A General principles Certain unique aspects of liver disease in infancy and childhood must be considered before specific hepatic disorders can be evaluated.

1. Estimation of liver **size.** In healthy children younger than 2 years of age, both the liver and spleen are usually palpable below the costal margins due to the relatively large size of these organs at this age. In older children, standards have been established for liver span as measured by percussion in the midclavicular line.
2. **Jaundice** is the most important manifestation of a variety of hepatic insults in infancy. **Dark urine** and **acholic stools** are often the most obvious clinical features of an obstructed biliary tract.
3. Key elements of the **history**
   a. The **family history** is important in the consideration of **metabolic** liver disease.
   b. Illness or exposure during pregnancy may suggest a **vertically transmitted** (i.e., from mother to infant) infectious cause of hepatitis.
   c. A **dietary history** is crucial in the diagnosis of hepatic disease resulting from the failure to metabolize galactose or fructose.
4. **Diagnostic tests.** Increased serum aminotransferase levels reflect hepatocyte **injury,** not liver dysfunction. On the other hand, blood glucose, serum albumin concentration, and prothrombin time are indirect measures of **function** because they are synthesized by the liver. The serum alkaline phosphatase level is usually elevated in children who have **obstructive** or **inflammatory** hepatic lesions. However, in infancy and adolescence, serum alkaline phosphatase levels from bone are normally elevated compared to adult values. Thus, other enzymes, such as γ-glutamyl transpeptidase (GGT), which is liver specific, are more useful. Enzymes originating from the biliary tract (GGT and alkaline phosphatase) are commonly more elevated than other enzymes in biliary obstruction.

B Neonatal jaundice **Direct hyperbilirubinemia** in the neonate is never "physiologic," and therefore this condition should always be thoroughly investigated. Direct hyperbilirubinemia is defined as a direct bilirubin level > 2 mg/dL or > 20% of the total bilirubin (see Chapter 2).

1. **Differential diagnosis.** Direct hyperbilirubinemia in the neonate is a **medical emergency** and must be expeditiously investigated to avoid permanent liver damage. The key distinction in the neonatal period is between **hepatocellular** and **obstructive** causes of direct hyperbilirubinemia. The primary hepatocellular cause of neonatal cholestasis is **idiopathic neonatal hepatitis.** Obstructive causes require prompt surgical therapy to relieve obstruction and reconstitute bile flow from the liver. Obstructive cholestasis results from an anatomic or functional obstruction

TABLE 11-5 Causes of Cholestasis with Direct Hyperbilirubinemia in the Infant

	Hepatocellular Causes		
Obstructive Causes	**Infectious**	**Metabolic**	**Miscellaneous**
Biliary atresia	Cytomegalovirus	Galactosemia	Neonatal hepatitis
Choledochal cyst	Toxoplasmosis	Hereditary fructose intolerance	Alagille syndrome
Common duct stenosis	Rubella	α_1-Antitrypsin deficiency	Progressive familial intrahepatic cholestasis (Byler disease)
Common duct stone	Herpes virus	Niemann-Pick disease	Zellweger syndrome
Obstructing tumor	Coxsackie virus	Gaucher disease	Trisomy (17, 18, 21)
Bile/mucus plug	Echovirus	Glycogen storage disease	Hypopituitarism
Spontaneous perforation of common duct	Syphilis		Hepatic hemangiomatosis
Cystic fibrosis	Hepatitis B		TPN-induced cholestasis
	Epstein-Barr virus		
	Urinary tract infection		

TPN, total parenteral nutrition.

of the biliary system. The principal causes of obstructive cholestasis in young children are presented in Table 11-5. **Biliary atresia** accounts for over 90% of cases. Cholestasis is frequently accompanied by the hallmark sign of alcoholic stools.

2. In a representative large study of neonatal cholestasis, the distribution of diagnoses in 1086 infants with neonatal cholestasis was biliary atresia, 34.7%; idiopathic neonatal hepatitis, 30.7%; α_1-antitrypsin deficiency, 17.4%; other hepatitis, 8.7%; Alagille syndrome, 5.6%; and choledochal cyst, 3.1%.
   a. **Tests** for specific causes of neonatal cholestasis
      (1) **Serum tests,** including total and direct bilirubin; aminotransferases and GGT; complete blood count; titers of toxoplasmosis, rubella, cytomegalovirus, and herpes simplex organisms (see Chapter 8); Venereal Disease Research Laboratories (VDRL); hepatitis B surface antigen (HbsAg); α_1-antitrypsin level and phenotyping; amino acids; blood culture (if clinically indicated); albumin; prothrombin time; and partial thromboplastin time
      (2) **Urine tests,** including urinalysis, reducing substances, urine culture, and organic and amino acids
      (3) Sweat test
      (4) Abdominal ultrasound to rule out a choledochal cyst, choledochocele, or common duct stone
      (5) Radionuclide biliary imaging to document patency of the extrahepatic biliary system
      (6) Liver biopsy
   b. Differentiation of **hepatocellular** vs **obstructive** idiopathic causes (Table 11-6)
      (1) Often, the tests for neonatal cholestasis reveal no specific cause. However, **neonatal hepatitis** and **biliary atresia** are the most common causes of persistent direct hyperbilirubinemia. No serum test (including aminotransferases, GGT, bilirubin, and alphafetoprotein) reliably distinguishes between these two entities. Further testing is directed at differentiating between these two entities, including percutaneous **liver biopsy,** which can reliably differentiate more than 90% of the time, when read by an experienced pediatric pathologist.
      (2) Ultimately, if there are features of biliary obstruction on the liver biopsy, it may be necessary to perform a **laparotomy** and **intraoperative cholangiography** to accurately delineate the patency of the extrahepatic biliary system.

3. **Therapy**
   a. **Neonatal hepatitis.** The treatment for neonatal hepatitis and other causes of prolonged hepatocellular cholestasis is **supportive,** including:
      (1) Administration of ursodeoxycholic acid, a secondary bile acid, to increase bile flow and reduce hypercholesterolemia

TABLE 11-6 Features of Neonatal Cholestatic Disease

Feature	Hepatocellular Causes	Obstructive Causes
Clinical		
Gestation	Premature SGA	Full term AGA
Family history	15%–20%	None
Appearance	Ill	Well
Stool color	Intermittent acholic	Acholic
Organomegaly	Hepatosplenomegaly	Splenomegaly later
Liver texture	Soft	Firm to hard
Anomalies	Peripheral pulmonic stenosis Vertebral anomalies Posterior embryotoxon	Polysplenia Malrotation of gut
Laboratory		
GGT	$< 10 \times$ normal	$> 10 \times$ normal
Ultrasound	Gallbladder	No gallbladder or small
Hepatobiliary scan	Excretion into bowel	No excretion
Liver biopsy		
Bile ducts	Normal or decreased	Proliferating
Fibrosis	Minimal	Established, portal
Giant cells	Often	25% of the time
Cholestasis	Yes	Yes
Other	Hepatocellular necrosis Lobular disarray	Bile plugs, bile lakes

GGT, γ-glutamyl transpeptidase; SGA, small for gestational age; AGA, appropriate for gestational age.

(2) Supplementation of fat-soluble vitamins (A, D, E, K)

(3) Supplementation of the diet with medium-chain triglycerides that do not require bile acids for assimilation

(4) Use of antihistamines to treat pruritus

b. Biliary atresia

(1) **Surgical management.** In most patients, a **portoenterostomy** must be created between the cut surface of the liver at the porta hepatis and the bowel (Kasai procedure). Successful drainage of the biliary tract occurs most frequently when the operation is performed before the infant is 60 days old. Complications of surgery include failure to establish bile flow, loss of bile flow due to further injury to bile ducts, and ascending cholangitis.

(2) **Medical management.** *See IX B 3 a* for previously described treatment of cholestasis, with the addition of prophylactic antibiotics (e.g., trimethoprim-sulfamethoxazole), to help prevent cholangitis. Cholangitis is aggressively treated with intravenous antibiotics.

4. Prognosis

a. Neonatal hepatitis

(1) In most patients, the cholestasis resolves over the first year of life with no sequelae.

(2) A few infants develop progressive liver disease and **cirrhosis,** with its complication of ascites, portal hypertension, esophageal varices, and liver failure. These children may be candidates for liver transplantation.

b. Biliary atresia

(1) Without surgical correction, biliary cirrhosis and its complications supervene, and most patients die in the first 2 years of life.

(2) After successful portoenterostomy and with normalization of serum bilirubin levels, the 5-year survival rate is 60% to 90%. Patients may continue to do well, but many eventually develop cirrhosis, especially if the course includes recurrent cholangitis.

(3) **Liver transplantation** is available for patients with biliary atresia who fail corrective surgery. The 5-year survival rate for liver transplantation recipients who have biliary atresia is > 85%.

TABLE 11-7 Comparison of Viral Hepatitis Types A, B, C, D, and E in the United States

Virus	Hepatitis A	Hepatitis B	Hepatitis C	Hepatitis D	Hepatitis E
Features	RNA	DNA	RNA	Defective RNA[a]	RNA
Age group	Primarily young	All ages	All ages	All ages	All ages, primarily 15–40 y
Onset	Abrupt	Insidious	Insidious	Insidious, fulminant	Abrupt
Incubation	21–42 d	50–180 d	42–56 d	Variable[b]	30–45 d
Transmission					
Feces	+	–	–	–	+
Water, food	+	–	–	+	+
Semen	–	+	?	+	–
Saliva	–	+	+	+	–
Transfusion	–	+	+	+	–
Needlestick	–	+	+	+	–
Drug abuse	–	+	+	+	–
Dialysis	–	+	+	+	–
Sexual contact	+	+	+	+	–
Household contact	+	–	–	–	+
Mother-infant	–	+	+	+	–
Secondary cases	10%–20%	Rare	Rare	Rare	2.5%
Prevalence	5%–10%	> 2%	0.6%	1%–10% of HBV	Rare
Symptoms					
Anorexia	Common	Common	Common	Common	Common
Nausea, vomiting	Common	Common	Common	Uncommon	Common
Fever	Common before jaundice	Uncommon	Uncommon	Uncommon	Common
Jaundice	Uncommon in children	More common	Uncommon	More common	Uncommon
Rash, arthritis	Rare	Common	Rare	Rare	Rare
Outcome					
Severity	Mild	Mild to severe	Intermediate	Mild to severe	Mild to severe
Mortality	Low (< 1%)	Low (1%–3%)	Low (1%–3%)	Low-moderate	High (pregnant women ≤ 20%)
Chronic hepatitis	No	Yes (5%–10%)	Yes (30%–50%)	Yes	No
Chronic carrier	No	Yes	Yes	Yes	No
Liver cancer	No	Yes	Yes	?	No

[a] Replicates and causes hepatitis only in patients who concurrently are infected with hepatitis B virus (HBV).
[b] Incubation period typical of hepatitis B if infection with delta virus is simultaneous. Incubation period short (35 d) if hepatitis D is superimposed on chronic HBV carrier state.

C Acute viral hepatitis (Table 11-7)

1. **Diagnosis** (Table 11-8). Typically, children with acute viral hepatitis have elevated serum levels of aminotransferases with or without icterus. In severe cases, hepatic synthetic function may be affected, with resulting prolongation of the prothrombin time. Care must be taken in establishing a diagnosis because of infectivity issues and to rule out other liver disease.
   a. **Hepatitis A virus (HAV, infectious hepatitis).** The diagnosis of acute hepatitis A is established by the finding of hepatitis A antibodies of the immunoglobulin M (IgM) class (IgM antibody is present for 1–3 months; IgG antibody is longer lasting). Anti-HAV IgG may represent past, not present, infection.
   b. **Hepatitis B virus (HBV, serum hepatitis)**
      (1) The standard marker for hepatitis B is the presence of hepatitis B surface antigen (HBsAg). The presence of antibodies directed against HBsAg (anti-HBs) usually indicates immunity.
      (2) IgG antibodies directed against hepatitis B core antigen (anti-HBc) may indicate acute infection, chronic infection, or past infection. IgM antibodies against HBcAg (anti-HBc IgM) are more indicative of acute infection.

TABLE 11-8 Understanding Serology in Viral Hepatitis

Hepatitis Marker	Abbreviation	Meaning
A antibody (IgM)	Anti-HAV (IgM)	Recent hepatitis A infection
B surface antigen	HbsAg	Infection with HBV (acute or chronic)
B surface antibody	Anti-HBs	Clinical recovery from HBV (protective)
B core antibody	Anti-HBc	Active HBV infection (acute-chronic)
	Anti-HBc (IgM)	Active HBV infection
B e antigen	HBeAg	Active HBV infection, high infectivity (> 6–8 wk suggests chronic carrier)
B e antibody	Anti-HBe	Resolving infection
B virus DNA	HBV DNA	Active HBV infection (high levels of infectivity)
C virus RNA	HCV RNA	Transfusion-related non-A, non-B is detectable in serum or liver by PCR; confirms infection with HCV
C virus antibody	Anti-HCV	Present in acute and chronic infection (not protective—up to 12 mo to seroconvert)
Delta antigen	HD Ag	Acute HDV infection
Delta antibody	Anti-HDV	Exposure to HDV; may transmit infection

HBV, hepatitis B virus; HCV, hepatitis C virus; HDV, hepatitis D virus; Ig, immunoglobulin; PCR, polymerase chain reaction.

(3) **Hepatitis B e antigen (HBeAg)** is a marker of viral replication and infectivity and chronic infection if it is present for more than 2 months. It almost guarantees transmission of hepatitis B virus from mother to infant when appropriate prophylaxis is absent.

c. **Hepatitis C virus (HCV, transfusion-related hepatitis).** IgG antibodies to hepatitis C virus have been developed. Reverse polymerase chain reaction to detect HCV RNA in the serum or liver is the most sensitive marker of infection with HCV.

(1) Anti-HCV antibody is a marker for hepatitis C, not for immunity. Its appearance may be delayed for up to 6 to 12 months after infection if the first-generation tests for anti-HCV are used. With the newer assays (second and third generation), HCV infection can usually be detected within 3 months of the time of exposure.

(2) Anti-HCV antibody persists in chronic hepatitis C but eventually disappears after recovery from acute hepatitis C.

d. **Hepatitis D (delta hepatitis)**

(1) Delta antigen in the serum is only briefly detectable (first 2 weeks of the disease). Antibodies to delta virus (anti-HDV) become detectable in more than 90% of patients within 3 to 8 weeks of infection with acute hepatitis D.

(2) The highest titers of anti-HDV are found in patients who have chronic hepatitis D.

2. **Therapy.** No specific therapy exists for acute viral hepatitis. Strict bed rest is not necessary, but vigorous activity should be avoided.

3. **Prognosis.** The prognosis is excellent for full recovery from nonfulminant hepatitis A. Chronic active or chronic persistent hepatitis develops in 5% of patients who have hepatitis B. Without prophylactic treatment (described below), vertical transmission at birth results in infection in more than 90% of exposed infants. Many of these infants become chronic carriers of HBV. Hepatitis C results more frequently in chronic hepatitis, with up to half of patients developing chronic active disease.

4. **Prevention**

a. **Hepatitis A.** Family members, children, and staff exposed at day care centers, as well as their sexual contacts, should receive immune globulin (0.02 mL/kg) within 2 weeks of contact. A **vaccine** is now available and is effective in preventing infection with hepatitis A in endemic areas (see Chapter 1).

b. **Hepatitis B**

(1) **Hepatitis B immune globulin (HBIG).** People who have had sexual, percutaneous, or mucosal exposure should receive HBIG (0.06 mL/kg) plus full vaccination. The dose of HBIG should be repeated in 1 month.

(2) **Hepatitis B vaccine** is a recombinant vaccine that is effective in infants as well as older children, with few side effects. It is given as three doses, 1 and 6 months following the first dose. The vaccine is now recommended for all infants, family contacts of chronic carriers, and other high-risk populations. These populations include all health care workers engaged in patient care or contact with laboratory specimens from patients, residents, and staff of institutions that care for cognitively impaired individuals; seronegative homosexual men; intravenous drug abusers; dialysis patients; and recipients of high-risk blood products (e.g., hemophiliacs).

(3) **Prophylaxis in infants.** All infants born in the United States should be immunized against hepatitis B (see Chapter 1). Infants of women who are serum HBsAg positive in the third trimester of pregnancy, especially if they are also HBeAg positive, should also receive 0.5 mL HBIG within 12 hours of birth and start the vaccine series. With the proper and timely administration of HBIG and hepatitis B vaccine, 90% of the cases of chronic HBV infection that would have resulted from perinatal transmission can be prevented.

(4) **Booster doses.** Anti-HBs that are generated by exposure to the vaccine appear to diminish with time. Long-term studies of children and adults indicate protection against chronic HBV infection for 10 years or more, even though anti-HB concentrations may become low. At present, routine booster doses of vaccine are not recommended, except for people continuously exposed to hepatitis B (e.g., health care workers) and immunocompromised patients (e.g., hemodialysis patients, those who have human immunodeficiency virus [HIV] infection).

D **Fulminant hepatitis** is severe acute hepatitis resulting in progressive liver failure and hepatic encephalopathy.

1. **Etiology**

   a. **Viral infection.** Fulminant hepatitis may follow any of the hepatitis viral infections described earlier, although acute liver failure from hepatitis A, B, or C is extremely rare in the western world. In underdeveloped countries, hepatitis A is the most common cause of reported fulminant hepatitis. Hepatitis B is an uncommon cause but is usually seen in infants of HBsAg-positive, anti–HBe-positive mothers, or in children exposed to blood products from donors who have that same serologic profile. Delta hepatitis infection superimposed on chronic hepatitis B may convert a stable or chronic persistent hepatitis B patient to one who has severe chronic active or even fulminant hepatitis. Hepatitis E is particularly virulent in pregnant women, causing fulminant hepatitis in approximately 20% of patients. Other important viral causes of fulminant hepatitis in infancy include herpes virus, echovirus, cytomegalovirus (CMV), and Epstein-Barr virus (EBV).

   b. **Metabolic causes.** Tyrosinemia, galactosemia, hereditary fructose intolerance, neonatal iron storage liver disease, α_1-antitrypsin deficiency, Zellweger syndrome, disorders of fatty acid oxidation, and bile acid synthetic defects in the neonate may lead to fulminant hepatic failure in infants or young children. Wilson disease may lead to this condition in the older child.

   c. **Hepatotoxic drugs** can cause fulminant hepatic failure by overdosage (e.g., acetaminophen) (see Chapter 2), through a genetic proclivity to slow metabolism (e.g., isoniazid), or through an idiosyncratic hypersensitivity reaction to a normal dose of the drug (e.g., halothane, phenytoin). In some patients, valproic acid is converted to toxic metabolites that disrupt various intramitochondrial pathways, which results in hyperammonemia, hypoglycemia, and hepatic steatosis and failure.

   d. Plant toxins have also been implicated (e.g., *Amanita phalloides* mushrooms).

   e. **Autoimmune chronic active hepatitis**, especially the type 2 form (positive antiliver/kidney microsomal antibodies)

   f. Infiltrative diseases (leukemia, hemophagocytic lymphohistiocytosis, hemangioendothelioma)

   g. Ischemia

   h. Irradiation

   i. Cryptogenic hepatitis of unknown cause

2. **Clinical features**

   a. Early symptoms include persistent anorexia and fever, progressive jaundice, and mental status changes.

b. On sequential physical examinations, a shrinking liver size despite a worsening clinical status may be noted, as may hyperventilation and the development of ascites.
c. Laboratory tests reflect **hepatic failure,** as indicated by vitamin K–resistant coagulopathy (low factor V and VII activity), hypoglycemia, hypokalemia, hypoalbuminemia, low blood urea nitrogen, low cholesterol, and high blood ammonia levels.
d. Central nervous system signs, including agitation, stupor, and eventually coma, with diffuse slowing of activity on electroencephalogram are seen.

3. **Complications**
   a. Gastrointestinal bleeding due to coagulopathy
   b. Secondary bacterial or fungal infection
   c. Renal dysfunction
   d. Increased intracranial pressure (ICP)
4. **Therapy.** The use of sedatives (especially benzodiazepines) and barbiturates should be avoided.
   a. **Supportive care** consists of:
      (1) Maintenance of fluid and electrolyte balance with correction of hyponatremia and hypokalemia
      (2) Correction of hypoglycemia, hypokalemia, and hypophosphatemia
      (3) Administration of H_2-receptor antagonists to prevent upper gastrointestinal bleeding and the use of fresh frozen plasma to correct clotting abnormalities when there is clinical evidence of bleeding
      (4) Endotracheal intubation and assisted ventilation as required by deepening coma and to hyperventilate the patient to reduce cerebral blood flow and ICP
      (5) Treatment of ICP, including ICP monitoring and the use of mannitol
      (6) Use of broad-spectrum antibiotics and antifungals
   b. Measures to **minimize encephalopathy.** Treatment involves measures to lower serum ammonia levels by decreasing protein available as substrate and eliminating ammonia-producing bacteria in the bowel, including:
      (1) Restriction of oral and intravenous protein
      (2) Use of cathartics
      (3) Oral or nasogastric administration of neomycin or lactulose
   c. Interventions such as plasmapheresis, exchange transfusion, charcoal hemoperfusion, and dialysis alone have not improved survival rates. However, as adjunctive measures to stabilize and maintain a patient before liver transplantation, these modalities appear to have a definite role.
   d. **Liver transplantation.** Children with fulminant hepatic failure have undergone transplantation with a 60% to 89% survival rate. This compares favorably with the 20% to 40% survival rate previously obtained with intensive conservative management.

E. **Chronic hepatitis** can be defined as an inflammatory process of the liver lasting longer than 6 months. Chronic hepatitis has been differentiated on the basis of pathology into **chronic persistent hepatitis** and **chronic active hepatitis.** Chronic persistent hepatitis is defined by an inflammatory reaction limited to the portal zone, with little or no fibrosis. Chronic active hepatitis is defined by an inflammatory reaction that is not limited to the portal area and periportal fibrosis. Patients with chronic persistent hepatitis have an improved chance of complete resolution and decreased progression to chronic active hepatitis. Although this distinction may be important for progression of disease and prognosis, chronic hepatitis is now more commonly grouped on the basis of underlying cause.

1. **Etiology**
   a. **Infectious. Chronic HBV** is still the most common cause of chronic liver disease in most of the world. In the United States, **chronic HCV** is now more common. Coinfection with other viruses such as HCV/HBV and HBV/HIV may also lead to chronic liver disease. Other viral causes include EBV and CMV.
   b. **Autoimmune chronic active hepatitis** is believed to be the result of either a primary or secondary defect in T-cell function that leads to injury. Often these patients are initially seen with hypergammaglobulinemia and a number of autoantibodies (e.g., antinuclear, anti–smooth muscle, antimitochondrial antibody). Autoimmune hepatitis may be classified on the basis of antibodies. **Type 1** (antinuclear antibody positive) tends to be more common and occurs in older patients. **Type 2** (antiliver/kidney microsomal [LKM] antibody positive) is less common;

it occurs in younger patients and has a poorer response to treatment. Further classifications based on clinical presentation and antibodies are being developed.

c. **Metabolic/genetic:** Wilson disease, α_1-antitrypsin deficiency, and cystic fibrosis

d. **Toxins/drugs**

2. **Clinical features**

a. Patients with chronic persistent hepatitis usually have symptoms similar to acute hepatitis, such as fever, malaise, anorexia, and abdominal pain.

b. The presentation in chronic active hepatitis is more severe, with jaundice, hepatosplenomegaly, and right upper quadrant abdominal pain. Ascites, digital clubbing, cutaneous stigmata of chronic liver disease (spider angioma, prominent abdominal wall venous pattern), and arthritis or glomerulonephritis may also occur.

c. **Laboratory studies.** The evaluation of a patient who has chronic hepatitis usually begins with a general chemistry panel (including levels of fractionated bilirubin, aminotransferases, γ-glutamyl transferase), complete blood count, and prothrombin time. In order to evaluate for an underlying cause, serologic tests for hepatitis A, B, C, and D; CMV; and EBV are helpful. Further evaluation for metabolic/autoimmune disease includes α_1-antitrypsin, ceruloplasmin, 24-hour urine copper collection, sweat chloride testing, and autoantibodies (antinuclear antibody, anti–smooth muscle antibody, and anti-LKM antibody). An ultrasound is often performed to evaluate the underlying anatomy of the liver.

d. **Laboratory findings**

(1) The serum bilirubin level is elevated but is usually < 5 mg/dL. The serum levels of aminotransferases are typically elevated at least 10-fold. Of the plasma proteins, serum albumin is low and γ-globulin is elevated. The erythrocyte sedimentation rate is likewise elevated.

(2) Approximately 25% of patients have detectable levels of serum HBsAg. Serum HBsAg-negative patients may have antinuclear antibodies, anti–smooth muscle antibodies, anti-LKM antibodies, or other serologic evidence of autoimmune disease. It is important to test for anti-HCV or HCV RNA in the serum to rule out hepatitis C as a cause.

(3) Hypersplenism may result in anemia, leukopenia, and thrombocytopenia.

e. **Therapy and prognosis**

(1) Until recently, there was no effective therapy for HBsAg-positive or anti–HCV-positive patients who have chronic hepatitis.

(a) **Hepatitis B**

(i) Treatment with **recombinant interferon alfa** results in a disappearance of viral markers of replication, decreased infectivity, normalization of levels of aminotransferases, and improved liver histology in approximately 50% of patients who have chronic hepatitis B. Long-term follow-up reveals that some of these patients relapse after therapy, but approximately one third of treated patients achieve a sustained response. Side effects include fever, fatigue, headaches, muscle aches, abdominal discomfort, neutropenia, and thrombocytopenia.

(ii) Although not yet routinely used in pediatric patients, **lamivudine**—a nucleoside analogue that inhibits DNA replication—has shown great promise in the treatment of chronic hepatitis B. In a recent study, lamivudine led to a sustained improvement of levels of aminotransferases in 68% of patients. Side effects were similar to those of interferon alfa and included respiratory tract infections, headache, cough, abdominal discomfort, diarrhea, malaise, and fatigue.

(b) **Hepatitis C**

(i) For patients who have hepatitis C, the initial response to therapy is equivalent to that of hepatitis B, but the relapse rate is very high. Patients who have the highest risk for progressing to cirrhosis may best benefit from **interferon alfa therapy.** This includes patients who have persistently elevated aminotransferase levels, positive HCV RNA, and portal or bridging fibrosis and moderate inflammation or necrosis on biopsy.

(ii) **Ribavirin** is a nucleoside analogue that, when used in combination with interferon alfa for a 6-month course, leads to improved sustained response rates compared to those seen with interferon alfa alone. The most common side effect is a reversible hemolytic anemia, with a decrease in hemoglobin by 10% to 20% of baseline.

(2) **Autoimmune hepatitis** is treated with **immunosuppression.** Prednisone is usually the first-line medication and is tapered very gradually in association with close monitoring of liver function. In patients unable to be weaned from prednisone, azathioprine may be helpful. Cyclosporine may be helpful in cases of treatment failure with other immunosuppressants. In one recent series, immunosuppressant therapy was able to be stopped in 19% of patients after a median of 3 years of treatment.

(3) **Liver transplantation** may be necessary for patients in whom cirrhosis develops, with its attendant complications (e.g., portal hypertension, esophageal varices, ascites, liver failure).

F Metabolic liver disease The metabolic diseases affecting liver function are numerous and varied in presentation. For example, α_1-antitrypsin deficiency can occur in neonates as cholestasis and in older children as cirrhosis. The remainder of this section focuses on two metabolic liver diseases of particular importance to the pediatrician: α_1-antitrypsin deficiency and Wilson disease.

1. **α_1-Antitrypsin deficiency**

a. **Pathogenesis**

(1) α_1-Antitrypsin is a serum protease inhibitor synthesized in the liver. Codominant alleles dictate the type and concentration of α_1-antitrypsin inherited.

(2) Deficiency of α_1-antitrypsin results from homozygous inheritance of the z-type α_1-antitrypsin gene (mapped to chromosome 14). This results in low serum α_1-antitrypsin levels and an abnormally slow-moving protein (**PiZZ protein**) on acid-starch electrophoresis compared with the normal protein.

(3) The mutated PiZZ protein has altered three-dimensional relationships that lead to polymerization of the molecules and accumulation of abnormal α_1-antitrypsin within the endoplasmic reticulum of the hepatocytes. The exact mechanisms by which this accumulation leads to hepatocyte injury are poorly understood.

b. **Clinical features**

(1) Approximately 10% to 20% of individuals who have the PiZZ protein will develop liver disease.

(a) PiZZ α_1-antitrypsin deficiency is the most common metabolic disease to cause neonatal hepatitis and for which children require liver transplantation.

(b) Approximately 5% to 10% of PiZZ patients have neonatal cholestasis. Jaundice resolves in most cases. Occasionally, severe disease causes death in the first year of life.

(2) Older infants and children may initially be seen with failure to thrive, hepatomegaly, or cirrhosis.

(3) In the adolescent and adult, the deficiency may cause early pulmonary disease (emphysema), cirrhosis, and hepatocellular carcinoma.

c. **Diagnosis**

(1) There are low serum levels of α_1-antitrypsin (usually < 100 mg/dL) and an abnormal protein phenotype (PiZZ).

(2) Liver biopsy shows characteristic periodic acid-Schiff (PAS)-positive, diastase-resistant eosinophilic cytoplasmic granules in periportal hepatocytes.

d. **Treatment.** Cigarette smoking accelerates the onset of lung disease and should be avoided. In patients who have liver disease and poor synthetic function, liver transplantation has been successful with 1-year survival of 80%. However, the progression to liver dysfunction may be gradual, and some patients do not require transplantation unless deterioration is present.

2. **Wilson disease** is a treatable, autosomal recessive disorder, which is the result of a mutation in a gene that maps to chromosome 13 (13q14.3-q21.1) and appears to encode a copper-binding, membrane-spanning protein. This diagnosis needs to be considered in the differential diagnosis of any liver disease in children 5 or older.

a. **Pathogenesis.** Organ damage occurs as the result of toxicity from copper deposition. Although levels of the copper-binding protein, ceruloplasmin, are low in 95% of patients, the exact mechanism underlying Wilson disease is not known.

b. **Clinical features.** Wilson disease has many unusual modes of presentation, so there is often a delay in diagnosis.

(1) **Liver disease** is the primary mode of presentation in pediatric patients, but it is rarely clinically evident before 5 years of age. The presentation may include an episode of acute hepatitis, fulminant hepatitis, chronic hepatitis, or cirrhosis.

(2) **Neurologic symptoms** (e.g., tremor, dysarthria, loss of fine motor control, chorea, ataxia, seizures) (see Chapter 18) usually occur in young adulthood. Psychiatric symptoms can be very striking, leading to a diagnosis of obsessive-compulsive disorder, schizophrenia, manic-depressive disorder, or antisocial behavior.
(3) Coombs-negative hemolytic anemia occurs.
(4) There is renal involvement, usually a Fanconi-like syndrome.
(5) Corneal deposition of copper causes the formation of characteristic Kayser-Fleischer rings.

c. Diagnosis
(1) **Kayser-Fleischer rings** are pathognomonic when present (a slit lamp may be required to see them).
(2) The **ceruloplasmin** level is usually below 20 mg/dL in 95% of patients who are heterozygous for Wilson disease, but it may be low in other disorders as well.
(3) Patients with Wilson disease have elevated urinary copper excretion ($> 100\ \mu g/24$ hours).
(4) Quantification of liver copper by biopsy demonstrates levels $> 250\ \mu g/g$ by dry weight.

d. Therapy
(1) **Dietary restrictions.** Chocolate, nuts, liver, shellfish, mushrooms, and other foods rich in copper should be avoided.
(2) Lifelong treatment with **chelating agents** is necessary. Such agents include D-penicillamine, trientine (if penicillamine is not tolerated), and oral zinc (to reduce intestinal copper absorption and help maintain negative copper balance).

e. Prognosis. The prognosis is excellent with early treatment. However, fulminant hepatitis continues to be associated with a poor prognosis.

G Liver transplantation Orthotopic liver transplantation has become the accepted therapy for end-stage liver disease and metabolic liver disease in children. With the use of reduced-size grafts and living related donors, organs are more readily available for the smaller pediatric patient.

1. **Major indications** for liver transplantation in children include:
   a. Biliary atresia (particularly after an unsuccessful Kasai procedure)
   b. α_1-Antitrypsin deficiency
   c. Tyrosinemia, Wilson disease, and other inborn errors of metabolism
   d. Cryptogenic cirrhosis and chronic active hepatitis
   e. Fulminant hepatitis
2. **Postoperative management.** Chronic immunosuppression with a calcineurin inhibitor (FK506 [Prograf; Fujisawa] or cyclosporine), prednisone, and azathioprine is necessary to prevent rejection.
3. **Prognosis.** One-year survival rates are nearly 90% and 5-year survival rates are approximately 80%. Children younger than 12 months of age experience a significantly poorer prognosis.
4. **Postoperative complications** include:
   a. Primary allograft nonfunction
   b. Vascular thrombosis (especially the hepatic artery in children)
   c. Biliary complications such as anastomotic stricture with primary biliary reconstruction, bile leak after removal of the T-tube, ischemic injury to the bile duct, and recurrent cholangitis
   d. Acute cellular rejection
5. **Long-term complications** of liver transplantation and chronic immunosuppression include:
   a. Growth impairment if high doses of corticosteroids are required
   b. Nephrotoxicity and hypertension
   c. Biliary strictures, obstruction, or leak
   d. Susceptibility to infection, including viral (e.g., Epstein-Barr virus, cytomegalovirus, and herpes simplex virus), *Pneumocystis carinii,* bacterial, and fungal infections
   e. Chronic rejection. This process occurs in approximately 10% of transplantation cases and leads to progressive cholestasis and decreased numbers of bile ducts. Retransplantation may be required.
   f. Lymphoproliferative disease is a potentially fatal disorder associated with the intensity of immunosuppression and EBV infection (either primary or reactivation). Treatment includes decreasing immunosuppression and antivirals (ganciclovir/acyclovir).

X DISORDERS OF THE PANCREAS

A Pancreatic insufficiency

1. **Cystic fibrosis (CF)** is the major cause of pancreatic insufficiency in the United States, Canada, and western Europe. The general aspects of cystic fibrosis and its pulmonary complications are discussed in Chapter 13. The following discussion focuses on pancreatic insufficiency and other gastrointestinal manifestations of cystic fibrosis.
   a. Pancreatic disease due to cystic fibrosis
      (1) **Pancreatic insufficiency.** Of patients who have cystic fibrosis, 85% to 90% have evidence of exocrine pancreatic dysfunction.
         (a) **Pathogenesis.** The pancreas seems to be affected in utero. Decreased ductal water flow is present because of decreased anion secretion by CF cells, which leads to a rise in the protein concentration of the pancreatic ducts. This in turn causes microprecipitation of protein and plugging of the ductal lumens. Later, exocrine pancreatic elements are replaced by fibrous tissue and fat.
         (b) **Clinical features**
            (i) Malnutrition and failure to thrive may begin in the first few months of life.
            (ii) Steatorrhea occurs, and stools are bulky, foul smelling, and pale and greasy in appearance.
            (iii) Complications due to malabsorption of fat-soluble vitamins or calcium may occur (e.g., hemorrhagic diathesis, rickets, neurologic abnormalities).
         (c) **Diagnosis** of pancreatic insufficiency is made on the basis of the following:
            (i) Quantitative determination of **fecal fat excretion**
            (ii) Serum levels of **pancreatic trypsinogen** (increased before the age of 8 years, but then subnormal)
            (iii) Duodenal intubation and **cholecystokinin-secretin stimulation** to assay enzymes and bicarbonate produced by the pancreas (gold standard)
            (iv) Bentiromide (*N*-benzoyl-L-tyrosyl-para-aminobenzoic acid) test. After oral administration of bentiromide, plasma para-aminobenzoic acid levels are low in patients who have steatorrhea.
         (d) **Therapy** (see Chapter 13) consists of:
            (i) Pancreatic extracts given before meals to supplement enzyme activity
            (ii) A balanced but high-caloric diet
      (2) **Pancreatitis** may occur in some patients who retain some pancreatic exocrine function.
   b. Other gastrointestinal and hepatic disorders associated with cystic fibrosis
      (1) Meconium ileus involving neonatal intestinal obstruction due to abnormal meconium (see Chapter 13)
      (2) Intestinal impaction in older children (distal intestinal obstruction syndrome)
      (3) Intussusception
      (4) Rectal prolapse
      (5) Liver disease, including neonatal cholestatic syndrome; fatty liver; and focal biliary fibrosis (in older children), which may progress to biliary cirrhosis
      (6) Abnormal gallbladder function and cholelithiasis

2. Other conditions associated with pancreatic insufficiency include:
   a. Malnutrition, which is the most common cause of childhood pancreatic insufficiency worldwide
   b. Shwachman-Diamond syndrome (pancreatic insufficiency and bone marrow dysfunction)
   c. Isolated pancreatic enzyme defects
   d. Johanson-Blizzard syndrome

B Pancreatitis

1. **Etiology.** A variety of factors may lead to activation of pancreatic enzymes, causing autodigestion and inflammation of the pancreas. Such factors include:
   a. Abdominal **trauma** (including surgery and endoscopic retrograde cholangiopancreatography)
   b. **Infections** (e.g., mumps and other viruses, *Mycoplasma* species)

c. **Biliary obstruction:** Stones, parasites, tumors
d. Congenital anomalies of the pancreatic ducts (e.g., pancreas divisum)
e. Drugs (e.g., L-asparaginase, azathioprine)
f. Systemic diseases (e.g., collagen vascular disease, Henoch-Schönlein purpura, hemolytic uremic syndrome, Kawasaki disease, inflammatory bowel disease, hyperlipidemia, hypercalcemia)
g. Cystic fibrosis
h. Penetrating duodenal ulcer
i. Metabolic abnormalities (e.g., organic acidemias)
j. Structural anomalies: Choledochal cyst, pancreas divisum, biliary stenosis
k. Unidentified factors (30% of cases are idiopathic; some of these factors may be familial)

2. **Clinical features**
   a. More than 75% of patients have epigastric pain, which may radiate to the back and is frequently exacerbated by eating.
   b. Nausea and vomiting are common.
   c. On examination, the abdomen is slightly distended and is tender on palpation. Bowel sounds are diminished.
   d. Severe cases may result in shock.
3. **Diagnosis**
   a. The serum amylase and lipase levels are usually elevated. However, normal values do not exclude the diagnosis. The degree of elevation of serum amylase and other pancreatic enzymes does not correlate with the severity of pancreatic inflammation or the clinical course.
   b. Abdominal ultrasound is the imaging method of choice for the diagnosis of pancreatitis in children.
4. **Complications** include:
   a. Hypocalcemia
   b. Hyperglycemia
   c. Pseudocyst formation, which occurs in 5% of patients and is heralded by an epigastric mass and recurrent pain (pseudocysts are easily detected and monitored by ultrasound)
   d. Pancreatic phlegmon, with a potential for secondary bacterial infection and abscess formation
   e. Peritonitis
5. **Therapy** is aimed at minimizing pancreatic stimulation and includes:
   a. Nothing by mouth. However, recent studies in adults suggest that early feeding in acute pancreatitis may improve the clinical course.
   b. Nasogastric suction for patients who have persistent vomiting secondary to ileus
   c. Administration of adequate intravenous fluids and electrolytes, with appropriate hemodynamic monitoring of patients who have severe cases
   d. Meperidine for pain
   e. With recovery, gradual introduction of a high-carbohydrate, low-fat diet
   f. Surgical drainage, which eventually may be needed for pseudocysts
6. **Prognosis**
   a. Fulminant hemorrhagic pancreatitis has a high mortality rate.
   b. Episodes may recur if the cause is not identified and remedied.

BIBLIOGRAPHY

Alvarez F: Autoimmune hepatitis and primary sclerosing cholangitis. *Clin Liver Dis* 10(1):89–107, 2006.

Bourke B, Ceponis P, Chiba N, et al.: Canadian Helicobacter Study Group Consensus Conference: update on the approach to Helicobacter pylori infection in children and adolescents—an evidence-based evaluation. *Can J Gastroenterol* 19(7):399–408, 2005.

Bucuvalas J, Yazigi N, Squires RH Jr: Acute liver failure in children. *Clin Liver Dis* 10(1):149–168, 2006.

Chaudry G, Navarro OM, Levine DS, et al.: Abdominal manifestations of cystic fibrosis in children. *Pediatr Radiol* 36(3):233–240, 2006.

Dennehy PH: Acute diarrheal disease in children: epidemiology, prevention, and treatment. *Infect Dis Clin North Am* 19(3):585–602, 2005.

Elisofon SA, Jonas MM: Hepatitis B and C in children: current treatment and future strategies. *Clin Liver Dis* 10(1):133–148, 2006.

Emerick KM, Whitington PF: Neonatal liver disease. *Pediatr Ann* 35(4):280–286, 2006.

Ferenci P, Caca K, Loudianos G, et al.: Inflammatory bowel disease. *Pediatr Rev* 26(9):314–320, 2005.

Hyman PE, Milla PJ, Benninga MA, et al.: Childhood functional gastrointestinal disorders: neonate/toddler. *Gastroenterology* 130(5):1519–1526, 2006.

Kay M, Wyllie R: Pediatric foreign bodies and their management. *Curr Gastroenterol Rep* 7(3):212–218, 2005.

Liacouras CA, Spergel JM, Ruchelli E, et al.: Eosinophilic esophagitis: a 10-year experience in 381 children. *Clin Gastroenterol Hepatol* 3(12):1198–1206, 2005.

McCollough M, Sharieff GQ: Abdominal pain in children. *Pediatr Clin North Am* 53(1):107–137, 2006.

North American Society for Pediatric Gastroenterology, Hepatology and Nutrition: Evaluation and treatment of constipation in children: summary of updated recommendations of the North American Society for Pediatric Gastroenterology, Hepatology and Nutrition. *J Pediatr Gastroenterol Nutr* 43(3):405–407, 2006.

Nydegger A, Couper RT, Oliver MR: Childhood pancreatitis. *J Gastroenterol Hepatol* 21(3):499–509, 2006.

Rasquin A, Di Lorenzo C, Forbes D, et al.: Childhood functional gastrointestinal disorders: child/adolescent. *Gastroenterology* 130(5):1527–1537, 2006.

Rufo PA, Bousvaros A: Current therapy of inflammatory bowel disease in children. *Paediatr Drugs* 8(5):279–302, 2006.

Schilsky M, Cox D, Berr F: Diagnosis and phenotypic classification of Wilson disease. *Liver Int* 23(3):139–142, 2003.

Tiao G, Ryckman FC: Pediatric liver transplantation. *Clin Liver Dis* 10(1):169–197, 2006.

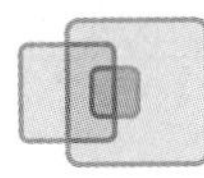

Study Questions

Directions: *Each of the numbered items or incomplete statements in this section is followed by answers or completions of the statement. Select the ONE lettered answer or completion that is BEST in each case.*

1. A 28-month-old boy is initially seen with increasing irritability, decreased appetite, and an episode of vomiting with streaks of red blood in the emesis. He underwent repair of a tracheoesophageal fistula and esophageal atresia in his first year of life. Findings from the physical examination are unremarkable. The patient undergoes barium swallow, and there is no evidence of an esophageal stricture at the level of the prior esophageal anastomosis. Which of the following diagnoses is most likely in this child?

- A Gastric ulcer
- B Esophageal varices
- C Peptic esophagitis
- D Ingestion of an unknown caustic substance
- E Achalasia

2. A 12-year-old boy who has cerebral palsy, moderate cognitive impairment, and a seizure disorder is brought to your office from his residential home because of an inability to swallow solids and increased vomiting, choking, and gagging. Before this visit, he had been on a regular diet, but now he can only take pureed foods. His physical examination findings are unremarkable, but his initial laboratory data show a hematocrit of 31%; a mean corpuscular volume of 67, with normal white blood cell and platelet counts; and stool that is positive for occult blood. Which of the following tests is most appropriate for discovering the cause of this child's problem?

- A Hemoglobin electrophoresis, followed by a bone marrow examination
- B Prolonged intraesophageal pH probe and gastric emptying scan
- C Esophageal manometry
- D Barium swallow (upper gastrointestinal series) and upper gastrointestinal endoscopy
- E Iron and total iron-binding capacity

3. A 3-year-old child is brought to the emergency department after being found with a lye-containing, hair-straightening cream on his hands, face, and lips. He is crying, is drooling, and has erythematous patches noted on his lips, buccal mucosa, and soft palate. Although frightened, the child does not appear to be in respiratory distress, and he has no stridor. His mother has given him water to drink before coming to the emergency department. Which of the following actions is the most appropriate first step in management?

- A Perform an immediate barium swallow
- B Give 8 ounces of milk and then induce vomiting
- C Prepare the child for an upper gastrointestinal endoscopy within 12 to 24 hours
- D Immediately order a chest radiograph
- E Administer a bolus of intravenous corticosteroids

4. An 8-week-old, full-term male infant with appropriate development for his gestational age is first seen with jaundice. He went home 5 days after birth, during which time he spent 2 days undergoing phototherapy for a total bilirubin level of 13.8 mg/dL. His bilirubin level when discharged was 9.5 mg/dL. At his 2-week check-up, the infant was still jaundiced, but the jaundice was attributed to breastfeeding. Weight gain was appropriate. The infant next returned at 2 months of age. By then, the jaundice had deepened, the stools were noted to be pale green or clay colored, and the urine was dark. Although the infant had grown and still appeared vigorous, the liver was enlarged with a firm, sharp edge, and the spleen was palpable 3 cm below the left costal margin. Laboratory tests revealed a total bilirubin level of 14.5 mg/dL, direct bilirubin of 8.8 mg/dL, aspartate aminotransferase of 243 U/L, alanine aminotransferase of 184 U/L, γ-glutamyl transferase of 487 U/L (normal is up to 40 U/L), and absence of reducing sugars from the urine. An abdominal ultrasound showed a small gallbladder, no gallstones, no choledochal cysts, and no dilated intrahepatic bile ducts. A radionuclide biliary imaging study showed concentration in the liver but no excretion into the gallbladder or small intestine. Which of the following next steps in management are most appropriate?

- A Stop breastfeeding, send the baby home, and recheck the bilirubin level in 4 weeks
- B Check the serum of both the infant and mother for hepatitis B
- C Test the serum for α_1-antitrypsin deficiency and await the results
- D Check the prothrombin and partial thromboplastin times; if they are normal, perform an immediate percutaneous liver biopsy
- E Test the serum for galactose 1-uridyl transferase, which is the defective enzyme in galactosemia

5. A sexually active 17-year-old boy comes to the clinic asking for a test for acquired immunodeficiency syndrome. On further questioning, he admits to being sexually promiscuous and having intercourse with multiple partners in the last 6 months. He vehemently denies intravenous drug use but does say that he "hangs out" with several girls who use intravenous drugs. One of his previous sexual partners recently became ill and was diagnosed with acute hepatitis B. In addition to testing this adolescent for hepatitis B and hepatitis C, which of the following diagnostic and/or therapeutic actions should the physician do first?

- A Give hepatitis B immune globulin (HBIG) and initiate the hepatitis B vaccine series immediately
- B Screen for elevations in levels of aminotransferases and follow-up the patient's levels of liver enzymes for the next 6 months
- C Test the patient for human immunodeficiency virus and inform him of the results
- D Give HBIG alone
- E Wait for all the serologic results before deciding whether to give immunoprophylaxis

6. A 15-year-old girl is first seen with recent persistent epigastric abdominal pain and vomiting. She states that the pain is burning in nature and is made worse by eating. It awakens her from her sleep. She has lost 5 lbs (2.25 kg). No hematemesis or melena has been noted. Family history is positive for peptic disease. Upper gastrointestinal endoscopy reveals diffuse micronodular antral gastritis but no ulceration. A rapid urease test performed on a gastric biopsy is positive. Which of the following results is most likely to be revealed in this patient on gastric antral mucosal biopsy?

- A Intense eosinophilic infiltration
- B Granuloma from Crohn disease
- C *Helicobacter pylori*
- D Vasculitis
- E G-cell hyperplasia

Directions: *Each set of matching questions in this section consists of a list of 4 to 6 lettered options followed by several numbered items. For each numbered item, select the ONE lettered option that is most closely associated with it. Each lettered option may be selected once, more than once, or not at all.*

QUESTIONS 7–10

For each patient below with lower gastrointestinal bleeding, select the most likely diagnosis.

- A Allergic proctocolitis
- B Hemolytic-uremic syndrome
- C Ulcerative colitis
- D Juvenile polyp in the rectum
- E Meckel diverticulum

7. A 6-year-old child who has streaks of bright red blood on the side of normal-formed stool and drops of bright red blood in the toilet, but no complaints of abdominal or rectal pain

8. A 3-year-old child who has bloody diarrhea, crampy abdominal pain, a low hematocrit, and a low platelet count

9. A 6-week-old child who has scant streaks of red blood mixed with normal stool

10. An 18-month-old child with painless passage of large amounts of maroon stool who is anemic and in shock

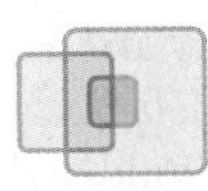

Answers and Explanations

1. The answer is C (*II A 2*). Children who have undergone repair of tracheoesophageal fistula and esophageal atresia all have some degree of gastroesophageal reflux. If not prophylactically treated, many of these children will have complications of gastroesophageal reflux, especially peptic esophagitis secondary to chronic reflux. The occurrence of this problem is often signaled by nonspecific signs (e.g., irritability, anorexia, failure to thrive) as opposed to more specific findings (e.g., vomiting, hematemesis, iron deficiency anemia, and occult blood in the stool). Toddlers do not complain of classic symptoms such as heartburn, dysphagia, or chest pain. Chronic vomiting is not always present before the discovery of peptic esophagitis.

Of the other choices, only gastric ulcer and caustic ingestion may be associated with blood-streaked emesis. Esophageal varices bleed more profusely. Caustic ingestions can result in the previously described symptoms, but they would be acute and often associated with drooling, inability to swallow, and oropharyngeal burns. Gastric ulcers can cause these symptoms, but in the setting of tracheoesophageal fistula repair, the physician should always be aware of chronic gastroesophageal reflux as a long-term complication.

2. The answer is D (*II A 3*). This child has an esophageal stricture most likely caused by chronic peptic esophagitis secondary to gastroesophageal reflux. Children who have severe spasticity and neurologic handicaps are at greater risk for chronic unremitting gastroesophageal reflux and the development of significant complications associated with reflux. If the patient can swallow liquids safely, the barium swallow is the best test for outlining the anatomy of the esophagus and defining both the tightness and location of the stricture. Peptic strictures tend to be in the distal third of the esophagus, close to the gastroesophageal junction. An upper gastrointestinal endoscopy with biopsy is important both to document the expected findings in peptic esophagitis and rule out other causes of esophagitis and stricture. This modality is also used to ascertain whether the patient has developed the histologic changes consistent with Barrett esophagus. The metaplastic change seen with Barrett esophagus increases the risk of adenocarcinoma of the esophagus and usually indicates the need for consideration of antireflux surgery. A prolonged intraesophageal pH probe is a very useful test to document chronic gastroesophageal reflux. However, acid may not reflux above a tight stricture, and the probe may not easily pass below the stricture. Esophageal manometry is the procedure of choice when trying to diagnose a primary motility disorder of the esophagus such as achalasia.

3. The answer is C (*II D 1*). The most important piece of information needed in any case of ingestion of caustic material is the presence and extent of mucosal burns to the upper gastrointestinal tract, particularly the esophagus. This information can be reliably obtained only by performing an upper gastrointestinal endoscopy. The absence of burns in the mouth or oropharynx should not exclude performing this examination, because patients can have esophageal mucosal burns without face, lip, or oropharyngeal pathology. The presence and degree of esophageal and gastric mucosal damage dictates management, including whether the patient is allowed to drink or eat, whether the patient needs parenteral nutrition, and whether treatment with corticosteroids or antibiotics should be considered. The decision as to whether a follow-up barium study is necessary to screen for the possibility of stricture formation can be made when the presence and degree of mucosal damage is determined. Vomiting should never be induced in patients who have ingested a caustic substance. Diluting or neutralizing the caustic substance with milk or water may be hazardous, and will delay endoscopy until the stomach is empty. A barium study is not an appropriate initial examination, but may be useful several weeks later to determine whether there is stricture formation. A chest radiograph is important if an esophageal perforation and mediastinitis are suspected.

4. The answer is D (*IX B*). Direct hyperbilirubinemia in an infant is a medical emergency and must be investigated without delay because of the possibility of an obstructive biliary tract lesion, such as biliary atresia or a choledochal cyst. If bile flow from the liver to the intestine is not re-established by 8 weeks of age, the damage may already be extensive and the liver may already be cirrhotic.

Infants with biliary atresia may have a rudimentary gallbladder not in continuity with the liver or intestine, and thus the presence of a gallbladder seen on the ultrasound does not rule out biliary atresia.

The nonexcreting biliary imaging scan does not automatically establish the diagnosis of biliary atresia, because severe intrahepatic cholestatic lesions (e.g., Alagille syndrome) and α_1-antitrypsin deficiency may occasionally result in the absence of biliary excretion of the radionuclide. A liver biopsy should distinguish between intrahepatic and extrahepatic cholestasis by either the paucity or proliferation of bile duct elements and other findings. If the biopsy shows bile duct proliferation, which suggests the presence of an obstructive lesion such as biliary atresia, an immediate exploration, intraoperative cholangiogram, and a procedure to re-establish biliary continuity with the bowel should be performed.

Breast milk jaundice causes indirect hyperbilirubinemia. Hepatitis B is rarely evident in an infant this young and would not cause acholic stools. Because there is a medical emergency in this patient, waiting for the results of the α_1-antitrypsin test cannot delay the investigation of the possibility of biliary atresia. Since the urine is negative for reducing sugars while the infant is consuming lactose-containing human milk, the possibility of galactosemia is highly unlikely.

5. The answer is A (*IX C 4*). With multiple sexual partners, many of whom may be in a high-risk group for hepatitis B, and recent sexual exposure to someone who has acute hepatitis B, there is a high likelihood that this patient has acquired hepatitis B. Postexposure prophylaxis with HBIG and hepatitis B vaccine has proved effective at modifying the infection and preventing the development of the chronic carrier state. Accelerated induction of protective antibody levels may be facilitated by an accelerated vaccine schedule. There is no decrease in the acquisition of effective immunity by giving HBIG and the first dose of vaccine simultaneously. There is no danger in giving the vaccine to a person who is already HBsAg positive. Giving HBIG alone may ameliorate the infection but may not prevent the development of chronic hepatitis B. This adolescent is in a high-risk group and needs to receive the hepatitis B vaccine regardless of whether he has already been exposed, so there is no rationale for waiting to get the results of testing before starting the vaccine series. Likewise, the sooner HBIG is given after exposure, the more effective it is, and so there is no valid reason to wait.

6. The answer is C (*III B*). Infection with *H. pylori* is usually asymptomatic, but may cause peptic ulcer disease in some individuals. Micronodules secondary to lymphoid hyperplasia can be seen on upper endoscopy, especially in the antrum, and biopsies confirm inflammation and the presence of *H. pylori*. *H. pylori* produce urease, which breaks down urea, releases ammonium and bicarbonate, and buffers the bacterial microenvironment. Antral gastritis in infants may be associated with eosinophilic infiltration in the setting of eosinophilic gastroenteritis. Mucosal granuloma may be seen in gastroduodenal Crohn disease. Vasculitis is associated with disorders such as Henoch-Schönlein purpura. G-cell hyperplasia (gastrin-producing cells) is a rare finding in children with refractory peptic inflammation who have increased gastric acid secretion.

7–10. The answers are 7-D, 8-B, 9-A, and 10-E (*IV A, Table 11-2*). The differential diagnosis of lower gastrointestinal bleeding in children depends on the child's age, the color and amount of blood, the presence or absence of diarrhea, and the presence or absence of abdominal and rectal pain or signs of peritonitis and a surgical abdomen. Certain disease entities that have a presentation of lower gastrointestinal bleeding are almost always confined to particular age groups. Allergic proctocolitis is usually a manifestation of cow's milk or soy protein allergy seen in infants younger than 6 months of age. Ulcerative colitis rarely affects children younger than 3 years of age. Juvenile polyps usually occur between 2 and 12 years of age, whereas the bleeding associated with Meckel diverticulum is usually first manifest when the patient is younger than 2 years of age.

The color and amount of blood are also characteristic of several of these lesions. Both allergic proctocolitis and juvenile polyps give rise to streaks of bright red blood. Most juvenile polyps are solitary and found in the rectosigmoid, and thus the blood seen is still red. In contrast, bleeding from a Meckel diverticulum located in the terminal ileum is usually painless, copious, and maroon or melanotic (purple clots). The presence or absence of diarrhea in the history of a child who has lower gastrointestinal bleeding is extremely important. Both ulcerative colitis and hemolytic-uremic syndrome involve abdominal cramps; tenesmus; and bloody, mucus-filled diarrhea. The bleeding from juvenile polyps is usually seen in the presence of otherwise normal stools.

Whether the child is sick or has signs of peritonitis or bowel obstruction is also a key element in evaluating the patient who has lower gastrointestinal bleeding. Children who have intussusception or volvulus, both of which can be accompanied by the passage of blood via the rectum, usually appear ill and have physical signs such as vomiting, abdominal distention, high-pitched or decreased bowel sounds, or even peritoneal signs. Patients who have ulcerative colitis and hemolytic-uremic syndrome often appear pale and ill, and have diffuse abdominal tenderness. In contrast, patients who have eosinophilic colitis and juvenile polyps almost always look well and have no significant physical signs.

The 6-year-old child has a juvenile polyp. Hemorrhoids are very unusual in children. Anal fissures are common but are often associated with anorectal pain and constipation. The 3-year-old child with bloody diarrhea could have ulcerative colitis, but he is young and has a low platelet count. Because platelets are acute-phase reactants, they are often elevated or at least normal in ulcerative colitis, and rarely are they decreased. In contrast, a low platelet count is an early sign of the intravascular coagulation and hemolysis that accompanies hemolytic-uremic syndrome. The 6-week-old child has allergic proctocolitis. The other common cause of this presentation in a young infant is anal fissures. The 18-month-old with maroon stool, anemia, and shock has a Meckel diverticulum until proved otherwise. Other rare possibilities for this presentation include colonic arteriovenous malformation, isolated ileal ulcer, or duodenal ulcer.

chapter **12**

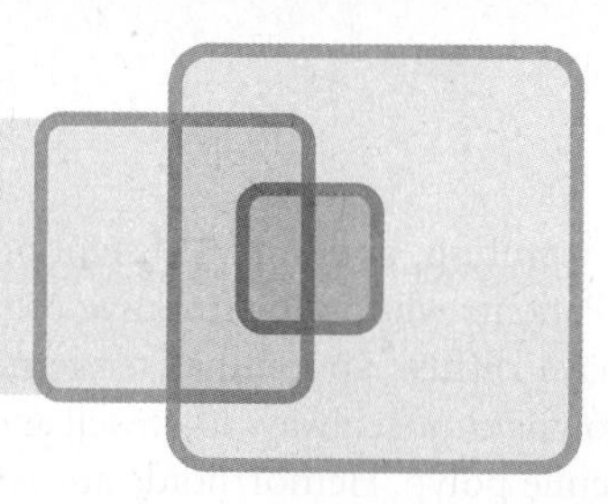

Cardiovascular Diseases

LEON CHAMEIDES • DANIEL J. DIANA • HARRIS B. LEOPOLD •
FELICE A. HELLER

I EVALUATION OF THE CARDIOVASCULAR SYSTEM

A History

1. **Cyanosis**
   a. Peripheral cyanosis (i.e., bluish discoloration **around** the mouth, eyelids, hands, and feet—but not of the mucous membranes) is common in normal newborns and is not abnormal (see Chapter 6).
   b. Cyanosis of the mucous membranes, also called central cyanosis, is diagnostic of a right-to-left shunt; it may be present at rest or only with exertion, such as crying.
2. **Shortness of breath.** A history of shortness of breath, exercise intolerance (manifested in infants as feeding difficulty), dyspnea, or syncope with exertion may be due to abnormal cardiac function.
3. **Familial disorders.** Some cardiovascular disorders (e.g., hyperlipidemia, hypertension), as well as some congenital heart abnormalities (e.g., atrial septal defect, aortic valve disease), may be familial.
4. **Chest pain** is common in the pediatric age group, particularly in adolescents, but is **rarely of cardiac origin,** especially if it occurs at rest. Analysis of specific features (e.g., quality, distribution, relationship to level of activity) helps to distinguish anginal pain from pain due to more benign causes.

B Physical examination

1. **General observations**
   a. **Weight.** Subnormal weight gain may indicate the presence of cardiac disease.
   b. **Cyanosis** and **clubbing** of the fingers and toes are diagnostic of a right-to-left shunt. Cyanosis should be confirmed by pulse oximetry and arterial blood gas analysis and, when present in a newborn, should be considered an urgent problem. Hypoxemia of **pulmonary** origin can usually be improved with oxygen administration, whereas hypoxemia of **cardiac** origin does not respond to oxygen.
   c. Other signs pointing to a **syndrome** or **genetic disorder** (Table 12-1; see Chapter 8) that includes congenital heart disease as one of its components should be looked for in the general examination.
2. **Pulses.** The presence and quality of peripheral pulses should be noted. It is important to palpate brachial (or radial) arteries in both arms simultaneously in order to determine timing and volume. If pulse volume in both upper extremities seems to be of equal magnitude, then a brachial (or radial) and femoral artery should be palpated simultaneously to rule out coarctation of the aorta. The quality and timing of the femoral pulse should be noted; the pulse may appear delayed and weaker if the arteries are filled via collateral vessels.
3. **Blood pressure** should be measured over the brachial and popliteal arteries with a cuff that has a bladder approximately two-thirds the size of the extremity and that completely covers its circumference. The diastolic pressure is recorded at the disappearance of Korotkoff sounds. Pressure in the lower extremities should normally be the same or slightly higher than in the upper. Lower pressure in the legs than the arms suggests a coarctation of the aorta and a wide pulse

TABLE 12-1 Cardiovascular Manifestations and Genetic Defects of Selected Congenital Disorders

Disorder	CV Manifestations	Gene Defect Locus
Marfan syndrome	Mitral valve prolapse; aortic root dilatation and rupture	Fibrillin gene, 15q22
Williams syndrome	Supravalvular aortic stenosis; diffuse vascular stenoses	Elastin gene, 7q11.23
CATCH-22 syndromes (includes DiGeorge and velocardiofacial syndromes)	Conotruncal defects (interrupted aortic arch, truncus arteriosus, tetralogy of Fallot)	?, 22q11
Hypertrophic cardiomyopathy	Marked hypertrophy of interventricular septum; sudden death	β-myosin heavy chain, 14q11; α-tropomyosin, 15q2; troponin T, 1q3; myosin binding protein C, 11p1?, 7q1; SCN5A (Na channel), 3p21–24; HERG (K channel), 11p15.5?, 4q25–27
Long QT syndrome	Prolonged QT interval, torsade de pointes, sudden death	
Duchenne and Becker muscular dystrophy	Dilated cardiomyopathy	Dystrophin Xp21
Down syndrome	Endocardial cushion defect	Trisomy 21 or translocation
Turner syndrome	Coarctation of aorta	XO
Trisomy 18 syndrome	Ventricular septal defect	Trisomy 18

CV, cardiovascular.

pressure (low diastolic) may indicate a "run-off" lesion such as aortic insufficiency or a patent ductus arteriosus.

4. **Precordial palpation.** A thrill or "palpable murmur" defines an area of maximal turbulence. A diffuse impulse in the parasternal region (heave) may indicate right ventricular enlargement.

5. **Cardiac auscultation**
   a. **Heart sounds (Figure 12-1)**
      (1) The **first heart sound (S_1)** may be single or split.
      (2) The **second heart sound (S_2)** is split during inspiration; abnormally wide splitting occurs with right ventricular overload, right ventricular conduction delay, right bundle branch block, and prolonged right ventricular emptying (Table 12-2).
         (a) The **pulmonary component** of S_2 is accentuated in pulmonary hypertension.
         (b) The **aortic component** of S_2 is accentuated in systemic hypertension or if the aortic valve is close to the chest wall, as in transposition of the great arteries.
      (3) **A third heart sound (S_3)** is usually a normal finding in children but may represent a pathologic condition if it is associated with other abnormal findings.
      (4) **A fourth heart sound (S_4)** is always an abnormal finding in children.

TABLE 12-2 Abnormally Wide Splitting of the Second Heart Sound (S_2)

Mechanism	Diagnosis
Increased right ventricular pressure	Pulmonary valve stenosis
Increased right ventricular volume	Pulmonary valve regurgitation; atrial septal defect; anomalous pulmonary venous return; ventricular septal defect
Right ventricular conduction delay	Right bundle branch block
Premature left ventricular emptying	Mitral valve regurgitation; ventricular septal defect

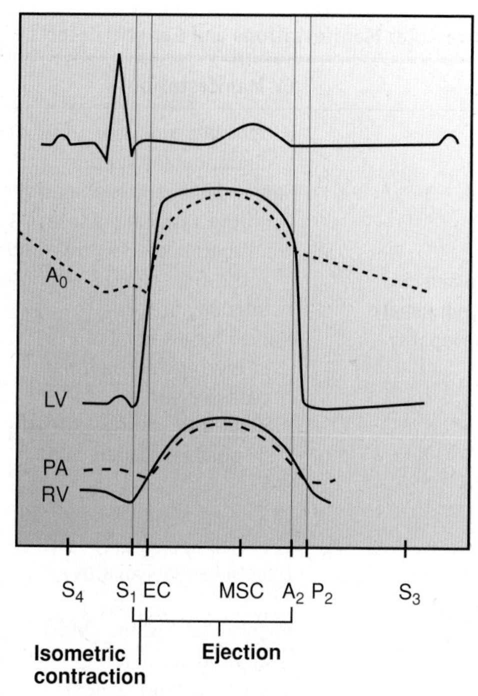

FIGURE 12-1 Relationship of the electrocardiogram, heart sounds, and pressures in the aorta (A_0), left ventricle (LV), pulmonary artery (PA), and right ventricle (RV). EC, ejection click; MSC, midsystolic click.

b. Clicks

(1) An **ejection click** occurs shortly after S_1; it originates from the opening of a stenotic but mobile semilunar valve or the sudden distention of an enlarged or hypertensive pulmonary artery.

(2) A **mid- or late systolic click** occurs when the ventricle reaches its peak pressure and originates from prolapse of the mitral or tricuspid valve.

c. Murmurs

(1) **Functional murmurs** (i.e., physiologic sounds of turbulence) are almost universally present at some time during childhood and are often age related (Table 12-3; see Chapter 1).

(2) **Pathologic murmurs** may occur during systole or diastole.

(a) **Systolic murmurs**

(i) Murmurs that begin during isovolumic contraction start with S_1 and are called regurgitant murmurs. They are caused by regurgitation through the atrioventricular (AV) valves or left-to-right flow through a ventricular septal defect. A regurgitant murmur may extend through all of systole (also called a pansystolic or holosystolic murmur) or may terminate before the end of systole.

TABLE 12-3 Functional Murmurs

Murmur	Approximate Age (Y)	Timing	Origin
PPS	Newborn	Systolic ejection	Division of pulmonary arteries
Vibratory (Still's)	3–8	Systolic ejection	Unknown
Carotid bruit	3–8	Systolic ejection	Carotid artery
Venous hum	3–8	Continuous	Jugular vein and superior vena cava
Pulmonary flow	6–18	Systolic ejection	Pulmonary valve

PPS, peripheral pulmonary artery stenosis.

(ii) Murmurs that begin immediately after isovolumic contraction are called ejection murmurs; they coincide with opening of the semilunar valves. Ejection murmurs may be caused by right or left ventricular outflow obstruction, but may also be functional.

(iii) Murmurs that begin late in systole are characteristic of mitral valve prolapse with mitral insufficiency.

(b) **Diastolic murmurs** beginning with S_2 are caused by semilunar (aortic or pulmonary) valve regurgitation; middiastolic murmurs are caused by increased flow across one of the AV valves or AV valve stenosis.

(c) **Continuous murmurs** start at the beginning of systole and continue into diastole.

C Laboratory evaluation

1. **Chest radiograph** permits evaluation of the location of the heart and abdominal organs; the size of the heart; and whether the pulmonary vasculature is normal, diminished, or increased.
2. The **electrocardiogram (ECG)** permits diagnosis of cardiac rhythm and the potential for abnormal rhythms (e.g., Wolff-Parkinson-White [WPW] syndrome, long QT syndrome), may reflect anatomic changes (e.g., ventricular or atrial hypertrophy), and may indicate the presence of myocardial ischemia.
3. The **echocardiogram** permits a systematic evaluation of cardiac structure and function. Direction and velocity of flow are visualized with pulse, continuous wave, and color flow mapping, thus permitting visualization of shunt direction and valve regurgitation. Doppler echocardiographic evaluation guided by color flow mapping permits fairly accurate estimation of pressure gradients across valves and defects.
4. **Cardiac catheterization** is an invasive procedure that provides much useful information and can be used therapeutically.

   a. **Pressure. Systolic pressure** in cardiac chambers and great vessels quantifies gradients across stenotic valves or vessels, whereas ventricular **end-diastolic pressure** is related to myocardial compliance. Pulmonary and systemic artery pressures are used to calculate pulmonary and systemic vascular resistances.

   b. **Oxygen** analysis in heart chambers and vessels permits detection and quantification of left-to-right and right-to-left shunts, measurement of cardiac output, and calculation of systemic and pulmonary vascular resistances.

   c. **Selective angiography** permits the visualization of cardiac and vascular anatomy.

   d. **Therapeutic catheter interventions** include balloon atrial septostomy, balloon angioplasty of stenotic valves and vessels, occlusion of communications such as shunts and collateral arteries, closure of atrial septal defects, and insertion of stents to maintain dilatation of stenotic vessels.

II FETAL AND NEONATAL CIRCULATION

Patency of three structures—the foramen ovale, ductus arteriosus, and ductus venosus—is a critical feature of the cardiovascular anatomy and physiology of the fetus.

A Normal physiology (see also Chapter 6)

1. **Fetal circulation** (see also Chapter 6)

   a. Fetal blood is oxygenated in the **placenta** and then enters the umbilical vein.

   (1) One portion of the oxygenated blood perfuses the liver and proceeds to the inferior vena cava via the hepatic veins.

   (2) Another portion enters the ductus venosus, which empties directly into the inferior vena cava.

   b. Together with venous return from the lower part of the body, this blood flows into the **right atrium.**

   (1) Approximately one third is shunted via the foramen ovale to the left atrium, left ventricle, and ascending aorta.

   (2) The remainder joins the venous return from the upper part of the body and enters the right ventricle and pulmonary artery. A small portion (< 10%) of this blood enters the

lungs; the remainder, because of high pulmonary vascular resistance and low systemic vascular resistance, crosses the ductus arteriosus to the descending aorta.

2. **Transition to neonatal circulation** (see also Chapter 6)
   a. At birth, the infant's first breaths cause an increase in arterial oxygen tension (PO_2); this lowers pulmonary vascular resistance, resulting in increased pulmonary blood flow. The increased pulmonary venous return to the left atrium causes the pressure to rise and results in **functional closure of the foramen ovale.**
   b. Systemic vascular resistance is increased by the elimination of the low-resistance vascular circuit of the placenta at birth.
   c. Closure of the ductus arteriosus occurs shortly after birth, first functionally as a result of a rise in PO_2 and a decline in circulating prostaglandin E, and then anatomically as a result of fibrosis.
   d. The neonatal circulation, with the ventricles working in series, is thus established.
3. **Normal changes in pulmonary vascular resistance.** Pulmonary vascular resistance drops dramatically within the first 24 hours and then continues to fall slowly, reaching normal adult levels by approximately 6 weeks; it is inversely related to the diameter of the small pulmonary arterioles.
   a. In the fetus, high pulmonary vascular resistance is maintained by constriction of the muscular tunica media of these arterioles.
   b. The arterioles dilate after birth as a result of a rise in PO_2 and synthesis of nitric oxide by the vascular endothelium. Further enlargement of these arterioles occurs as the muscular tunica media gradually atrophies. (In the average adult, cardiac output can increase fourfold without causing an increase in pulmonary artery pressure.)

B Abnormalities of the pulmonary circulation

1. **Persistent pulmonary hypertension of the newborn.** Pulmonary vascular resistance can remain high after birth if constriction of the arteriolar lumina by a pathologic process occurs (e.g., due to hypoxemia, acidosis, or some unidentified factor). The resultant pulmonary hypertension leads to right-to-left shunting at the ductus or foramen ovale.
2. **Other arteriolar abnormalities**
   a. **Anatomic changes.** If stimuli to pulmonary arteriolar constriction, such as pulmonary or venous hypertension, continue into infancy, the tunica media remains thickened instead of atrophying with age. Progressive pathologic changes may develop in a small number of infants and children, including cellular intimal proliferation, fibrosis of the intima and media, angioma formation, and arteriolitis.
   b. **Physiologic changes.** A rise in pulmonary vascular resistance causes diminution in left-to-right shunting (e.g., through a patent ductus or ventricular septal defect) and then, as pulmonary vascular resistance surpasses systemic resistance, a reversal of the shunt. Once fibrosis of the arterioles occurs, the process is irreversible. The combination of an irreversibly high pulmonary vascular resistance (culminating in pulmonary vascular obstructive disease) and a right-to-left shunt is known as **Eisenmenger reaction.**

III CONGENITAL STRUCTURAL ABNORMALITIES

A General considerations

1. **Etiology**
   a. The cause of congenital heart disease is usually unknown. Evidence points to a **multifactorial etiology.** A specific gene abnormality has been identified for several cardiac lesions (see Table 12-1). Several mutations may cause the same phenotype, whereas mutations in one gene can cause different phenotypes (e.g., severity of Marfan syndrome).
   b. Most congenital heart lesions are **sporadic.** However, their incidence is slightly higher in families that include one member who has such an abnormality. There are families with several affected members.
   c. Congenital heart disease is a **component of several syndromes** (see Table 12-1 and Chapter 8), such as Down syndrome and other trisomies.

d. Congenital heart disease has been associated with several **teratogenic factors:**

(1) **Medications** including thalidomide, folic acid antagonists, dextroamphetamine, anticonvulsants, estrogens, trimethadione, and retinoic acid

(2) **Excessive maternal alcohol ingestion**

(3) **Maternal infections,** such as antenatal **rubella** and possibly antenatal **cytomegalovirus** and **coxsackievirus** infections

(4) **Maternal diabetes** (not gestational) is associated with a higher incidence of congenital heart disease and is related to maternal HbA_{1C} levels at the time of organogenesis. **Maternal lupus** with the presence of anti-Ro antibodies can cause fetal congenital heart block.

2. Clinical considerations. Children with congenital heart abnormalities involving high- to low-pressure turbulent lesions such as ventricular septal defect, valve or subvalve stenosis, and valve insufficiency, may develop **subacute bacterial endocarditis** as a result of bacteremia such as may occur during dental procedures and should therefore practice excellent dental and gum hygiene. Those with turbulent lesions who are cyanotic, including patients with shunts and conduits, those with a prosthetic valve, and children who postoperatively have a residual turbulent shunt adjacent to prosthetic material, should also receive prophylactic antibiotics prior to dental procedures.

B Examples of left-to-right shunts

1. Atrial septal defect (ASD)

a. Description. ASD (Figure 12-2) can occur high in the septum, in the midportion, and low in the septum primum **(ostium primum defect**, also known as **partial endocardial cushion defect).** In ostium primum atrial septal defect, the **anterior leaflet** of the **mitral valve** is often **cleft** and **incompetent.**

b. Pathophysiology. Greater right than left ventricular compliance and low pulmonary vascular resistance result in a left-to-right shunt at the atrial level, thus increasing flow across the tricuspid and pulmonary valves. As a result, the right ventricle and the pulmonary artery are usually enlarged.

c. Clinical features. Most children are asymptomatic but symptoms can include slow weight gain and frequent lower respiratory tract infections.

d. Diagnosis

(1) **Physical examination.** The precordium is hyperdynamic and a right ventricular heave is present. A systolic ejection murmur in the pulmonic area and a middiastolic rumble in the lower right sternal area reflect the increased flow across the pulmonary and tricuspid valves. S_2 is widely and constantly split during inspiration and expiration. Occasionally, the physical examination may be completely normal.

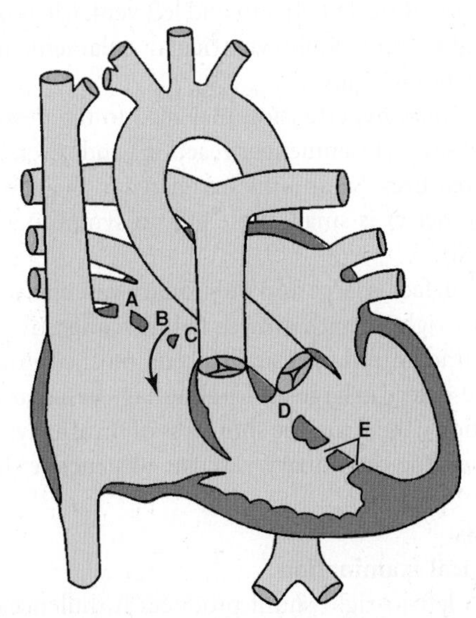

FIGURE 12-2 Anatomy of atrial and ventricular septal defects. *A* and *B*, high and midsecundum defects; *C*, ostium primum atrial defect; *D*, membranous ventricular defect; *E*, muscular ventricular defect.

(2) **Laboratory evaluation**

(a) **Chest radiograph.** The heart and main pulmonary artery segment are enlarged; pulmonary vascularity is increased.

(b) **ECG.** Right-axis deviation is often seen in secundum defects; the hallmark of a primum defect is an extreme left-axis deviation. Right ventricular enlargement is represented by an rsR′ in the right precordial leads. First-degree block may be present in primum and secundum atrial defects.

(c) **Echocardiogram.** The right ventricle is enlarged, and the septum often moves in a paradoxical fashion in diastole. The defect can usually be visualized, and the anatomy of the mitral valve can be assessed on a two-dimensional study. Color flow mapping demonstrates the direction of flow and competence of the mitral valve.

(d) **Cardiac catheterization** is not necessary for diagnosis. The presence and size of a left-to-right shunt are indicated by an increase in oxygen saturation at the atrial level. Pressure in the pulmonary artery is normal or slightly elevated, and a small pressure gradient may be present across the pulmonary valve. Severe pulmonary hypertension is rare in children. Mitral regurgitation is often found in ostium primum defects.

e. **Therapy**

(1) **Medical management.** Selected secundum atrial defects can be closed with a device in the catheterization laboratory.

(2) **Surgical closure** of all types of atrial septal defects can be accomplished with minimal risk.

2. **Ventricular septal defect (VSD)**

a. **Description** (see Figure 12-2). VSD (persistent patency of the interventricular septum) is the most commonly diagnosed congenital heart abnormality, accounting for 26% of all congenital cardiac lesions. A VSD may be single or multiple and may be found anywhere along the septum; it is most common in the membranomuscular portion. Inflow VSDs, also called **endocardial cushion defects,** often have associated abnormalities of the tricuspid and mitral valves and are most commonly present in children with Down syndrome.

b. **Pathophysiology**

(1) In small defects, the size of the shunt is determined by resistance at the defect; small defects result in small shunts. If the defect is large, both the size and direction of the shunt are dependent on the relative resistances in the pulmonary and systemic circuits.

(2) As long as pulmonary vascular resistance is lower than systemic vascular resistance, the shunt is left to right. If pulmonary vascular resistance rises above systemic vascular resistance, the shunt reverses.

(3) Large defects tend to result in pulmonary hypertension, whereas in small defects pulmonary vascular dynamics remain normal.

(4) The size of the left atrium and left ventricle is directly proportional to the size of the left-to-right shunt. Right ventricular enlargement occurs only when pulmonary vascular resistance increases.

(5) Pulmonary hypertension may lead to the development of pulmonary vascular obstructive disease (Eisenmenger reaction) and reversal of the shunt (right to left).

c. **Clinical features.** Symptoms are related to the size of the shunt.

(1) If the defect is small, there are no symptoms. Many of the small defects close spontaneously.

(2) If the defect is large and pulmonary vascular resistance is not significantly elevated (large left-to-right shunt), growth failure, congestive heart failure, and repeated lower respiratory tract infections usually occur, most commonly beginning at 1 to 2 months of age.

(3) If the defect is large and pulmonary vascular resistance is very high (i.e., Eisenmenger reaction), there may be shortness of breath, dyspnea on exertion, chest pain, and cyanosis. Irreversible pulmonary vascular obstructive disease is uncommon in children younger than 2 years of age.

d. **Diagnosis**

(1) **Physical examination**

(a) A left-to-right shunt produces turbulence during isovolumic contraction; the murmur therefore begins with S_1 and ends in midsystole in small defects, and extends to S_2 in large left-to-right shunts. The murmur is harsh and is best heard at the midsternal or lower left sternal border. In large left-to-right shunts, a middiastolic rumble resulting from increased flow across the mitral valve (relative mitral stenosis) is also heard, and tachypnea may be present.

(b) As pulmonary vascular resistance increases, and the left-to-right shunt decreases, the middiastolic murmur disappears, the systolic murmur becomes shorter, and the pulmonary component of S_2 increases in intensity.

(c) In the presence of pulmonary vascular obstructive disease, a right ventricular heave, ejection click, short systolic ejection murmur, diastolic murmur of pulmonary valve insufficiency, and loud S_2 are heard.

(2) **Laboratory evaluation**

(a) **Chest radiography.** In small defects, the chest radiograph may be normal or show mild cardiomegaly and a slight increase in pulmonary vascularity. In large left-to-right shunts, cardiomegaly, increased pulmonary vascularity, and enlargement of the left atrium and left ventricle are seen. As a rule, the size of the heart is directly proportional to the magnitude of the left-to-right shunt. As pulmonary vascular resistance rises and the left-to-right shunt decreases, the heart and distal pulmonary arteries become smaller, but the proximal pulmonary arteries enlarge.

(b) **ECG.** In small defects, the ECG findings are normal. In large left-to-right shunts, left atrial, left ventricular, or biventricular hypertrophy is seen. Right ventricular hypertrophy predominates when pulmonary vascular resistance is high. An extreme left-axis deviation is characteristic of VSDs in the endocardial cushion region.

(c) **Echocardiogram.** Chamber size can be determined and moderate to large defects can be identified with a two-dimensional study. Color flow mapping can localize defects that are too small for two-dimensional resolution. Continuous-wave Doppler allows estimation of right ventricular and pulmonary artery pressures.

(d) **Cardiac catheterization.** Measurement of oxygen content in the cardiac chambers and the great vessels makes it possible to calculate the magnitude and direction of the intracardiac shunt. Pulmonary arterial pressure can be measured, and pulmonary and systemic vascular resistances can be calculated. Left ventricular angiography defines the interventricular septum and can show the size as well as the number of defects.

e. **Therapy**

(1) **Medical management.** Congestive heart failure is treated with digoxin, diuretics, and afterload-reducing medications.

(2) **Surgical management.** A large VSD should be repaired in infancy. Small defects do not require surgical repair.

3. **Patent ductus arteriosus (PDA)**

a. **Description.** The ductus arteriosus connects the pulmonary artery and descending aorta in the fetus and normally closes shortly after birth. Patency of the ductus constitutes approximately 10% of congenital heart defects. It is especially common in very-low-birth-weight babies with pulmonary disease.

b. **Pathophysiology**

(1) The **direction of flow** through a large PDA depends on the relative resistances in the pulmonary and systemic circuits. As long as the former is lower than the latter, a left-to-right shunt is present. If pulmonary vascular resistance rises above systemic vascular resistance, a right-to-left shunt develops.

(2) The **size of the shunt** depends on the size of the PDA and the relative resistances in the pulmonary and systemic circuits. The left atrium and ventricle enlarge in direct proportion to the magnitude of the left-to-right shunt. If the PDA is large, pulmonary vascular obstructive disease (Eisenmenger reaction) can develop. The right ventricle enlarges with an increase in the pulmonary vascular resistance. If the PDA is small, its size limits the left-to-right shunt, and pulmonary vascular disease does not develop.

c. **Clinical features.** Symptoms are related to the size of the defect and the direction of flow. A small PDA causes no symptoms. A large PDA with a large left-to-right shunt may result in congestive heart failure, slowed growth, and repeated lower respiratory tract infections. Even small left-to-right shunts may cause severe compromise in low-birth-weight infants with coexistent pulmonary disease. Reversal of flow as a result of high pulmonary vascular resistance causes cyanosis, shortness of breath, and dyspnea on exertion.

d. Diagnosis

(1) Physical examination

(a) Pulse volume is related to the pulse pressure, which in turn is related to the volume of the left-to-right shunt. If the flow is small, pulses are normal. If the left-to-right shunt is large, diastolic runoff causes a wide pulse pressure, which translates clinically into bounding pulses.

(b) The murmur is continuous: It begins after S_1, peaks with S_2, and trails off in diastole. If pulmonary vascular resistance rises, first the diastolic murmur and subsequently the systolic murmur become softer and shorter, and S_2 increases in intensity.

(2) Laboratory evaluation

(a) Chest radiograph. Heart size, pulmonary vascularity, and left atrial and left ventricular size are all directly related to the magnitude of the left-to-right shunt. In a small PDA, the radiographic findings may be normal. If the PDA and left-to-right shunt are large, cardiomegaly and left heart enlargement are pronounced.

(b) ECG. The ECG findings are normal if the PDA is small. Left ventricular or biventricular hypertrophy is seen if the left-to-right shunt is large. Right ventricular hypertrophy predominates in the presence of increased pulmonary vascular resistance.

(c) Echocardiogram. The PDA can usually be visualized with color flow mapping, which also demonstrates the direction of flow. Doppler ultrasonography shows diastolic turbulence in the pulmonary artery and diastolic runoff in the aorta. If the shunt is large, the left atrium and ventricle are enlarged.

(d) Cardiac catheterization is not usually necessary for diagnosis. It will show a step-up in pulmonary arterial oxygen saturation and define pulmonary artery pressure. The ductus often can be traversed with the catheter, and angiography with selective injection in the descending aorta shows the ductal anatomy.

e. Therapy

(1) Medical management. Indomethacin is often effective in closing a PDA in the preterm newborn infant. Ductal closure may be achieved in the catheterization laboratory in selected patients with a variety of occlusive devices.

(2) Surgical management. Division or ligation of the ductus is curative.

C Examples of right-to-left shunts

1. Tetralogy of Fallot (Figure 12-3) is the most common cyanotic congenital cardiac abnormality, accounting for approximately 10% of all congenital cardiac lesions.

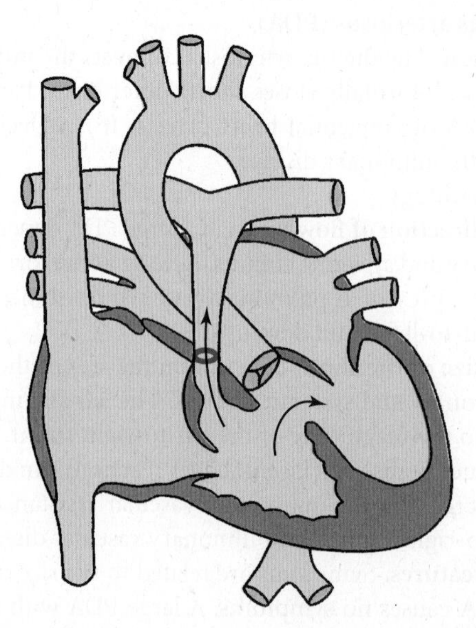

FIGURE 12-3 Anatomy of tetralogy of Fallot. The pulmonary annulus is hypoplastic, and the aorta straddles the ventricular septum. *Arrows* indicate the usual direction of flow.

a. Description

(1) The primary lesion appears to be underdevelopment of the infundibulum, which leads to:

(a) Variable degree of right ventricular outflow tract obstruction (pulmonary stenosis)

(b) Dextroposition of the aorta (override of the ventricular septum)

(c) VSD

(d) Right ventricular hypertrophy

(2) A **right aortic arch** is not uncommon, and a varying degree of hypoplasia of the pulmonary arteries is often present.

b. Pathophysiology. Of the four components of tetralogy of Fallot, only the VSD and the right ventricular outflow obstruction are physiologically important. This combination equalizes right and left ventricular pressures. The magnitude of the right-to-left shunt is directly related to the degree of right ventricular outflow obstruction.

c. Clinical features reflect the degree of hypoxemia, which is governed by the severity of right ventricular outflow obstruction. Signs include cyanosis, squatting posture, hyperpnea, and dyspnea on exertion. **Hypoxemic spells** consist of episodes of increasing irritability, hyperpnea, cyanosis, and syncope. These spells are often paroxysmal, may be fatal, and are not necessarily related to the severity of the obstruction.

d. Diagnosis

(1) **Physical examination**

(a) Cyanosis is variable and may be absent (acyanotic tetralogy).

(b) Digital clubbing and hyperpnea at rest are directly related to the degree of cyanosis.

(c) A right ventricular heave is present, S_2 is often single, and a harsh systolic ejection murmur is heard along the sternal border; its length and loudness are inversely proportional to the degree of outflow obstruction.

(2) **Laboratory evaluation**

(a) **Chest radiograph.** The heart size is normal. The apex is uptilted, and a concavity is noted in the pulmonary segment, which gives the heart the appearance of a boot. The pulmonary vascular markings are diminished according to the severity of outflow obstruction. The aortic arch is right-sided in approximately 25% of patients.

(b) **ECG** shows right-axis deviation and right ventricular hypertrophy.

(c) The two-dimensional **echocardiogram** is diagnostic. It demonstrates the location and size of the VSD, the outflow obstruction, the size of the pulmonary annulus, the size of the pulmonary arteries, and the degree of aortic override. Doppler ultrasonographic analysis makes estimation of the right ventricular outflow pressure gradient possible, and color flow mapping demonstrates the direction of flow through the VSD.

(d) **Cardiac catheterization** is useful in measuring the degree of desaturation and the pressures in the ventricles and aorta. Angiography is used to evaluate the pulmonary and coronary arteries, the ventricular septal defect, and the anatomy of the right ventricular outflow obstruction.

e. Therapy

(1) **Medical management**

(a) Bacterial endocarditis prophylaxis is necessary. Good oral hygiene must be maintained.

(b) Hypoxemic spells are acutely treated by placing the child in a knee-chest position to increase systemic vascular resistance and diminish right-to-left shunting. Morphine sulfate is given to depress the respiratory center, and oxygen is administered. α-Adrenergic agonists (e.g., phenylephrine) and β-adrenergic receptor blocking agents (e.g., propranolol) are also useful. Surgery is urgently recommended for children who experience a hypoxemic spell.

(2) **Surgical management**

(a) **Palliative surgery.** Pulmonary blood flow can be increased with a systemic artery-to-pulmonary artery shunt.

(b) **Corrective surgery** consists of closing the VSD and resecting the right ventricular outflow obstruction and, if necessary, enlarging the area with a patch.

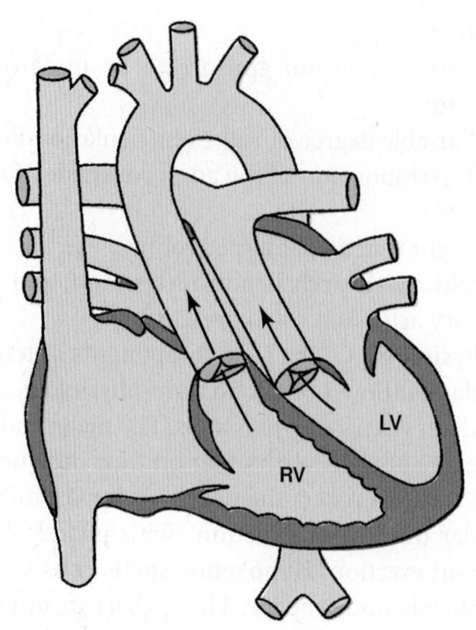

FIGURE 12-4 Anatomy of transposition of the great arteries. *Arrows* indicate the usual direction of flow. RV, right ventricle; LV, left ventricle.

2. **Transposition of the great arteries** (Figure 12-4)
   a. **Description.** This lesion, also known as **simple transposition,** accounts for 5% of congenital heart defects and is more common in boys than in girls. The aorta arises from the right ventricle anteriorly and to the right of the pulmonary artery, which arises posteriorly from the left ventricle. Associated abnormalities may include VSD, PDA, pulmonary stenosis, or a combination of these.
   b. **Pathophysiology.** Systemic venous (unoxygenated) blood is recirculated through the body, and pulmonary venous (oxygenated) blood is recirculated through the lungs. A lesion that allows mixing of the systemic and pulmonary circulations (e.g., ASD, VSD, PDA) is necessary for survival.
   c. **Clinical features.** Cyanosis is present from birth, the degree varying with the associated mixing lesion.
   d. **Diagnosis**
      (1) **Physical examination.** Intense cyanosis is noted in the absence of mixing lesions. In addition, a right ventricular heave and a single loud S_2 are usually found, and a soft flow murmur may be heard.
      (2) **Laboratory evaluation**
         (a) **Chest radiograph.** Pulmonary vascularity is increased or may be normal. Slight cardiomegaly and a narrow base produced by the anterior-posterior arrangement of the great arteries give the heart the shape of an egg on its side.
         (b) **Arterial blood gas analysis** shows severe hypoxemia (PO_2 is often in the low 20s); increasing the ambient FIO_2 to 100% does not significantly alter the arterial PO_2.
         (c) **ECG** findings are normal in the newborn.
         (d) **Echocardiogram** shows the anterior-posterior arrangement of the great arteries and the chamber from which they originate, the normal anatomy of the ventricles, and the presence of associated abnormalities. Color flow mapping shows the direction of flow through associated abnormalities.
         (e) **Cardiac catheterization.** Right ventricular pressure is systemic. Left ventricular pressure may be systemic in the newborn but decreases with a decline in pulmonary vascular resistance. Angiography confirms the anatomy and indicates the direction of blood flow. Balloon atrial septostomy (Rashkind procedure) allows creation of an ASD, through which the mixing of oxygenated and deoxygenated blood can occur.
   e. **Therapy**
      (1) **Medical management.** Creation of an ASD by balloon atrial septostomy is life saving in the absence of a PDA or VSD. Prostaglandin E_1 is also used to maintain patency of the ductus arteriosus while awaiting surgical repair.

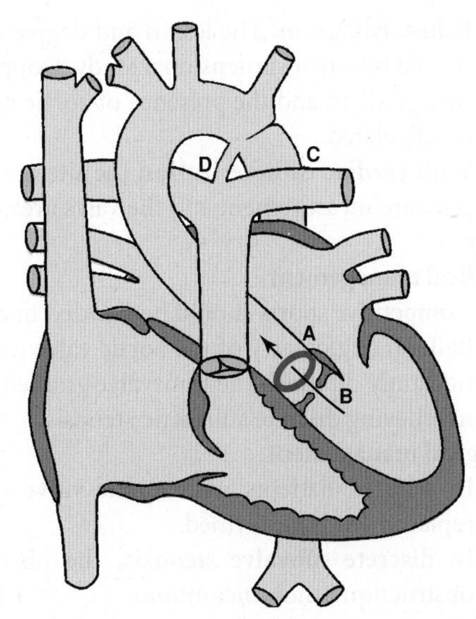

FIGURE 12-5 Anatomy of coarctation of the aorta, aortic valve stenosis, and discrete subvalve stenosis. The ductus arteriosus is patent. *A,* aortic valve stenosis; *B,* discrete subaortic stenosis; *C,* coarctation of the aorta; *D,* patent ductus arteriosus.

(2) **Surgical management.** An **arterial switch procedure** with **coronary artery reimplantation** is best performed in the first 2 weeks of life and involves moving the arteries, but not the valves, into their "normal" position. Two atrial switch procedures, the **Senning** and **Mustard,** have been used in the past.

D Examples of left-sided obstructions

1. **Aortic valve and discrete subaortic stenosis** (Figure 12-5)
   a. **Description**
      (1) In **aortic valve stenosis,** the valve tissue is thickened and often bicuspid, with fused commissures and an eccentric orifice.
      (2) In **discrete subaortic stenosis,** a membranous diaphragm or fibrous ring encircles the left ventricular outflow tract just beneath the base of the aortic valve.
   b. **Pathophysiology.** Left ventricular outflow obstruction causes a rise in the systolic pressure in the left ventricle that is proportional to the degree of obstruction. The resulting left ventricular hypertrophy and the high intracavitary pressure may lead to inadequate coronary filling and result in a mismatch between myocardial supply and demand. Left ventricular end-diastolic pressure rises if left ventricular function is impaired or if hypertrophy is severe enough to reduce myocardial compliance.
   c. **Clinical features.** Symptoms are often absent but may include fatigability and exertional dyspnea due to lowered cardiac reserve and angina due to inadequate coronary blood flow to meet the needs of the hypertrophied left ventricle (mismatch between supply and demand). Syncope and sudden death may occur with exercise.
   d. **Diagnosis**
      (1) **Physical examination**
         (a) A harsh systolic ejection murmur is heard at the right base and, in aortic valve stenosis, is preceded by an ejection click that is heard best at the lower left sternal border.
         (b) A systolic thrill is often felt in the jugular notch, and a diastolic murmur of aortic regurgitation, heard best at the mid-left sternal border, may be heard in both valve and discrete subvalve stenosis.
      (2) **Laboratory evaluation**
         (a) **Chest radiograph.** Poststenotic dilatation of the ascending aorta is present in aortic valve, but not subvalve, stenosis.
         (b) The **ECG** may show left ventricular hypertrophy by voltage criteria and/or T-wave inversion, but correlation with the severity of the stenosis is lacking. Left ventricular ischemia, shown by ST-segment depression and T-wave inversion, is indicative of severe stenosis, but absence of left ventricular ischemia does not exclude severe stenosis.

(c) **Echocardiogram.** The lesion and degree of left ventricular hypertrophy are demonstrated by a two-dimensional study. Doppler ultrasonography can estimate the pressure gradient and the presence of aortic valve insufficiency. The aortic valve area can be calculated.

(d) With **cardiac catheterization** the site and degree of obstruction can be assessed by pressure measurement and the valve area can be calculated.

e. Therapy

(1) Medical management

(a) Competitive sports should be avoided in all but the mildest cases.

(b) Balloon angioplasty of the aortic valve can decrease the severity of stenosis and significantly diminish the transvalve gradient. Angioplasty has not been found effective in relieving discrete subaortic stenosis.

(2) Surgical management

(a) In selected patients with **aortic valve stenosis,** open valvotomy or aortic valve replacement is performed.

(b) In **discrete subvalve stenosis,** the obstructive tissue is resected. Recurrence of obstruction is not uncommon.

2. Coarctation of the aorta (see Figure 12-5)

a. Description. Coarctation of the aorta accounts for 8% of congenital heart defects and is twice as common in boys as in girls. When it occurs in a girl, Turner syndrome must be considered (see Chapter 8). The obstruction is usually located in the descending aorta, just opposite the ligamentum arteriosum. This condition may coexist with tubular hypoplasia of the aortic arch. The aortic valve is bicuspid in more than 50% of patients. Mitral valve abnormalities (stenosis, regurgitation, or both) may also be present.

b. Pathophysiology. Coarctation represents a mechanical obstruction between the proximal and distal aorta. The proximal aortic pressure and left ventricular afterload are elevated, whereas the distal aortic pressure is low. Collateral vessels, usually involving the internal mammary and intercostal arteries, develop in response to the pressure differential.

c. Clinical features. Congestive heart failure develops in infancy in approximately 10% of patients. Most children are asymptomatic. Leg cramps, headaches, and chest pain may occur in older children.

d. Diagnosis

(1) Physical examination

(a) Signs typically seen in the older infant and child include weak, delayed, or absent femoral pulses compared to upper extremity pulses, upper extremity hypertension, and blood pressure differential between the arm and leg. These signs may not be present in the newborn when the aortic end of the duct is open.

(b) Flow across the coarctation or via collateral vessels may produce a systolic ejection murmur heard at the apex, left sternal border, and interscapular area. Collateral pulsations may be palpable around the scapula in older patients. If the aortic valve is bicuspid, an ejection click is heard.

(2) Laboratory evaluation

(a) **Chest radiograph.** Notching of the fourth through eighth ribs, caused by erosion from collateral vessels, may be seen in children older than 5 years of age.

(b) **ECG** findings may be normal or show left ventricular hypertrophy.

(c) **Echocardiogram.** The coarctation may be visualized, and a pressure can be estimated by Doppler ultrasonography. Left ventricular function and associated abnormalities can be evaluated.

(d) **Cardiac catheterization.** The aortic pressure gradient can be measured. Aortography allows visualization of the lesion and evaluation of the collateral vessels.

e. Therapy

(1) Medical management

(a) Treatment of hypertension may be necessary.

(b) Balloon angioplasty of native coarctation is still controversial, but it is the procedure of choice for the treatment of restenosis of the coarctation after its surgical correction. A stent may be needed to maintain the dilatation.

(2) **Surgical management.** Surgical repair is accomplished in one of several ways: Resection with end-to-end anastomosis, patch repair, or graft interposition.

E Example of right-sided obstruction

1. **Pulmonary valve stenosis**
   a. **Description.** Pulmonary valve stenosis accounts for 5% to 8% of congenital heart defects. The pulmonary commissures are fused, the valve is domed, and there is poststenotic dilatation of the main pulmonary artery. The pulmonary valve is occasionally bicuspid and is dysplastic in 10% of patients.
   b. **Pathophysiology.** To maintain cardiac output, right ventricular pressure rises. In severe stenosis, right ventricular end-diastolic pressure may also increase. A consequent increase in right atrial pressure may open the foramen ovale and cause a right-to-left shunt.
   c. **Clinical features.** Most patients are asymptomatic. Severe to critical pulmonary stenosis may cause exertional dyspnea, fatigability, and exertional chest pain. Congestive heart failure is unusual except in infants who have critical stenosis.
   d. **Diagnosis**
      (1) **Physical examination**
         (a) An ejection click, whose loudness varies with respiration, and a harsh systolic ejection murmur are present at the upper left sternal border.
         (b) In moderately severe stenosis, a thrill and right ventricular heave are palpable; the pulmonary component of S_2 is diminished; the ejection click merges with S_1; and the murmur becomes longer and louder.
         (c) If the stenosis is critical, cyanosis may become evident and an S_4 gallop may be heard.
      (2) **Laboratory evaluation**
         (a) **Chest radiograph.** Heart size and pulmonary vascularity are usually normal, but the pulmonary artery segment is prominent because of poststenotic dilatation. In critical stenosis, cardiomegaly and diminished pulmonary blood flow may be seen.
         (b) **ECG.** The degree of right-axis deviation and right ventricular hypertrophy highly correlates beyond the neonatal period with right ventricular pressure and, therefore, with severity of the stenosis.
         (c) **Echocardiogram.** Right ventricular hypertrophy, or dilatation, doming of the pulmonary valve, and poststenotic dilatation of the pulmonary artery can all be seen. The integrity of the interatrial septum can be assessed. Doppler ultrasonography can estimate the transvalve gradient.
         (d) **Cardiac catheterization.** Right ventricular function and the transvalve gradient can be accurately assessed. Severity of stenosis is defined by right ventricular pressure: In mild stenosis, right ventricular pressure is $< 50\%$ of systemic pressure; in moderate stenosis, it is 50% to 80% of systemic pressure; and in severe stenosis, it is $> 80\%$ of systemic pressure.
   e. **Therapy**
      (1) **Medical management.** Percutaneous balloon valvuloplasty of the pulmonary valve may be performed at the time of cardiac catheterization and is highly effective.
      (2) **Surgical management.** Surgical resection of the pulmonary valve is reserved for those patients in whom balloon angioplasty has failed, including patients who have dysplastic valves.

IV ACQUIRED STRUCTURAL ABNORMALITIES

A **Rheumatic heart disease** (see also Chapter 9) is a result of single or multiple episodes of acute rheumatic fever. **Mitral valve insufficiency** is the most common lesion, followed by **aortic valve insufficiency. Mitral valve stenosis** is less common and is usually the end result of multiple attacks of acute rheumatic fever. Least common is **aortic valve stenosis.** The tricuspid and pulmonary valves are virtually never affected. Symptoms are proportional to the degree of valve damage. Daily penicillin prophylaxis for patients who have had an episode of acute rheumatic fever is mandatory to prevent recurrent episodes of acute rheumatic fever and increased valve damage.

B **Kawasaki disease** (see also Chapter 9). Cardiac effects may include pericarditis, myocarditis, and transient rhythm disturbances. However, it is the development of **coronary artery aneurysms,** with their potential for occlusion or rupture, that makes this disease potentially life threatening. Coronary artery aneurysms develop during the subacute phase (11th–25th day) of the disease in approximately 30% of patients but regress in most. Echocardiography is used to assess the presence of coronary artery aneurysms, ventricular function, and pericardial fluid. Early therapy with γ-globulin decreases the incidence of coronary artery aneurysms to $< 5\%$. Low-dose salicylate therapy lessens the likelihood of aneurysm occlusion.

C **Endocarditis** (see also Chapter 10) usually occurs on the low-pressure side of a turbulence-producing lesion (e.g., VSD, semilunar valve stenosis, AV valve regurgitation, semilunar valve regurgitation) and artificial valve. This condition does not usually occur with abnormalities lacking turbulence (e.g., ASD). Good dental hygiene and preventive dental care is especially important for children with congenital heart disease. Antibiotic prophylaxis prior to dental procedures is used in situations where the risk of developing endocarditis is greater than the risk of taking antibiotics. These include children with turbulent lesions and cyanosis, children with prosthetic valves, and during the first 6 months following surgical repair if a residual turbulent lesion remains adjacent to foreign material such as a patch.

D **Coronary artery disease** is rare in childhood, but the atherosclerotic process begins early in life. There is evidence that progression of atherosclerosis is adversely influenced by genetic factors (e.g., coronary artery disease or familial hypercholesterolemia; see Chapter 17) and lifestyle (e.g., cigarette smoking; high-cholesterol, high-saturated-fat diet, sedentary lifestyle, and hypertension). Because many lifetime habits are formed during childhood, an opportunity exists to influence young people to adopt healthful habits. Children with high cholesterol levels need a change in lifestyle and may need cholesterol-lowering medications.

V DISORDERS OF CARDIAC FUNCTION

A **Myocarditis** (inflammation of the myocardium) is most commonly of **infectious** etiology (see also Chapter 10). **Noninfectious** inflammatory lesions are primarily associated with collagen vascular diseases. Some patients may be asymptomatic, and the diagnosis is made only by observing changes in the ST-segment and T-wave on serial ECGs. Other patients may manifest signs of congestive heart failure, low cardiac output, or rhythm disturbances. Myocardial inflammation can be fatal or progress to congestive cardiomyopathy and chronic congestive heart failure. Myocardial biopsy can help establish an etiology and guide initial therapy. Cardiac transplantation may be necessary for patients who have chronic and unremitting myocardial failure resistant to medical therapy.

B **Cardiomyopathies** are a group of idiopathic myocardial disorders that affect function of the heart. Possible causes such as abnormalities of coronary arteries must be ruled out. Cardiomyopathies have been classified into several types:

1. **Congestive cardiomyopathy**
   a. **Description.** Congestive, or **dilated,** cardiomyopathy is characterized by myocardial dysfunction and ventricular dilatation. Although this condition is usually a primary disorder, it may be associated with neuromuscular disease (e.g., Duchenne muscular dystrophy) or result from drug toxicity (e.g., doxorubicin).
   b. **Pathophysiology.** Failure of the left ventricle causes an increase in end-diastolic volume, which results in increases in left atrial, pulmonary venous, and pulmonary capillary pressures. Mitral valve regurgitation may result from papillary muscle dysfunction or severe dilatation of the valve annulus.
   c. **Clinical features.** Initially, dyspnea on exertion is present. As left ventricular failure progresses, small increases in left ventricular volume occur, followed by a marked increase in pulmonary capillary pressure. This results in orthopnea, paroxysmal nocturnal dyspnea, and bronchospasm. Eventually, right heart failure—characterized by dependent edema—occurs.
   d. **Diagnosis**
      (1) **Physical examination** depends on the stage of the disease but may include tachypnea, tachycardia, a right ventricular heave, prominent second pulmonary sound, gallop

rhythm, and murmurs of mitral or tricuspid valve regurgitation. In advanced stages, blood pressure may be low and pulse pressure narrow; pulsus alternans may be present.

(2) **Laboratory evaluation**

(a) **Chest radiograph** may show cardiomegaly, an enlarged left atrium, pulmonary venous congestion, and pleural effusions.

(b) **ECG** defines rhythm disturbances. Left ventricular hypertrophy as well as nonspecific ST-segment and T-wave changes may be present.

(c) Left ventricular **function** can be assessed by **echocardiography, radionuclide studies,** and, if necessary, **cardiac catheterization.** Myocardial biopsy may be helpful in defining the pathologic process.

e. **Therapy** is directed at improving left ventricular function with inotropic agents and unloading the left ventricle with vasodilators. Preload is decreased with diuretics, and antiarrhythmic medications are used to control potentially fatal rhythm disturbances. In the event of clinical deterioration, cardiac transplantation may be needed.

2. **Hypertrophic cardiomyopathy**

a. **Description.** This disorder, also known as **idiopathic hypertrophic subaortic stenosis** and **hypertrophic obstructive cardiomyopathy,** is an autosomal dominant genetic disorder with a high degree of penetrance, but it can also be sporadic. The septum is usually thickened out of proportion to the left free ventricular wall, which may also be thickened.

b. **Pathophysiology.** In the thickened, stiff left ventricle, systolic function is well preserved, but diastolic function is compromised. Thickening of the septum may result in left ventricular outflow obstruction and abnormal motion of the mitral valve. This abnormal motion may result in mitral regurgitation.

c. **Clinical features.** Symptoms include dyspnea on exertion because of an inability to significantly increase cardiac output with exercise, chest pain due to myocardial ischemia, and syncope. Death may result from rhythm disturbances.

d. **Diagnosis**

(1) **Physical examination.** The pulse is often biferious (double peaked) because ejection is interrupted by septal obstruction. A forceful left ventricular impulse may be present, and an S_3 or S_4 may be audible at the apex. Murmurs of left ventricular outflow obstruction or mitral regurgitation may be heard. Decreasing left ventricular volume (Valsalva maneuver, standing) increases left ventricular outflow obstruction and with it, the intensity of the murmur.

(2) **Laboratory evaluation**

(a) **ECG** often shows left-axis deviation, left ventricular hypertrophy, deep Q waves, ST-segment depression, and T-wave inversion. Rhythm disturbances are best defined by Holter monitoring.

(b) **Echocardiogram** is diagnostic. It allows measurement of the septum and left ventricular free wall. In addition, the small diastolic left ventricular cavity size and the anterior motion of the mitral valve in systole can be seen. Doppler ultrasonography and color flow mapping allow evaluation of mitral valve regurgitation and estimation of the left ventricular outflow gradient.

e. **Therapy** is aimed at preventing fatal arrhythmias and decreasing the stiffness of the left ventricle with negative inotropic medications (calcium channel and β-adrenergic blockers). Avoidance of competitive sports is recommended because of the risk of sudden death with exertion.

VI RHYTHM ABNORMALITIES (SEE ALSO CHAPTER 7)

A **Premature beats** may originate from either the atrium or ventricle.

1. **Premature atrial beats** (Figure 12-6A) are characterized by an abnormally shaped P-wave that occurs prematurely, a normal QRS complex, and usually no compensatory pause. Premature atrial beats are common and usually benign.

2. **Premature ventricular beats** (Figure 12-6B) are characterized by a wide QRS complex, lack of a relationship between the P and QRS waves, an inverted T-wave, and a compensatory pause.

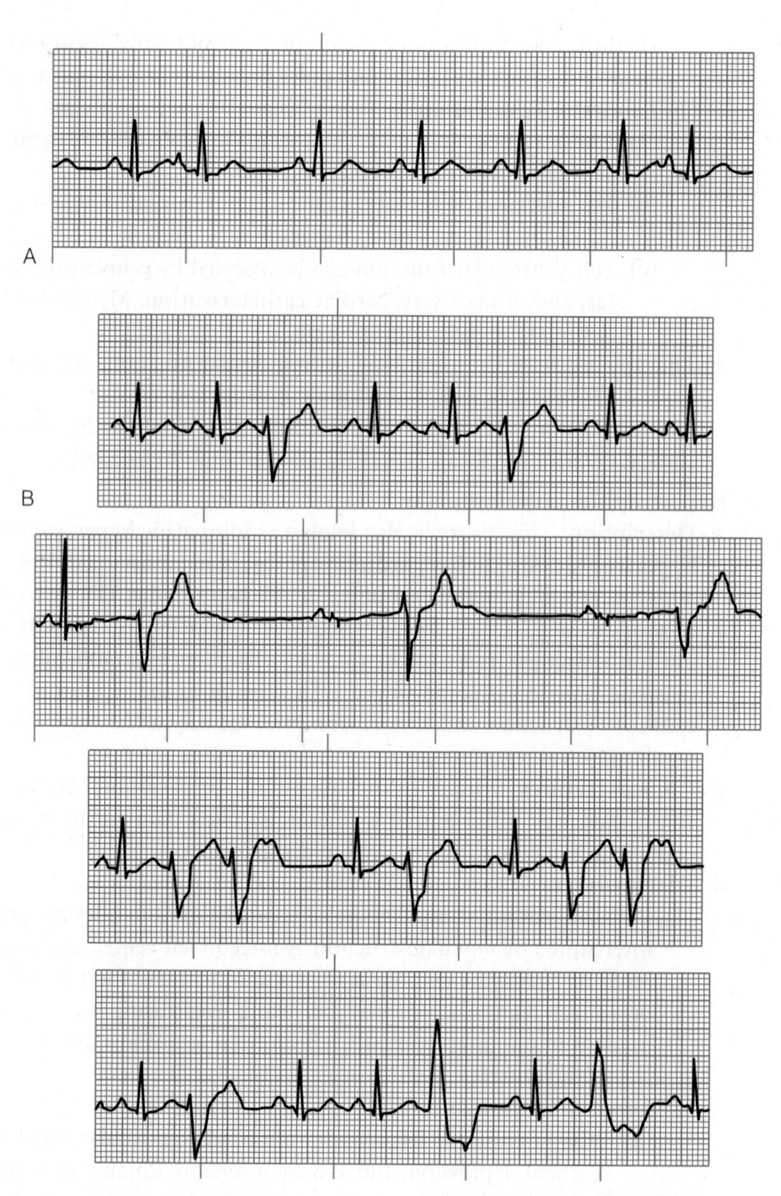

FIGURE 12-6 **A:** Premature atrial beats. In the second and seventh beats, the P waves and PR intervals are different from other beats. QRS waves are the same. **B:** Premature ventricular beats. The first strip shows two similar premature ventricular beats (uniform). In the second strip, each premature beat is coupled with a normal beat (bigeminy). The third strip shows two consecutive premature ventricular beats (couplets). The fourth strip shows three different premature ventricular beats (multiform).

Premature ventricular beats are usually benign, unless they are multiform, increase with exercise, or are associated with a prolonged QT interval or cardiomyopathy.

B **Supraventricular tachycardia (SVT)** (Figure 12-7A) is the most common symptomatic arrhythmia in the pediatric age group; it is usually caused by a re-entrant mechanism, is often paroxysmal, and may occur at any age—including the fetus and newborn. A bypass tract (concealed or evident on the ECG) is sometimes one path of the re-entry circuit. The ECG manifestation of the most common bypass tract is the **Wolff-Parkinson-White syndrome,** which consists of a short PR interval and a wide QRS complex with a slurred upstroke (delta wave) (Figure 12-7B).

1. During a paroxysm of SVT, the R-R interval is uniform; the heart rate is usually approximately 160 beats per minute (bpm) in adolescents, and it may be as high as 300 bpm in infants (Figure 12-7A). Hemodynamic consequences depend on the heart rate, age of the child, and presence of underlying heart disease. Symptoms of low cardiac output may develop in infants who have very rapid heart rates, especially if they also have heart disease.

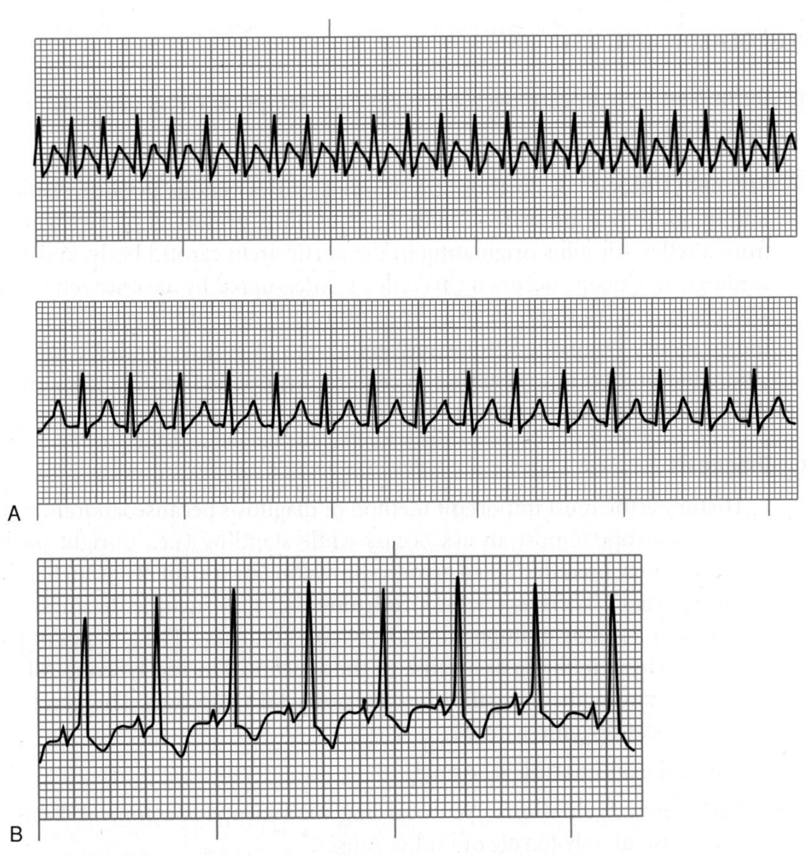

FIGURE 12-7 **A:** Supraventricular tachycardia in an infant (*top*) at a rate of 240 beats per minute (bpm) and in an adolescent (*bottom*) at a rate of 160 bpm. **B:** Wolff-Parkinson-White conduction disturbance.

2. **Therapy** includes vagal maneuvers and intravenous administration of adenosine, digoxin, or β-blocking agents. Infants in imminent danger of cardiovascular collapse should be treated with synchronized electric cardioversion. If the paroxysms of tachyarrhythmia are difficult to control, radiofrequency ablation eliminates the re-entry circuit.

C **In complete heart block** (Figure 12-8), there is loss of conduction from atria to ventricles. The ensuing idioventricular rhythm is slower than normal. Congenital heart block may be caused by maternal Ro antibodies in mothers who have collagen vascular diseases such as systemic lupus erythematosus (SLE). These antibodies cross the placenta early in pregnancy and produce fibrosis of the conduction system. The pathophysiology and clinical symptoms are related to the level of the block. The lower the block is, the slower the heart rate, and the greater the symptoms of inadequate cardiac output. In symptomatic patients, therapy involves pacemaker implantation.

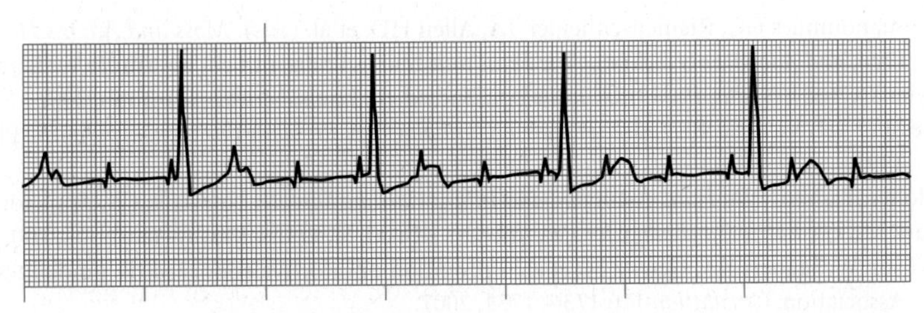

FIGURE 12-8 Congenital complete heart block. The atrial rate is 140 beats per minute (bpm), and the ventricular rate is 45 bpm.

VII NEUROCARDIOGENIC SYNCOPE

A Definition Neurocardiogenic syncope is a temporary loss of consciousness caused by cerebral hypoperfusion.

B Pathophysiology An orthostatic stimulus causes venous pooling resulting in decreased cardiac output and blood pressure. Cerebral perfusion is preserved by tachycardia and vasoconstriction from a reflex stimulus originating in the aortic arch, carotid body, and cardiac chambers. Neurocardiogenic syncope occurs if this reflex is interrupted by another reflex that originates in the cardiac chambers as a response to a hypercontractile state of the ventricles. The sudden withdrawal of the excitatory sympathetic tone and an increase in parasympathetic tone cause peripheral vasodilation and bradycardia, resulting in cerebral hypoperfusion. The abnormal reflex is relaxed when the patient becomes horizontal.

C Diagnosis

1. **History** is the most important method of diagnosis because laboratory findings are usually negative. Syncope almost always occurs while standing (i.e., upright **posture**) and is sometimes immediately preceded by an anxiety-provoking or fearful event such as blood drawing (**precipitating** event). There is often a **prodrome** that may include dizziness, light-headedness, loss of vision, or a feeling of impending loss of consciousness. The absence of **palpitations** helps to rule out a tachyarrhythmia as a cause of the syncope. During syncope, which is self-limited and of short duration, there is **pallor** but few **postictal** symptoms. This can be remembered as the **6 Ps** of neurocardiogenic syncope.
2. **Physical examination is** normal.
3. **Laboratory evaluations.** Neurocardiogenic syncope is a clinical diagnosis. Laboratory evaluation is useful only to rule out other causes.
   a. **ECG** is characteristically normal. It is helpful in ruling out the prolonged QT interval syndrome and pre-excitation, and may be helpful in the diagnosis of hypertrophic cardiomyopathy.
   b. **Chest radiographic** findings are normal.
   c. **Echocardiogram** is normal, but is helpful in ruling out other diagnoses, especially hypertrophic cardiomyopathy.
   d. The usefulness of reproducing the syncope with **head-up tilt table testing** is controversial because of the many false-positive and false-negative results and the lack of reproducibility. Some clinicians consider the test useful in confusing circumstances.

D Therapy

1. Avoiding hypovolemia is often sufficient to prevent syncope. If the prodrome is long enough, sitting or lying down may abort the reflex.
2. Fluorohydrocortisone—a safe, mild salt- and water-retaining hormone—is useful to help prevent hypovolemia.
3. Metoprolol has been found to be clinically safe and effective. Its exact mechanism of action is unknown, but it is theorized that this agent blunts the hypercontractile state or blocks sensitization of the C fibers to catecholamines.

BIBLIOGRAPHY

Emmanouilides GC, Riemenschneider TA, Allen HD, et al. (eds): *Moss and Adams Heart Disease in Infants, Children, and Adolescents including the Fetus and Young Adults,* 6th ed. Baltimore, Williams & Wilkins, 2000.

Fyler DC (ed): *Nadas' Pediatric Cardiology,* 2nd ed. St. Louis, Mosby-Yearbook, 2002.

Gessner IH, Victoria BE (eds): *Pediatric Cardiology: A Problem Oriented Approach.* Philadelphia, WB Saunders, 1993.

Moller JH, Neal WA: *Fetal, Neonatal, and Infant Cardiac Disease.* Norwalk, CT, Appleton & Lange, 1990.

Park MK: *Pediatric Cardiology for Practitioners,* 4th ed. St. Louis, Mosby-Yearbook, 2002.

Wilson W, Taubert KA, Gewitz M, et al.: Prevention of infective endocarditis: guidelines from the American Heart Association. *Circulation* 116:1736–1754, 2007.

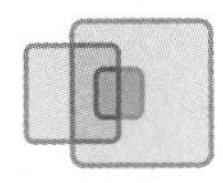

Study Questions

Directions: *Each of the numbered items or incomplete statements in this section is followed by answers or completions of the statement. Select the ONE lettered answer or completion that is BEST in each case.*

1. A 2-year-old, active, asymptomatic boy is examined by a physician for the first time. His blood pressure is 130/86 in the right arm and 95/60 in the right leg with a barely palpable right femoral pulse. An ejection click is heard at the upper left sternal border followed by a grade 2/6 systolic ejection murmur. Which of the following is the most likely diagnosis?

- A Isolated aortic valve stenosis
- B Coarctation of the aorta with a bicuspid aortic valve
- C Pulmonary valve stenosis
- D Ventricular septal defect
- E Isolated coarctation of the aorta

2. A 3-month-old infant has mild cyanosis with crying. She has a grade 3 long harsh systolic ejection murmur at the mid-left sternal border. The second heart sound is single. Which of the following is the most likely diagnosis?

- A Transposition of the great arteries
- B Atrial septal defect
- C Tetralogy of Fallot
- D Ventricular septal defect with high pulmonary vascular resistance (Eisenmenger)
- E Patent ductus arteriosus with high pulmonary vascular resistance

Directions: *Each set of matching questions in this section consists of a list of 4 to 6 lettered options followed by several numbered items. For each numbered item, select the ONE lettered option that is most closely associated with it. Each lettered option may be selected once, more than once, or not at all.*

QUESTIONS 3–6

For each patient described below, select the most likely diagnosis.

- A Ventricular septal defect
- B Aortic valve stenosis
- C Patent ductus arteriosus
- D Atrial septal defect
- E Transposition of the great arteries

3. A 2-year-old asymptomatic child has a systolic ejection murmur at the upper left sternal border and a middiastolic rumble at the lower left sternal border

4. An asymptomatic 14-year-old girl has a systolic ejection click at the midsternal border and a systolic ejection murmur at the upper right sternal border

5. A 3-month-old baby has signs of congestive heart failure and a pansystolic murmur at the mid-left sternal border and a middiastolic murmur at the apex

6. An asymptomatic 3-year-old has a pansystolic murmur that spills into diastole at the upper left sternal border

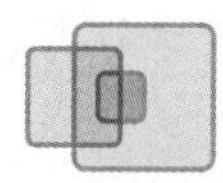

Answers and Explanations

1. The answer is B (*III D 2 d [1]*). The arm hypertension with low pressure in the leg and weak pulses are characteristic of coarctation of the aorta. The ejection click and systolic ejection murmur are characteristic of aortic valve abnormality and turbulence across the valve. A bicuspid aortic valve is frequently associated with coarctation of the aorta. Ventricular septal defect produces a regurgitant murmur without an ejection click.

2. The answer is C (*III C 1 d*). Transposition of the great arteries produces no turbulence and therefore no murmur and the cyanosis is severe in the newborn period. Atrial septal defect would be expected to produce a wide split of the second heart sound and would not be accompanied by cyanosis. If pulmonary vascular resistance were high, the second sound would be loud and there would only be a soft murmur or none at all.

3–6. The answers are 3-D (*III B 1 d*), **4-B** (*III D 1 d*), **5-A** (*III B 2 d*), and **6-C** (*III B 3 d*). Atrial septal defect: The systolic ejection murmur is from increased turbulence across the right ventricular outflow and the middiastolic murmur is due to increased flow across the tricuspid valve. Aortic valve stenosis: The ejection click is caused by opening of a stenotic semilunar valve and the systolic ejection murmur is caused by turbulence across the outflow tract. The fact that the murmur is best heard over the aortic area makes it most likely that it comes from the aortic valve. In none of the other choices is an ejection click heard. Ventricular septal defect: The pansystolic murmur is characteristic of a ventricular septal defect and the middiastolic rumble from increased flow across the mitral valve tells us that the left-to-right shunt is large, thus accounting for the congestive failure. Patent ductus arteriosus: A pansystolic murmur that spills into diastole is characteristic of a patent ductus. This sound is not heard in any of the other choices.

chapter **13**

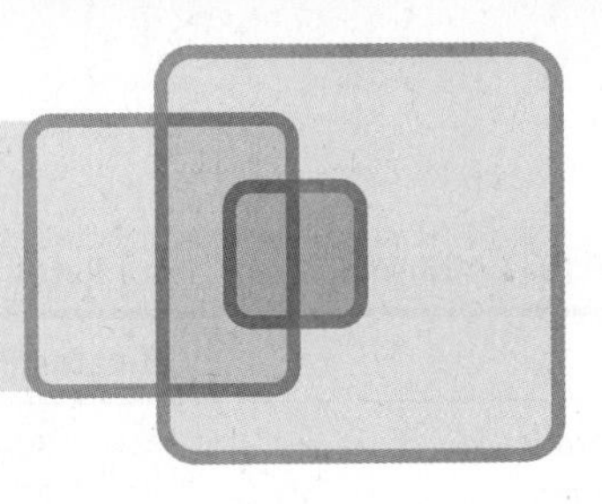

Pulmonary Diseases

KAREN L. DAIGLE

I GENERAL PRINCIPLES OF PULMONARY DISEASE IN CHILDREN

A Common pathologic features of pulmonary disease Acute and chronic pulmonary disease or symptoms are among the most common causes for visits to pediatric health care providers. Asthma, bronchiolitis, and pneumonia are the leading diagnoses for hospital admission, especially in children younger than 5 years.

1. **Underlying pathologic process.** Most lung diseases in children are classified as obstructive or restrictive.
   a. **Obstruction** (i.e., airway narrowing) may be caused by intraluminal secretions, edema or inflammation of the airway wall, hypertrophy or contraction of the bronchial smooth muscle, or extrinsic compression.
   b. **Restriction** (i.e., decreased lung volume) may be caused by decreased lung compliance (stiff lungs), atelectasis or pneumothorax causing lung collapse, neuromuscular disease, or disorders of the chest wall.
2. **Pathophysiology**
   a. **Hypoxemia** (i.e., deficient oxygenation of blood) most commonly is caused by ventilation-perfusion abnormalities but also may be due to intracardiac or intrapulmonary shunts, hypoventilation, or diffusion problems.
   b. **Hypercapnia** (i.e., excess carbon dioxide in blood) most commonly is caused by primary hypoventilation (due to upper airway obstruction, neuromuscular weakness, or central nervous system depression), but also may be seen with severe lower airway obstruction.
3. **Pathogenic factors**
   a. The **small airways** of the child result in high airway resistance and put the child at great risk to develop obstruction.
   b. The young child lacks **specific immunity** (organism-specific antibody) and is relatively defenseless against invading microorganisms.
   c. In children, most pulmonary disease has a **single cause,** whereas in adults, pulmonary disease is often multifactorial in etiology.

B Evaluation of pulmonary disease

1. **History.** Diagnosis of pulmonary disease is typically based on a careful history, focusing on the following questions:
   a. **Is the disorder acute, chronic, or recurrent?** The physician must determine whether the condition is acute and self-limited; chronic (i.e., with symptoms occurring daily for more than 4 weeks); or recurrent (i.e., with disease-free intervals).
   b. **Is the disorder immediately or eventually life threatening?**
      (1) Cyanosis, respiratory distress, or severe stridor indicate the need for immediate action.
      (2) Problems such as progressive weight loss or a progressive pulmonary opacification imply a serious long-term outlook.
   c. **What are the symptoms?** Specific pulmonary symptoms should be sought, such as:
      (1) Presence of a cough and its characteristics

TABLE 13-1 Normal Respiratory Rates in Children	
Age	**Breaths Per Minute**
Newborn	30–75
6–12 mo	22–31
1–2 y	17–23
2–4 y	16–25
4–10 y	13–23
10–14 y	13–19

(2) Labored or noisy breathing and its interference with activities
(3) Presence of wheezing, chest pain, or sputum production

d. **What factors affect the severity of symptoms?** Identify factors that improve or worsen symptoms. Asthma is suggested when symptoms are exacerbated by changes in weather, viral infections (e.g., common colds), exercise, laughing or crying, or exposure to allergens.

e. **Is there a family history of pulmonary disease?** Some diseases such as cystic fibrosis and asthma have a genetic or familial basis.

f. **Have any treatments been given?** Inquire about types, dosages, and duration of therapy the child has received, and response of symptoms to treatment.

2. **Physical examination**

a. **Respiratory rate** (Table 13-1) is the best indicator of pulmonary function in young infants. As the respiratory rate is influenced by activity when the child is awake, the most reliable and reproducible rate is the sleeping respiratory rate.

b. **Effort of breathing** is a guide to pulmonary dysfunction.

(1) **Grunting** is heard when vocal cords are adducted during exhalation, in an effort to maintain lung volume. It is frequently heard in neonatal respiratory distress syndrome and pulmonary edema.
(2) **Chest retractions** (suprasternal, supraclavicular, intercostal, subcostal) occur when airway resistance is increased. In infants, **head bobbing** may also be seen.
(3) **Nasal flaring** is a sign of increased airway resistance.

c. **Breath sounds** are also informative.

(1) **Crackles** are heard primarily on inspiration. They are produced by the opening of small airways that closed on the previous breath.
(2) **Wheezing** is produced by partial airway obstruction. It usually is expiratory in origin but can be inspiratory when the airway obstruction is fixed and rigid, as in airway edema. Wheezing is usually a sign of asthma, but it can occur in any critical narrowing of the airways.
(3) **Stridor** is a harsh, inspiratory wheeze produced by obstruction of extrathoracic airways, usually at the laryngeal level.
(4) **Rhonchi** are sonorous sounds produced by secretions in large airways.

d. **Anatomic changes** of significance include the following:

(1) **A change in tracheal position** signals mediastinal shift and an inequality between the two sides of the chest, as with a pneumothorax or atelectasis.
(2) **A change in thoracic configuration.** A barrel-chest deformity suggests hyperinflation and overdistention of the lungs due to chronic airway obstruction.
(3) **Clubbing of the fingers and toes** is caused by lifting of the nail base by tissue proliferation on the dorsal surface of the terminal phalanx. As a sign of pulmonary disease in children, clubbing most often is caused by cystic fibrosis.

3. **Laboratory studies**

a. **Imaging procedures**

(1) **Chest radiograph** is indicated if pulmonary disease is suspected.
(2) **Fluoroscopy** is useful for dynamic studies (e.g., to evaluate diaphragmatic movements, identify tracheal collapse).
(3) **Ultrasonography** is used to confirm pleural effusion and to guide thoracentesis; it can be used instead of fluoroscopy to evaluate diaphragmatic motility.

TABLE 13-2 Pulmonary Function Tests

Measurement	Definition
FVC: Forced vital capacity	Total volume forcefully exhaled following maximal inspiratory effort
FEV_1: Forced expiratory volume, 1 second	Total volume exhaled in the first second of a forced expiratory maneuver; approximately 85% of FVC in normal children
$FEF_{25\%-75\%}$: Forced expiratory flow over 25%–75% of FVC	Average flow during the midportion of the forced expiratory maneuver; effort independent
PEFR: Peak expiratory flow rate	Highest recorded flow; effort dependent

(4) **Barium swallow** can identify gastroesophageal reflux, aspiration, and lesions causing extrinsic compression of the large intrathoracic airways.

(5) **Computed tomography (CT) scanning** of the chest differentiates pulmonary lesions that cannot be distinguished on chest radiograph (e.g., to differentiate a collapsed lung from a mediastinal mass, or pleural fluid from a consolidated lung). Chest CT scanning may also show the extent of cystic lesions and bronchiectasis not visualized on routine chest radiographs.

b. **Pulmonary function tests** are used to evaluate obstructive and restrictive abnormalities. They cannot diagnose specific diseases.

(1) **Commonly used tests** in children are **spirometry and flow-volume curves**. Table 13-2 includes a description of the important elements of these tests.

(a) Testing requires a child to be cooperative by taking a deep breath to total lung capacity and then exhaling completely. Therefore, the test cannot be performed in most children younger than age 5 to 6 years of age or in children with cognitive impairment.

(b) Tests can be performed before and after inhalation of a bronchodilating agent (to determine whether abnormalities are reversible) or before and after exercise (as a challenge to elicit airway obstruction). Exercise testing is also used to evaluate cardiopulmonary fitness.

(2) In **obstructive lung disease,** the pertinent findings are reductions in the forced expiratory volume in 1 second (FEV_1) and FEV_1/forced vital capacity (FVC) and a concave or "scooped" appearance of the flow-volume loop.

(3) In **restrictive lung disease,** the FVC is reduced with a proportional reduction in FEV_1; this results in a normal FEV_1/FVC. The shape of the flow-volume loop is normal.

(4) **Examples** of different types of lung disorders are listed in Table 13-3 according to pulmonary function.

c. **Analysis of gas exchange**

(1) **Arterial oxygen tension (PO_2)** is a sensitive indicator of overall pulmonary function. The arterial PO_2 and arterial carbon dioxide tension (PCO_2) provides information about the adequacy of alveolar gas exchange.

(2) **Capillary pH and PCO_2.** If obtaining a sample of arterial blood is difficult, an alternative is to determine the pH and PCO_2 of capillary blood and monitor oxygen saturation by pulse oximetry.

(3) **Pulse oximetry** is a noninvasive technique that uses the principle of differential light absorption spectra for saturated oxyhemoglobin compared with reduced hemoglobin to record oxygen saturation.

d. **Tests for specific situations**

(1) In children suspected of having **asthma,** pulmonary function tests before and after bronchodilator inhalation and allergy skin tests to specific environmental allergens are helpful.

(2) In children suspected of having **cystic fibrosis,** sweat testing for chloride levels is diagnostic (*see IV D 1*).

(3) In children suspected of having **immunodeficiency disorders,** immunoglobulin levels and tests of immune function can be determined (see Chapter 9).

TABLE 13-3 Types of Pulmonary Disorders in Children

Type of Pulmonary Disease	Pulmonary Function Test Results	Examples of Disorders
Obstructive	FVC: Normal FEV_1: ↓ FEV_1/FVC: ↓ $FEF_{25\%-75\%}$: ↓ PEFR: ↓ or normal	Asthma Cystic fibrosis Foreign body aspiration Pneumonia Drowning
Restrictive	FVC: ↓ FEV_1: ↓ FEV_1/FVC: Normal $FEF_{25-75\%}$: ↓ or normal PEFR: ↓	Duchenne muscular dystrophy Respiratory distress syndrome Pleural effusion Acute pneumothorax Atelectasis Obesity

$FEF_{25-75\%}$, forced expiratory flow over 25%–75% of FVC; FEV_1, forced expiratory volume in 1 second; FVC, forced vital capacity; PEFR, peak expiratory flow rate.

(4) In children who have had a significant episode of **apnea, are unstable, are premature, or have unexplained bradycardia, a polysomnogram** may be helpful.

(a) In this study, heart rate and rhythm, airflow at the nose, chest wall motion, and oximetry are recorded during sleep or over a 12-hour period. Polysomnography can be combined with other testing, such as pH probe monitoring, electroencephalography, or eye movement.

(b) Polysomnography can distinguish central from obstructive apnea, and it identifies cardiac arrhythmias and oxygen desaturation.

e. **Endoscopic procedures**

(1) **Laryngoscopy** is useful in patients who have stridor or laryngeal disorders. The exam can be done indirectly by mirror or directly with sedation or general anesthesia.

(2) **Flexible bronchoscopy** is useful for dynamic airway studies in patients who have stridor or airway obstruction; it is also used for obtaining culture specimens. It is performed with conscious sedation or general anesthesia.

(3) **Rigid bronchoscopy** is used for foreign body removal and other airway surgery. It requires general anesthesia and usually is performed by a surgeon.

f. **Thoracentesis** is used to obtain pleural fluid for culture and analysis.

II ACUTE RESPIRATORY FAILURE (SEE CHAPTER 7)

A Definition Respiratory failure occurs when dysfunction of the respiratory tract leads to abnormal gas exchange, resulting in hypoxemia (i.e., arterial PO_2 below 50 mm Hg) and/or hypercapnia (i.e., arterial PCO_2 above 50 mm Hg).

B Etiology Acute respiratory failure can be caused by many disorders. It is critical to try to identify the cause and the underlying pathophysiology to direct appropriate management in an individual case. Representative examples of the many causes are shown in Table 13-4.

C Clinical features Table 13-5 lists the clinical features of acute respiratory failure.

D Therapy depends on the underlying pathophysiology, the degree of hypoxemia, and the arterial pH value. Ultimate recovery requires correction of the underlying causes of respiratory failure.

1. **Adequate oxygenation** (arterial PO_2 above 60 mm Hg) should be achieved at the lowest concentration of supplemental oxygen, to avoid oxygen toxicity. Positive-pressure ventilation (invasive or noninvasive) may be necessary to treat refractory hypoxemia.
2. **Securing a patent airway** may call for removal of bronchial secretions and use of bronchodilators, as well as intubation or mechanical ventilation. **Endotracheal or nasotracheal intubation** may be sufficient in upper airway obstruction.

TABLE 13-4 Causes of Acute Respiratory Failure in Children

Obstructive disorders
- Upper airway obstruction
  - Anomalies
    - Choanal atresia, Pierre Robin syndrome, laryngeal webs, subglottic stenosis, vascular rings
  - Aspiration of gastric secretions or a foreign body
  - Infections (peritonsillar or retropharyngeal abscess)
  - Allergic laryngospasm
  - Growths (tumors, cysts, tonsillar and adenoidal hypertrophy)
- Lower airway obstruction
  - Anomalies (bronchomalacia, lobar emphysema)
  - Aspiration (due to tracheoesophageal fistula, pharyngeal incoordination)
  - Infection (pertussis, bronchiolitis, pneumonia)
  - Inflammation and bronchospasm (asthma, bronchopulmonary dysplasia)

Restrictive disorders of the lung parenchyma
- Pulmonary hypoplasia
- Respiratory distress syndrome
- Pneumothorax
- Hemorrhage
- Pulmonary edema
- Pleural effusion

Inefficient alveolar–capillary gas transfer
- Diffusion defects
  - Pulmonary edema
  - Adult respiratory distress syndrome secondary to shock, sepsis, and near-drowning
  - *Pneumocystis carinii* pneumonia
- Respiratory center depression
  - Cerebral trauma
  - Central nervous system infection
  - Sedative overdose
  - Severe asphyxia

3. **Intubation and positive-pressure ventilation** may be required for an elevated arterial PCO_2 with respiratory acidosis.

III ASTHMA

A Definition. Asthma is a lung disease characterized by the following features:

1. **Variable airway obstruction** that is reversible (partially or completely) either spontaneously or with treatment

TABLE 13-5 Clinical Features of Respiratory Failure

Pulmonary Features	Cardiac Features	Neurologic Features
Tachypnea	Tachycardia	Headache
Altered depth and pattern of respiration	Hypertension	Restlessness
Chest retractions	Bradycardia	Irritability
Nasal flaring	Hypotension	Seizures
Cyanosis	Cardiac arrest	Coma
Diaphoresis		
Decreased air movement		
Grunting		

TABLE 13-6 Asthma Triggers in Children

Respiratory infections (viral, mycoplasma)	Changes in weather
Irritants (cigarette smoke, ozone, air pollution)	Emotional stress (crying, laughing)
Exercise	Medications (aspirin)
Allergens	Gastroesophageal reflux
Inhaled	Chemicals (tartrazine, sulfites,
Ingested (rare)	monosodium glutamate)

2. **Chronic airway inflammation**
3. **Airway hyperresponsiveness** to a variety of stimuli

B **Incidence** Asthma is the most common chronic lung disease of childhood, affecting 6.5 million children with an overall prevalence in the United States of 9% in 2005.

1. Non-Hispanic Black and Puerto Rican children are at greatest risk with prevalence as high as 12% and 19%, respectively.
2. Boys have higher prevalence rates and death rates throughout childhood.
3. Asthma is more severe in young children and health care utilization is highest in this group.

C **Triggering mechanisms** for acute episodes of asthma are numerous (Table 13-6).

D **Pathophysiology** Symptoms of an acute asthma exacerbation are the result of bronchospasm, increased mucus production, and acute and chronic inflammation of the airway mucosa resulting in airway edema.

E **Clinical features** Typical symptoms include cough, chest tightness, wheezing, and dyspnea (tachypnea in young children). Symptoms may change in severity both spontaneously and as a result of therapy, necessitating frequent clinical reassessment. During an acute exacerbation, hypoxemia results from airway obstruction, and arterial PO_2 continues to drop as the obstruction progresses. Initially, because of hyperventilation, arterial PCO_2 is low. During severe attacks, PCO_2 rises as hypoventilation and respiratory failure ensue.

F **Risk factors** for asthma are shown in Figure 13-1.

G **Diagnosis**

1. **Clinical diagnosis.** A description of the child's typical recurrent symptoms is often diagnostic. Diagnosis is more difficult when symptoms are atypical (e.g., chronic cough without wheezing or dyspnea) or when asthma begins in infancy.
2. **Differential diagnosis.** Wheezing can occur in any process that results in sufficient airway narrowing. Those likely to be confused with asthma include bronchiolitis, cystic fibrosis, tracheomalacia, foreign body aspiration, and congestive heart failure.
3. **Assessment of severity** is based on the frequency of symptoms and the degree of abnormality on pulmonary function tests, if available. Asthma severity is divided into four categories: Mild, intermittent; mild, persistent; moderate, persistent; and severe persistent. It is recommended that patients with moderate or severe persistent asthma be evaluated by an asthma specialist.

H **Therapy**

1. **Management of the acute attack**
   a. **Emergency therapy.** Table 13-7 describes emergency therapy procedures.
      (1) Inhaled β-adrenergic agonists (e.g., albuterol) are rapidly effective and have minimal side effects in most patients. They are the drugs of choice in acute asthma management.
      (2) In children older than 5 years of age, peak expiratory flow rate (PEFR) measurements can be obtained and used to follow up effectiveness of therapy. PEFR $< 25\%$ predicted can be associated with elevated PCO_2 levels.

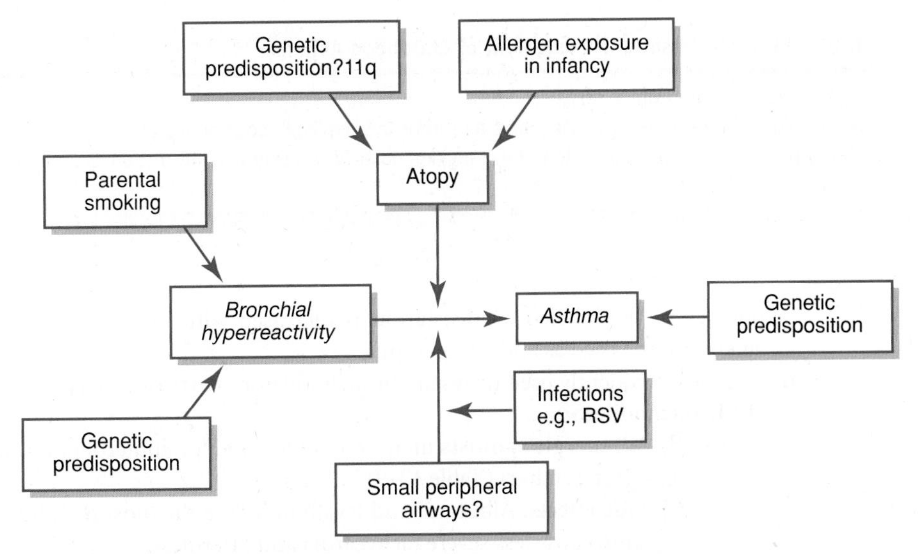

FIGURE 13-1 Possible risk factors for the development of asthma. RSV, respiratory syncytial virus. (Reprinted from Loughlin GM, Eigen H: *Respiratory Disease in Children: Diagnosis and Management.* Baltimore, Williams & Wilkins, 1994, p. 225.)

(3) Addition of an inhaled anticholinergic (ipratropium bromide) may be beneficial if there is severe obstruction (PEFR $< 50\%$).

(4) Failure to respond to inhalation therapy is an indication for hospital admission. By definition, this condition is **status asthmaticus.**

b. **In-hospital therapy** (Table 13-8). Blood gas analysis is indicated for a patient with severe obstruction. Hypercapnia ($PCO_2 > 42$ mm Hg in this circumstance) warrants admission to an intensive care unit. Serum electrolytes should be checked to monitor for albuterol-induced hypokalemia. A chest radiograph is advisable if there are localized abnormalities on pulmonary auscultation.

2. **Maintenance therapy.** Three approaches are used in the management of chronic asthma.
   a. **Avoidance,** if possible, of allergens and other triggers (except exercise) is the simplest, most direct method of treatment. Children with exercise-associated symptoms may need pretreatment but should be encouraged to exercise.
   b. **Desensitization** may be helpful when certain allergens (e.g., ragweed) cannot be avoided, but such immunotherapy is not a panacea.
   c. **Drugs** are the keystone of therapy. The key principle of therapy is to match therapy to severity. All children with asthma should have access to bronchodilator rescue. Short bursts of oral steroids may be required for acute symptoms in patients with asthma of any severity. Children who have persistent asthma require treatment with daily controller therapy. Preferred agents are inhaled corticosteroids, long-acting β_2-adrenergic agonists, and antileukotrienes. Inhaled corticosteroids are the most effective therapy for persistent asthma. The dose and

TABLE 13-7 Emergency Management of Childhood Asthma
O_2 to keep O_2 saturation $> 90\%$
Aerosolized albuterol (with O_2 6-liter flow)
0.15 mg/kg/dose (max. 5 mg/dose) q20 min $\times$ 3
plus
Prednisone (1–2 mg/kg/dose bid) if no response after first aerosol or recent steroid use
Good response: Discharge on additional medication
Inadequate response: Admit

TABLE 13-8 In-Hospital Management of Childhood Asthma

O_2 to keep O_2 saturation > 90%
Aerosolized albuterol (0.15 mg/kg/dose q1–2h or 0.5 mg/kg/h continuously)
Methylprednisolone or prednisolone (1–2 mg/kg/dose IV or PO q6h × 48 h then 1–2 mg/kg/d in 2 divided doses)

potency of the inhaled corticosteroid is increased with increasing asthma severity. Other agents may be used as add-on therapy.

d. The most frequently used drugs are bronchodilators, corticosteroids, and antileukotrienes.

(1) Bronchodilators

(a) β_2-Adrenergic agonists include albuterol and levalbuterol (short acting) and salmeterol (long acting) (Table 13-9).

(i) Side effects. Albuterol and levalbuterol are the most β_2-adrenergic specific and, thus, cause less severe tachycardia and jitteriness.

(ii) Short-acting inhaled β_2-adrenergic agonists are preferably administered by air compressor with nebulizer (for young children or patients in significant respiratory distress) or by a metered-dose inhaler (MDI). Holding chambers should be used for all children. Failure to respond to an MDI usually is the result of improper technique. Salmeterol, a **long-acting β_2-adrenergic agonist,** is administered by a dry powder inhaler. It should not be used for acute asthma episodes because it has an onset of action of approximately 20 minutes.

(b) The **anticholinergic** ipratropium bromide has a slower onset of action and provides less maximal bronchodilation, but has a longer duration of action than β_2-adrenergic agonists.

(2) Corticosteroids inhibit the late asthmatic response and the subsequent increase in airway reactivity induced by allergen challenge. They have significant side effects when used orally for long periods. Oral preparations are extremely effective as short-term therapy (usually 3–5 days) for acute exacerbations. Due to their high levels of topical anti-inflammatory activity but low systemic absorption, inhaled corticosteroids are highly effective and can be used safely for chronic asthma therapy. They are first-line therapy for persistent asthma. They are administered by MDI, dry powder inhaler, and aerosol.

TABLE 13-9 Bronchodilators Used for Treating Asthma

Medication	Formulations	Dose
β-Adrenergic Agonist		
Albuterol	5 mg/mL (0.5% solution) 2.5 mg/3 mL (0.083% solution)	0.5 mg/kg (maximum 2.5 mg), up to 4 times daily
	MDI 90 μg/puff	2 puffs, 3–4 times daily PRN
Levalbuterol	1.25 mg/3 mL solution 0.63 mg/3 mL solution	0.025 mg/kg (minimum dose 0.63 mg) q4–8h
Salmeterol	DPI 50 μg/inhalation	1 inhalation q12h
Anticholinergics		
Ipratropium bromide	0.5 mg/2.5 mL (0.02% solution)	0.25–0.5 mg q6h
	MDI 18 μg/puff	1–2 puffs q6h

DPI, dry powder inhaler; MDI, metered-dose inhaler.

Modified from NAEPP Expert Panel Report: Guidelines for the Diagnosis and Management of Asthma—Update on Selected Topics 2002. Publication No. 02-5074, Bethesda, MD, 2002.

(3) **Leukotriene modifiers.** The most commonly used type is the leukotriene receptor antagonist montelukast. The drug is administered orally as sprinkles or a chewable tablet. Although typically used as an add-on agent, antileukotriene therapy may be useful in children who have mild, persistent asthma in lieu of inhaled anti-inflammatory therapy.

(4) **Other controller agents** are used much less frequently. The **cromones (cromolyn sodium and nedocromil)** are mast cell stabilizers that inhibit pulmonary histamine release. They can also be used to prevent exercise- or allergen-associated symptoms. Theophylline is administered in a long-acting oral form and has both anti-inflammatory and bronchodilator effects. It may be used for select patients as add-on therapy or for those with steroid or other medication side effects.

IV CYSTIC FIBROSIS

Cystic fibrosis (CF) is a life-shortening inherited disease, primarily of whites. Approximately 30,000 of people in the United States have CF and the estimated carrier rate is 1 in 31. This section will review the general aspects of cystic fibrosis and its pulmonary complications. Pancreatic insufficiency and other gastrointestinal manifestations of cystic fibrosis are covered in Chapter 11.

A Definition Cystic fibrosis is a disease of the exocrine glands that causes viscid secretions. The gastrointestinal and respiratory systems are most commonly and most severely affected.

B Underlying defect

1. Cystic fibrosis is inherited as an **autosomal recessive trait.** The CF gene is located on chromosome 7, and it codes for a protein that is named the **cystic fibrosis transmembrane regulator (CFTR).** In 70% of patients in the United States, there is an absence of a three-base pair that encodes for the amino acid phenylalanine (Δ508).
2. The defect in cystic fibrosis is thought to be a **blocked or closed chloride channel** in the cell membrane of epithelial cells. This blockage traps chloride ions inside the cell and draws sodium ions and water into the cell. This results in dehydration of mucous secretions and an abnormal airway environment that may inactivate cell defense mechanisms and promote bacterial growth.

C Clinical features of CF vary considerably in nature and severity.

1. **Most common and most severe manifestations**
   a. **Respiratory insufficiency** occurs eventually in more than 95% of all patients and is caused by abnormal mucous gland secretion in the airways, producing airway obstruction and secondary infection, cough, dyspnea, bronchiectasis, and pulmonary fibrosis.
   b. **Malabsorption** of fats and protein due to pancreatic insufficiency and abnormal mucous gland secretions in the gastrointestinal tract occurs in 85% of patients (see Chapter 11). This malabsorption results in fatty stools, fat-soluble vitamin deficiencies, failure to gain weight, and retarded growth.
2. **Other manifestations and complications**
   a. **Electrolytes in sweat.** Concentrations of sodium and chloride in sweat are abnormally high in all patients. This can lead to a hyponatremic, hypochloremic metabolic alkalosis.
   b. **Respiratory complications** include hemoptysis, pneumothorax, and cor pulmonale.
   c. **Other intestinal problems**
      (1) **Meconium ileus,** in which abnormally viscid meconium completely obstructs the ileum, occurs in 10% to 15% of all infants born with cystic fibrosis.
      (2) A comparable fecal obstruction called distal intestinal obstruction syndrome (DIOS) can occur in older children as a result of dietary indiscretion or insufficient enzyme replacement therapy.
   d. **Hepatic effects.** Steatosis (fatty liver) and focal biliary cirrhosis are common findings (10%–70% of patients). The latter may be severe enough to produce portal hypertension and esophageal varices.
   e. **Pancreatic effects.** Abnormal glucose tolerance and CF-related diabetes mellitus occur in pancreatic insufficient patients. The incidence of diabetes increases with increasing age, with median age of onset at 20 years.

f. **Nasal effects**
   (1) Chronic sinusitis with opacification of the sinuses occurs in all patients.
   (2) Nasal polyposis occurs in 5% to 40% of patients.
g. **Reproductive effects**
   (1) Virtually all males with CF are sterile because of congenital obliteration of the vas deferens.
   (2) Females who have CF produce thick, spermicidal cervical mucus and have reduced fertility.

D Diagnosis The diagnosis of cystic fibrosis is made in 65% of patients in the first year of life, but in 10% of patients, the diagnosis is not made until after the age of 10 years. Diagnostic criteria for cystic fibrosis include a **positive sweat test or genetic testing** and **typical clinical findings and/or a positive family history of CF.**

1. The **sweat test** result is positive if the chloride concentration of sweat exceeds 60 mEq/L before age 20 years and 80 mEq/L in adults. Normal sweat chloride values are below 40 mEq/L.
   a. The test must be done correctly. The method of choice is quantitative pilocarpine iontophoresis by the Gibson and Cooke or Westcor method.
   b. False-positive results can occur in patients who have nephrogenic diabetes insipidus, hypothyroidism, mucopolysaccharidosis, adrenal insufficiency, ectodermal dysplasia, severe malnutrition, and anorexia nervosa.
2. **DNA testing** is available for all cystic fibrosis mutations and is indicated:
   a. If adequate amounts of sweat for analysis cannot be collected
   b. If sweat test results are borderline or equivocal
   c. If sweat tests do not correlate with clinical symptoms
   d. For in utero diagnosis, such as a fetus with ultrasound evidence suggestive of meconium ileus, or in a fetus with a family history of CF
3. Evidence of meconium ileus is virtually diagnostic of cystic fibrosis. Failure to pass a stool in the first 24 hours of life, combined with small bowel obstruction and evidence of a microcolon, strongly suggests meconium ileus.
4. Without evidence of meconium ileus, a **high index of suspicion** is required to make the diagnosis. Any of the following initial signs and symptoms should suggest the possible need for a confirmatory sweat test:
   a. **Respiratory signs and symptoms** include chronic cough; recurrent pneumonia and atelectasis; hyperinflation; digital clubbing; persistent crackles on lung auscultation; the presence of pathogens such as *Pseudomonas aeruginosa* or *Staphylococcus aureus* in sputum; hemoptysis; and nasal polyposis.
   b. **Gastrointestinal signs and symptoms** include steatorrhea, chronic diarrhea, rectal prolapse, biliary cirrhosis, and DIOS.
   c. **Other signs and symptoms** include failure to thrive; hyponatremic, hypochloremic metabolic alkalosis; and the symptom complex of hypoproteinemia, anemia, and edema in infants.
5. **Neonatal screening** using blood spots collected shortly after birth to detect elevated levels of immunoreactive trypsin is available in some states. Preliminary studies suggest that early diagnosis improves growth early on and may favorably affect outcome.

E Therapy

1. **Treatment of respiratory problems**
   a. **Antibiotics** are given either continuously or intermittently to prevent or treat pulmonary bacterial infection.
      (1) **Oral therapy** usually consists of antistaphylococcal drugs, cephalosporins, and trimethoprim-sulfamethoxazole. In older patients, oral quinolones are used.
      (2) **Aerosolized aminoglycoside therapy** is used to decrease chronic lung infection and reduce the need for hospitalization.
      (3) **Intravenous therapy** lasting 10 to 21 days may be needed for established infections. Usually, an aminoglycoside (e.g., tobramycin) and either a semisynthetic penicillin (e.g., piperacillin) or third-generation cephalosporin (e.g., ceftazidime) are given.
   b. **Other drugs.** Inhaled **bronchodilators** are used frequently to improve clearance of airway secretions. The **mucolytic** DNAse, administered by aerosol, breaks down the DNA from

necrotic neutrophils and thins mucus, produces modest improvements in pulmonary function, and decreases hospitalization rates.

c. **Chest physiotherapy** is critical to removal of viscid airway secretions. When performed on a regular basis, it helps to maintain lung health. Intensification during an acute pulmonary infection can contribute to recovery. Forms of therapy include breathing exercises, chest percussion (manual or mechanical), active cycle of breathing, and use of oscillatory devices.

d. **Lung transplantation** is available to some patients who have CF, with risks similar to those faced by other lung transplantation recipients.

2. **Treatment of digestive problems**
   a. **Pancreatic enzymes** (freeze-dried extracts of animal pancreas) are given before each meal or snack. The dosage is adjusted on the basis of growth and stool pattern.
   b. A **high-calorie, high-protein diet** should be provided. For anorectic children, an oral, enteral, or parenteral supplement may be needed to improve caloric consumption.
   c. **Vitamin supplementation** is given, especially the fat-soluble vitamins A, E, and K.

3. **Treatment of complications**
   a. **Meconium ileus** usually requires surgery, although the obstruction sometimes can be cleared by instilling an enema composed of radiocontrast agent (meglumine diatrizoate) or acetylcysteine.
   b. **Distal intestinal obstruction** usually can be relieved with enemas.
   c. **Pneumothorax** is usually treated by closed-tube thoracostomy if it is symptomatic or large. Persistent leaks require procedures such as stapling, sclerosis, or pleural stripping and abrasion.
   d. **CF-related diabetes** requires nutritional management and sometimes insulin, if there is fasting hyperglycemia.

4. **Future therapy**
   a. **Gene replacement** may prove to be promising; very early work suggests at least localized feasibility.
   b. In lieu of gene replacement, development of therapeutic agents that **correct or modify the chloride channel defect** has been a focus of research.

F Prognosis The outlook for cystic fibrosis patients has improved significantly with advances in therapy. In 2005, the predicted median age of survival for people with CF was 36.5 years; some individuals live into the sixth or seventh decade. Most patients (95%) die of respiratory failure; others die of liver failure or other complications.

V BRONCHOPULMONARY DYSPLASIA

A Definition Bronchopulmonary dysplasia (BPD) is a chronic pulmonary disease of infants characterized by the need for oxygen therapy beyond 28 days of life, chronic respiratory signs and symptoms, and an abnormal chest radiograph. BPD typically develops in preterm infants (usually < 32 weeks' gestation) who receive oxygen therapy and mechanical ventilation.

B Pathology BPD is the manifestation of inadequate repair of acute lung injury to the immature lung, resulting in arrested lung development. The most prominent features are:

1. **Alveolar oversimplification** with fewer, larger alveoli with decreased septation
2. **Reduced vascular growth** with fewer, dysmorphic arteries

C Pathogenesis

1. **Important pathogenetic factors** in BPD include:
   a. **Deficiency of lung surfactant** leads to atelectasis and impaired gas exchange.
   b. **Decreased host antioxidant defenses** against the stress of hyperoxia and infection result in inflammation and lung injury.
2. **Other factors** that may play a role include lung structural immaturity, volutrauma, and inadequate nutrition. Familial predisposition to asthma may contribute to the severity of disease.

D Clinical features include retractions, tachypnea, wheezing, and cyanosis, especially with stress. Infants are also at risk for pulmonary and systemic hypertension.

E Diagnosis

1. **Pulmonary physical examination** should emphasize sleeping respiratory rate, signs of breathing effort, and auscultation to determine the presence of crackles and wheezes.
2. **Chest radiographic findings** are not sensitive or specific for BPD and do not correlate with disease severity. Findings might include increased interstitial markings, atelectasis, hyperinflation, and evidence of pulmonary edema.
3. **Blood gas analysis** reflects increased dead space and ventilation-perfusion mismatch with hypercapnia and hypoxemia.
4. **Electrocardiography** and **echocardiography** help to identify the presence of ventricular hypertrophy and pulmonary hypertension.

F Therapy

1. **Supplemental oxygen,** the mainstay of therapy, is given to maintain an oxygen saturation > 92% during all daily activities. Complications of chronic hypoxemia include pulmonary hypertension, poor growth, and apnea. Some infants require oxygen for 6 to 12 months.
2. **Pharmacologic therapy** has largely been studied in the acute and evolving phases of BPD. Inadequate data are available about the long-term effectiveness of commonly used therapies.
   a. **Diuretics** such as furosemide, hydrochlorothiazide, and spironolactone can be used acutely to treat pulmonary edema. They also have a direct effect on improving lung mechanics.
   b. **Bronchodilator therapy,** typically β_2-agonists, can reverse acute bronchospasm and improve lung mechanics. They are useful for older infants with evidence of asthma.

G Prognosis

Most outcome data available are for infants born in the presurfactant era, with few studies available on adolescents and young adults.

1. **Early childhood.** Despite growth of the airways during early childhood, many patients with BPD have evidence of persistent airflow obstruction. Episodic respiratory distress, usually due to viral respiratory tract infections, frequently leads to hospitalization.
2. **Later childhood and adolescence.** Older children with BPD, especially those with respiratory symptoms during the first 2 years, are at greater risk for wheezing and persistent pulmonary function abnormality (obstruction, ventilation-perfusion mismatch, exercise intolerance).

VI APNEA (SEE ALSO CHAPTER 6)

A Definition

Apnea is the cessation of breathing for longer than 20 seconds or for any duration if the apnea is associated with pallor, limpness, cyanosis, or bradycardia.

B Types of apnea and their causes

1. **Central apnea.** When there is no central neurologic drive to breathe, there is no chest wall or abdominal movement. Central apnea is a common symptom of disease in infants; it is not a disease itself. This condition may also be idiopathic. Causes of central apnea are listed in Table 13-10.
2. **Obstructive apnea.** When airway obstruction results in apnea, chest wall and abdominal movements will be present in the absence of airflow at the nose and mouth. (See Table 13-10 for causes of obstructive apnea.) **Obstructive sleep apnea syndrome** is a disorder of older children that disrupts normal ventilation during sleep and interferes with normal sleep patterns.

C Evaluation of the infant who has apnea

1. **History.** Obtaining a thorough history is the critical part of the evaluation. Questions should focus on the circumstances of the event, including sleep/wake state; relation to feeding; limb and chest wall movements; duration of the event; and need for stimulation or resuscitation.
   a. An **apparent life-threatening event** (**ALTE**) is an episode of apnea associated with color change (pallor or cyanosis), marked change in muscle tone (usually limpness, rarely rigidity), or choking and gagging.

TABLE 13-10 Causes of Apnea in Infancy

Central Apnea	Obstructive Apnea
Prematurity (see Chapter 6)	Macroglossia (e.g., Down syndrome, hypothyroidism, or Pierre Robin syndrome)
Medications to mother or infant	Enlarged tonsils and adenoids
Infections, bacterial or viral	Posterior pharyngeal muscle incoordination (e.g., from cerebral palsy or trauma)
Anemia	Laryngospasm
Cardiac arrhythmias (especially Wolff-Parkinson-White syndrome)	Cleft lip repair
Seizures	Achondroplasia
Gastroesophageal reflux or aspiration (vagally mediated)	Obstructed tracheostomy
Hypoxemia	
Hypoglycemia	
Central alveolar hypoventilation	

b. Observers may fear the child will die and intervene with vigorous stimulation or cardiopulmonary resuscitation.

2. **Physical examination.** Special attention should be paid to the neurologic and cardiac examinations as well as to the airway examination.

3. **Laboratory studies.** The history and physical examination may suggest a specific diagnosis; if so, appropriate diagnostic studies can be pursued. If the clinical findings are unrevealing, the following might be considered the minimum diagnostic evaluation:
   a. Analysis of oxygenation and acid-base status (blood gas analysis or serum electrolytes, pulse oximetry)
   b. Complete blood count with differential

4. **Subsequent laboratory studies.** If the initial diagnostic evaluation is inconclusive, careful review of the history should be undertaken. If there are no additional clues, more extensive diagnostic studies might include:
   a. Chest radiography
   b. Polysomnography with/without pH probe monitoring (for reflux)
   c. Electroencephalography
   d. Electrocardiography/echocardiography
   e. Barium swallow

D **Therapy** is directed at the cause of apnea, if it can be identified (e.g., correction of anemia or arrhythmias, treatment of seizures or gastroesophageal reflux). Several diagnoses warrant special consideration:

1. **Central apnea with bradycardia** may be helped by the stimulant effects of theophylline or caffeine.

2. **Obstructive sleep apnea syndrome** is usually corrected by removal of tonsils and/or adenoids. Nocturnal continuous positive airway pressure (CPAP) should be considered for nonsurgical candidates and those with persistent findings after surgery.

3. Evaluation of the infant with **an apparent life-threatening event** may not identify a cause. Use of a home monitor may be recommended if the apneic episode is thought to be significant and if a recurrence is potentially fatal.

VII SUDDEN INFANT DEATH SYNDROME

A **Definition** Sudden infant death syndrome (SIDS) is the sudden and unexpected death of an infant whose history or postmortem examination cannot demonstrate a specific cause of death. SIDS is the leading cause of death in infants after the neonatal period.

B **Incidence** In 2001, the rate of SIDS deaths in the United States was 0.6 per 1000 live births. This represents a > 50% decrease over the preceding 10 years. Peak incidence is age 2 to 4 months; 90% of deaths occur by age 6 months.

C **Etiology and pathogenesis** of SIDS remain unclear. Infants at risk may have abnormal arousal and hypoxic drive, associated with inadequate airway protective mechanisms.

D **Prevention** The most effective way to reduce the incidence of SIDS in the United States is to put infants to sleep on their backs.

VIII CONGENITAL MALFORMATIONS

Congenital malformations that cause respiratory problems during the neonatal period are discussed in Chapter 6. The following discussion is focused on those congenital malformations that do not cause symptoms until after the neonatal period or that have late complications.

A **Laryngomalacia (infantile larynx)** This congenital disorder is the most common cause of inspiratory stridor in infancy. The larynx appears disproportionately small, and the supporting structures may be abnormally soft.

1. **Clinical features**
   a. Stridor begins within the first 4 weeks of life and is accentuated by increased ventilation (e.g., from crying or excitement) or upper respiratory tract infections.
   b. Stridor usually resolves by age 12 months but may recur with respiratory tract infections until approximately 3 years of age.
2. **Diagnosis** is by fiberoptic bronchoscopy or direct laryngoscopy.
3. **Therapy** is usually not needed. Rarely, laser therapy of redundant tissue or a tracheostomy is required when stridor occurs in association with failure to thrive or with life-threatening apnea or airway obstruction.
4. **Other causes** of stridor in children include subglottic stenosis associated with inspiratory and expiratory stridor, and vocal cord paralysis associated with inspiratory stridor and hoarseness.

B **Vascular rings** Congenital anomalies of the aortic arch or its branches can create a ring around the airway that compromises respiration (see also Chapter 12).

1. **Types.** Vascular anomalies most likely to compress the trachea are:
   a. A right aortic arch with a left ligamentum arteriosum or patent ductus arteriosus
   b. A double aortic arch
   c. An anomalous innominate or left carotid artery
   d. A pulmonary artery sling
2. **Clinical features**
   a. Many of these infants have stridor.
   b. Other respiratory symptoms can include raucous respirations, intercostal retractions, tachypnea, and dyspnea with prolonged exhalation. The child may prefer an opisthotonic position to decrease airway collapse.
   c. Respiratory symptoms may become worse with feeding.
3. **Therapy** is surgical correction of the anomaly.

C **Tracheoesophageal fistula (see also Chapter 11)** Children born with a tracheoesophageal fistula are prone to development of chronic pulmonary disease, particularly tracheomalacia, airway hyperreactivity, or bronchiectasis. Chronic aspiration is believed to be a major factor resulting from uncoordinated esophageal peristalsis.

IX OTHER PULMONARY DISEASES

Other pulmonary diseases not discussed in this chapter but found elsewhere in the book include aspiration of foreign bodies (see Chapter 2), aspiration of hydrocarbons (see Chapter 2), drowning (see Chapter 2), upper and lower respiratory tract infections (see Chapter 10), and pulmonary neoplasms (see Chapter 16).

A Pulmonary tuberculosis

1. **Incidence**
   a. Approximately 6% of annually reported tuberculosis cases are in children younger than 15 years of age.
   b. Risk factors include age younger than 5 years, being foreign born or of nonwhite race or ethnic groups, living in an urban area, being immunocompromised, or having chronic illness or malnutrition.
2. **Etiology and pathogenesis**
   a. The etiologic agent, *Mycobacterium tuberculosis,* is usually transmitted via mucous droplets from a symptomatic adult family member.
   b. Following infection, all children have an asymptomatic incubation period (median 3–4 weeks). The primary lesion occurs in the lung, involving the parenchyma and regional lymph nodes. If the acquired immune response is inadequate, hematogenous spread of bacilli can result in disseminated tuberculosis and extrapulmonary disease.
3. **Clinical features and laboratory findings**
   a. **Latent tuberculosis infection (LTBI).** The majority of children remain asymptomatic; they have a positive tuberculin skin test but no clinical or radiographic findings of disease.
   b. **Tuberculosis disease**
      (1) **Pulmonary disease** is present when there is clinical or radiographic evidence of infection. Symptoms include cough, fever, and weight loss. **Radiographic findings** evolve from the primary complex (parenchymal or Ghon focus with enlarged regional lymph nodes) and may advance to multilobar involvement, cavitation, and pleural involvement.
      (2) **Extrathoracic diseases** of note include meningitis (the most severe form and more likely to occur in young children) and infection of superficial lymph nodes or scrofula (the most common form).
4. **Diagnosis.** In childhood tuberculosis, important diagnostic points include:
   a. A history of contact with the disease
   b. A positive **tuberculin skin test** result; the amount of induration at 48 to 72 hours that constitutes a positive test finding varies with the clinical history and degree of suspicion
      (1) Induration $\geq$ 15 mm is a positive finding in a child older than 4 years of age with no risk factors.
      (2) Induration of $\geq$ 10 mm is a positive finding in a child at risk for disseminated disease (age younger than 4 years or with a chronic medical condition) or at risk for exposure (homeless, exposure to adults at risk, born or travel in high prevalence countries).
      (3) Induration of $\geq$ 5 mm is a positive finding in a child who is immunosuppressed, has known or suspected contagious household contacts, or has clinical evidence of infection (including a chest radiograph compatible with previously active tuberculosis).
   c. Recovery of *M. tuberculosis* in sputum or gastric washings
5. **Therapy**
   a. **Latent tuberculosis infection** is treated with isoniazid (INH) for 9 months. Rifampin is used when there is a contraindication to INH or the child has exposure to a person with INH-resistant tuberculosis.
   b. **Tuberculosis disease** is treated with two or more drugs for at least 6 months; drugs typically used are INH, rifampin, ethambutol, and pyrazinamide. Specific regimens are based on susceptibility testing and the site of infection.
6. **Control and prevention.** Administration of **bacille Calmette-Guérin** (bCG) vaccine decreases the risk of developing more severe forms of disease in high prevalence countries; it does not prevent primary infection. It is not administered in the United States.

BIBLIOGRAPHY

American Academy of Pediatrics: *2006 Red Book: Report of the Committee on Infectious Diseases,* 27th ed. Elk Grove Village, IL, American Academy of Pediatrics, 2006.

Chernick V, Boat T, Wilmott R, et al.: *Kendig's Disorders of the Respiratory Tract in Children,* 7th ed. Philadelphia, WB Saunders, 2006.

Loughlin GM, Eigen H: *Respiratory Disease in Children: Diagnosis and Management.* Baltimore, Williams & Wilkins, 1994.

NAEPP Expert Panel Report: Guidelines for the Diagnosis and Management of Asthma—Update on Selected Topics 2002. Publication No. 02-5074, Bethesda, MD, 2002.

National Heart, Lung and Blood Institute, National Institutes of Health: National Asthma Education and Prevention Program Expert Panel Report 2: Guidelines for the Diagnosis and Management of Asthma. Publication No. 97-4051, Bethesda, MD, 1997.

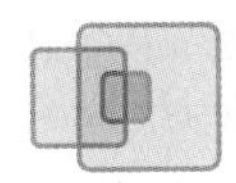

Study Questions

Directions: *Each of the numbered items or incomplete statements in this section is followed by answers or completions of the statement. Select the ONE lettered answer or completion that is BEST in each case.*

1. A 6-week-old infant has a history of noisy breathing. The noise was first noted shortly after birth, is inspiratory in nature, is worse now that the infant has a viral respiratory illness, and remits almost completely when the child is asleep. Which of the following is the most likely etiology of this child's noisy breathing?

A Asthma
B Bronchopulmonary dysplasia
C Cystic fibrosis
D Laryngomalacia
E Tuberculosis

2. A 3-year-old girl has a history of recurrent pneumonia. On physical examination, wheezing and crackles are heard, and digital clubbing is evident. Which of the following is the most likely diagnosis for this child?

A Asthma
B Bronchopulmonary dysplasia
C Cystic fibrosis
D Pulmonary embolus
E Tracheoesophageal fistula

3. A 2-month-old with bronchopulmonary dysplasia is described as irritable and feeding poorly. His weight has decreased since his visit 3 weeks ago. Physical exam findings are sleeping respiratory rate of 80 breaths per minute and clear breath sounds on auscultation. Oxygen saturation on room air is 89%. Which of the following is the most appropriate therapy?

A Administer albuterol 2.5 mg aerosol × 3
B Give supplemental oxygen to maintain oxygen saturation > 92%
C Give furosemide 1 mg/kg orally
D Increase the caloric density of the infant's formula
E Start a 5-day course of prednisolone 1 mg/kg daily

4. A 15-year-old adolescent who has asthma wakes up in the middle of the night with an acute asthma attack. He comes to the emergency room for therapy. On physical examination he is afebrile and has a normal respiratory rate, but is noted to be wheezing. His peak expiratory flow rate is 70% of predicted. Which of the following is the most appropriate inhaled therapy to administer?

A Albuterol 5 mg
B Budesonide 200 μg
C Ipratropium bromide 2 mg
D Levalbuterol 320 μg
E Salmeterol 100 μg

Directions: *Each set of matching questions in this section consists of a list of 4 to 6 lettered options followed by several numbered items. For each numbered item, select the ONE lettered option that is most closely associated with it. Each lettered option may be selected once, more than once, or not at all.*

QUESTIONS 5–9

For each patient who requires investigation of a pulmonary problem, select the appropriate imaging study

- A Chest radiography
- B Chest computed tomography
- C Barium swallow
- D Chest ultrasonography

5. To evaluate an infant who has apnea

6. To rule out the diagnosis of diaphragmatic paralysis in a child

7. To evaluate a child who has chronic cough and wheezing

8. To differentiate a mediastinal mass lesion from a collapsed lung in a child

9. To guide needle thoracentesis to sample a pleural effusion in a child

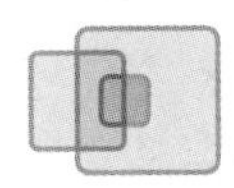

Answers and Explanations

1. The answer is D (*VIII A*). This infant's history and physical examination demonstrate stridor, which is inspiratory and is sensitive to changes in airflow. Of the causes of stridor in children, laryngomalacia is the most common.

2. The answer is C (*IV D 4 a*). In children who have a history of pulmonary disease, the presence of digital clubbing suggests cystic fibrosis until proved otherwise. Asthma, pulmonary sequestration, laryngomalacia, and bronchopulmonary dysplasia are not usually associated with clubbing.

3. The answer is B (*V F 1*). Maintaining an adequate level of oxygenation is critical to the overall health and growth of an infant with bronchopulmonary dysplasia. The tachypnea, irritability, poor feeding, and weight loss are due to hypoxemia. Although airway edema and inflammation contribute to airway obstruction, there is no evidence of an acute exacerbation that would warrant dosing with diuretic, bronchodilating, or corticosteroid therapy. Increasing the caloric density of the formula should be considered after the hypoxemia is corrected.

4. The answer is A (*III H 1 a*). Emergency management of acute asthma should focus on aggressive use of bronchodilating therapy. Based on his age and presumed weight, the dose of albuterol 5 mg would be appropriate as initial therapy. The appropriate dose of levalbuterol recommended is 630 μg (0.63 mg). Ipratropium bromide can be added early in emergency management at a dose of 0.5 mg per treatment. Salmeterol is a long-acting bronchodilator with delayed onset of activity and is not recommended for use in acute asthma.

5–9. The answers are 5-C, 6-D, 7-A, 8-B, and 9-D (*I B 3 a*). A barium swallow or gastrointestinal pH probe may be useful in evaluating the possibility of gastrointestinal reflux as a cause of apnea in an infant. Chest ultrasonography is useful for evaluating diaphragmatic motility. It also can be used to distinguish pleural effusion from adjacent lung and to guide needle thoracentesis. With chest ultrasonography, the high levels of radiation exposure associated with chest fluoroscopy are avoided. Chest radiography is indicated in the evaluation of a child who has chronic cough and wheezing in order to rule out chronic pneumonia, atelectasis, and hyperinflated lungs. In a child who has asthma, increased peribronchial lung markings and air trapping are signs of chronic, poorly treated disease. Computed tomography (CT) scanning of the chest helps to differentiate among pulmonary lesions of differing radiographic densities that cannot be distinguished on chest radiograph (e.g., a collapsed lung vs. a mediastinal tumor). CT scanning of the chest is also useful in determining the extent of pulmonary cysts and in detecting signs of bronchiectasis.

chapter **14**

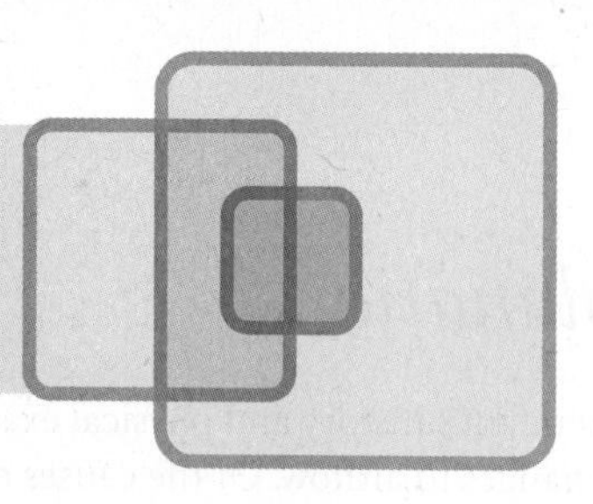

Renal Diseases

THOMAS L. KENNEDY

I GENERAL PRINCIPLES OF RENAL DISEASE IN CHILDREN

A Introduction Renal disease and dysfunction are generally considered in terms of the kidney's role in filtration, clearance, and excretion of nitrogenous waste. Equally important considerations, however, are the kidney's roles in fluid and electrolyte balance, blood pressure regulation, and acid-base homeostasis, and as an endocrine organ elaborating many hormones including erythropoietin, prostaglandins, renin, kinins, and vitamin D's most active metabolite. Other important and unique aspects of renal disease in childhood are the limitations of normal function that exist at birth and the growth and maturational changes that occur through infancy and childhood, as well as congenital anomalies of the kidney and urinary tract.

B Evaluation of renal function

1. **Urinalysis,** although not totally specific or sensitive, is a useful, noninvasive indicator of renal function and disease. Urine bags can be used to collect urine in small infants, although they should never be used to obtain a culture.
   a. **Urine concentration** and **dilution** can be measured by specific gravity or osmolality. Specific gravity is best determined using a refractometer, which requires only a drop of urine. Also, dipsticks roughly estimate specific gravity. Although in general it correlates well with urine osmolality, urine specific gravity measures the density of the solution and is disproportionately increased by high-molecular-weight substances, including protein, glucose, mannitol, and intravenous contrast agents.
      (1) Maximally diluted urine has a specific gravity of 1.002 (osmolality of 50 mOsm/kg).
      (2) Maximally concentrated urine has a specific gravity of 1.035 (osmolality of 1200 mOsm/kg).
      (3) Urine that is neither diluted nor concentrated (isosthenuria) has a specific gravity of 1.010 (osmolality of 300 mOsm/kg).
   b. **Urine dipsticks**
      (1) The dipstick provides a general estimate of **acidity (pH)** and detects **albumin, glucose, ketones, urobilinogen, bilirubin, blood** (including free hemoglobin or myoglobin), white blood cells (pyuria), and Gram-negative infection.
   c. **Urine microscopy.** A freshly voided urine specimen is centrifuged, and the sediment is examined for **bacteria, cells, casts,** and **crystals.**
      (1) **Bacteria.** It is difficult to distinguish infecting organisms from amorphous material (e.g., phosphates, urates) in the unstained sediment. A careful **Gram stain,** however, may help to identify bacteria. Also, pyuria is not a reliable indicator of infection because significant bacteriuria may occur in the absence of leukocytes, and pyuria may occur with acute illness in the absence of infection. Therefore, a **culture** must be obtained to confirm the diagnosis of a urinary tract infection and establish the antimicrobial sensitivities.
      (2) **Cells.** The **morphology** of red blood cells (RBCs) in urine may help to distinguish glomerular bleeding from blood loss elsewhere in the urinary tract. Crenated, dysmorphic RBCs in fresh urine suggest a glomerular origin.
      (3) **Casts** of compacted red blood cells extracted from the tubular lumen **(RBC casts)** are the result of glomerular bleeding and are usually diagnostic of glomerulonephritis. **Leukocyte casts** are occasionally seen in pyelonephritis and interstitial nephritis. **Hyaline**

casts and **granular casts** are not diagnostic of renal disease and may occur in the sediment of children who have oliguria of any cause.

(4) **Crystals** of many varieties may be present in the urine. They are rarely diagnostic of disease. In fact, they reflect factors such as the amount and concentration of solute and solubilizers as well as urinary pH and osmolarity. An exception is the hexagonal **cystine** crystal, which is diagnostic of cystinuria.

2. **Tests of glomerular function** have traditionally used timed urine collections. Ideally, urine should be collected over 24 hours, but 8- to 12-hour collections are usually acceptable for small children.

a. **Glomerular filtration rate (GFR).** Endogenous **creatinine clearance** is usually used to measure GFR; this measurement is accurate unless the GFR is very low (< 20 mL/minute), where it overestimates GFR because of a small component of tubular secretion.

(1) The **normal GFR** in children 2 years of age or older is 120 mL/minute/1.73 m^2 (range: 80–140 mL/minute/1.73 m^2).

(2) Because timed urine collections are frequently difficult to obtain (e.g., in an infant or toddler), GFR can be estimated as follows:

$$CC = \frac{K\ (\text{height in cm})}{\text{serum creatinine (mg/dL)}}$$

where CC = creatinine clearance and K = 0.45 in infants younger than 1 year of age, 0.55 in infants/ children older than 1 year of age, 0.33 in low-birth-weight infants, and 0.7 in adolescent boys.

(3) Because it is produced and excreted in a smooth and consistent manner, creatinine should be measured to verify the accuracy of any timed urine collection. Young children should excrete at least 10 mg/kg/day, and older children and adolescents should excrete 15 to 20 mg/kg/day (females) and 20 to 25 mg/kg/day (males).

b. **Urinary protein excretion**

(1) **Total urinary protein** should be < 150 mg/24 hours, or < 4 mg/m^2/hour. Random urine specimens expressing the protein-to-creatinine ratio may be used to accurately estimate proteinuria.

(2) **Protein-to-creatinine ratio** should be < 0.2 to 0.3. A ratio exceeding 2.0 to 3.0 suggests the heavy proteinuria that defines the nephrotic syndrome.

3. **Tests of renal tubular function**

a. **Concentrating, diluting,** and **acidifying capacity.** Useful information is provided by tests that determine the kidney's capacity to concentrate, dilute, and acidify the urine. Renal concentrating capacity is accomplished by a well-monitored overnight fluid deprivation test, with serial determinations of body weight, serum osmolality, urine flow rate, and urine specific gravity. Dilution is determined by water loading. Urinary acidification is assessed by urine pH in the presence of metabolic acidosis.

b. **Reabsorptive capacity**

(1) **Tubular dysfunction** is suggested by **detection of compounds in the urine that are normally reabsorbed completely by the renal tubules.** Such substances include glucose, amino acids, β_2-microglobulin, and many others.

(2) The **tubular reabsorption of phosphate (TRP)** can be calculated using a small serum sample and random urine specimen. The TRP is normally > 80% to 85%. It is determined as:

$$TRP = 1 - (\text{urine phosphate} \times \text{serum creatinine/serum phosphate} \times \text{urine creatinine}) \times 100\%$$

4. **Tests of bladder function** and **anatomy**

a. **Cystometry.** Bladder function can be assessed using the urodynamic test, cystometry. Because this procedure is invasive (use of catheters, rectal pressure balloons, and needle electrodes), and because it requires patient cooperation, cystometry is not used frequently in children. It is indicated in the evaluation of voiding difficulty (e.g., overflow incontinence, urine retention) or urinary incontinence with a suspected neurologic cause. The test provides a profile of intravesical volume, pressure, and contractility. Pediatric-sized ultrasound bladder scanners help in the assessment of a child with possible residual urine.

b. Cystoscopy is the most direct method of visualizing the urethra and bladder. Because cystoscopy is invasive, requires general anesthesia, and adds little to other imaging techniques, it has limited usefulness in children. Indications include preoperative evaluation of vesicoureteral reflux, investigation of congenital bladder anomalies, and suspicion of bladder neoplasia.

5. Imaging procedures

a. Ultrasonography is the least invasive and most useful renal **anatomic imaging** technique for children. However, it cannot assess renal function and cannot accurately detect mild renal scarring.

(1) Ultrasonography provides information on kidney location, size, shape, and echogenicity.

(a) Serial studies are useful for evaluating renal growth and scarring.

(b) Ultrasonography can be used to diagnose obstruction, malformations, cysts, calcifications, and tumors.

(2) Ultrasonography is safe, and, because the equipment is portable, it can be performed on the most critically ill of patients.

(3) When combined with color Doppler imaging, blood flow velocity in the renal artery and renal vein can be evaluated, as well as urine flow in the ureters.

b. Retrograde voiding cystourethrography (VCUG). In this procedure, the contrast material is instilled by urethral catheter, and the bladder is visualized using fluoroscopy. The test defines the presence and magnitude of vesicoureteral reflux and provides information about the capacity and anatomy of the bladder and urethra, as well as postvoid residual.

c. Radionuclide scanning is a useful test of renal function. Although it involves the intravenous injection of a radiolabeled tracer, radiation exposure is low.

(1) **Evaluation of renal function.** Renal scanning can provide an estimate of total renal function, including GFR (with the use of technetium 99m [Tc 99m]-labeled diethylenetriamine penta-acetic acid) as well as tubular function (with the use of mercaptoacetyltriglycine [MAG_3]). Renal scanning can also quantitate the contribution of each renal unit to total function.

(2) **Evaluation of vesicoureteral reflux.** Radionuclide scanning can be used to provide cystograms in the assessment of vesicoureteral reflux.

(a) For cystography alone, the tracer is instilled directly into the bladder by catheter. For cystography in conjunction with a renal scan, the nuclide MAG_3 is given by intravenous injection to a child who is able to cooperate by storing urine until instructed to void.

(b) The major **advantage** of radionuclide cystography over standard radiographic cystography is the much lower radiation dose. This is important because the child who has reflux frequently needs one or more repeat studies.

(c) The major **disadvantages** of radionuclide cystography are its relatively poor structural delineation and its inability to evaluate the urethra. For these reasons, a radiographic VCUG is initially recommended, with follow-up studies done by radionuclide cystography.

(3) **Evaluation of kidney infection.** Tc 99m-labeled dimercaptosuccinic acid (DMSA), a radionuclide that localizes to tubular cells of functioning nephrons, is very valuable as an aid in the diagnosis of renal parenchymal infection and scarring by demonstrating focal areas of decreased uptake.

d. Other renal imaging techniques

(1) **Computed tomography** (CT) can be used to evaluate tumors, calcification of the renal parenchyma, nephrolithiasis, trauma, or perinephric abscess. Its main disadvantage is relatively high radiation exposure.

(2) **Arteriography** is the definitive study to evaluate for renal artery narrowing and vascular malformations. The ability to achieve selective renal artery catheterization and fully visualize the renal arterial distribution may be limited in small infants.

(3) **Magnetic resonance imaging (MRI)** is used as an adjunct in tumor evaluation. When administered with contrast (magnetic resonance angiography [MRA]), it is useful in evaluation of vasculitis.

6. **Renal biopsy** is the definitive study for **histologic diagnosis** of renal disease. It provides tissue for examination by light, immunofluorescence, and electron microscopy.

a. **Procedure.** Renal biopsy is usually performed as a percutaneous procedure under ultrasonic guidance. In infants, renal biopsy is most safely carried out under general anesthesia. For older patients, moderate sedation and analgesia are adequate.

b. **Risks and contraindications.** The risks of the procedure include obtaining insufficient tissue for diagnosis, causing bleeding or infection, and creating an arteriovenous fistula within the kidney. Contraindications to a percutaneous biopsy include bleeding disorders and the presence of a single kidney.

c. **Indications.** Renal biopsy is not commonly indicated and is reserved for situations where there is significant uncertainty regarding issues of prognosis and therapeutic intervention.

C Common presenting signs of renal disease

1. **Hematuria** (blood in the urine) may be gross (macroscopic) or microscopic.

a. **Causes.** Virtually any congenital anomaly, injury, or inflammatory disease of the kidney or urinary tract may cause hematuria.

(1) Isolated microscopic hematuria is relatively common and is usually not indicative of serious renal disease. Most cases are idiopathic. However, when microscopic hematuria occurs in association with proteinuria, it is more likely to be a sign of significant disease.

(2) A common cause of microscopic hematuria in childhood is **idiopathic hypercalciuria,** which may be documented by a timed urine collection (normal urine calcium is < 4 mg/kg/day) or a random urine sample for calcium-to-creatinine ratio (normally < 0.2) in children older than 6 years old.

(3) Isolated hematuria rarely indicates a bleeding disorder or coagulopathy.

b. **Evaluation**

(1) **Microscopic examination** of a fresh urine specimen is essential in evaluating a child with hematuria detected by dipstick. Microscopic hematuria is significant if it is persistent and there are more than 5 to 10 RBCs per high-powered field. Urine that is brown or tea-colored suggests glomerular bleeding; more specific indicators are the presence of misshapen, dysmorphic red blood cells (best seen using phase contrast microscopy) or RBC casts.

(2) Persistent, unexplained microscopic hematuria for longer than 6 to 12 months or a single episode of gross hematuria should be evaluated by **ultrasonography** to exclude abnormalities such as obstruction, renal cysts, or calcifications.

2. **Proteinuria** refers to protein, generally albumin, in the urine.

a. Causes

(1) Asymptomatic proteinuria, discovered in a random urine specimen, is most commonly the result of protein excreted when the patient is ambulatory and active. This **postural or orthostatic proteinuria** occurs in 5% to 10% of adolescents and young adults. It is less common in younger children.

(a) Because postural proteinuria disappears when the patient is recumbent, it is identified by comparing the first morning urine with urine obtained later in the day.

(b) Although isolated postural proteinuria is almost always a harmless finding, patients who have significant renal disease may also show increased proteinuria when ambulatory. Therefore, adolescents with orthostatic proteinuria should be followed for several years.

(2) Heavy proteinuria indicates **glomerulopathy.** Proteinuria that exceeds 960 mg/m^2/day defines the protein loss associated with nephrotic syndrome.

b. **Evaluation.** The **urine dipstick** is specific for albumin and does not detect tubular glycoproteins or globulins. **Sulfosalicylic acid precipitation and urine protein immunoelectrophoresis** are seldom-used tests that estimate total urinary protein.

3. **Oliguria** is defined as urine output < 300 $mL/m^2/day$ (urine volume insufficient to excrete even a minimal renal solute load in maximally concentrated urine). In a child receiving intravenous fluids, oliguria generally translates to urine flow < 1 mL/kg/hour in infants and < 0.5 mL/kg/hour in older children.
   a. **Causes.** Oliguria is frequently a manifestation of **acute renal failure,** but it may also occur as an appropriate renal response to **hypovolemia** and **hypotension (prerenal oliguria).**
   b. **Evaluation**
      (1) Differentiation of oliguric renal failure from prerenal oliguria (appropriate renal salt and water retention as a result of decreased renal perfusion) is often evident from the **history** and **physical examination.**
      (2) When volume depletion is suspected, differentiation is aided by response to an adequate **fluid challenge** with an intravascular volume expander, such as isotonic saline infusion (20 mL/kg given over 30 minutes). Repeat boluses may be indicated after the patient is carefully assessed.
      (3) **Laboratory tests,** in addition to urine specific gravity, may also help to differentiate prerenal oliguria from renal failure.
         (a) The **blood urea nitrogen (BUN)-to-serum creatinine ratio** may be elevated (the normal ratio is 10:1 to 20:1; in prerenal oliguria the ratio exceeds 40:1) because urea is reabsorbed with water in prerenal states.
         (b) Also helpful is a **random urine sodium concentration,** which is very low (< 20 mEq/L) in prerenal oliguria but usually high (> 50 mEq/L) in renal failure.
         (c) Likewise, the **fractional excretion of sodium (FENa)** is low (< 1%) in prerenal oliguria and higher (> 3%) in renal failure. The FENa is determined as follows:

$$\text{FENa} = \frac{\text{urine sodium} \times \text{serum creatinine}}{\text{urine creatine} \times \text{serum sodium}} \times 100\%$$

4. **Polyuria** (excessive urine output) usually causes thirst and therefore is accompanied by **polydipsia** (excessive fluid intake). When free access to fluids is not possible, as with infants or the vomiting child, polyuria may contribute to dehydration and electrolyte disturbances.
   a. **Causes** (Table 14-1; see also Chapter 17). Polyuria most commonly is caused by disorders of renal concentrating ability or by the use of diuretics, although it occasionally results from an abnormal desire for fluids **(psychogenic polydipsia).**
   b. **Evaluation** of polyuria involves a **fluid deprivation test** under close supervision in the hospital. Serum osmolarity, urine osmolarity, and body weight are monitored.
      (1) Failure to achieve an adequate increase in urine osmolarity (> 750 mOsm/L) indicates a concentrating defect (e.g., maximum urinary concentration should occur with a serum osmolality exceeding 300 or with an acute 3% weight loss).

TABLE 14-1 Causes of Polyuria

Central diabetes insipidus (ADH deficiency)
Complete or partial ADH deficiency
Congenital or acquired ADH deficiency
Nephrogenic diabetes insipidus (ADH resistant)
Inherited vs. acquired (e.g., sickle cell disease, interstitial nephritis, hypokalemia)
Diuretic-induced polyuria
Osmotic agents (glucose, mannitol)
Volume expansion (intravenous fluids, resolution of acute renal failure)
Diuretic agents (furosemide)
Abnormal fluid ingestion (psychogenic polydipsia)

ADH, antidiuretic hormone (vasopressin).

(2) The defect can be further categorized as vasopressin deficient or vasopressin resistant by the response to administration of vasopressin (also called antidiuretic hormone), or its analogue, desmopressin.

II NEPHROTIC SYNDROME

A General considerations

1. **Definition.** Nephrotic syndrome is characterized by heavy **proteinuria** (urinary protein excretion exceeding 960 mg/m^2/day). This leads to hypoalbuminemia, edema, and hyperlipidemia. Nephrotic syndrome is not a single disease entity. It may accompany any glomerular disease or injury.
2. **Pathogenesis.** Nephrotic syndrome develops when the glomerular basement membrane shows a marked, prolonged increase in permeability to anionically charged plasma proteins, mainly albumin. The underlying pathogenesis is unknown, but evidence strongly supports the importance of immune mechanisms.

B **Minimal change nephrotic syndrome** is so named because the histologic changes visible on electron microscopy are limited to effacement of epithelial foot processes.

1. **Incidence** and **etiology.** Although uncommon, minimal change disease accounts for 80% of all cases of nephrotic syndrome in children. It occurs at all ages, but most commonly between 2 and 5 years of age. The cause is unknown.
2. **Clinical features** and **course**
   a. The affected child usually has edema, which may be generalized and severe. Although frequently asymptomatic, fatigue, anorexia, abdominal pain, diarrhea, infection, and intravascular volume depletion may be present.
   b. Minimal change disease usually has a relapsing course. Acute infections frequently trigger relapses, which may be detected promptly by urine testing for albumin with dipsticks.
3. **Diagnosis.** The typical patient with minimal change disease has normal renal function, normal blood pressure and serum complement levels, and no hematuria, although exceptions are not uncommon.
   a. The best diagnostic indicator of minimal change disease, short of a renal biopsy, is the response to steroid therapy. A full **response to a trial of steroid therapy** leads the clinician to a presumptive diagnosis of minimal change disease.
   b. Table 14-2 lists other tests that are useful in establishing the diagnosis of nephrotic syndrome, excluding other renal disease, and monitoring for complications.
4. **Therapy**
   a. **Steroids. Prednisone** is administered daily, generally for 4 to 8 weeks (2 mg/kg; maximum 60 mg) in the initial episode. Alternate-day therapy is given to minimize steroid side effects and administered as a single, morning dose to mimic endogenous glucocorticoid release. The dose is slowly tapered over many weeks to prevent a rapid recurrence of proteinuria as well as untoward steroid withdrawal effects.
   b. **Alkylating agents.** A child who has minimal change disease who fails to respond to steroids or who manifests intolerable steroid toxicity may be treated successfully with **cyclophosphamide.** Because of its potentially serious side effects, this agent is used only when absolutely necessary.
   c. **Diuretics.** In the acute, edematous phase of minimal change disease, aggressive diuretic therapy may worsen the intravascular volume depletion. However, diuretics do have a role in controlling the edema of chronic nephrotic states when intravascular volume depletion is not present.
   d. **Cyclosporine.** Cyclosporine is effective in inducing remission of nephrotic syndrome for children in whom steroid therapy is contraindicated. Its usefulness is limited by its failure to maintain remission when it is discontinued and potential nephrotoxicity.
   e. **Supportive measures.** Edema is managed by restricting sodium but not fluid intake. Dietary protein intake does not have to be increased above normal recommended levels.

TABLE 14-2 Tests Useful for Evaluating Nephrotic Syndrome

Purpose	Test
Establish the presence of nephrotic syndrome	Timed urinary protein excretion
	Total serum protein
	Serum albumin
	Serum cholesterol and triglycerides
Exclude other renal disease[a]	Kidney function tests
	Blood urea nitrogen
	Serum creatinine
	Creatinine clearance
	Urinalysis (examine for cellular casts)
	Serologic tests
	Complement components C3 and C4
	Total hemolytic complement (CH_{50})
	Antinuclear antibodies
	Hepatitis A, B, and C antigen and antibodies
	HIV screen
	Renal ultrasonography
	Renal biopsy
Monitor for complications (including those related to steroid therapy)	Complete blood count
	Appropriate cultures
	Serum electrolytes, Ca^{H}, phosphate, and Mg^{H}
	Bone densitometry (for steroid-induced demineralization)
	Eye examinations (for steroid-induced cataracts)

HIV, human immunodeficiency virus.
[a]Not all tests are necessary in all children.

Pneumococcal vaccine should be given to lessen the risk of serious infection, ideally when the child is in remission and not taking steroids. Because nephrotic syndrome is a hypercoagulable state, deep venipuncture as well as intravascular volume depletion should be avoided.

5. **Prognosis.** The long-term outlook is good because most cases of minimal change disease eventually remit permanently. The greatest concern is for steroid-related morbidity, especially growth retardation and osteopenia. Controversy surrounds the possibility that minimal change disease may rarely transform to another glomerulopathy, such as focal glomerulosclerosis.

C **Other forms of nephrotic syndrome** (Table 14-3). The remaining 20% of cases of childhood nephrotic syndrome (i.e., those not associated with minimal change disease) occur with primary glomerulopathies, systemic diseases, or secondary to toxic injuries. Accurate diagnosis is based on renal biopsy. These patients are less likely to be steroid responsive and are more apt to develop renal insufficiency than those patients who have minimal change disease.

III GLOMERULOPATHIES

Glomerulopathies are a heterogeneous group of diseases involving the glomerulus, which vary greatly in cause, presentation, course, and outcome. Most are immunologically mediated and are accompanied by varying degrees of hematuria, proteinuria, and azotemia. A large proportion of glomerulopathies are inflammatory and thus are referred to as **glomerulonephritis.**

TABLE 14-3 Representative Causes of Childhood Nephrotic Syndrome

Representative Causes of Childhood Nephrotic Syndrome
Primary Nephrotic Syndrome
Without glomerulonephritis
Minimal change disease
Focal segmental glomerulosclerosis
Congenital nephrotic syndrome
With glomerulonephritis
Mesangial proliferative glomerulonephritis
Membranoproliferative glomerulonephritis
Membranous nephropathy
IgA nephropathy
Acute postinfectious glomerulonephritis
Systemic Diseases Associated with Nephrotic Syndrome
Infections
Viral (e.g., HIV, hepatitis B or C, cytomegalovirus, and Epstein-Barr virus infections)
Bacterial (e.g., subacute bacterial endocarditis, shunt nephritis)
Parasitic (e.g., malaria)
Malignant diseases
Lymphoma and leukemia
Solid tumors (e.g., Wilms tumor, carcinomas)
Metabolic diseases
Diabetes mellitus
Hypothyroidism
Inflammatory diseases
Systemic lupus erythematosus
Systemic vasculitis
Henoch-Schönlein purpura
Other disorders
Sickle cell disease
Renal venous thrombosis
Hemolytic-uremic syndrome
Exogenous Agents Associated with Nephrotic Syndrome
Allergens (e.g., pollens, venoms)
Vaccines (e.g., DTP)
Toxic agents (e.g., heavy metals, heroin)
Medications (e.g., captopril, penicillamine)

DTP, diphtheria and tetanus toxoids with pertussis; HIV, human immunodeficiency virus; Ig, immunoglobulin.

A **Postinfectious glomerulonephritis** may follow many viral, bacterial, fungal, and parasitic infections.

1. **Acute poststreptococcal glomerulonephritis**
   a. **Pathogenesis.** This prototype of postinfectious glomerulonephritis is mediated by the inflammatory response to immune complex deposition.
      (1) Glomerulonephritis usually **follows infection with several specific types of streptococci,** the so-called **nephritogenic strains.** There is a latent period of approximately 10 days (range, 1–4 weeks) between the streptococcal illness and the onset of glomerulonephritis. There are no data supporting the concept that appropriate antistreptococcal therapy will prevent the nephritis.
      (2) **Hypocomplementemia** (decreased levels of complement component C3) develops transiently along with the nephritis in 90% of patients. (Other renal diseases associated with hypocomplementemia include membranoproliferative glomerulonephritis and glomerulonephritis that occurs in association with systemic lupus erythematosus, chronic infection, or inherited complement deficiencies.)
   b. **Clinical features** and **course.** The presentation may vary from mild, asymptomatic microscopic hematuria to gross hematuria, nephrotic syndrome, or severe renal failure. The typical

TABLE 14-4 Types of Chronic Childhood Glomerulonephritis

Types	Progression to Chronic Renal Failure	Therapy	Comments
Mesangial proliferative nephritis	Variable	Prednisone	Often steroid dependent or steroid resistant
Membranoproliferative nephritis	Common (decreased with treatment)	Chronic alternate-day prednisone	Three histologic types
Membranous nephritis	Variable	None	Spontaneous remission common; much more common condition in adults
IgA nephritis	Uncommon	Fish oil for heavy proteinuria	Presentation and recurrences associated with acute infections
Henoch-Schönlein nephritis	Uncommon	None	Histologically identical to IgA nephropathy
Rapidly progressive nephritis (crescentic glomerulonephritis)	Common	Intravenous high-dose prednisone	May be idiopathic or associated with other forms of glomerulonephritis
Lupus nephritis	Variable	Prednisone, cyclophosphamide, MMF	Several histologic types
Diabetic nephropathy	Rare in childhood	Preventive (e.g., good glycemic control)	Most common cause of end-stage renal disease in adults with antecedents in childhood
Sickle cell nephropathy	Unusual in childhood	None	Concentrating and acidifying defects most often seen

Ig, immunoglobulin; MMF, mycophenodate mofetil.

affected child has a brief period of brownish urine, a sediment showing RBC casts, and mild renal insufficiency with volume-dependent hypertension and edema. The interval of azotemia (increased BUN) is short, and complete recovery of renal function is the rule. Microscopic hematuria, however, may persist as long as 2 years.

2. **Other infections that may lead to glomerulonephritis** include:
   - **a.** Bacterial (staphylococcal infection)
   - **b.** Viral (hepatitis B, infectious mononucleosis)
   - **c.** Fungal (histoplasmosis)
   - **d.** Parasitic (toxoplasmosis, falciparum malaria)

B Table 14-4 lists other forms of glomerulopathies that occur in childhood. None is commonly seen. All may be associated with the nephrotic syndrome.

IV URINARY TRACT INFECTION

A Incidence Urinary tract infection is common in infants and children. In newborns, it is twice as common in boys, but in childhood, it is ten times more common in girls. Approximately 5% to 10% of school-age girls will have a urinary tract infection, and up to 60% of these patients experience a recurrence.

B Localization A urinary tract infection is frequently classified based on involvement of the renal parenchyma **(pyelonephritis)** or the bladder **(cystitis).** Because no laboratory study can conclusively localize the infection, diagnosis is usually based on clinical findings (Table 14-5). Unfortunately, the

TABLE 14-5 Clues to the Localization of Urinary Tract Infections

Sign or Symptom	Pyelonephritis	Cystitis
Fever > 39°C (~102°F)	Common	Very unusual
Constitutional symptoms	Common (anorexia, vomiting, abdominal pain)	Unusual
Leukocytosis	WBC frequently > 20,000	WBC usually normal
Elevated erythrocyte sedimentation rate	Virtually always	Unusual
Dysuria, frequency, urgency	Variable	Common
Abnormal DMSA radionuclide scan	Areas of decreased uptake	Normal
Flank pain and costovertebral angle tenderness	Common (except in infants)	Absent

DMSA, dimercaptosuccinic acid; WBC, white blood cell.

symptoms of a urinary tract infection in infants and young children are frequently nonspecific and vague. Urinary tract infection is present in 5% to 10% of febrile infants with no obvious source. Thus, a high index of suspicion is important.

C Etiology and pathogenesis

1. **Role of fecal flora.** In virtually all cases, a urinary tract infection results from fecal flora, especially coliform bacteria that ascend the urethra to the bladder (Table 14-6). Factors important to the development of urinary tract infection include the ability of organisms to adhere to the urinary epithelium, surface immunoglobulins, completeness and frequency of bladder emptying, and urine pH. Pyelonephritis implies that organisms have ascended the ureters, as can occur in vesicoureteral reflux (retrograde flow of urine up the ureters from the bladder).
2. **Vesicoureteral reflux** (VUR) is present in 35% of children who have a urinary tract infection; this condition is much less common in the general population, but the precise incidence at various ages is unknown. A causal relationship between VUR and urinary tract infection is uncertain, but VUR definitely increases the risk of pyelonephritis.
   a. VUR results either from a congenitally abnormal insertion of the ureter into the bladder or dysfunctional voiding patterns. Mild VUR may occur transiently with urinary tract infection and resolve when the infection is treated.
   b. **Renal scarring** is found in 50% of children who have VUR and infection. Scarring most likely results from reflux of infected urine into the renal parenchyma **(intrarenal reflux).** In most cases, scarring occurs before age 4 years, which indicates the need for prompt diagnosis and treatment of urinary tract infection in infants. It is not known if VUR, in the absence of infection or obstruction, can injure the kidney.

TABLE 14-6 Organisms Causing Urinary Tract Infections in Infants and Children

Organism	Comments
Gram-Negative Organisms	
Escherichia coli	Accounts for 80% of urinary tract infections
Proteus species	Urea splitters; urine often has a high pH
Klebsiella	More common following recent use of antibiotics
Haemophilus influenzae	Uncommon; does not grow well on usual media
Pseudomonas species	Urinary tract anomalies (e.g., duplication, obstruction) are often a contributing factor
Gram-Positive Organisms	
Staphylococcus saprophyticus	Common cause in adolescents
Enterococcus species	As with other Gram-positive organisms, does not convert nitrates to nitrites
Group B *Streptococcus*	Unusual

D Clinical features Recognizing urinary tract infection in children, particularly infants, may be difficult. The classic symptoms of cystitis (i.e., dysuria, urgency, frequency) are often absent, as are the flank pains and shaking chills associated with pyelonephritis in adults. Children with urinary tract infection may have unexplained fever, failure to thrive, vague gastrointestinal and abdominal complaints, and enuresis.

E Diagnosis

1. **Urine culture.** The diagnosis must be based on culture results, not on symptoms or urinalysis. Urine cultures should be obtained only in children in whom urinary tract infection is suspected, not as a screen in asymptomatic individuals. Reliable urine screening culture kits are available in outpatient settings.
   a. **Definitive results.** A count of 10^5 colony-forming units per milliliter for a single organism usually is accepted as proof of infection, although counts of 5×10^4 or less should not be discounted as contaminants, particularly in newborns.
   b. **Methods of urine collection**
      (1) **Clean-catch,** midstream samples are reliable and are acceptable in toilet-trained children.
      (2) **Catheterization** and **suprapubic aspiration** are more specific means of obtaining samples, but these methods may cause discomfort and involve minimal risk. They are the methods of choice in infants.
   c. **Repeat culture** is required if symptoms do not improve within 48 to 72 hours of initiating antimicrobial therapy.
   d. **Follow-up culture,** if obtained, should be delayed at least 72 hours after completion of antimicrobial therapy.
2. **Urinary white blood cells.** Pyuria is neither a sensitive nor specific sign of urinary tract infection.
3. **Imaging** is indicated for all culture-documented first urinary tract infections in all children younger than 2 years of age, in all boys and girls who have parenchymal infection, and in all children in whom localization of the infection is in doubt. Uncomplicated cystitis in school-age girls does not require radiologic evaluation if follow-up is ensured.
   a. **Ultrasonography** should be performed to look for obstruction or urinary tract anomalies. It can be repeated serially to monitor renal growth.
   b. **Voiding cystourethrography** identifies vesicoureteral reflux and establishes the degree of reflux. The optimal time to obtain the cystogram remains unknown, but 4 to 6 weeks after completing treatment is most common.

F Therapy

1. **Uncomplicated cystitis.** Antimicrobial therapy is based on the results of urine culture and sensitivity testing. Usually, 7 to 10 days of therapy is effective and well tolerated. Short-course therapy is established, effective therapy in adults. In children, 3 to 4 days of therapy for lower tract urinary tract infection is sufficient.
2. **Pyelonephritis**
   a. The same drugs used orally for cystitis yield antimicrobial urinary levels that are adequate to treat renal parenchymal infections. Often, however, the child who has pyelonephritis is vomiting and severely ill. Furthermore, until the organism is identified, parenteral broad-spectrum antibiotics may be desirable, and hospitalization for initial parenteral antibiotic and fluid therapy is then indicated.
   b. A single episode of pyelonephritis may be treated with 10 to 14 days of oral therapy.
   c. **Nephronia.** Occasionally, an acute lobar infection may occur in the kidney and be detected on ultrasound as hyper- or hypoechogenic areas. A minority of these focal infections progress to abscess formation.
3. **Preventive therapy**
   a. **Risk factors** for urinary tract infections should be **investigated** and **eliminated.** These factors include:
      (1) **Congenital anomalies of the urinary tract** (e.g., diverticula of the bladder)
      (2) **Conditions associated with incomplete emptying of the bladder.** Prominent among them are chronic constipation and dysfunctional voiding patterns, especially those associated with urinary incontinence.

(3) **Habits that lead to chronic infection or irritation of the perineal area** (e.g., bubble baths, wiping "back to front")

(4) There is a 30% to 40% risk for VUR in siblings of a child who has reflux. Families and physicians should be aware of this risk and obtain urine cultures promptly when these siblings develop fever. Routine VCUGs performed on all siblings of a child with VUR are not recommended.

(5) The risk for **uncircumcised males** is controversial. Although their risk of urinary tract infection is approximately ten times higher, urinary tract infection is still so uncommon that 99 circumcisions must be performed to prevent one urinary tract infection.

(6) Other risk factors are sexual activity and immunocompromised states.

b. The child who has vesicoureteral reflux, other urinary tract anomalies, or a recurrent urinary tract infection requires **continuous antimicrobial therapy.** A single daily low dose of nitrofurantoin is effective and well tolerated. Alternate-day therapy with trimethoprim-sulfamethoxazole is also effective.

G Complications and prognosis Although urinary tract infection is frequently recurrent, the risk of progression to chronic renal insufficiency, even with pyelonephritis, is very low (estimated to be $<$ 1 in 10,000 in the United States).

1. **Hypertension** is the most common long-term sequela of recurrent pyelonephritis.
2. **Renal scarring** can also result from pyelonephritis.
   - **a.** Renal scarring occurs in infants and young children; it uncommonly develops in older children and adults. The variability in progression of renal scars is immunologically mediated and not completely understood.
   - **b.** Renal scarring is frequently focal, and hypertrophy of normal surrounding renal tissue maintains normal overall function.
3. **Severe vesicoureteral reflux.** Most VUR in childhood resolves spontaneously, but severe reflux (e.g., reflux with marked dilatation of the ureters, the renal pelvis, or both) may require surgery to reimplant the ureter (**ureteroneocystostomy**). However, there is no evidence that surgery alters renal function outcome. Serial cystograms, preferably with radionuclides, are obtained every 18 to 24 months to monitor the resolution of vesicoureteral reflux. Antimicrobial prophylaxis should be continued as long as reflux is present.

V HYPERTENSION

A Definition and incidence

1. **Definition.** Hypertension in childhood is defined as a blood pressure reading greater than the 95th percentile for age obtained on at least three separate occasions. Approximately 1% of the pediatric population and 3% of adolescents are hypertensive by this definition.
2. **Blood pressure norms.** Figure 14-1 shows age-specific percentiles of blood pressure measurements in boys and girls, 1 to 13 years of age. Blood pressure values progressively increase from infancy to adolescence. A "normal value" does not imply freedom from the long-term risk of cardiovascular disease and therefore is not necessarily a "healthy value." Blood pressure normal values are more relevant when expressed in terms of body mass index (kg/m^2) or height rather than age.
3. Blood pressures should be obtained routinely in children ages 3 and older, because early recognition and therapy of hypertension will prevent long-term sequelae. However, it remains uncertain how well early childhood blood pressure ultimately correlates with adult levels or predicts later hypertension. Hypertension is classified as prehypertension (90th–95th percentile or readings in the 120s/80s at any age), stage I (95th–99th percentile), and stage 2 ($>$ 99th percentile + 5 mm Hg).

B Etiology

1. **Primary hypertension** (also called **idiopathic** or **essential hypertension**) is the most common form of hypertension (as defined earlier) in childhood. As in adults, primary hypertension is a heterogeneous group of disorders. The blood pressure elevation is usually mild to moderate and asymptomatic. If sustained for long periods, it becomes an important risk factor in the develop-

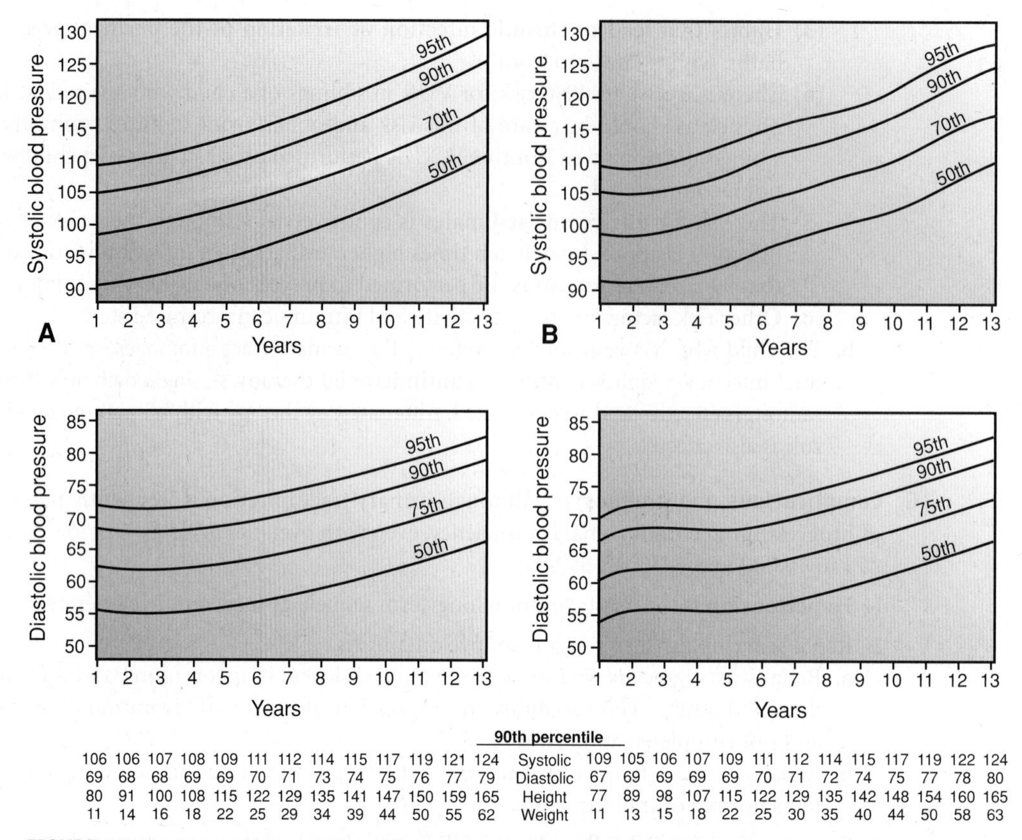

													90th percentile													
106	106	107	108	109	111	112	114	115	117	119	121	124	Systolic	109	105	106	107	109	111	112	114	115	117	119	122	124
69	68	68	69	69	70	71	73	74	75	76	77	79	Diastolic	67	69	69	69	69	70	71	72	74	75	77	78	80
80	91	100	108	115	122	129	135	141	147	150	159	165	Height	77	89	98	107	115	122	129	135	142	148	154	160	165
11	14	16	18	22	25	29	34	39	44	50	55	62	Weight	11	13	15	18	22	25	30	35	40	44	50	58	63

FIGURE 14-1 Age-specific percentiles of blood pressure measurements in **(A)** boys and **(B)** girls, 1 to 13 years of age; Korotkoff phase IV sounds were used for determining diastolic blood pressure. Height is measured in centimeters, and weight is measured in kilograms.

ment of cardiovascular disease and stroke. Often, a strong family history of high blood pressure exists and is an important risk factor. The risk to the child of one parent who is hypertensive is about 25% and if both parents are hypertensive, the risk rises to almost 50%.

2. **Secondary hypertension**
   a. **Renal disease** is the most common cause of secondary hypertension. Virtually any renal disease, glomerular or interstitial, may be the cause. The hypertension may be transient or sustained and may be out of proportion in severity to the degree of renal insufficiency. Renal hypertension is caused by salt and water retention with volume expansion and/or a renin-mediated increase in vascular resistance.
   b. **Vascular causes** of hypertension (e.g., coarctation of the aorta, renal artery stenosis, renal artery occlusion), although uncommon, are important to identify because they may cause severe, symptomatic hypertension and they may be curable. Anatomic vascular abnormalities are identified by angiography. In addition to vascular narrowing, all forms of vasculitis may be associated with elevated blood pressure (e.g., Henoch-Schönlein purpura) (see Chapter 9).
   c. **Endocrine causes** of hypertension are very uncommon and are conditions associated with excess levels of catecholamines or aldosterone. These include pheochromocytoma, primary or secondary aldosteronism, and congenital adrenal hyperplasia with 11-hydroxylase or 17-hydroxylase deficiency (see also Chapter 17). Diagnosis is based on serum and urine concentrations of catecholamines and their metabolites, aldosterone, and (in the case of congenital adrenal hyperplasia) 17-hydroxysteroids and 17-ketosteroids. Hyperthyroidism may also cause hypertension.
   d. **Neurologic disease** as a cause of hypertension is often hard to document. Increased intracranial pressure and the Guillain-Barré syndrome are well-recognized causes (see also Chapter 18). Conditions such as cerebral palsy and seizure disorders are less definitely associated with

TABLE 14-7 Medications and Illicit Drugs That May Cause Hypertension

Adrenocorticotropic hormone (ACTH)
Corticosteroids (both glucocorticoids and mineralocorticoids)
Amphetamines
Birth control pills
Sympathomimetic agents (including phenylephrine eye drops in young children)
Phencyclidine (PCP, angel dust)
Cocaine

hypertension. In the latter conditions, spasticity and hypertonicity may make accurate blood pressure determination difficult.

e. **Miscellaneous causes**
   (1) **Obesity** is an independent risk factor for blood pressure elevation in children.
   (2) Acute, significant **rises in serum calcium** may increase blood pressure. Hypercalcemia and hypertension may develop in children who are suddenly and completely immobilized.
   (3) Hypertension independent of hypercalcemia may develop in children who are placed in **traction.**
   (4) A variety of **medications** and **illicit drugs** may cause hypertension in some people. Table 14-7 lists agents that may cause hypertension in children and adolescents.
   (5) **Renin-secreting juxtaglomerular tumors** are very rare.

C Diagnosis Most children who have high blood pressure do not need an extensive or invasive evaluation.

1. **Basic evaluation.** The evaluation of any child who has elevated blood pressure should focus on three areas: (a) identification of a secondary cause, (b) identifying risk factors for hypertension and cardiovascular disease (because hypertension is an important risk factor for the latter), and (c) recognizing the complications of hypertension already present.
   a. **History.** Significant items include previous growth and state of health; urinary tract symptoms or infections; medications; tobacco use; dietary intake; level of activity; and family history of hypertension, stroke, or premature cardiovascular disease. Symptoms are usually absent, but if present are nonspecific and may include dizziness, headache, or abdominal pain.
   b. **Physical examination**
      (1) **Blood pressure readings** should be obtained when the heart rate is stable and repeated until values are consistent. This minimizes the child's anxiety and helps eliminate "white coat hypertension." Diastolic values are best expressed by both the phase 4 (muffling) and phase 5 (disappearance) Korotkoff sounds since some children's heart sounds may be heard all the way to "0" (e.g., 90/60/10). Blood pressure readings should be obtained in all extremities, and pulses should be checked.
      (2) **Auscultation** for murmurs and bruits and **funduscopic examination** of retinal vessels are important.
      (3) Erroneously high blood pressure readings are frequently obtained because the **size of the cuff** is too small. An appropriate blood pressure cuff is the largest cuff that comfortably fits around the arm. The inflatable bladder should almost completely encircle the arm. The bladder width should be approximately 40% of the circumference of the arm's midpoint.
      (4) The use of **continuous ambulatory blood pressure monitoring,** employed for many years in hypertensive adults, is now used in pediatrics and may prove valuable, especially in the evaluation of children who have labile hypertension.
   c. **Laboratory studies** should include a urinalysis, serum electrolytes, uric acid, BUN and creatinine, chest radiograph, and an electrocardiogram. There should be strong consideration for an echocardiogram, especially if ventricular hypertrophy is suspected. Total cholesterol and a lipid profile are important indicators of additional risk for cardiovascular disease.

2. **Further evaluation for secondary hypertension** is indicated by findings on the initial evaluation or any of the following:
   a. **Very high blood pressure readings** (e.g., above 120/80 mm Hg in infants, 140/90 mm Hg in children, 160/100 mm Hg in adolescents)
   b. Any level of blood pressure that causes symptoms (e.g., headache, vomiting, signs of congestive heart failure)
   c. Hypertension that is **progressive and severe**
   d. Hypertension that is **refractory to therapy**

D Therapy

1. **Initial therapy** for mild hypertension should be nonpharmacologic, namely, reduction of hypertension risk factors such as salt intake and, if indicated, weight reduction and increased physical activity.
2. **Drug therapy** is given when the preceding measures do not suffice.
   a. **Approach.** Drugs chosen should be those that can be taken infrequently and that will allow an active lifestyle, including competitive sports. The lowest possible effective dose is determined by starting with a small, recommended dose and increasing it until the desired control has been attained or side effects intervene and/or a maximum recommended dose is reached.
   b. **Agents** used most often to treat childhood hypertension are listed in Table 14-8. Many of the newer, more effective agents are not officially approved for pediatric patients, but

TABLE 14-8 Drugs Commonly Used to Treat Childhood Hypertension

Drug	Comments
Diuretics	
Hydrochlorothiazide	Very effective in mild and moderate hypertension; ineffective in patients who have a low GFR; may cause hypokalemia or hyperuricemia
Furosemide	Potent diuretic used to reduce intravascular volume; long-term effectiveness is limited
β-Adrenergic Blockers	
Propranolol	First and most commonly used of a large family of drugs; not β-receptor selective; may cause bronchospasm
Atenolol	Cardioselective; once-daily dosing
Adrenergic Agonist	
Clonidine	Often effective in hypertensive "urgencies"; may be applied to the skin as a patch
α-Adrenergic Blockers	
Prazosin	Infrequently ordered; commonly used with β-adrenergic blocker; well tolerated
Vasodilators	
Hydralazine	Causes salt and water retention and is no longer commonly used; flushing; headache
Minoxidil	Very effective; severe hypertrichosis and fluid retention limit its use
Angiotensin-Converting Enzyme (ACE) Inhibitors	
Captopril	Effective in children who have high renin states; may decrease renal function in renovascular disease; may cause hyperkalemia
Enalapril	Once-daily dosing; may reduce proteinuria
Calcium Channel Blockers	
Nifedipine Amlodipine	Effective; well tolerated; use with caution with other vasodilators
Angiotensin-Receptor Blockers	
Losartan	May be given once a day; antiproteinuric effect

GFR, glomerular filtration rate.

TABLE 14-9 Drugs Used to Treat Childhood Hypertensive Emergencies

Drugs	Comments	Side Effects
Vasodilators		
Nitroprusside	Immediate effect; titrate to desired blood pressure; continuous administration necessary	Hypotension, thiocyanate toxicity
Hydralazine	Administered slowly intravenously; not predictably effective	Headache, nausea
Calcium Channel Blockers[a]		
Nifedipine, isradipine	Administered orally or sublingually; safe and effective	Dizziness, headache
Nicardopine	May be given intravenously	
α-Adrenergic Blockers		
Phentolamine	Used only when pheochromocytoma is suspected	Tachycardia, dysrhythmias
β- and α-Adrenergic Blockers		
Labetalol	Administered intravenously	Bradycardia, bronchospasm

[a]Calcium channel blockers also act through vasodilation.

nevertheless are used by pediatricians who treat hypertension. One practical limitation regarding these medications in small children is the fact that they are unavailable in liquid or appropriate low-dose pill form.

3. **Therapy for secondary hypertension** involves eliminating the cause when possible as well as administering antihypertensive medication to stabilize the blood pressure and the patient. Surgery or angioplasty is indicated for coarctation of the aorta and renal artery stenosis.

E **Hypertensive emergencies** When the blood pressure is severely elevated (e.g., 180/110 mm Hg), producing symptoms, or increasing rapidly, treatment must be given promptly (Table 14-9), and the child must be monitored continuously.

VI FLUID AND ELECTROLYTE DISTURBANCES

Fluid and electrolyte disturbances in children commonly are the result of gastrointestinal illness (i.e., diarrhea, vomiting, or both) and involve some degree of dehydration. Most cases are mild and may be treated with oral fluids. When choosing among the several acceptable approaches to therapy, it is best to keep the approach as simple as possible.

A **Maintenance water** and **electrolyte requirements** (Table 14-10) are the amounts required daily to maintain homeostasis in a person in a resting, basal state.

TABLE 14-10 Daily Maintenance Requirements for Water and Electrolytes

Substance	Requirement/24 Hours
Water	1500 mL/m^{2}[a]
Sodium	2–3 mEq/kg
Potassium	2–3 mEq/kg
Chloride	2–3 mEq/kg

[a]Amount of water is for patients weighing more than 3.4 lb (1.5 kg).

TABLE 14-11 Approximate Composition of Gastrointestinal Fluids[a]

Fluid	Sodium (mEq/L)	Potassium (mEq/L)	Chloride (mEq/L)	Bicarbonate (mEq/L)
Gastric	75	20	100	0
Small intestinal	135	15	100	30
Large intestinal	60	40	80	50
Diarrhea (in infants)	60	45	60	45

[a]These may be quite variable.

1. **Water.** Maintenance water requirements can be calculated as 1500 $mL/m^2/day$ for children weighing more than 1.5 kg. Surface area (SA) may be obtained from a nomogram or calculated as follows:

$$SA = \frac{(4W + 7)}{(W + 90)}$$

where W is the weight in kilograms. More commonly, maintenance water is estimated by body weight:

100 mL/kg for body weight kilograms 1–10
50 mL/kg for body weight kilograms 11–20
20 mL/kg for body weight kilograms > 20

Maintenance water balances the following **natural losses:**

a. **Insensible water loss.** Approximately 40% of maintenance water replaces evaporative, electrolyte-free water lost from the skin and lungs.
b. **Fecal loss.** Approximately 5% to 10% of maintenance water replaces fecal loss.
c. **Urinary loss.** The remaining 50% to 55% of maintenance water replaces urinary water loss. The amount of water lost in the urine is the amount necessary to excrete a basal renal solute load as urine that is neither concentrated nor diluted (i.e., with specific gravity of 1.010).

2. **Electrolytes.** Maintenance electrolytes include sodium, potassium, and chloride; the daily requirements for these are shown in Table 14-10.

B Dehydration states

1. **Etiologic considerations**

a. Dehydration in the pediatric age group is usually the result of **acute gastrointestinal illness,** in which losses from diarrhea, vomiting, or both are combined with inadequate oral fluid intake. The serum electrolyte concentrations in a child who has dehydration reflect the electrolyte composition of the intake and losses. Table 14-11 lists the approximate composition of gastrointestinal fluids. Table 14-12 shows the composition of oral fluids used to treat mild or early cases of gastrointestinal illness.

TABLE 14-12 Composition of Oral Fluids Commonly Used to Treat Gastroenteritis

	Carbohydrate (g/dL)	Sodium (mEq/L)	Potassium (mEq/L)
Pedialyte[a]	2.5	45	20
Gatorade	4.6	23	3
Kool-Aid[b]	10.5	3	0.1
Ginger ale[b]	9.0	3.5	0.1
Rehydralyte[a]	2.5	75	20

[a]Oral rehydration solution.
[b]Not recommended for use.

TABLE 14–13 Signs and Symptoms of Dehydration

Signs	Symptoms
Sunken eyes (if subtle, may be noted only by parents)	Thirst
Dry mucous membranes	Lethargy, irritability
Decreased tears	Decreased urine output
Poor skin turgor	
Postural blood pressure change	
Sunken fontanelle (in quiet, sitting infants)	

b. The increased water requirements induced by various disease states may be exacerbated by such factors as fever, hyperventilation, ambient humidity, sweating, and increased metabolic rate.

2. **Diagnosis.** Table 14-13 lists the signs and symptoms of dehydration.

3. **Types of dehydration.** Although the classification of dehydration states by plasma osmolality is based on serum sodium levels, it is simplest to consider the water deficit and sodium deficit separately.

   a. **Isotonic dehydration.** Net sodium and water losses are proportionate. This form of dehydration is found in approximately 75% of children hospitalized for dehydration.

      (1) Serum sodium values are within the broad range of normal (130–150 mEq/L).

      (2) Although extracellular fluid (ECF) tonicity remains normal, gastrointestinal losses are unevenly hypotonic, and there is a net loss of water from the intracellular fluid (ICF) as well.

   b. **Hypertonic dehydration.** Water is lost in excess of sodium.

      (1) **Hypernatremia** (serum sodium level above 150 mEq/L) results when there is little oral intake, ongoing insensible water loss, and hypotonic diarrheal losses. For example, giving a child with significant diarrhea and little intake due to vomiting a high osmolar, high carbohydrate oral solution can worsen diarrheal water loss and contribute to hypernatremia. Gastrointestinal water loss is increased with intake of relatively high carbohydrate-containing fluid. With hypernatremia, the water loss is primarily from the ICF, and the ECF is relatively well preserved.

      (2) **Signs.** The classic signs of dehydration are frequently diminished. Instead, neurologic signs (e.g., irritability, lethargy, seizures) are prominent, and the skin may feel doughy.

      (3) **Associated abnormalities** include hyperglycemia, metabolic acidosis, and hypocalcemia.

   c. **Hypotonic dehydration.** Sodium is lost in excess of water. A child might be expected to develop hyponatremia if there are large diarrhea losses but significant intake of fluids containing low sodium (e.g., tea).

      (1) **Hyponatremia** is defined by a serum sodium level below 130 mEq/L.

      (2) **Signs**

         (a) Because the losses are mainly from the ECF, the classic signs of dehydration and intravascular volume depletion (i.e., decreased skin turgor, decreased tearing, dry mucous membranes, sunken anterior fontanelle, tachycardia and orthostatic hypotension, low jugular venous pulsation) occur early.

         (b) Neurologic signs, including seizures, may occur and are directly related to both the severity of hyponatremia and the rapidity with which it develops.

      (3) **Associated abnormalities.** The various causes of hyponatremia (Table 14-14) must be considered.

4. **Degree of dehydration**

   a. The extent of dehydration can be estimated from the change in body weight if the prior weight or growth parameters are available. Acute weight loss may be assumed to equal water loss (i.e., 1 g = 1 mL).

   b. Reasonable clinical estimates of dehydration can be made on the basis of history and physical assessment: A loss of 5% generally correlates with subtle evidence of dehydration, a loss of 10% with obvious evidence, and a loss of 15% with signs of severe intravascular deficits or shock.

TABLE 14-14 Causes of Hyponatremia

Pseudohyponatremia	**Dilutional Hyponatremia**
Hyperlipidemia	Hyperglycemia
Hyperproteinemia	Congestive heart failure
Depletional Hyponatremia	Nephrotic syndrome
Gastrointestinal loss	Liver disease
Sweat loss	Water intoxication
Renal loss (adrenal insufficiency, chronic renal insufficiency, diuretics)	SIADH
	Reset osmostat

SIADH, syndrome of inappropriate antidiuretic hormone secretion.

5. **Electrolyte deficits**
   a. **Sodium deficit** occurs in all forms of dehydration, although the deficit is greatest in hyponatremic and smallest in hypernatremic states.
      (1) **Isotonic dehydration.** The losses reflect uneven hypotonic losses, so that the net water deficit from the ICF approximates the loss from the ECF. Therefore, a 1-L deficit in a child who has a normal serum sodium concentration consists of 0.5 L of ECF (sodium, 140 mEq/L) and 0.5 L of ICF (sodium, 5–10 mEq/L).
      (2) **Hypertonic dehydration.** In hypernatremic states, the sodium deficit is smaller because water losses from the ICF, where the sodium content is very low, represent approximately three fourths of the total water loss.
      (3) **Hypotonic dehydration.** In hyponatremic states, ECF losses are accentuated, because the hypotonic ECF causes fluid to shift from the ECF into the ICF.
   b. **Potassium deficit** is difficult to estimate but in general approximates the sodium deficit found in isotonic states. The amount administered is usually limited by the concentration of potassium in intravenous fluids and should not exceed 40 mEq/L when infused into a peripheral vein.
6. **Treatment of dehydration**
   a. **Shock.** When signs of shock are present (e.g., weak, rapid pulse; cool, mottled extremities; delayed capillary refill; hypotension), intravascular volume should be re-expanded promptly without regard to electrolyte status. An isotonic volume expander such as 0.9% (normal) saline is given at 20 mL/kg over 15 to 30 minutes. Further fluid resuscitation is often necessary and should be given as indicated by reassessing the child.
   b. **Isotonic dehydration.** Fluids that correct the deficit and provide daily maintenance requirements are given over 24 hours, with half of the total administered in the first 8 hours. Rehydration may be carried out with either intravenous fluids or oral rehydration solution. However, no matter which method is used, prompt reinstitution of enteral nutrition is important. Treatment of a 10% dehydrated child who weighs 10 kg (when well) and whose surface area is 0.6 m^2 is as follows:
      (1) The child should receive 1 L of water for maintenance (100 mL/kg) and 1 L of water for deficit replacement (10% of 10 kg). The child should also receive 20 to 30 mEq each of sodium and potassium for maintenance and 70 mEq each of these electrolytes for deficit replacement. (The sodium deficit represents the sodium concentration in the 0.5 L of deficit water estimated to come from the ECF. Again, the potassium deficit approximates the sodium deficit.)
      (2) Half of the total, or 1 L, of one-third normal saline in 5% dextrose should be given in the first 8 hours, and the remainder given over the next 16 hours.
      (3) The child must be re-evaluated at regular intervals, with monitoring for sources of ongoing losses (e.g., continued diarrhea).
   c. **Hypertonic dehydration.** To avoid too rapid a reduction in sodium concentration, the deficit amounts should be given slowly and evenly over 48 hours, along with maintenance fluids. The sodium concentration should fall at a rate no greater than ½ mEq/hour or 15 mEq/day.

d. Hypotonic dehydration

(1) The sodium required to convert a hyponatremic dehydrated state to an isonatremic one may be calculated as follows:

$$\text{required Na}^+ \text{ (mEq)} = 0.6 \times \text{body wt (kg)} \times [\text{desired Na}^+ \text{ (mEq/L)} - \text{observed Na}^+ \text{ (mEq/L)}]$$

(2) The total sodium deficit should not be corrected completely because of the risk of neurologic injury, including **central pontine myelinolysis** (the osmotic demyelinization syndrome), which is rare in children.

(a) In general, sodium should be corrected only to a level safe from neurologic manifestations. Generally, a sodium level of 125 mEq/L is reasonable.

(b) When the initial serum sodium level is very low (e.g., < 110 mEq/L), the correction should be more modest (e.g., correct to 115–120 mEq/L).

(c) The correction may be made with 3% saline (1 mL = 0.5 mEq of sodium) given at a rate to increase serum sodium about 2 mEq/L/hour.

(3) Further correction of the dehydration may then proceed as with isotonic dehydration, including administering both maintenance and deficit water and electrolytes.

VII ACID-BASE DISTURBANCES

A Normal acid-base homeostasis

1. Acid-base balance is maintained by the pulmonary excretion of carbon dioxide plus the renal excretion of excess hydrogen ions.
2. Acute changes in acid-base status are prevented by the body's buffer systems. The most important of these in the ECF is bicarbonate because it is plentiful, can be conserved and generated by the kidney, and links the lungs and kidneys by carbonic acid dissociation:

$$CO_2 + H_2O \rightleftharpoons H_2CO_3 \rightleftharpoons H^+ + HCO_3^-$$

3. The growing child excretes approximately 2 to 3 mEq of hydrogen ions per kilogram daily. Most of this net acid is derived from dietary protein. The kidney excretes net acid by acidifying the urine via the following mechanisms:
   a. Reclaiming all filtered bicarbonate
   b. Excreting urinary anions (e.g., phosphate), which combine with hydrogen ions to form titratable acid
   c. Producing ammonia in proximal renal tubular cells, which may bind hydrogen ions to form ammonium ions

B Assessing acid-base status

Measuring a patient's serum electrolytes, blood pH, and blood gases provides the data for determining acid-base status.

1. **Serum electrolyte levels** provide the total carbon dioxide and permit calculation of the anion gap.
   a. The **total carbon dioxide** is almost identical to the serum bicarbonate plus small contributions of dissolved carbon dioxide and carbonic acid.
   b. The **anion gap** [serum sodium − (chloride + total carbon dioxide)] is normally < 12 in older children and < 17 in infants. A large anion gap means there is an excess of one or more unmeasured anions such as lactate or acetoacetate.
2. **Blood pH** indicates the net acid-base status and identifies **acidemia** (pH < 7.35) or **alkalemia** (pH > 7.45). The pH may be within the normal range in acid-base disorders if there is compensation for the primary disturbance or if there is a mixed disorder. Reasonable estimates of the pH change expected in an uncompensated, primary acid-base disturbance are as follows:
   a. For every change in the arterial partial pressure of carbon dioxide ($PaCO_2$) of 10 mm Hg, the pH will change inversely by 0.08.
   b. For every change in serum bicarbonate of 10 mmol/L, the pH will change 0.15.
   c. In situations in which the expected changes are not observed, there is either a mixed acid-base disturbance or compensation (or both).

3. **Arterial blood gas analysis** provides the carbon dioxide partial pressure (PCO_2) that allows assessment of pulmonary ventilation. Analysis of blood gases also provides the amount of buffer base excess or deficit (negative excess), which is calculated by determining how much of a change in pH cannot be explained by a change in $PaCO_2$. The base excess (or deficit) equals 0.67 multiplied by the multiple of 0.01 pH unit unexplained by the $PaCO_2$. The base deficit can be used to estimate the total bicarbonate deficit using the following formula:

(base deficit) × (body weight in kg) × (0.3)

C. **Acidosis** results from any process that reduces the body's pH.

1. **Respiratory acidosis**
   a. **Causes.** Respiratory acidosis is caused by the accumulation of carbon dioxide as the result of pulmonary hypoventilation. It may occur with any cause of respiratory failure, including pulmonary disease, neuromuscular disease, and central nervous system depression.
   b. **Compensation.** The body attempts to compensate for respiratory acidosis by the renal conservation of bicarbonate and increased excretion of hydrogen ion.
   c. **Therapy** is directed at restoring adequate ventilation. Alkalinizing agents (e.g., bicarbonate) should not be used.
2. **Metabolic acidosis**
   a. **Causes.** Metabolic acidosis is caused by the accumulation of net acid or the excessive loss of bicarbonate.
      (1) **Accumulation of net acid** occurs with ingestion of acid (e.g., salicylate intoxication, which also causes respiratory alkalosis by stimulating central hyperventilation), excess production of acid (e.g., lactic acidosis, diabetic ketoacidosis), or decreased excretion of acid (e.g., in renal failure). These forms of acidosis usually have a wide anion gap.
      (2) **Excess loss of bicarbonate** commonly occurs with diarrhea. It may also occur in renal disease, although renal failure affects all phases of urine acidification. Metabolic acidosis resulting from bicarbonate loss usually has a **normal anion gap** and is called **hyperchloremic metabolic acidosis.**
   b. **Compensation.** The body's compensation for metabolic acidosis is increased respiratory minute ventilation (hyperventilation), leading to a reduction in PCO_2 and returning pH toward normal. Maximum hyperventilation can lower the PCO_2 to 10 to 12 mm Hg (occasionally < 10), which keeps the pH in the normal range, with a bicarbonate concentration as low as 8 mmol/L.
   c. **Renal tubular acidosis** is the term given to a heterogeneous group of disorders, all of which are characterized by hyperchloremic metabolic acidosis and tubular dysfunction, but usually not by renal insufficiency. Renal tubular acidosis is classified broadly into three types. Table 14-15 lists representative causes for each type. Children with renal tubular acidosis may have growth failure and episodes of vomiting and dehydration.
      (1) **Distal renal tubular acidosis (type I)** is characterized by failure of the distal nephron to secrete the 2 to 3 mEq/kg/day of dietary acid (hydrogen ion) necessary to maintain acid-base homeostasis. The urine cannot be maximally acidified and new bicarbonate cannot be generated. Chronic positive hydrogen ion imbalance results in buffering by bone. This leads to increased skeletal calcium resorption, hypercalciuria, and increased risk of nephrocalcinosis and stones. In most children, there is also a urinary bicarbonate leak, which has implications in determining the amount of therapy needed to correct the acidosis.
      (2) **Proximal renal tubular acidosis (type II)** is characterized by decreased proximal tubular reabsorption of bicarbonate. A reduction in the normally variable renal threshold for bicarbonate causes a marked bicarbonate leak, which disappears when the serum bicarbonate falls below the threshold level (e.g., to 15 mmol/L). The defect may be isolated or may occur with other proximal tubular abnormalities, such as glycosuria, aminoaciduria, or depressed phosphate reabsorption. Diffuse proximal tubular dysfunction is termed **Fanconi syndrome.**
      (3) **Type IV renal tubular acidosis** includes a group of disorders, all of which are characterized by defects in distal tubular hydrogen ion and potassium secretion, leading to hyperchloremic metabolic acidosis and hyperkalemia.

TABLE 14-15 Types of Renal Tubular Acidosis in Children and Representative Causes

Distal Renal Tubular Acidosis (type I)	Proximal Renal Tubular Acidosis (type II)
Isolated, primary	Isolated, primary
Inherited	Inherited
Acquired	Acquired
Associated with heritable disorders	Associated with carbonic anhydrase deficiency
Sickle cell disease	Inherited
Marfan syndrome	Acquired
Wilson disease	Acetazolamide administration
Ehlers-Danlos syndrome	Associated with Fanconi syndrome
Associated with renal disease	Inherited
Renal transplantation	Cystinosis
Obstructive uropathy	Lowe syndrome
Chronic pyelonephritis	Tyrosinemia
Acute tubular necrosis	Galactosemia
Associated with other systemic disease	Glycogen storage disease type I
Systemic lupus erythematosus	Associated with renal disease
Chronic active hepatitis	Renal transplantation
Malnutrition	Nephrotic syndrome
Induced by drugs or poisons	Medullary cystic disease
Amphotericin B	Associated with other systemic disease
Vitamin D	Rubella syndrome
Toluene	Sjögren syndrome
	Amyloidosis
	Medullary cystic disease
	Induced by poisons
	Heavy metals
	Lindane
	Type IV Renal Tubular Acidosis
	Primary aldosterone deficiency
	Hyporeninemic hypoaldosteronism
	Mineralocorticoid-resistant hyperkalemia
	Transient renal tubular acidosis in newborns

d. Therapy

(1) **Renal tubular acidosis** is treated with alkalinizing agents. Doses of either bicarbonate or citrate must be sufficient to correct the acidosis completely. As little as 2 mEq/kg/day to as much as 20 mEq/kg/day may be required to return the serum bicarbonate to a normal concentration. Adequate therapy restores normal growth in affected children.

(2) **Metabolic acidosis other than renal tubular acidosis** is sometimes treated with alkalinizing agents, although such treatment is controversial.

(a) In mild to moderate acidosis in which respiratory compensation has occurred and renal function is normal, therapy directed at the underlying cause of the acidosis is sufficient.

(b) Although controversial, in severe acidemia ($pH < 7.0$), alkali therapy may be given to increase the serum bicarbonate concentration and decrease the energy expended by compensatory respiratory effort. The amount of bicarbonate given should correct the pH to no greater than 7.2; it is essential to avoid fully correcting the base deficit, which places the patient at risk for **overshoot alkalosis.** Alkali should **never** be given unless adequate ventilation can be ensured.

D **Alkalosis** results from any process that increases the body's pH through either a reduction in PCO_2 or an increase in bicarbonate buffer base.

1. Respiratory alkalosis

a. **Causes.** Respiratory alkalosis is caused by the excessive loss of carbon dioxide as the result of hyperventilation, which is usually centrally mediated (e.g., salicylate intoxication, head injury, hysteria).

b. **Compensation.** The body's attempt at renal compensation is through increased bicarbonate excretion.

c. **Therapy** is directed at the cause of the hyperventilation.

2. **Metabolic alkalosis**

a. **Causes** and **compensation.** Metabolic alkalosis is caused by a loss of hydrogen ions or an increase in base. Compensation is through a small and unpredictable decrease in minute volume to allow the $PaCO_2$ to rise slightly.

(1) The **most common cause** of metabolic alkalosis in children is the use of diuretics, which leads to volume contraction and potassium and chloride depletion. These changes, in turn, lead to increased bicarbonate reabsorption and aldosteronism, with increased hydrogen ion secretion. Volume contraction with significant chloride and potassium loss as a result of recurrent vomiting is another common cause. A gain of base can be the result of excessive alkali administration.

(2) **Less common causes** of metabolic alkalosis in children include Bartter syndrome, familial chloride diarrhea, chronic steroid administration, dietary chloride deficiency, chronic potassium depletion, and posthypercapnic states.

b. **Therapy.** Metabolic alkalosis is treated by restoring intravascular volume and replacing potassium and chloride deficits. Correction of the underlying cause of the alkalosis (e.g., surgery for pyloric stenosis, discontinuing diuretic therapy) is essential. The use of acid to correct alkalosis through the infusion of ammonium chloride or dilute hydrochloric acid is rarely indicated and should be reserved for patients who have severe alkalosis and those who cannot tolerate volume repletion.

VIII RENAL FAILURE

A Definition

Renal failure occurs when the kidneys no longer meet the body's need to maintain water, electrolyte, and acid-base balance and eliminate the end products of protein metabolism.

1. Renal failure may be **acute or chronic.**

a. Differentiation is important for prognosis and therapy.

b. Differentiation is not always obvious because chronic renal insufficiency may evolve from acute signs and symptoms.

2. Renal failure may be **oliguric or nonoliguric.**

a. Just as renal failure is not always oliguric, oliguria does not always indicate renal failure. Differentiation is aided by history, physical examination, urine indices (*see I C 3 b*), and, if indicated, response to a fluid challenge.

b. Nonoliguric and oliguric renal failure are equally significant, but nonoliguric failure is easier to manage because fluid restriction need not be so severe and the patient can more easily be given medications, electrolytes, and calories.

B Acute renal failure

1. **Etiology** and **pathogenesis.** In childhood, acute renal failure frequently occurs as a component or complication of serious systemic illness (e.g., septic shock) or multiorgan injury (e.g., severe trauma). The pathogenesis is not completely understood but is multifactorial, involving hemodynamic, cellular, hormonal, and metabolic factors.

a. **Categories.** Acute renal failure (ARF) is divided into three categories, based on the nature of the insult or disease.

(1) **Prerenal failure,** most common in children, results from factors that decrease renal perfusion and impair the delivery of oxygen and energy substrate to the kidney. Prerenal factors include hypotension, severe hypertension, hypovolemia, hypoxemia, renal artery occlusion, decreased cardiac output, and hypoglycemia. Causes include dehydration, shock, septicemia, and heart failure.

(2) **Renal parenchymal failure.** Intrinsic renal parenchymal injury can affect glomerular function, tubular function, or both. Causes include all forms of glomerulonephritis,

nephrotoxicity (e.g., from heavy metals, uric acid, myoglobin, or aminoglycoside antibiotics), and renal venous obstruction.

(3) **Postrenal failure** is very uncommon in children, and results from factors that are bilateral and injure the kidney by obstructing urine flow. Causes include stones, Wilms tumor, and congenital anomalies (e.g., obstructed ureteropelvic junction, posterior urethral valves).

b. **Acute tubular necrosis** (ATN) is the term applied to acute renal failure following severe or prolonged underperfusion or a nephrotoxic insult. The term accurately reflects that energy consumption and metabolic work are greatest in the tubules, whereas energy for filtration is derived from the left ventricle. If prerenal, parenchymal, or postrenal insults are mild or promptly reversed, ARF may not develop. ATN is usually self-limited and reversible, although chronic renal impairment and hypertension may be sequelae.

2. **Complications**

a. **Water retention** may lead to dilutional hyponatremia and possible neurologic symptoms ranging from lethargy to seizures or coma.

b. **Sodium retention** causes a compensatory expansion of the ECF, which can lead to edema, hypertension, or congestive heart failure.

c. **Renal ischemia** causes hyperreninemia, which can also lead to hypertension.

d. **Hyperkalemia** results from diminished filtration and failure of the distal nephron to secrete potassium. Hyperkalemia is usually not a serious problem unless the ARF is sudden, unless there is a high potassium load (e.g., from tumor lysis syndrome), or until the GFR has fallen to < 5 mL/minute.

e. **Metabolic acidosis** develops from failure of renal acidification mechanisms and bicarbonate wasting.

f. **Uremic syndrome,** with anorexia, pruritus, lethargy, and encephalopathy, results from the failure to excrete uremic toxins and requires renal replacement therapy (dialysis).

3. **Therapy**

a. **Initial treatment** of acute renal failure is aimed at:

(1) Reversing or removing the underlying cause

(2) Minimizing the excretory work of the kidneys, especially reducing the nitrogen load by limiting protein intake and renal solute load

(3) Limiting fluids to replacement of insensible water loss (approximately one third of maintenance fluids, or 500 mL/m^2/day) plus additional measured losses

(4) Assessing medications that are potentially nephrotoxic or eliminated by the kidney for change in dose or frequency and discontinuing them, if possible.

(5) Treating the previously mentioned complications

(6) Providing adequate caloric intake and restricting sodium, potassium, and phosphate

b. **Dialysis** is indicated when the preceding measures are inadequate. There is no specific BUN or creatinine level at which dialysis should be instituted.

4. **Recovery** from acute renal failure often involves a period of brisk urine output, the so-called **diuretic phase** or **recovery phase** of acute renal failure. Most often, this diuresis is appropriate and reflects excretion of water that was retained in the earlier oliguric phase.

C Hemolytic-uremic syndrome

1. **Definition.** Hemolytic-uremic syndrome (HUS) is acute nephropathy characterized by the triad of microangiopathic hemolytic anemia, thrombocytopenia, and acute renal failure. Although the kidney is often the only organ affected, other organs may also be involved, including the central nervous system, gastrointestinal tract, lungs, and myocardium. With systemic involvement, it is impossible to differentiate hemolytic-uremic syndrome from thrombotic thrombocytopenic purpura (TTP).

2. **Incidence.** Hemolytic-uremic syndrome may occur at any age. It is a leading cause of acquired acute renal failure in infants and children. Although it is usually sporadic, clusters of cases occur.

3. **Etiology** and **pathogenesis**

a. **Etiology.** Hemolytic-uremic syndrome is usually preceded by diarrhea, most commonly the verotoxin-secreting, enterohemorrhagic *Escherichia coli* 0157:H7, which has caused food-borne outbreaks.

b. Pathogenesis. Endothelial injury leads to platelet aggregation and depletion. Platelet thrombi damage erythrocytes, causing hemolysis. The vascular injury leads to renal ischemia and acute renal failure.

4. Clinical features and **course**

a. The anemia and thrombocytopenia may be mild or profound. Renal insufficiency varies from mild, nonoliguric renal failure to severe oliguria lasting several days to many weeks. Progression to end-stage renal failure is uncommon.

b. Long-term sequelae may include hypertension and varying degrees of renal insufficiency. Recurrences are uncommon but are seen in some individuals, even after renal transplantation.

5. Therapy is supportive with careful attention to nutrition.

a. The acute renal failure and hematologic problems are the targets of therapy. Transfusions (red cell) may be required.

b. Dialysis may be needed if prolonged acute renal failure occurs.

D **Chronic renal failure** (CRF) is a significant and irreversible reduction in GFR. CRF is severity graded from 1 to 5 where 1 is renal injury with a normal GFR and 5 is a GFR < 15 mL/minute (end-stage renal disease [ESRD]).

1. Etiology. Although any renal disorder can lead to chronic renal failure, congenital nephropathies are the most common cause of chronic renal failure in childhood. Renal dysplasia, which may be a consequence of prenatal urinary tract obstruction, is the most common cause of progressive renal insufficiency in the first decade of life. Glomerulopathies of all types are the second most common cause in the pediatric population and the most frequent cause in adolescents.

2. Course. CRF progresses at different rates in different individuals. Although the GFR generally progressively declines, it may plateau for periods of time. It usually does not improve.

3. Complications and **their management.** Besides the complications seen with acute renal failure, several additional problems occur with chronic renal failure.

a. **Problems with nutrition** and **growth** are the most significant complications seen in children.

(1) **Nutrition.** The goal of dietary management is to maximize caloric intake, reduce excretory solute load, and preserve residual renal function. The diet should be high in carbohydrates and fat, with mildly restricted protein (2 g/kg/day) and phosphorus intake. There are special formula drinks for children with chronic renal failure.

(2) **Growth.** Most children who have chronic renal failure grow poorly due to a number of factors, including inadequate calories, acidosis, anemia, and renal osteodystrophy. The use of **recombinant human growth hormone** has been very encouraging as children demonstrate increased growth rates without significant side effects.

b. **Renal osteodystrophy** results from several factors, including impaired vitamin D metabolism, decreased intestinal calcium absorption, phosphate retention, secondary hyperparathyroidism, and metabolic acidosis. The combination of skeletal demineralization and hyperparathyroidism retards growth and leads to rickets.

(1) Therapy with vitamin D metabolites (e.g., calcitriol [1,25-dihydroxyvitamin D_3]) prevents or heals the skeletal abnormalities but does not dramatically improve growth.

(2) Calcium carbonate is given to provide extra calcium for gastrointestinal absorption and to act as a binder of dietary phosphate.

(3) To prevent hyperphosphatemia, it is often necessary to limit phosphorus intake and give phosphate binders such as semelaver or calcium carbonate.

c. **Hyperkalemia.** Dietary potassium limitation is usually not needed until the child reaches ESRD. Potassium balance is maintained in chronic renal failure by increased excretion from remaining nephrons and the large intestine. A potassium-binding resin (e.g., sodium polystyrene sulfonate) may be given orally or rectally to remove potassium.

d. **Anemia**

(1) Normochromic, normocytic anemia is common in chronic renal failure, and most commonly results from decreased erythropoiesis due to decreased erythropoietin levels and uremic inhibition of bone marrow.

(2) Other causes include nutritional anemia resulting from iron or folate deficiency, or both. To prevent or treat the anemia, erythropoietin and iron are administered.

E End-stage renal disease When the progression of chronic renal failure is no longer adequately managed by medical means (i.e., when the GFR is < 15 mL/minute), replacement therapy is required, using hemodialysis, peritoneal dialysis, or transplantation.

1. **Incidence.** The incidence of ESRD in the pediatric age group (birth to 19 years) in the United States is approximately 13 per million annually. The incidence increases with age through childhood and adolescence.
2. **Transplantation.** Renal transplantation is the therapy of choice for children who have end-stage renal disease because it provides the best opportunity for a normal, active lifestyle and achieving good physical and cognitive growth. Approximately 800 renal transplantations are done annually in children in the United States; approximately 85% of these procedures are first-time transplantations. Results are excellent, continue to improve, and remain slightly better with transplantations from living, related donors (slightly more than 50% of pediatric transplantations and an 80% 5-year graft survival vs. 66% from a deceased donor). Although renal transplantation may be carried out on a child at any age, infants and adolescents have the lowest graft survival rate, the former because of technical limitations and the latter for reasons of disease recurrence and nonadherence.
   a. **Improvements in pretransplantation care** include the use of erythropoietin, which negates the need for transfusions and the risk of pretransplantation sensitization to human leukocyte antigens.
   b. **Advances in immunosuppressive therapy** include better recognition and treatment of rejection, the routine use of the calcineurin inhibitors tacrolimus and mycophenolate mofetil (MMF), the significantly reduced use of corticosteroids, the selective administration of the monoclonal antibody OKT3, and the development of other potent immunosuppressives such as rapamycin.
   c. **Problems.** Posttransplantation growth acceleration ("catch-up growth") remains disappointing, particularly in older children and adolescents, but is best in children with good graft function and with minimal or no steroids. Other problems that persist include:
      (1) The continued shortage of donor kidneys
      (2) Complications of immunosuppressive drug use, such as drug toxicity, susceptibility to infection, and a small, but definite, risk of posttransplant lymphoproliferative disorder or a malignancy
      (3) The absence of effective therapy to reverse chronic rejection
      (4) Hypertension, which may persist or develop in more than half of transplantation recipients
      (5) Persistent problems with pre-existing urologic abnormalities
      (6) Recurrence of disease in the transplanted kidney
3. **Dialysis**
   a. **Methods** (Table 14-16)
      (1) **Peritoneal dialysis** has been used for many years to treat acute renal failure, as well as for effective and well-tolerated renal replacement therapy (RRT) in ESRD.
         (a) **Continuous peritoneal dialysis** involves the placement of a permanent, intraperitoneal, silicon rubber (Tenckhoff) catheter that exits through a subcutaneous tunnel on the abdominal wall. Fluid is instilled into the peritoneal cavity, where solute diffuses from the extracellular fluid compartment to achieve dynamic equilibrium with the dialysate. The fluid is drained and the process repeated eight to ten times overnight by a mechanical cycler while the child sleeps. By increasing the percent glucose and osmolarity of the dialysate, net volume may be removed (i.e., ultrafiltration).
      (2) **Hemodialysis** has been used successfully to treat ESRD in children.
         (a) **Process.** In the pediatric age group, hemodialysis is virtually always performed at a dialysis center and usually requires three sessions per week, lasting 3 to 5 hours each.
         (b) **Major improvements in the success of pediatric hemodialysis** include the development of smaller and more efficient dialyzers, dialysis prescriptions better tolerated by children, and the use of chronically implanted, double-lumen Silastic catheters (e.g., in the internal jugular vein).
   b. **Disadvantages**
      (1) **Neither** peritoneal dialysis nor hemodialysis addresses the problem of **osteodystrophy** or **is capable of reversing the poor growth** associated with chronic renal failure.

TABLE 14-16 Comparative Advantages of Peritoneal Dialysis and Hemodialysis[a]

Peritoneal Dialysis
More easily carried out in infants
May be done entirely at home; proximity to dialysis center not required
Less expensive
Peritoneal cavity vs. vascular access easier to achieve and maintain
Less restriction of dietary intake and physical activity
Improved sense of well-being
Hemodialysis
More efficient form of dialysis; less total time commitment
Carried out by nursing staff; does not require participation of family
Less chance of fatigue ("burnout") by child and family

[a]Both procedures carry an acceptably low long-term mortality rate and are well established in the clinical setting.

(2) **Infections at the catheter site** are a problem with both procedures. Additionally, peritonitis is common in peritoneal dialysis, and thrombosis may occur in hemodialysis catheters.

IX HEREDITARY RENAL DISEASES

Although most renal diseases in childhood do not demonstrate single gene autosomal dominant or recessive patterns, it is clear that many renal diseases have a genetic basis. Genetic testing is now a reality for several nephropathies. Table 14-17 presents a representative list of heritable renal disease. Several examples are considered in this section.

A **Hereditary nephritis (Alport syndrome)** is a progressive disorder with variable severity.

1. **Clinical features.** It is most commonly acquired via X-linked inheritance, although it also has autosomal recessive or dominant patterns.

TABLE 14-17 Types of Heritable Renal Disease

Cystic Diseases
Polycystic kidney disease
Autosomal dominant (adult type)
Autosomal recessive (infantile type)
Medullary cystic disease
Autosomal dominant
Autosomal recessive (nephronophthisis)
Noncystic Diseases
Glomerular
Hereditary nephritis (Alport syndrome)
Nail-patella syndrome (hereditary onycho-osteodysplasia)
Tubulopathies
Fanconi syndrome (may also be acquired)
Renal glycosurias
X-linked hypophosphatemic rickets
X-linked nephrolithiasis
Cystinuria
Bartter syndrome
Gitelman syndrome
Liddle syndrome

a. The most common presentation in childhood is asymptomatic hematuria. Hypertension is also common. Renal insufficiency usually does not begin until the second decade.

b. The nephropathy may occur alone or with auditory or visual problems. High-frequency sensorineural hearing loss occurs in one third of patients. Diverse eye problems, usually involving the lens, occur in 15% of patients.

2. **Diagnosis** is made by renal biopsy showing characteristic abnormalities, notably lamellation and thinning of the glomerular basement membrane visible on electron microscopy.

3. **Therapy.** The only effective therapy is transplantation.

B Polycystic kidney disease Two types exist that differ in pattern of inheritance and age at onset.

1. **Autosomal recessive polycystic kidney disease** is a disorder usually detected at birth. Mutations in the PKHD1 gene occur in most cases.

a. **Clinical features**

(1) The infant has large kidneys and oliguria. Ultrasound reveals echogenic kidneys. (If the oliguria is present during intrauterine life, severe pulmonary hypoplasia may result, and the condition may be incompatible with life.) Renal insufficiency is slowly progressive, although it varies in severity.

(2) The condition is virtually always associated with hepatomegaly due to **congenital hepatic fibrosis,** which eventually causes portal hypertension and secondary varices.

b. **Therapy** for infantile polycystic disease includes renal transplantation, some form of portosystemic vascular shunt, and occasionally liver transplantation.

2. **Autosomal dominant polycystic kidney disease** is mainly a disorder in adults but may present in childhood.

BIBLIOGRAPHY

Andreoli SP: Acute renal failure in the newborn. *Semin Perinatol* 28(2):112–123, 2004.

Chan J, Williams D, Roth K: Kidney failure in infants and children. *Pediatr Rev* 23(2):47–59, 2002.

Daschner M: Drug dosage in children with reduced renal function. *Pediatr Nephrol* 20:1675–1686, 2005.

Mesrobian HG, Pan C: Recent advances in pediatric urology and nephrology. *Pediatr Clin North Am* 53(3):379–400, 2006.

National High Blood Pressure Education Program Working Group: The Fourth Report on the Diagnosis, Evaluation, and Treatment of High Blood Pressure in Children and Adolescents. *Pediatrics* 114(2):555–576, 2004.

Patel HP: The abnormal urinalysis. *Pediatr Clin North Am* 53(3):325–337, 2006.

Schwaderer A, Schwartz GJ: Acidosis and alkalosis. *Pediatr Rev* 25(10):350–356, 2004.

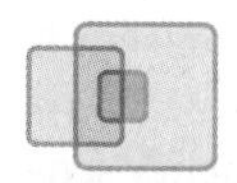

Study Questions

Directions: *Each of the numbered items or incomplete statements in this section is followed by answers or completions of the statement. Select the ONE lettered answer or completion that is BEST in each case.*

1. A 5-year-old boy has a 1-day history of cola-colored urine with RBCs and RBC casts. Two weeks ago, he had culture-positive group A β-hemolytic streptococcal tonsillitis. You suspect acute poststreptococcal glomerulonephritis. Which of the following is the single best diagnostic test result short of a renal biopsy?

- A Blood pressure determination greater than the 95th percentile for age
- B Positive antistreptolysin O (ASO) titer
- C Increase in his blood urea nitrogen and creatinine levels
- D Negative findings from antinuclear antibody, human immunodeficiency virus, anti–double-stranded DNA, and hepatitis screening
- E A very low complement component C3 level

2. A 6-month-old usually healthy girl has a fever of 102°F (39.8°C). There are no accompanying symptoms. A urinalysis shows "1+" leukocyte esterase, 10 white blood cells per high-powered field, and moderate bacteria. Which of the following is the most reasonable next step in management?

- A Obtain a renal ultrasound
- B Begin broad-spectrum, intravenous antibiotics
- C Obtain a dimercaptosuccinic acid renal scan
- D Obtain a urine culture by catheter and consider starting antibiotics
- E Check for costovertebral angle tenderness and if absent, exclude the diagnosis of urinary tract infection

3. A 6-year-old girl is discovered to have microscopic hematuria on a routine urinalysis. Her physical examination findings are entirely normal. History reveals that her mother and maternal grandmother both have microscopic hematuria and mild hypertension. Three maternal uncles have renal disease, including renal insufficiency and hypertension. One uncle is undergoing hemodialysis. Which of the following is the most appropriate next step(s) in evaluation?

- A Obtain blood urea nitrogen, creatinine, ASO, and complement component C3 determinations
- B Obtain a renal ultrasound, and if there are no cysts, conclude that the condition is not hereditary nephritis
- C Obtain an audiogram and eye examination, and if these findings are normal, conclude that this condition is not hereditary nephritis
- D Ask the family to attempt to obtain the medical records from other affected family members
- E Obtain a kidney biopsy as soon as possible

4. A 15-month-old girl has a history of poor oral fluid intake, occasional vomiting, rapid breathing, and decreased urine output. Physical examination reveals a pulse rate of 150 beats per minute, blood pressure of 120/80 mm Hg, and a respiratory rate of 60/minute. There are bibasilar rales, and the liver is palpable 4 cm below the right costal margin. Which of the following is the most appropriate next step in caring for this child?

- A Give a fluid challenge with isotonic saline, 20 mL/kg
- B Give Zofran and Imodium
- C Give fluid boluses with oral rehydration solution via nasogastric tube
- D Give a dose of intravenous furosemide
- E Calculate the fractional excretion of sodium

Directions: *Each set of matching questions in this section consists of a list of 4 to 6 lettered options followed by several numbered items. For each numbered item, select the ONE lettered option that is most closely associated with it. Each lettered option may be selected once, more than once, or not at all.*

QUESTIONS 5–6

For each of the following patients, select the most likely associated laboratory finding for complement level

- [A] Low C3
- [B] Normal C3
- [C] Elevated C3

5. 5-year-old, apparently healthy child has had three episodes of painless, grossly dark urine and is diagnosed with membranoproliferative glomerulonephritis

6. A 5-year-old, apparently healthy child presents with fatigue, anorexia, and generalized edema and is diagnosed with minimal change nephrotic syndrome

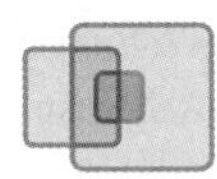

Answers and Explanations

1. The answer is E (*III A 1*). At least 90% of children with acute poststreptococcal glomerulonephritis have a reduced complement component C3 at the time of presentation. Although several other forms of glomerulonephritis are associated with complement activation and a low C3, the clinical presentation in this child suggests acute poststreptococcal glomerulonephritis (APSGN). A follow-up C3, to document return to normal, is indicated in 6 to 8 weeks. Both elevation in blood pressure and transient renal insufficiency are common in APSGN, but there is nothing specific to the diagnosis about either. A positive antistreptolysin O titer is evidence of a recent streptococcal infection, but does not add any additional information already known. A serologic screen helps to rule out other causes of glomerulonephritis, that is, systemic lupus erythematosus, human immunodeficiency virus infection, and chronic hepatitis, but their exclusion does not diagnose APSGN.

2. The answer is D (*IV E*). Definitive diagnosis of urinary tract infection depends on results of appropriately collected urine for culture and sensitivity. Not all pyuria is the result of urinary tract infection, and white blood cells may be seen in the urine of children who have other febrile illnesses. The report of "moderate bacteria" by the microscopic examination of a routine urinalysis is unreliable, because amorphous phosphates and urates may easily be mistaken for bacteria. However, a Gram stain of the urine sediment is useful. The renal ultrasound is indicated if the diagnosis of urinary tract infection is established. Likewise, a DMSA renal scan may be considered appropriate to help localize the site of infection, once the diagnosis of urinary tract infection is made. Starting antibiotics empirically without the possibility of knowing the causative organism will prevent the logical choice of an appropriate oral agent. The presence or absence of costovertebral angle tenderness in an infant is not a reliable sign of renal inflammation.

3. The answer is D (*IX A*). The family history suggests a dominantly inherited renal disease in which males are more severely affected than females. This is certainly compatible with hereditary nephritis, so-called Alport syndrome. Renal cysts are not a usual finding in Alport syndrome and therefore a renal ultrasound showing no cysts is perfectly compatible with Alport syndrome. Although polycystic kidney disease is also an autosomal dominant condition, gender differences are not usually observed. Also, hearing loss is peculiar to Alport syndrome, although it is seen in only a minority of patients, and its absence does not exclude the diagnosis. Evaluation of this child's renal function would probably not show any abnormality and would be useful only as "baseline" data. A renal biopsy would not be needed at present and perhaps not at all, especially if other family members already had a biopsy-proven diagnosis.

4. The answer is D (*I C 3*). Despite the history of poor intake of oral fluid, this infant shows signs of congestive heart failure and fluid overload. In view of these findings, a fluid challenge could be dangerous whether administered by IV or nasogastric tube. If the oliguria is the result of congestive heart failure and poor renal perfusion, the urine sodium concentration and fractional excretion of sodium should be low, the blood urea nitrogen and serum creatinine should be normal or slightly elevated, and the child may respond well to furosemide.

5–6. The answers are 5-A (*III A 1 a [2]*) and **6-B** (*II B 3*). Several renal diseases are associated with a low C3 including poststreptococcal glomerulonephritis, membranoproliferative glomerulonephritis, the nephritis associated with chronic infections, and lupus nephritic nephritis. Congenital C3 deficiency is associated with glomerulonephritis but is very uncommon. Patients with minimal change disease typically have normal serum complement levels, although exceptions are not rare.

chapter **15**

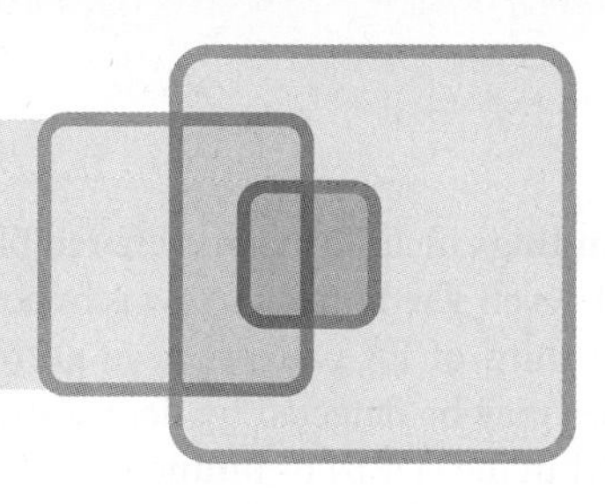

Hematologic Diseases

J. NATHAN HAGSTROM

I GENERAL PRINCIPLES

A Definition Hematologic disorders are those that produce either quantitative or qualitative defects in the cellular elements of the blood or in those soluble elements related to hemostasis. In evaluating hematologic data in the pediatric patient, it is important to recognize the normal developmental variations that are essential to proper interpretation of a particular blood response in infancy and childhood.

B Hematopoietic homeostasis Compared with most normal cells in the body, those in the peripheral blood have a relatively short lifespan—120 days for red blood cells (RBCs), 10 days for platelets, and only 8 to 20 hours for neutrophils. Maintenance of adequate blood counts, therefore, requires continuous replenishment in massive quantities from the bone marrow. It has been estimated that the average adult must produce approximately 100 to 200 billion each of new RBCs, neutrophils, and platelets daily to meet this demand.

1. **Assessment of hematopoiesis.** When quantitative abnormalities of any of the cellular elements are encountered, it is useful to distinguish between disorders of **production** and disorders of **destruction.**
2. Production of red blood cells can be estimated by means of the reticulocyte count, whereas neutrophil and platelet production are usually evaluated by **examination of the bone marrow.**

II DISORDERS OF THE HEMATOPOIETIC STEM CELL

A **Pancytopenia** is a reduction of RBCs, white blood cells (WBCs), and platelets. It is not a disease itself, but it may result from specific disease processes. The patient with pancytopenia may have the pallor and lethargy of anemia, the infectious complications of neutropenia, or the hemorrhagic diathesis of thrombocytopenia. **Bone marrow examination** is often required to distinguish among bone marrow aplasia, bone marrow replacement (e.g., by leukemic cells), and peripheral autoimmune destruction (Evans syndrome).

B **Bone marrow aplasia** severe enough to produce pancytopenia may be **congenital** or **acquired.** The congenital form is frequently associated with characteristic phenotypic and cytogenetic abnormalities. Certain metabolic diseases are also associated with bone marrow failure (e.g., Pearson syndrome).

1. **Constitutional (congenital) aplastic anemia (e.g., Fanconi anemia)**
   a. **Pathogenesis.** Fanconi anemia (FA) is an autosomal recessive cancer predisposition syndrome associated with chromosome fragility, congenital abnormalities, and bone marrow failure.
   b. **Clinical features.** Although it is a congenital disorder, Fanconi anemia does not usually produce significant anemia or thrombocytopenia until the affected child is 3 to 8 years of age.
      (1) There are a **variety of associated phenotypic abnormalities** that are of diagnostic value. Among these are abnormal skin pigmentation, retarded growth, renal abnormalities, and skeletal deformities (e.g., absent or hypoplastic thumbs, aplasia of the radii, aplasia of the first metacarpals).

(2) **Other abnormal findings** include macrocytic red blood cell indices and an elevated fetal hemoglobin (Hb) F level. The bone marrow is hypoplastic.

(3) Approximately one third of FA patients have no obvious clinical abnormalities. These clinically silent cases may be detected by demonstrating chromosomal instability in the presence of diepoxybutane (DEB) or bifunctional alkylating agents.

(4) At least 20% of FA patients will develop malignancies. The most common neoplasm is acute myelogenous leukemia; however, cancers of the skin, gastrointestinal system, and gynecologic system are also seen with increased frequency.

c. **Therapy** involves appropriate supportive care with RBC and platelet transfusions until an appropriate donor source of hematopoietic stem cells (HSCs) can be identified.

d. **Prognosis.** As HSC transplant technology improves, the survival for FA has also improved. Secondary malignancies continue to be a concern, however, even after successful HSC transplantation.

2. **Acquired aplastic anemia**

a. **Etiology**

(1) Acquired aplastic anemia may result from **exposure** to chemicals (e.g., benzene), drugs (e.g., chloramphenicol, sulfonamides), infectious agents (e.g., viral hepatitis), and ionizing radiation.

(2) In many instances, no clear-cut etiologic agent is identified, and the case is classified as **idiopathic.** In most patients who have acquired aplastic anemia, bone marrow failure is the result of immunologically mediated destruction of hematopoietic stem cells. A variety of events (drugs, viruses, pregnancy, graft vs. host disease) can activate the immune system to produce bone marrow aplasia. Immune destruction may then be mediated by either T or B lymphocytes.

b. **Clinical features.** The hypocellular marrow distinguishes acquired aplastic anemia from other forms of pancytopenia, such as leukemia and Evans syndrome, in which the marrow is not aplastic.

c. **Therapy** and **prognosis.** Bone marrow transplantation is the treatment of choice when there is a human leukocyte antigen (HLA)-matched sibling available for hematopoietic stem cell transplant. The prognosis for severe aplastic anemia is poor: Without effective treatment, 60% to 70% of patients die within 3 to 6 months of diagnosis. Patients who do not have appropriate matched donors may be considered for immunosuppressive therapy with agents such as cyclosporine and antithymocyte globulin (ATG).

III ANEMIA

A General considerations

1. **Definition.** Anemia is an abnormal decrease in the number of circulating RBCs, the hemoglobin concentration, and the hematocrit. It is not a disease itself but is a symptom of another disorder.

2. **Normal red blood cell values** in the pediatric years are listed in Table 15-1. It is important to consider the following developmental variations when evaluating an infant or child for anemia.

a. **Hemoglobin level** and **hematocrit** are relatively high in the newborn; these values subsequently decline, reaching a nadir at approximately 7 weeks of age for the premature infant and at 2 to 3 months of age for the term infant. (This condition is referred to as the "physiologic anemia" of infancy.) Total hemoglobin concentration and hematocrit rise gradually during childhood, reaching adult values after puberty.

b. **Hb F** is the major hemoglobin of prenatal and early postnatal life. Hb F values decline postnatally; by 9 to 12 months of age, the Hb F values represent $< 2\%$ of the total hemoglobin concentration.

c. **Mean corpuscular volume (MCV)** is relatively high during the neonatal period but declines during the latter part of infancy. The MCV is lowest during infancy, gradually increasing with age during childhood, reaching adult levels during adolescence.

3. **Classification** (Table 15-2). In clinical practice, anemias are classified according to the morphologic appearance (i.e., color and size) of the red blood cells on peripheral smear as well as the

TABLE 15-1 Normal Red Blood Cell Values in the Pediatric Years

Age	Hemoglobin g/dL		Hematocrit (%)		Mean Corpuscular Volume (fL)		Mean Corpuscular Hemoglobin (pg per cell)	
	Mean[a]	Lower Limit[a]	Mean	Lower Limit	Mean	Lower Limit	Mean	Lower Limit
1–3 d (term infant)	18.5	14.5	56	45	108	95	34	31
1 mo	14.0	10.0	43	31	104	85	34	28
2 mo	11.5	9.0	35	28	96	77	30	26
3–6 mo	11.5	9.5	35	29	91	74	30	25
½–2 y	12.0	11.0	36	33	78	70	27	23
2–6 y	12.5	11.5	37	34	81	75	27	24
6–12 y	13.5	11.5	40	35	86	77	29	25
12–18 y								
Female	14.0	12.0	41	36	90	78	30	25
Male	14.5	13.0	43	27	88	78	30	25

[a]Mean and lower limit of normal. Lower limit is 2 standard deviations below the mean.
Adapted from Dallman PR, Siimes MA: Percentile curves for hemoglobin and red cell volume in infancy and childhood. *J Pediatr* 94:26, 1979.

MCV. The suffix "chromic" refers to color, and the suffix "cytic" refers to size. The primary classifications are:

a. **Hypochromic, microcytic** (small, pale RBCs; a low MCV)
b. **Macrocytic** (large RBCs; a high MCV)
c. **Normochromic, normocytic** (cells of normal size and shape; a normal MCV)

B Hypochromic, microcytic anemias

1. **General considerations**
   a. **Defect.** Hypochromic, microcytic red blood cells indicate impaired synthesis of the heme or globin components of hemoglobin.
      (1) **Defective heme synthesis** may be the result of iron deficiency, lead poisoning, chronic inflammatory disease, pyridoxine deficiency, sideroblastic anemia, or copper deficiency.
      (2) **Defective globin synthesis** is characteristic of the thalassemia syndromes.
   b. **Evaluation.** Laboratory studies that are useful in evaluating the hypochromic, microcytic anemias include determinations of ferritin, total iron-binding capacity, and soluble transferrin receptor (sTR), as well as quantitative measurements of the Hb A_2 and Hb F levels.
2. **Iron deficiency anemia** is by far the **most common cause of anemia in children.** Most cases result from inadequate intake of iron; however, loss of iron through hemorrhage must be considered in the differential diagnosis.
   a. **Pathogenesis**
      (1) **Nutritional iron deficiency** usually develops when rapid growth puts excessive demands on iron stores. This is seen mainly during:
         (a) **Infancy,** when iron stores at birth are inadequate due to low birth weight or when the diet is composed exclusively of milk or cereals with low iron content
         (b) **Adolescence,** when a rapid growth spurt often coincides with a diet of suboptimal iron content (this is a particular problem in girls, who also lose iron with menses)
      (2) **Iron deficiency resulting from blood loss** can occur prenatally, perinatally, or postnatally.
         (a) **Prenatal iron loss** can result from extrusion of fetal blood either into the maternal circulation (fetomaternal transfusion) or into the circulation of a twin (twin-to-twin transfusion).

TABLE 15-2 Classification of Anemias of Infancy and Childhood

Microcytic Anemias	Normocytic Anemias
Defects of heme synthesis	Hemolytic disorders
Iron deficiency	Disorders of the external milieu
Nutritional	Antibody mediated
Through blood loss (chronic)	Microangiopathic
Chronic inflammation	Due to toxins
Sideroblastic anemia	Due to infectious agents
Due to lead poisoning	Due to hypersplenism
Due to pyridoxine deficiency or dependency	Disorders of the red blood cell membrane
Defects of globin synthesis	Hereditary spherocytosis
Classic thalassemias	Hereditary elliptocytosis
Thalassemic hemoglobinopathies	Hereditary stomatocytosis
Hemoglobin Lepore	Paroxysmal nocturnal hemoglobinuria
Hemoglobin E	Hemoglobinopathies
Hemoglobin Constant Spring	Hemoglobin S
Macrocytic Anemias	Hemoglobin C
With megaloblastic bone marrow	Unstable hemoglobins
Vitamin B_{12} deficiency	Other hemoglobinopathies
Folic acid deficiency	Enzymopathies
Hereditary oroticaciduria	Disorders of the hexose monophosphate shunt (e.g., G6PD deficiency)
Without megaloblastic bone marrow	Disorders of the Embden-Meyerhof pathway (e.g., PK deficiency)
Liver disease	Hemorrhage (acute or subacute)
Hypothyroidism	Hypoproduction disorders
Bone marrow failure states	Pure red blood cell aplasia
Acquired aplastic anemia	Transient erythroblastopenia of childhood
Fanconi anemia	Drug-induced aplasia
Diamond-Blackfan syndrome	Chronic renal disease
Myelodysplasia	Pancytopenia
	Acquired aplastic anemia
	Fanconi anemia
	Bone marrow replacement (e.g., by leukemic cells)

G6PD, glucose-6-phosphate dehydrogenase; PK, pyruvate kinase.

(b) **Perinatal bleeding** may result from obstetric complications such as placental abruption or placenta previa.

(c) **Postnatal blood loss** may be of an obvious cause (e.g., after surgery or due to trauma) or may be occult, as occurs in idiopathic pulmonary hemosiderosis, parasitic infestations, or inflammatory bowel disease.

b. Clinical features. Iron deficiency is most commonly seen between 6 and 24 months of age. The typical patient is on a diet consisting almost exclusively of milk.

(1) **Symptoms.** Although mild iron deficiency is relatively asymptomatic, as it becomes more severe, the infant manifests irritability, anorexia, lethargy, and easy fatigability.

(2) **Signs.** On physical examination, the milk-fed infant is fat, pale, and sallow; other findings include tachycardia and a systolic murmur. If the anemia is very severe (i.e., hemoglobin < 3 g/dL) or if the patient has complications that put added stress on the cardiovascular system, there may be signs of congestive heart failure (i.e., a gallop rhythm, cardiomegaly, distended neck veins, hepatomegaly, and rales).

c. Diagnosis

(1) Anemia may vary from very mild to very severe, depending on the degree and duration of iron deficiency. Small, pale RBCs are evident on the peripheral smear; the reduction in

MCV, mean corpuscular hemoglobin (MCH), and mean corpuscular hemoglobin concentration (MCHC) is usually proportional to the severity of the anemia.

(2) The serum iron level is decreased, whereas the iron-binding capacity (transferrin level) is increased, and the percentage of saturation is low (usually $< 15\%$). The serum ferritin level is decreased (which is a reflection of low iron stores in the bone marrow), and the sTR level is increased.

d. Therapy

(1) **Mild to moderate anemia** (i.e., hemoglobin > 3 g/dL without signs of cardiac decompensation) can be managed by administration of iron. This can be provided by the oral route at a dosage of 6 mg/kg/day of elemental iron. Therapy is continued for a period of 2 to 3 months after the hemoglobin level has returned to normal; this allows replenishment of tissue iron stores. Dietary counseling must be simultaneously provided to caregivers to give the patient adequate amounts of dietary iron. Parenteral administration of iron is sometimes used when there is a gastrointestinal problem that would interfere with iron absorption or if there is concern about the reliability of administration.

(2) **Severe anemia.** Although infants can tolerate remarkable degrees of anemia, particularly if the decline in the hemoglobin concentration is gradual, patients with extremely severe anemia in whom signs of cardiac decompensation have developed should undergo slow transfusion with packed RBCs until the clinical condition has stabilized.

3. Anemia of inflammation and chronic disease

a. Pathogenesis

(1) The anemia of chronic disease is associated with a variety of disorders, including:

(a) Chronic inflammatory disease (e.g., Crohn disease, juvenile inflammatory arthritis)

(b) Chronic infection (e.g., tuberculosis)

(c) Malignancy

(2) Iron is not released from its storage sites in the macrophages; thus, it is unavailable for hemoglobin synthesis in developing erythroblasts.

(3) A modest decrease in the survival of RBCs and a relatively limited erythropoietin response to the anemia also contribute to the development of anemia.

(4) A mild and transient form of anemia of inflammation may occur following infections, including common viral infections.

b. Diagnosis

(1) The anemia is mild in degree (i.e., hemoglobin concentration is 7–10 g/dL) often with hypochromic, microcytic indices.

(2) As in iron deficiency anemia, the serum iron level is reduced. However, in contrast with iron deficiency anemia, the iron-binding capacity is normal or reduced, and the serum ferritin level is increased or normal.

c. Therapy. The anemia resolves when the underlying disease process is treated adequately. Therapy with medicinal iron is unnecessary unless concomitant iron deficiency is present.

4. Sideroblastic anemia

a. Pathogenesis

(1) Among the conditions that produce sideroblastic anemia in childhood are:

(a) Pyridoxine deficiency

(b) Pyridoxine dependency

(c) Lead poisoning

(2) Iron enters the erythroblast freely; however, because of a metabolic block, it cannot be incorporated into hemoglobin. Instead, it accumulates in the mitochondria, giving the cell a characteristic appearance (a ringed sideroblast) when stained for iron content.

b. Diagnosis

(1) All sideroblastic anemias are associated with hypochromic, microcytic indices. Stippled RBCs may be found on the peripheral smear.

(2) The bone marrow shows micronormoblastic hyperplasia. Ringed sideroblasts and increased iron stores are evident when the cells are stained with Prussian blue.

c. Therapy

(1) A trial of pyridoxine (50–300 mg/day) should be instituted for several weeks.

(2) If the anemia is not responsive to the pyridoxine or related to a toxin that can be eliminated, the patient may require support with red blood cell transfusions.

5. Thalassemias

a. Definition. Thalassemias are hereditary hemolytic anemias characterized by decreased or absent synthesis of one or more globin subunits of the hemoglobin molecule. **α-Thalassemia** results from reduced synthesis of α-globin chains, and β-**thalassemia** results from reduced synthesis of β-globin chains.

b. Epidemiology. Approximately 3% to 8% of Americans of Greek or Italian ancestry and 0.5% of Blacks carry a gene for β-thalassemia. The α-thalassemia gene is seen with increased frequency in individuals from southeast Asia.

c. Pathogenesis

(1) Among the mechanisms responsible for producing thalassemias are:

(a) **Gene deletion,** which is the most common abnormality in α-thalassemia

(b) **An abnormality in the transcription or processing of messenger RNA,** which occurs more frequently in β-thalassemia

(c) **Thalassemic hemoglobinopathy,** in which a structurally abnormal globin chain is produced in subnormal amounts (e.g., Hb Lepore, Hb E, Hb Constant Spring)

(2) An imbalance in globin chain production is a hazard to the RBC because excess unpaired globin chains produce insoluble tetramers that precipitate, causing membrane damage. This makes RBCs susceptible to destruction within the reticuloendothelial system of the bone marrow (resulting in ineffective erythropoiesis) as well as the reticuloendothelial system of the liver and spleen (resulting in hemolytic anemia).

d. α-Thalassemias are usually the result of gene deletion.

(1) α-Thalassemia variants are found most often in populations of African or East Asian ancestry.

(2) Normally there are four α-globin genes; clinical manifestations of α-thalassemia variants reflect the number of genes affected (Table 15-3).

TABLE 15-3 Clinical Manifestations of α-Thalassemia Variants

Variant of Disease	Number of Genes Deleted	Characteristic Hb Pattern	Clinical Features
α-Thalassemia major	Four	γ_4F (Hb Bart)	Hb Bart has high O_2 affinity—does not release it to tissues Hb Bart has poor solubility—forms inclusions in RBC Ineffective erythropoiesis Hemolytic anemia Hydrops fetalis/death in utero
Hemoglobin H disease	Three	γ_4F (Hb Bart)—fetus and early infancy β_4A (Hb H)—beyond early infancy	Sufficient α-globin chains produced in utero to allow fetus to come to term, albeit with severe anemia Anemia persists throughout life
α-Thalassemia minor	Two	Normal	Mild anemia No clinical symptoms
Silent carrier	One	Normal	No anemia Normal RBC indices

Hb, hemoglobin; RBC, red blood cell.

e. **β-Thalassemias.** The clinical phenotype of β-thalassemia is related to the degree of globin chain imbalance.

(1) **Homozygous β-thalassemia (β-thalassemia major, Cooley anemia, and intermedia).** Patients who have this form of anemia are usually of Mediterranean background.

(a) **Defect.** Molecular defects range from complete absence of β-globin synthesis (genotype β^0/β^0) to partial reduction in the gene product from the affected locus (genotype β^+/β^+).

(b) **Clinical features** and **course.** Beginning in the middle of the first year of life, the infant manifests a progressively **severe hemolytic anemia** associated with marked **hepatosplenomegaly.** If untreated, the hepatosplenomegaly becomes progressive, and anemia, failure to thrive, and **bone marrow hyperplasia** develop. The bone marrow hyperplasia produces characteristic features such as tower skull, frontal bossing, maxillary hypertrophy with prominent cheekbones, and overbite. Death due to congestive heart failure usually occurs within the first few years of life unless the patient is supported with blood transfusions.

(c) **Diagnosis**

(i) Despite the severity of anemia, there is reticulocytopenia, which reflects ineffective erythropoiesis. Peripheral blood smear shows marked hypochromia, microcytosis, anisocytosis, and poikilocytosis. The red blood cell indices are significantly reduced.

(ii) On hemoglobin electrophoresis, Hb A is either markedly decreased or totally absent. Of the total hemoglobin concentration, 30% to 90% is Hb F.

(d) **Therapy.** The mainstay of treatment is **transfusion with packed RBCs.** Splenectomy is usually considered when transfusional requirements exceed 250 mL/kg/year.

(i) Even in the untransfused state, iron overload develops in thalassemic patients because of hyperabsorption of dietary iron. The iron load becomes even greater with chronic transfusion therapy. When the bone marrow storage capacity for iron is exceeded, iron accumulates in parenchymal organs such as the liver, heart, pancreas, gonads, and skin, producing the complications of **hemochromatosis** ("bronzed diabetes"). Many patients succumb to congestive heart failure in their late teens and early 20s.

(ii) In an effort to prevent hemochromatosis, patients who receive chronic transfusion regimens are treated with chelating agents (e.g., deferoxamine, deferiprone, deferasirox) that promote iron removal from the body.

(2) **Heterozygous β-thalassemia (β-thalassemia minor)**

(a) **Clinical features.** The growth and development of patients with this disorder are normal. The only abnormality is mild anemia (a hemoglobin level that is approximately 10 g/dL).

(b) **Diagnosis**

(i) Hypochromia, microcytosis, and anisocytosis are found disproportionately severe to the degree of anemia.

(ii) Hemoglobin electrophoresis shows elevation of the Hb A_2 level and, sometimes, elevation of the Hb F level.

(c) **Therapy.** No treatment is necessary. It is important, however, that thalassemia minor is distinguished from iron deficiency to prevent inappropriate therapy with medicinal iron. Genetic counseling is also important.

C Macrocytic anemias

1. **General considerations**

a. **Defect.** Macrocytic anemias are typified by large red blood cells (i.e., high MCV) in the peripheral blood. Some macrocytic anemias are associated with megaloblastic hematopoiesis (and often an elevated random distribution of weight [RDW]), whereas others are not.

(1) **Macrocytosis in association with megaloblastic hematopoiesis** indicates a **defect in DNA synthesis,** usually caused by a deficiency of vitamin B_{12}, folate, or both.

(2) **Macrocytosis in the absence of megaloblastic changes** is seen in **liver disease, hypothyroidism,** and **dysmyelopoietic states** (e.g., Diamond-Blackfan syndrome, Fanconi anemia, preleukemia).

b. Evaluation

(1) **Macrocytic anemia with megaloblastic marrow** is characterized by macroelliptocytes and hypersegmented neutrophils on the peripheral smear and bone marrow hypercellularity, with asynchrony between nuclear and cytoplasmic maturation. The nucleus remains relatively large, with poor condensation of chromatin as the cytoplasm matures.

(2) **Macrocytic anemia without megaloblastic** marrow may be associated with elevated fetal hemoglobin, which may be found in dyserythropoiesis and myelodysplasia. Because young RBCs are generally larger than mature cells, significant reticulocytosis due to any cause also produces macrocytes in the peripheral smear and elevates the MCV.

2. Folate deficiency

a. Etiology

(1) **Dietary deficiency of folic acid** is unusual in developed countries. However, folic acid deficiencies may develop in infants fed on boiled milk or goat's milk and in children who have severe anorexia.

(2) **Impaired absorption of folate** is seen in malabsorptive states (e.g., regional enteritis [Crohn disease], celiac disease) that affect the small bowel (primarily the jejunum; see Chapter 11). Patients usually have a history of weight loss, poor weight gain, irritability, lethargy, and abnormal stools.

(3) **Increased demand for folate** is seen in conditions characterized by an increased cell turnover (e.g., pregnancy, chronic hemolysis, malignancy). Relative folate deficiency may develop if the diet does not provide adequate folate to meet these needs.

(4) **Abnormal folate metabolism.** Certain anticonvulsant drugs (e.g., phenytoin and phenobarbital) interfere with folate metabolism.

b. Diagnosis of folic acid deficiency is confirmed by the demonstration of a decreased folate level and a hematologic response to a 50-mg test dose of folic acid.

c. Therapy. The patients should receive 5 to 10 mg of orally administered folic acid daily until the anemia and megaloblastosis are corrected. Unless a true dietary deficiency exists, therapy should also be directed toward the underlying disease process.

3. Vitamin B_{12} deficiency

a. Etiology. Dietary vitamin B_{12} deficiency is rare in developed countries; the one exception occurs in the infant who is breast-fed by a mother who is a strict vegetarian. The usual cause of vitamin B_{12} deficiency is a selective or generalized absorptive problem.

(1) Vitamin B_{12} is absorbed primarily in the terminal ileum; combination with a factor produced by the gastric parietal cells (**intrinsic factor**) is necessary for absorption to occur. Once absorbed into the bloodstream, vitamin B_{12} is transported in the plasma by means of a specific transport protein (**transcobalamin II**).

(2) Any condition that alters intrinsic factor production, interferes with intestinal absorption in the terminal ileum, or reduces transcobalamin II levels reduces the availability of vitamin B_{12}.

b. Clinical features. Vitamin B_{12} deficiency affects multiple tissues, including the gastrointestinal mucosa (exemplified by diarrhea and weight loss) and the nervous system (seen in subacute combined degeneration of the spinal cord).

c. Diagnosis is confirmed by the demonstration of a subnormal serum level of vitamin B_{12}. The mechanism of malabsorption can be demonstrated by the **Schilling test,** which measures the absorption and "flushing out" into the urine of a small dose of radioactive vitamin B_{12}.

d. Therapy for most forms of vitamin B_{12} deficiency requires intramuscular injection of a loading dose (1000 μg) of the vitamin followed by monthly maintenance of intramuscular doses (100 μg).

D Normochromic, normocytic anemias

1. General considerations. Normochromic, normocytic anemias are a heterogeneous group of disorders. The distinction between those associated with shortened survival of red blood cells and those due to impaired production of RBCs is facilitated by analysis of the reticulocyte count and analysis of the other cellular elements of the blood.

a. A **low reticulocyte count** usually suggests bone marrow failure.

(1) Anemia may be an isolated finding (pure RBC aplasia).

(2) Anemia may occur in association with neutropenia and thrombocytopenia (pancytopenia).

b. A **high reticulocyte count** with normal neutrophil and platelet counts is characteristic of a hemolytic or hemorrhagic disorder. Reticulocytosis following blood loss may take several days to peak.

2. Pure red blood cell aplasia

a. Congenital anemia (Diamond-Blackfan syndrome) is transmitted in an autosomal recessive fashion.

(1) **Clinical and laboratory features.** In many patients, anemia becomes apparent within the first few months of life, and most patients manifest signs of anemia within the first year. In addition to anemia, patients with this condition have reticulocytopenia, macrocytic RBC indices, and elevated Hb F levels.

(2) **Differential diagnosis.** The early appearance of anemia, the presence of neutropenia and thrombocytopenia, and a normal phenotypic expression differentiate Diamond-Blackfan syndrome from Fanconi anemia, the other congenital anemia of childhood (*see II B 1*). The early age at presentation, macrocytosis, and chronic course distinguish Diamond-Blackfan syndrome from transient erythroblastopenia of childhood (see below).

(3) **Therapy.** Approximately 50% of patients who have Diamond-Blackfan syndrome respond to corticosteroids; in some of these patients, red blood cell production can be maintained on remarkably low doses (e.g., 2.5–5.0 mg prednisone once or twice weekly). Other patients may require red blood cell transfusions to maintain hemoglobin at an adequate level. Hematopoietic stem cell transplantation may be used in cases that fail to respond to low-dose prednisone.

b. Acquired anemia (transient erythroblastopenia of childhood) is of unknown cause but may be a postviral autoimmune phenomenon.

(1) **Clinical features** and **diagnosis.** Transient erythroblastopenia of childhood is seen somewhat later in infancy than is Diamond-Blackfan syndrome. The anemia, which sometimes can be very severe, is normochromic and normocytic. Aside from reticulocytopenia, there are no other abnormalities in the peripheral blood. The Hb F level is normal until recovery begins.

(2) **Therapy.** Unless the anemia is severe enough to cause cardiac decompensation, no therapy is required. Most patients recover spontaneously within 2 to 4 weeks.

c. Other forms of acquired red blood cell aplasia

(1) **Disorders of the kidneys, liver,** and **thyroid gland** may result in hypoproliferation of the bone marrow.

(2) **Hypoproliferative** anemia may follow **bacterial** and **viral infections.** The etiologic agent that is documented most often is **parvovirus B19.** Usually, the anemia is not severe unless the patient has an underlying hemolytic disorder; failure of the bone marrow to meet the increased red blood cell turnover in this case may lead to an **aplastic crisis.** Acquired chronic pure red cell aplasia is rare in childhood, but has been described and is most often also an autoimmune phenomenon.

3. Hemolytic anemias are caused either by intrinsic defects of the red blood cell **(intracorpuscular)** or factors extrinsic to the red blood cell **(extracorpuscular).** In general, intracorpuscular defects are hereditary, and extracorpuscular defects are acquired.

a. Hemolytic anemia associated with extracorpuscular defects. The external milieu of the red blood cell consists of the plasma and the vascular endothelium. The presence of autoantibodies or isoantibodies, toxic chemicals, or infectious agents in the plasma may shorten red blood cell survival. Likewise, irregularities of the vascular endothelium (microangiopathic changes) may be damaging to the red blood cell.

b. Hemolytic anemia associated with intracorpuscular defects. Intracorpuscular defects reflect abnormalities of the membrane, hemoglobin, or enzymes. With the exception of paroxysmal nocturnal hemoglobinuria, these disorders are hereditary.

(1) **Membrane defects** include hereditary spherocytosis, hereditary elliptocytosis, hereditary stomatocytosis, and paroxysmal nocturnal hemoglobinuria.

(2) **Hemoglobinopathies** result from a qualitative change in the structure of one of the globin chains. This can result in one or more of the following consequences:

(a) No functional change

(b) Alteration in electrical charge, which allows identification by hemoglobin electrophoresis

(c) Alteration in solubility

(i) Paracrystalline gel may form when hemoglobin is deoxygenated (e.g., Hb S).

(ii) The hemoglobin may precipitate as Heinz bodies (e.g., unstable hemoglobins).

(d) Alteration in oxygen affinity

(i) High-affinity hemoglobins bind oxygen tightly, which results in erythrocytosis.

(ii) Low-affinity hemoglobins release oxygen easily and are associated with a physiologic anemia.

(e) Alteration in ability to maintain heme iron in a reduced (i.e., Fe^{2+}) state

(i) Methemoglobin (i.e., Fe^{3+}) forms.

(ii) The patient appears mildly cyanotic.

(3) **Enzymopathies** generally involve either the glycolytic (Embden-Meyerhof) pathway or the hexose monophosphate shunt.

(a) The most common glycolytic enzyme involved is **pyruvate kinase (PK).**

(b) The most common hexose monophosphate shunt enzyme involved is **glucose-6-phosphate dehydrogenase (G6PD).**

4. Antibody-mediated hemolytic anemias

a. General considerations

(1) Major types

(a) **Autoimmune hemolytic anemias** are the result of antibodies generated by an individual's immune system against his or her own red blood cells.

(b) **Isoimmune hemolytic anemias** result from antibodies produced by one individual against the red blood cells of another individual of the same species.

(2) Typical antibodies involved

(a) Antibodies of the **immunoglobulin (Ig) G** class, for the most part, are **warm reactive** (i.e., they have maximal activity at 37°C). They are detected using the direct antiglobulin (Coombs) test.

(i) These are **incomplete antibodies** in that they do not agglutinate red blood cells, although they coat the surface. These antibodies fix early complement components but cannot activate the complement cascade.

(ii) Hemolysis occurs extravascularly due to trapping of opsonized red blood cells by macrophages in the spleen and other reticuloendothelial organs.

(iii) IgG antibodies are associated clinically with autoimmune diseases, lymphomas, and viral infections. Occasionally, no underlying cause is demonstrable.

(b) Antibodies of the **IgM** class are usually **cold reactive** (i.e., most have maximal activity at low temperatures).

(i) These are **complete antibodies** in that they agglutinate red blood cells and activate the complement sequence through C9, causing lysis of red blood cells.

(ii) Hemolysis occurs intravascularly.

(iii) IgM antibodies are associated clinically with mycoplasmal pneumonia, Epstein-Barr virus, and transfusion reactions.

(c) **Donath-Landsteiner antibody**

(i) Donath-Landsteiner antibody is of the **IgG** type, but it is exceptional in that it reacts best in the cold and can activate complement, causing hemolysis to occur intravascularly.

(ii) Its clinical associations include syphilis and viral infections. It may also be idiopathic.

b. Autoimmune hemolytic anemias

(1) **Etiology.** Autoimmune hemolytic anemia may be idiopathic or the result of infectious agents, drugs, lymphoid neoplasms, or disorders of immune regulation (e.g., systemic lupus erythematosus, agammaglobulinemia).

(2) **Therapy** depends on the cause, clinical condition of the patient, and expected duration of the illness. Because most cases of childhood autoimmune hemolytic anemia are idiopathic or postinfectious and self-limited, supportive care and judicious use of transfusions and corticosteroids are the therapies most commonly used. Treatment modalities include:

(a) Supportive care with bed rest and oxygen

(b) Transfusion with packed red blood cells

(c) Corticosteroids
(d) Splenectomy
(e) Immunosuppressive agents

c. **Isoimmune hemolytic anemias** can be seen in hemolytic disease of the newborn (see Chapter 6). Hemolytic transfusion reactions are associated with isoimmune hemolytic anemias (e.g., the transfusion of type A blood into an individual who has type B blood).

5. **Microangiopathic hemolytic anemias**

a. **Defect and pathogenesis.** In these conditions, the red blood cells suffer mechanical damage due to irregularities in the vascular endothelium (e.g., in association with severe hypertension, chronic renal disease, artificial heart valves, hemolytic-uremic syndrome, giant hemangioma, or disseminated intravascular coagulation [DIC]). The resulting hemolytic anemia occurs because of red blood cell fragmentation in the presence of small vessel disease.

b. **Diagnosis** is supported by demonstration of RBC fragmentation on peripheral smear in the form of burr cells, helmet cells, and other irregularly shaped red blood cells.

c. **Therapy** involves supportive care and treatment of the underlying condition.

6. **Hereditary spherocytosis**

a. **Defect.** Hereditary spherocytosis is an autosomal dominant type of hemolytic anemia associated with a **defect in spectrin,** the major supporting protein of the RBC membrane. The defect leads to a loss of membrane fragments and the formation of small, spherical red blood cells with a high volume-to-surface ratio **(microspherocytes)** with less deformability than normal red blood cells and excessive permeability to sodium, which places a metabolic strain on the cell because energy in the form of adenosine triphosphate (ATP) is required to pump excess sodium out of the RBC.

b. **Pathogenesis.** The spleen plays a major role in the pathogenesis of hemolysis.

(1) The spleen has the smallest vessels in the body; thus, the rigid microspherocytes are trapped in its microvasculature.
(2) Glucose and oxygen levels are very low in the sluggish splenic sinusoids; thus, the excess metabolic demands of the microspherocyte for ATP cannot be met.

c. **Clinical features**

(1) Hereditary spherocytosis may manifest in the newborn as jaundice, which is sometimes severe enough to require exchange transfusions.
(2) Infants and children may have pallor or splenomegaly.
(3) Occasionally, patients may have severe hypoproliferative anemia due to an aplastic crisis after a viral infection (*see III D 2 c* [2]).
(4) Gallstones may develop in teenagers and adults with risk of **cholecystitis.**

d. **Diagnosis**

(1) **Physical examination** findings are usually positive for pallor, icterus, and mild to moderate splenomegaly.
(2) **Laboratory findings**
(a) Mild anemia and reticulocytosis are usually present. During aplastic episodes, the anemia may become severe and the reticulocyte count declines.
(b) Diagnosis is confirmed by the demonstration of increased osmotic fragility.

e. **Therapy**

(1) **Supportive care** involves folic acid supplementation (to meet the needs imposed by increased RBC turnover) and RBC transfusion (during aplastic crises).
(2) **Definitive therapy** is splenectomy, which alleviates anemia, reticulocytosis, and icterus; however, characteristic microspherocytes persist after splenectomy.
(3) Because the asplenic patient is susceptible to overwhelming sepsis caused by encapsulated Gram-positive cocci, special precautions should be taken (Table 15-4).

TABLE 15-4 Precautions Related to Splenectomy and the Hyposplenic State

1. Postpone splenectomy until older than 6 y of age
2. Immunize against pneumococci, meningococcus, and *Haemophilus influenzae* before splenectomy
3. Administer daily oral penicillin prophylaxis postsplenectomy
4. Treat febrile illnesses as potential sepsis (blood culture/intravenous antibiotics)

7. Hb S disorders

a. Epidemiology. This hemoglobinopathy is the most common cause of hemolytic anemia in the black population. It is also occasionally found in Greeks, Italians, Saudi Arabians, and Veddoids of southern India.

b. Defect and pathogenesis

(1) The molecular defect is the result of an abnormal autosomal gene that substitutes valine for glutamic acid in the sixth position of the β-globin chain. Under conditions of hypoxia, the hemoglobin aggregates into insoluble long polymers that align themselves into rigid paracrystalline gels (tactoids), which distort the RBC into a sickle shape.

(2) The clinical consequences of the solubility anomaly are:

(a) Shortened red blood cell survival (hemolytic anemia)

(b) Microvascular obstruction, which leads to tissue ischemia and infarction

c. Heterozygous state (sickle cell trait). Approximately 10% of blacks are heterozygous for the Hb S gene. Both Hb A and Hb S exist in individuals who have sickle cell trait; there is more Hb A than Hb S.

(1) **Clinical features.** Sickle cell trait is usually **asymptomatic,** unless the affected individual is subjected to hypoxemic stress. Otherwise, abnormalities may be limited to failure to concentrate urine, painless hematuria, or both.

(2) **Diagnosis.** Sickle cell trait may be diagnosed by hemoglobin electrophoresis or solubility tests (e.g., precipitation with dithionate and phosphate, sodium metabisulfite slide test). It is important to detect the trait for purposes of genetic counseling.

(3) **Therapy.** No specific treatment is required; however, precautions to avoid hypoxemia associated with severe pneumonia, unpressurized flying, exercise at high altitudes, and general anesthesia are in order. Tourniquet surgery and deep hypothermia should be avoided.

d. Homozygous state (sickle cell anemia)

(1) **Clinical features**

(a) In the **asymptomatic period,** the high levels of Hb F during fetal life and the first few months of postnatal life protect the patient.

(b) The **earliest clinical manifestation** may occur at 4 to 6 months of age, when symmetric, painful swelling of the dorsal surfaces of the hands and feet (dactylitis) develops. This is caused by avascular necrosis of the bone marrow of the metacarpal and metatarsal bones. During this same period, progressive anemia with jaundice and splenomegaly begins to develop.

(c) There are two major **life-threatening problems relating to the spleen** that affect infants.

(i) **Splenic sequestration crises.** The spleen may suddenly become engorged with red blood cells, trapping a significant portion of the blood volume. If not corrected rapidly, this can lead to hypovolemic shock and death.

(ii) **Overwhelming infection.** Despite its large size, in the early childhood years, the spleen does not efficiently perform its filtering function with respect to blood-borne microorganisms. Patients are very susceptible to overwhelming infection, particularly with encapsulated bacteria such as pneumococci and *Haemophilus influenzae*; *Salmonella* septicemia and osteomyelitis are also seen with increased frequency in patients who have sickle cell anemia.

(d) **Aplastic crises** can occur at any age when there is suppression of erythropoiesis in response to a viral infection such as parvovirus B19 (*see III D 2 c* [2]).

(e) **Vaso-occlusive episodes** can involve any tissue. Depending on the involved organ, a vaso-occlusive episode can produce abdominal pain, bone pain, cerebrovascular accident (CVA), pulmonary infarction, hepatopathy, or hematuria. These episodes are often precipitated by infection, dehydration, chilling, vascular stasis, or acidosis.

(i) The **acute chest syndrome** is characterized by fever, rales, pleuritic chest pain, and pulmonary infiltrates on chest radiography. Although frequently indistinguishable from an acute bacterial or viral pneumonitis, this syndrome may more often result from pulmonary vascular occlusion and ischemia/infarction.

(ii) Repeated vaso-occlusive episodes in the spleen lead to infarction and fibrosis of this organ; it gradually regresses in size and is usually no longer palpable after the age of 5 years.

(f) Late manifestations. By the time a patient reaches his or her late teens or early 20s, he or she is suffering the long-term consequences of chronic anemia, tissue hemosiderosis, and tissue infarction. Many succumb to progressive myocardial damage with congestive heart failure. Other long-term complications include gallstones, leg ulcers, renal damage, and aseptic necrosis of the long bones.

(2) Therapy

(a) Infections. Because these patients suffer from functional asplenia, the same precautions to protect them from overwhelming Gram-positive sepsis must be taken as for the patient whose spleen has been surgically removed (see Table 15-4). However, after the age of 5, there is little evidence to suggest that routine penicillin prophylaxis is required.

(b) Vaso-occlusive episodes. Prevention involves the avoidance of dehydration, hypoxia, chilling, and acidosis. Treatment is as follows:

(i) Analgesics should be given for pain.

(ii) When a vital organ (the brain, liver, or lung) is threatened, transfusion with packed red blood cells may be necessary.

(iii) After a documented CVA, the patient remains at high risk for recurrent CVAs for an indefinite period of time; such patients should be maintained on a chronic transfusion program designed to keep the Hb S level at $< 30\%$. As is the case with chronic transfusion programs for patients who have thalassemias, iron overload may eventually necessitate chelation therapy (*see III B 5 e (1) (d)* [ii]).

(c) Severe aplastic crises should be treated by transfusion with packed RBCs when the patient is asymptomatic.

(d) Use of agents that elevate Hb F levels. Because Hb F levels correlate inversely with disease severity, efforts have been made to identify medications that might increase Hb F levels in sickle cell anemia patients. Hydroxyurea has become the drug most commonly used for this purpose; early trials have indicated improvement in both laboratory and clinical parameters for children treated with this agent.

(e) HSC transplantation from healthy, HLA-matched sibling donors has proved to be potentially curative; however, this approach is limited by the paucity of HLA-matched siblings and the toxicity of the conditioning regimens.

8. Glucose-6-phosphate dehydrogenase deficiency is the most common RBC metabolic disorder. It is usually transmitted in an X-linked recessive fashion.

a. Defects. There are approximately 150 G6PD variants. The two prototypic forms are the A- variant and the Mediterranean variant.

(1) The A- variant is found mainly in the black population and is associated with an isoenzyme that deteriorates rapidly (it has a half-life of 13 days).

(2) The Mediterranean variant is found mainly in individuals of Greek and Italian descent and is associated with almost complete absence of enzyme activity, even in young cells, due to extreme instability (it has a half-life of several hours).

b. Pathogenesis

(1) G6PD-deficient cells do not generate an amount of reduced glutathione that is sufficient to protect the red blood cells from oxidant agents. Exposed sulfhydryl groups of hemoglobin are oxidized, predisposing the molecule to denaturation.

(2) The heme and globin moieties dissociate, with the globin precipitating as Heinz bodies, which form disulfide bridges to the red blood cell membrane. The damaged RBCs are then removed by the reticuloendothelial system; severely damaged cells may lyse intravascularly.

c. Clinical features

(1) The classic picture of G6PD deficiency is an **episodic hemolytic anemia** that is usually drug induced. However, this condition may also manifest as hemolysis precipitated by infection, neonatal jaundice, chronic nonspherocytic hemolytic anemia, or favism.

(2) When patients with either the A- or the Mediterranean variant of G6PD deficiency are exposed to **oxidant drugs** (e.g., sulfonamides, salicylates, phenacetin), there is a lag period of 1 to 3 days, after which a brisk hemolytic process ensues. The subsequent course differs for the two variants, however.

(a) Patients with the A- variant have self-limited hemolysis confined to the older red blood cell population. Recovery occurs as young RBCs with enzyme activity sufficient to resist oxidant stress emerge from the bone marrow.

(b) Patients with the Mediterranean variant have hemolysis that destroys most of their red blood cells and may require transfusions until the drug is eliminated from their bodies.

d. Therapy

(1) Patients with variants of G6PD deficiency that are associated with acute acquired hemolysis should avoid drugs that initiate hemolysis.

(2) Splenectomy does not benefit patients who have G6PD deficiency.

9. Pyruvate kinase deficiency is clinically heterogeneous and inherited in an autosomal recessive fashion.

a. Pathogenesis

(1) PK catalyzes the final step in the glycolytic pathway; the consequence of its deficiency is inadequate production of ATP. This puts metabolic stress on the red blood cells, because ATP is required to energize the pump that maintains intracellular sodium and potassium ions at the proper levels; thus, PK-deficient cells lose potassium and gain sodium.

(2) Reticulocytes, with their increased metabolic demands, are particularly vulnerable to destruction, especially in the sluggish splenic cords.

b. Clinical features

(1) The severity of hemolysis is variable; newborns may have jaundice, chronic anemia, or splenomegaly.

(2) Although the signs and symptoms of PK deficiency are the same as those of other chronic hemolytic anemias, because of selective destruction of reticulocytes, there may be an inappropriately low reticulocyte count in response to the anemia.

c. Therapy. Splenectomy has proved beneficial in individuals who have severe enzyme deficiency. Paradoxically, the reticulocyte count rises after splenectomy because the reticulocytes are then able to survive longer.

IV POLYCYTHEMIA (ERYTHROCYTOSIS)

refers to a greater-than-normal number of red blood cells in the blood.

A Etiology Erythrocytosis may be caused by an increase in red blood cell mass (**absolute erythrocytosis**) or a decrease in plasma volume, in which case the total number of circulating red corpuscles is unaffected, although their concentration is increased (**relative erythrocytosis**).

B Pathophysiology Abnormal elevation of hematocrit is usually considered to be a hematocrit of 55% and above. Cardiac work is increased by an excessively elevated hematocrit, which can increase blood viscosity, leading to diminished blood flow and decreased oxygen delivery to tissues.

C Relative erythrocytosis is commonly associated with **dehydration.**

D Absolute erythrocytosis may be the result of a primary defect of the hematopoietic stem cell (**polycythemia vera**) or secondary to **elevated erythropoietin levels.**

1. Polycythemia vera, in which leukocytes and platelets are also increased in number, is extremely rare in childhood.

2. Elevated erythropoietin levels, leading to erythrocytosis, may be seen in the following clinical situations:

a. Hypoxia

(1) The most common cause of erythrocytosis in childhood is cyanotic cardiac disease. Pulmonary disease and high altitudes may also produce sufficient hypoxia to induce erythrocytosis.

(2) Hemoglobins with a high affinity for oxygen do not release it readily to tissues. The consequent tissue hypoxia may be sufficient to induce an erythropoietin response, which can

be diagnosed by demonstrating a P_{50} (the partial pressure of oxygen at which half of the hemoglobin has oxygen bound to it) that is lower than normal.

b. Inappropriate erythropoietin production by renal cysts, renal tumors, and some other tumors (e.g., cerebellar hemangioblastoma)

V LEUKOCYTE DISORDERS

In most clinical settings, the status of the leukocyte population is assessed by measuring the total WBC count and the differential count. In evaluating these parameters, it is important to remember that for the first 4 years of life, there is a relative preponderance of lymphocytes.

A Neutropenia

1. General considerations

a. Definition. Although the absolute neutrophil count (ANC) varies somewhat according to age and race, a value of 1500/mm^3 is usually considered the lower limit of normal. However, an increased propensity to infection is not seen until the ANC falls below 1000/mm^3. With an ANC of 500 to 1000/mm^3, patients are at higher risk for cutaneous and mucous membrane infections (e.g., furunculosis, gingivitis, mouth ulcers, perianal cellulitis). When the ANC is below 500/mm^3, the risk for severe visceral infections (including septicemia) increases proportionally to the lowering of the ANC.

b. Etiology and classification. Neutropenia may occur in conjunction with anemia and thrombocytopenia as part of a generalized bone marrow dysfunction (e.g., aplastic anemia, malignancy) or as an isolated cytopenia. Isolated neutropenia may be the result of **either decreased production** or **increased destruction of neutrophils.** Determination of the cause of neutropenia routinely requires bone marrow aspiration.

2. Neutropenia due to decreased production of neutrophils

a. Congenital or **familial neutropenias.** Some chronic neutropenias appear to be of congenital origin or to follow a familial pattern. These vary in severity from benign disorders detected accidentally by routine blood count to disorders associated with frequent life-threatening infections. Neutropenia may be associated with metabolic or phenotypic abnormalities, as well as with immunologic disorders (see Chapter 9). It is not always possible to predict prognosis based on ANC or bone marrow examination; instead, a combination of family history and clinical follow-up is often the best guide to patient management.

(1) Cyclic neutropenia

(a) Clinical features. Cyclic neutropenia is characterized by regular development of marked neutropenia, usually at 21-day intervals. Coincident with the neutropenia, the patient has fever, oral ulcers, furunculosis, and other types of infection. Fatal infections are rare.

(b) Diagnosis. Twice-weekly blood counts for 6 to 8 weeks will show the cyclic pattern. Genetic testing for mutations in the neutrophil elastase gene (ELA2) is increasingly becoming available.

(c) Management

(i) The patient who has high fever in conjunction with ANC $< 500/mm^3$ should be treated with broad-spectrum intravenous antibiotics.

(ii) Patients who have severe episodes of neutropenia may benefit from use of granulocyte colony-stimulating factor (G-CSF) to stimulate neutrophil production.

(2) Chronic benign neutropenia

(a) Clinical features. This is a heterogeneous group of disorders, with variable inheritance patterns and morphologic features. Patients tend to have "nuisance" infections (i.e., mild furuncles, mouth ulcers) rather than life-threatening ones. The ANC is usually 500 to 1500/mm^3.

(b) Diagnosis. The bone marrow often shows adequate numbers of myeloid precursors associated with an apparent arrest in development at any stage of maturation from promyelocyte to band form.

(3) Severe congenital agranulocytosis (congenital neutropenia (CN); Kostmann syndrome) is inherited as a recessive disorder, a dominant disorder, or sporadically. The majority of mutations are found in severe CN are in the ELA2 gene. The bone marrow shows maturation arrest at the promyelocyte or early myelocyte stage. Severe and often lethal pyogenic infections of the skin and respiratory tract occur, often beginning in the first month of life. The outlook for these patients has improved markedly with the introduction of G-CSF to stimulate production of neutrophils. Some patients are at increased risk of developing acute myelogenous leukemia, which suggests an underlying genomic instability.

b. **Neutropenia caused by infection.** Various bacterial and viral agents are associated with neutropenia in children. The mechanisms responsible for the neutropenia are ill-defined and probably include myelosuppression as well as increased peripheral utilization, sequestration, and margination.

(1) **Viruses** commonly causing neutropenia include influenza (A and B), hepatitis, respiratory syncytial, rubella, varicella, and Epstein-Barr viruses.

(2) **Bacterial infections** that may produce neutropenia include those that cause typhoid, paratyphoid, brucellosis, and tularemia.

c. **Drugs and toxic agents**

(1) **Two patterns of drug-induced myelosuppression** are recognized.

(a) **Cytotoxic drugs,** such as methotrexate, cause regularly occurring, dose-dependent suppression of all bone marrow elements.

(b) **Idiosyncratic suppression** of neutrophil production can be caused by drugs such as sulfonamides, synthetic penicillins, antithyroid agents, and phenothiazines.

(2) **Heavy metals** and **benzene agents** can also suppress granulocytopoiesis.

3. **Neutropenia due to increased destruction of neutrophils**

a. **Immune-mediated neutropenia.** Antineutrophil antibodies may be self-produced (autoimmune) or transmitted to the patient from another individual (isoimmune).

(1) **Autoimmune neutropenia** may be idiopathic or occur secondary to drug sensitization, systemic disease (e.g., systemic lupus erythematosus), a neoplasm (e.g., lymphoma), or viral infection. Some patients respond to corticosteroid therapy. G-CSF has also been used to treat autoimmune neutropenia. Idiopathic autoimmune neutropenia is seen most commonly in young children.

(2) **Isoimmune neutropenia** results from the transfer of antineutrophil antibodies from the mother to the fetus. This may occur because the mother has been sensitized to an antigen on the fetal neutrophils or because the mother has an illness (e.g., systemic lupus erythematosus) that has induced an autoimmune process in her. When the neonatal neutropenia is severe, pyogenic infections of the skin, umbilical cord, respiratory tract, and bloodstream may develop. In most cases, the neutropenia resolves spontaneously when the maternal antibody is cleared from the infant's circulation.

b. **Drug-induced neutropenia.** In addition to their myelosuppressive effects, drugs may produce neutropenia by acting as haptens in immune neutropenia or directly damaging circulating neutrophils. Neutropenia may resolve after the withdrawal of the offending drug or through the use of steroids.

c. **Splenic sequestration (hypersplenism).** Splenomegaly from any cause can lead to neutropenia due to trapping of the neutrophils. Red blood cells and platelets may be affected as well. Treatment of the underlying illness or splenectomy (if clinically indicated) usually resolves this form of neutropenia.

B Disorders of neutrophil function (see Chapter 9)

VI HEMOSTASIS

Normal hemostasis (Figure 15-1) requires the integrity of three elements: **Blood vessels, platelets,** and **soluble factors.** Hemorrhage or thrombotic disease may result from deficiency, dysfunction, or imbalance of any of these elements.

A Hemorrhagic diathesis

1. **Clinical features.** Indications of significant hemorrhagic diathesis include:

a. Petechiae, large or spontaneous purpura, or unusual locations of ecchymoses

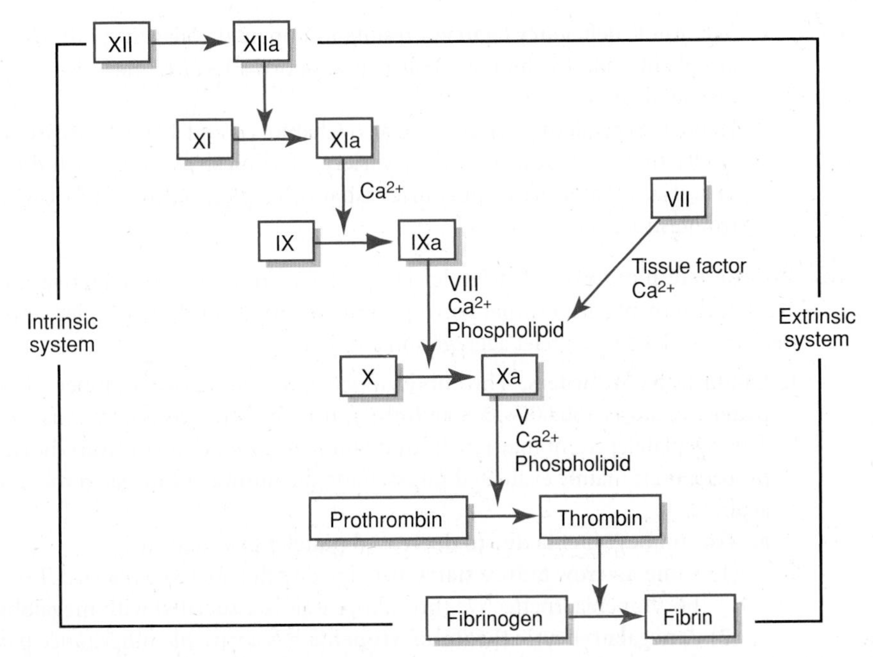

FIGURE 15-1 The coagulation cascade. The intrinsic pathway is initiated by activation of factor XII, whereas the extrinsic pathway is initiated by release of tissue factor and activation of factor VII. Both pathways converge with the activation of factor X. a, activated.

- **b.** Severe recurrent epistaxis (in the absence of an obvious local cause)
- **c.** Prolonged or excessive bleeding after dental extractions, surgical procedures, or major trauma
- **d.** Recurrent hemarthrosis
- **e.** Menorrhagia

2. **Screening** the patient who has a suspected hemorrhagic diathesis requires a battery of laboratory tests for assessing coagulation, including platelet count, partial thromboplastin time (PTT) (to measure intrinsic and common pathways), and prothrombin time (PT) (to measure extrinsic and common pathways). The only accurate method for assessing platelet function is platelet ATP release and aggregation testing.
3. **General approach to management**
   - **a.** Drugs that compromise platelet function (e.g., aspirin) must be avoided, as should deep venipunctures and intramuscular injections. The patient should be protected against trauma (especially to the head). Prolonged immobilization should be avoided.
   - **b.** When the nature of the defect is identified, specific replacement measures should be employed.
   - **c.** If the bleeding is life threatening, fresh frozen plasma (10–20 mL/kg) can be used as a temporizing measure for defects in coagulation factors until a specific factor deficiency is identified.

B Disorders of blood vessels

1. **Role of blood vessels in hemostasis.** Injury to a blood vessel elicits at least three responses that help to control bleeding:
   - **a. Vasoconstriction** reduces blood flow through the injured vessel.
   - **b.** Exposure of **subendothelial collagen** activates platelets and coagulation factors.
   - **c. Tissue factor,** which activates the extrinsic pathway of coagulation, is released.
2. **Vascular abnormalities** leading to a bleeding diathesis include **vasculitis** as well as the following conditions:
   - **a. Excessive capillary fragility** is seen in hereditary disorders of collagen synthesis (e.g., Ehlers-Danlos syndrome).
   - **b. Hereditary hemorrhagic telangiectasia** is an autosomal dominant disorder. Vascular abnormalities occur throughout the body, especially on mucosal surfaces. Gastrointestinal bleeding may be severe. Iron deficiency anemia invariably occurs.

c. **Vitamin C deficiency (scurvy)** results in impaired collagen synthesis. Walls of blood vessels are pliable due to the poor collagen support. Bleeding may also be caused by qualitative platelet defects.

d. **Henoch-Schönlein purpura** (see also Chapters 9 and 14) is a disease of children and young adults that is associated with a variety of clinical features, including arthritis, nephritis, urticaria, a characteristic purpuric rash involving the buttocks and lower extremities, and gastrointestinal pain.

C Disorders of platelets Platelet defects can be quantitative or qualitative. **Quantitative disorders** are detected by platelet estimate on a peripheral blood smear or platelet count. **Qualitative disorders** are detected by platelet aggregation studies.

1. **Quantitative disorders.** Thrombocytopenia is a decreased number of platelets (the normal platelet count is 150,000–350,000/mm^3); it is the most common cause of abnormal bleeding. The low platelet count may result from failure of production or from shortened survival. Platelet production is mainly evaluated by assessing the number of megakaryocytes in the bone marrow aspirate.

   a. **Thrombocytopenia due to decreased platelet production**

      (1) **Bone marrow failure** states associated with pancytopenia (*see II A*) are causes of thrombocytopenia. Ineffective thrombopoiesis is associated with megaloblastic hematopoiesis.

      (2) **Amegakaryocytic thrombocytopenia** has a variable inheritance pattern, although when it is caused by the **thrombocytopenia-absent radius (TAR) syndrome,** it is inherited as an autosomal recessive trait. The thrombocytopenia in TAR syndrome may be associated with renal disorders and congenital heart disease.

      (3) **Wiskott-Aldrich syndrome** (see also Chapter 9) has an X-linked recessive inheritance. Clinically, it is characterized by eczema, recurrent infections due to deficiencies in T-cell and B-cell immunity, and thrombocytopenia. The thrombocytopenia may be severe, and the bleeding is often aggravated by sepsis. Small platelets (**microthrombocytes**) are seen on peripheral smear.

   b. **Thrombocytopenia due to shortened survival**

      (1) **Immune-mediated thrombocytopenia** may be associated with **viral infection** or **drugs,** but most cases in childhood are **idiopathic.** The term **idiopathic thrombocytopenic purpura (ITP)** refers to a thrombocytopenia for which exogenous causes are not apparent. Opsonized platelets are trapped and destroyed in the reticuloendothelial system.

         (a) **Clinical features.** ITP may be seen after either a mild viral illness or an immunization. The onset is usually abrupt, with bleeding of the skin and mucous membranes. Bleeding is severe after trauma.

         (b) **Clinical course.** Severe internal hemorrhage is rare, despite a very low platelet count. In 80% to 90% of patients, ITP resolves spontaneously within 1 to 6 months. However, some cases become relapsing or chronic. The mortality rate is $< 1\%$.

         (c) **Therapy.** Conservative management is advisable because the acute form of ITP observed in children resolves spontaneously in most cases. Mild cases (platelet count $> 20{,}000/mm^3$ and minimal hemorrhagic manifestations) may be managed with observation alone. Primary management of more severe cases may include the use of intravenous γ-globulin, anti-RhD antibody, or corticosteroids. These agents presumably elevate the platelet count by interfering with splenic sequestration of antibody-coated platelets. Refractory or chronic cases may be treated with splenectomy or immunosuppressive agents.

      (2) **Hypersplenism** (*see V A 3 c*) is associated with thrombocytopenia as well as anemia and neutropenia.

      (3) **Disseminated intravascular coagulation** (*see VI D 3 c*) has also been associated with thrombocytopenia.

   c. **Thrombocytopenia in the newborn.** There are many causes of thrombocytopenia in the newborn. Among the most common are congenital infections (e.g., *Toxoplasma gondii,* rubella virus, cytomegalovirus, and herpes virus [TORCH] infections—see Chapter 8), bacterial sepsis, immune-mediated causes, and DIC. In **immune-mediated thrombocytopenia** in the newborn, antibody is formed by the mother against antigen on her own platelets

TABLE 15-5 Congenital Thrombocytopathies

Congenital Thrombocytopathy	Platelet Abnormality	Clinical Features
Bernard-Soulier syndrome	Glycoprotein 1_b membrane deficiency	Giant platelets Abnormal platelet adhesion to collagen Mild thrombocytopenia
Glanzmann thrombasthenia	Glycoprotein II_b-III_a membrane deficiency	Abnormal platelet aggregation
Gray platelet syndrome	Absent α-granules Decreased dense granules	Agranular platelets Normal aggregation reaction in response to exogenous ADP
Storage pool disease		Poor release of endogenous ADP

ADP, adenosine diphosphate.

(autoimmune antibodies) or on the fetus's platelets (isoimmune antibodies). IgG antibodies cross the placenta and opsonize the infant's platelets. Platelets are trapped and destroyed within the infant's reticuloendothelial system.

(1) **Autoimmune antibodies** are produced by women with ITP, systemic lupus erythematosus, and drug-induced thrombocytopenia. The mother is usually thrombocytopenic or has a history of thrombocytopenia.

(2) **Isoimmune antibodies** are produced by the mother whose fetus' platelets possess an antigen that her platelets lack. The mother's platelet count is normal.

(a) The most common platelet antigen to be affected is the platelet A^1 (Pl^{A1}) antigen.

(b) Sensitization to the Pl^{A1} antigen may involve the first pregnancy as well as all subsequent pregnancies.

(c) Severe thrombocytopenia may develop in utero and result in prenatal intracranial bleeding.

2. **Qualitative platelet disorders (thrombocytopathies)** may be congenital or acquired. Thrombocytopathies are associated with platelets that, although sufficient in number, are dysfunctional in hemostasis.

a. **Congenital (inherited) thrombocytopathies** (Table 15-5)

b. **Acquired thrombocytopathies**

(1) **Drug-induced** (specifically aspirin-induced) **thrombocytopathia** is the most common cause of platelet dysfunction. Aspirin inhibits the platelet release reaction. Normal amounts of the dense granule contents (e.g., adenosine diphosphate) are not released by platelets. The second wave of platelet aggregation is deficient.

(2) **Myeloproliferative disorders** (disorders of bone marrow production) are also implicated in acquired platelet dysfunction.

D Disorders of soluble procoagulant factors

1. **General considerations**

a. Deficiencies of factors involved in either the intrinsic or extrinsic pathways of coagulation can lead to a hemorrhagic diathesis.

b. Coagulopathies due to deficiency of a single factor are usually hereditary, whereas multiple factor deficiencies are usually acquired disorders.

2. **Disorders of single coagulation factors**

a. **Hemophilia A (factor VIII deficiency)**

(1) **Clinical features.** The most characteristic features of hemophilia A are spontaneous or traumatic hemorrhages, which can be subcutaneous, intramuscular, or within joints (hemarthrosis). In infants, excessive bleeding may occur after circumcision or after trauma; otherwise, hemophilia A is usually not a problem in the first year of life. Severely

affected individuals (i.e., those whose VIII:C activity is below 1%) show easy bruising and a propensity to hemarthrosis from the time they begin to walk. In later life, soft tissue, muscle, and joint bleeding dominate the clinical course; life-threatening internal hemorrhage may follow trauma.

(2) **Diagnosis.** The PTT is prolonged, indicating a deficiency in the intrinsic pathway. A decrease in VIII:C activity with a normal level of VIII:R is diagnostic. The bleeding time is normal.

(3) **Therapy**

(a) Supportive care measures include immobilization, local pressure on bleeding sites, and ice packs where appropriate.

(b) Desmopressin releases factor VIII from storage sites (Weibel-Palade granules) in endothelial cells. It may be used to treat soft tissue bleeds or hemarthroses in patients with mild to moderate hemophilia A, but the levels achieved are not adequate for major traumatic injuries or surgical procedures. Severely affected hemophilia A patients usually require infusion of product containing factor VIII.

(c) Clotting factors derived from human blood products (fresh frozen plasma, cryoprecipitate, factor concentrates) all convey the risk of transmission of infectious agents, primarily hepatitis B and C and human immunodeficiency virus (HIV). Current techniques for preparing factor concentrates (e.g., heat inactivation, solvent/detergent exposure) inactivate HIV.

(d) Recombinant factor VIII concentrates provide a safer (albeit more expensive) alternative to the use of blood-derived products.

b. von Willebrand disease

(1) **Clinical features.** As is true with hemophilia A, the severity of von Willebrand disease varies with the degree of deficiency of factor VIII. Usually, the bleeding is mild, with mucosal and cutaneous (platelet-type) bleeding most dominant. However, severe hemorrhage may occur after trauma.

(2) **Diagnosis.** There is prolonged bleeding time and prolonged PTT. Ristocetin cofactor activity is abnormal. Both factor VIII:C and VIII:R levels are low.

(3) **Therapy**

(a) **General supportive care** as per hemophilia A

(b) As previously mentioned, desmopressin can be used to release the factor VIII molecule from storage sites in endothelial cells.

(c) The lack of high-molecular-weight multimers of VIII:R in factor VIII concentrates makes these concentrates inappropriate for management of severe von Willebrand disease; such patients are usually treated with cryoprecipitate or a factor VIII concentrate, which contains high-molecular-weight von Willebrand factor (e.g., Humate P).

c. Hemophilia B (factor IX deficiency; Christmas disease) is inherited as an X-linked recessive disorder.

(1) **Clinical features.** Hemophilia B is a bleeding diathesis similar to hemophilia A (i.e., deep-muscle hematomas, hemarthroses, significant bleeding after trauma or surgery).

(2) **Diagnosis.** The PTT is prolonged. The activity of factor IX is decreased.

(3) **Therapy.** General supportive measures (as previously described for hemophilia A) are indicated for the bleeding diathesis. Until recently, replacement therapy with prothrombin complex concentrate (which is a mixture of coagulation factors II, VII, IX, and X) was the treatment of choice. However, recombinant factor IX concentrates are now available; these products are preferable to the prothrombin complex concentrates in that they are less likely to transmit infectious agents or promote thrombosis.

3. Disorders of multiple coagulation factors

a. Vitamin K deficiency. Coagulation factors II, VII, IX, and X (which are synthesized in the liver), as well as the antithrombotic factors protein C and protein S, are dependent on vitamin K. When the vitamin is deficient, normal coagulation does not occur.

(1) **Etiology**

(a) Vitamin K deficiency can occur in **malabsorption states** and other gastrointestinal disorders. **Drugs** (e.g., coumarin) that are vitamin K antagonists can interfere with metabolism of the vitamin.

(b) **Hemorrhagic disease of the newborn** can occur in neonates if the now routine administration of vitamin K at birth is omitted.

(2) **Therapy.** Nutritional disorders and malabsorption states respond to parenteral administration of vitamin K. Fresh frozen plasma or the prothrombin complex concentrate is indicated for severe bleeding.

b. **Liver disease.** All of the coagulation factors, with the exception of factor VIII, may be deficient in liver disease. In addition, hepatic clearance of activated clotting factors may be impaired. Thus, both PTT and PT are prolonged. Fresh frozen plasma is indicated as therapy (prothrombin complex concentrates are to be avoided because activated factors may produce intravascular coagulation).

c. **Disseminated intravascular coagulation**

(1) **Pathogenesis.** Intravascular activation of the coagulation cascade leads to fibrin deposition in the small blood vessels, tissue ischemia release of tissue thromboplastin, consumption of labile clotting factors (i.e., platelets; factors II, V, and VIII; and fibrinogen), and activation of the fibrinolytic system.

(a) **Damage to the vascular endothelium** occurs in patients who have renal disease, sepsis, and giant hemangioma.

(b) **Introduction of thromboplastic substances into the circulation** occurs in acute promyelocytic leukemia.

(c) **Impairment of clearance of activated clotting factors** occurs in patients who have liver disease.

(2) **Clinical features**

(a) The bleeding diathesis is diffuse. There is oozing from venipuncture sites and around indwelling catheters; gastrointestinal and pulmonary bleeding as well as hematuria occur; bleeding occurs from traumatized sites.

(b) Thrombotic lesions affect the extremities, skin, kidney, and brain.

(3) **Diagnosis.** The PTT and PT are prolonged. There is thrombocytopenia and hypofibrinogenemia. The levels of fibrin degradation products are elevated. Microangiopathic erythrocyte morphology is apparent on blood smear.

(4) **Therapy.** The primary disease process should be treated. Supportive measures are indicated for the bleeding diathesis. If bleeding persists or if thromboses are present, heparinization with replacement of platelets and clotting factors (i.e., fresh frozen plasma) should be considered.

4. **Thrombophilic disorders.** Predisposition to venous or arterial thrombosis may result from defects in proteins that inhibit coagulation or fibrinolysis. Table 15-6 lists congenital thrombophilic disorders. The two principle endogenous anticoagulant pathways are the **antithrombin-heparan sulfate** pathway and the **protein C/protein S** pathway.

a. The antithrombin (AT) system

(1) AT is a serine protease inhibitor that inactivates thrombin and the activated forms of factors IX, X, XI, and XII; its activity is markedly accelerated when it is bound to heparin.

(2) Defects of the AT gene may result in decreased production of AT (type I deficiency) or functional impairment of the molecule (type II deficiency).

TABLE 15-6 Congenital Thrombophilic Disorders

Defects in Inactivation of Activated Clotting Factors
Antithrombin III deficiency
Protein S deficiency
Protein C deficiency
Factor V Leiden
Miscellaneous
Dysfibrinogenemia
Prothrombin G20210A mutation
Hyperhomocystinemia

b. The protein C/protein S system

(1) Protein C is a vitamin K–dependent glycoprotein that inactivates activated factors V and VIII; protein S acts as a cofactor for protein C.

(2) Defects in either of these factors may predispose to thrombosis, as does a mutation in the structure of factor V (factor V Leiden) that promotes resistance to its inactivation by protein C.

c. Management of inherited thrombophilia encompasses primary prophylaxis, treatment of acute thrombotic events, and secondary postthrombotic prophylaxis.

(1) **Primary prophylaxis.** With the exception of newborns who have homozygous protein C deficiency, lifelong prophylaxis should not be routinely employed. However, patients exposed to thrombotic risk by virtue of surgical procedures or prolonged immobilization may benefit from treatment with heparin and/or warfarin sodium. The use of B-complex vitamins (folic acid/cobalamin/pyridoxine) may lower homocysteine levels in patients who have hyperhomocysteinemia.

(2) **Acute thrombotic events.** The management of acute thrombosis usually begins with heparin, followed by warfarin sodium after 1 to 2 days of full heparinization. Heparin is continued until the desired warfarin sodium response is achieved, that is, achieving an international normalization ratio (INR) of 2.0 to 3.0. Low-molecular-weight heparin is now the heparin of choice for deep venous thrombosis treatment.

(3) **Secondary postthrombotic prophylaxis.** Patients with inherited thrombophilia who have had a life-threatening thrombotic event or more than one episode of thrombosis should be considered for lifelong prophylaxis. Current recommendation is to use warfarin sodium, maintaining the INR between 2.0 and 3.0.

BIBLIOGRAPHY

Handin RI, Lux SE, Stossel TP (eds): *Blood: Principles and Practice of Hematology*, 2nd ed. Philadelphia, Lippincott Williams & Wilkins, 2002.

Nathan DG, Orkin SH: *Nathan and Oski's Hematology of Infancy and Childhood*, 6th ed. Philadelphia, WB Saunders, 2003.

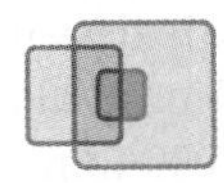

Study Questions

Directions: *Each of the numbered items or incomplete statements in this section is followed by answers or completions of the statement. Select the ONE lettered answer or completion that is BEST in each case.*

1. A 1-year-old girl is discovered to have a hemoglobin of 10.6 g/dL, an MCV of 65 fL, and an RBC count of 4 million/L. Iron studies are normal (ferritin, total iron-binding capacity). Hemoglobin Bart was identified on her newborn screen. Which of the following is the most likely diagnosis?

A Homozygous β-thalassemia
B Thalassemic hemoglobinopathy
C α-Thalassemia trait
D Double heterozygote α- and β-thalassemia
E Silent carrier of α-thalassemia

2. A 3-month-old infant has suffered recurrent episodes of fever, skin pustules, and pneumonia since the first week of life. Repeated blood counts have shown ANC to be $< 500/mm^3$, whereas hemoglobin and platelet count are normal. Which of the following is the most likely diagnosis?

A Aplastic anemia
B Congenital leukemia
C Kostmann disease (severe congenital neutropenia)
D Cyclic neutropenia
E Chronic granulomatous disease

3. A 3-day-old neonate develops significant bleeding after circumcision was performed at home following a home delivery. PT, PTT, factor VIII, and factor IX assays are performed. Which of the following is the correct pattern of coagulation test results for a patient with vitamin K deficiency?

	Prothrombin Time (PT)	Partial Thromboplastin Time	Factor VIII	Factor IX
A	Prolonged	Prolonged	Low	Low
B	Prolonged	Normal	Normal	Normal
C	Normal	Prolonged	Low	Low
D	Prolonged	Prolonged	Normal	Low
E	Prolonged	Prolonged	High	Normal

4. A healthy 3-year-old girl presents with acute onset of petechiae, purpura, and epistaxis. Her complete blood count is as follows: Hemoglobin 12 g/dL, white blood cell count $5550/mm^3$ with normal differential, and platelet count $2000/mm^3$. Which of the following is the most likely diagnosis?

A Idiopathic thrombocytopenic purpura
B Acute lymphocytic leukemia
C Aplastic anemia
D Disseminated intravascular coagulation
E Glanzmann thrombasthenia

5. A 7-year-old boy with hereditary spherocytosis has a high fever and is brought to the emergency department in a state of circulatory collapse. He has had no medical problems and has taken no medications since splenectomy was performed at 6 years of age. Which of the following is the most likely cause of his current condition?

A *Pseudomonas* sepsis
B Acute hemorrhage from splenic vessels
C *Haemophilus influenzae* meningitis
D Pneumococcal sepsis
E Acute hemolytic crisis

6. A 2-year-old child is brought to your office because of recent onset of pallor and icterus. He had been in good health except for a mild febrile illness. Complete blood count is as follows: Hemoglobin 5 g/dL, hematocrit 16%, white blood cell count 5300/mm^3 (normal differential), and platelets 300,000/mm^3. Microspherocytes and polychromatophilia are noted on peripheral blood smear. Reticulocyte count is 20%. Direct Coombs test is strongly positive. Which of the following is the most likely explanation for this child's anemia?

A Autoimmune hemolytic anemia
B Isoimmune hemolytic anemia
C Congenital spherocytosis
D Pyruvate kinase deficiency
E Diamond-Blackfan syndrome

7. A 3-year-old girl with sickle cell anemia presents with pallor, tachycardia, hypotension, and massive splenomegaly. Which of the following is the most likely explanation?

A Hemorrhagic shock
B Splenic sequestration
C Septic shock
D Cardiogenic shock
E Hemolytic crisis

8. A 12-year-old girl presents with progressive fatigue over the past few months and increasing bruising over the past few weeks. She has had no fevers or bone pain. The parents noted that she was quite pale. She has oral mucosal petechiae and cutaneous bruising mostly on the extremities, but also on the trunk. The CBC shows hemoglobin of 5.6 g/dL with a reticulocyte count of 0.9%, a platelet count of 10,000, and a WBC of 3000. The MCV is elevated and the review of the peripheral smear reveals no unusual looking cells. Which of the following is the most likely diagnosis?

A Acute lymphoblastic leukemia
B Acute myelogenous leukemia
C Aplastic anemia
D Evan syndrome
E ITP

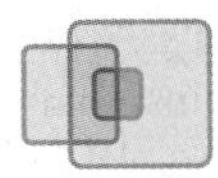

Answers and Explanations

1. The answer is C (*III B 5 c; Table 15-3*). Hemoglobin Bart is a tetramer composed of four γ-chains. It is found in fetuses with α-thalassemia genotypes whose red blood cells have decreased ability to produce α-chains, which would normally combine with the γ-chains to form fetal hemoglobin (Hb F). Hemoglobin Bart is not found in the silent carrier of α-thalassemia, which is associated with normal hemoglobin pattern and normal RBC indices. This patient has a profile most consistent with α-thalassemia trait because of the microcytic RBCs, borderline hemoglobin, but high RBC count. Iron deficiency is important to rule out with ferritin and total iron-binding capacity, which was done in this case.

2. The answer is C (*V A 2 a* [*3*]). The patient has a severe congenital cytopenia that is limited to the neutrophil lineage; thus, aplastic anemia and acute leukemia, which affect all hemic lineages, are very unlikely. Chronic granulomatous disease is characterized by dysfunction of neutrophils, but with a normal neutrophil count. Cyclic neutropenia is characterized by a periodicity in ANC rather than a constant lowering of ANC. The use of granulocyte colony-stimulating factor to stimulate neutrophil production has markedly improved the prognosis for patients with both Kostmann agranulocytosis and cyclic neutropenia.

3. The answer is D (*VI D 3 a*). The vitamin K–dependent factors are involved in maintaining integrity of the intrinsic (factor IX), extrinsic (factor VII), and common (factors II, X) pathways of coagulation. Thus, both PT and PTT will be prolonged in significant vitamin K deficiency. Factor VIII is not vitamin K dependent, and, therefore, its level will be normal.

4. The answer is A (*VI C 1 b* [*1*]). Idiopathic thrombocytopenic purpura is most commonly seen in previously healthy children who may have encountered a recent viral infection. Because the pathogenesis involves peripheral destruction of platelets, the bone marrow appears normal and other hemic lineages are not affected (unlike the case of acute leukemia or aplastic anemia). In contrast to the patient with ITP, the child with DIC usually is extremely ill. In Glanzmann thrombasthenia, the bruising diathesis is caused by qualitative dysfunction of platelets rather than a quantitative deficiency of platelets.

5. The answer is D (*III D 6 e* [*3*]*; Table 15-4*). In the absence of a functioning spleen, encapsulated organisms (e.g., pneumococci, *Haemophilus influenzae*) are not filtered from the bloodstream and may cause septicemia. To protect the asplenic patient from this complication, he or she should be immunized with pneumococcal and *H. influenzae* vaccines before splenectomy and placed on prophylactic penicillin indefinitely after surgery. Patients with congenital agammaglobulinemia are also at increased risk for pneumococcal or *H. influenzae* sepsis, whereas Gram-negative sepsis is seen more commonly as a complication of severe neutropenia.

6. The answer is A (*III D 4 b*). The presence of jaundice, polychromatophilia, and reticulocytosis indicates that the patient has a hemolytic anemia. The positive direct Coombs test confirms the presence of either complement components or antibody molecules on the surface of the patient's RBCs, thereby establishing the diagnosis of autoimmune hemolytic anemia. Because the patient is not a newborn and has not recently received blood products, this cannot be an isoimmune hemolytic anemia with anti-RBC membrane antibodies acquired passively. The microspherocytes seen in this patient's blood smear are generated by membrane damage resulting from removal of membrane components by reticuloendothelial macrophages; a patient with congenital spherocytosis would not have a positive direct Coombs test. Diamond-Blackfan syndrome produces a pure RBC aplasia with reticulocytopenia.

7. The answer is B (*III D 7 d* [*1*] [*c*] [*i*]). The key physical finding is the massively enlarged spleen. The sudden engorgement of the spleen with red blood cells can sequester a significant portion of the blood volume, leading to hypotension. Aggressive volume replacement with colloid or crystalloid products is essential to stabilize the patient's condition until the spleen releases the trapped red blood cells. Acute hemolysis produces lowering of hemoglobin and hematocrit, but blood pressure usually remains unaffected.

8. The answer is C (*II B 2 b*). Most patients with leukemia will present with bone pain and fever. Lymphadenopathy, hepatosplenomegaly, and visualization of blasts on a peripheral smear are also common with acute leukemia. This patient has pancytopenia of apparent gradual onset with a poor reticulocyte count, but is otherwise well. This is most consistent with aplastic anemia. ITP can be associated with anemia and leukocytopenia, but often the anemia is from blood loss and the reticulocyte count is elevated.

chapter **16**

Oncologic Diseases

MICHAEL S. ISAKOFF

I GENERAL PRINCIPLES OF CANCER IN CHILDREN

A Epidemiology Cancer is the most common cause of disease-related death in childhood and has an annual incidence of 1 in 600 for those younger than 15 years. The majority of children are cured of their disease with an estimated overall survival of 79%.

B Types

1. **Common types of cancer in children** (Table 16-1). **Leukemia and tumors** of the central nervous system represent the majority of childhood neoplasms, followed by a wide array of solid tumors. Typically, childhood tumors are derived from nonepithelial origins.
2. **Uncommon types of cancer in children.** Typical adult-type epithelial-derived tumors such as carcinomas of the lung, colon, and breast are extremely rare during childhood.

C Oncogenesis

1. Malignant cells proliferate and develop abnormally because they have escaped normal control mechanisms. The genetic alterations that lead to this escape are especially likely to **occur during periods of increased cell proliferation,** such as gestation, infancy, and early childhood, when many systems and organs are developing.
2. **Two well-characterized causes of transformation are activation of oncogenes and loss of tumor suppressor genes.**
   a. **Proto-oncogenes** are normal regulatory genes that control cellular proliferation, differentiation, and development. Upon genetic alteration, these proto-oncogenes are converted to **oncogenes that abnormally produce excessive or abnormal oncoproteins.** The oncoproteins that are produced behave in a dominant fashion, because their production predominates over the unaltered gene products from the other allele. **Oncogenes are commonly produced in the following ways.**
      (1) **Translocation** of proto-oncogenes to new locations in the genome. This leads to:
         (a) Escape of genes from their usual regulatory mechanisms that instead come under the influence of new genes that inappropriately activate them. For example, Ewing sarcoma typically involves a translocation of the EWS and FLI-1 gene t(11;22) that leads to an abnormal fusion protein. In this new product, there is replacement of the weak transcriptional activation domain of FLI-1 with the strong activation domain of EWS. The result is believed to lead to abnormal gene activation and cell proliferation.
         (b) The formation of novel gene fusion products, which alter normal cellular function
            (i) In chronic myelogenous leukemia, the t(9;22) **Philadelphia chromosome** produces a bcr-abl fusion gene that produces a novel protein with tyrosine kinase activity that inhibits apoptosis.
            (ii) In acute promyelocytic leukemia, the t(15;17) translocation produces a promyelocytic leukemia (PML)–retinoic acid receptor-α (RAR-α) fusion gene that codes for a novel protein that alters the retinoic acid receptor's function. Consequently, the normal differentiation and apoptosis of the cell are blocked, and therefore, abnormal promyelocytes accumulate rather than terminally differentiate and die.

TABLE 16-1 Common Types of Childhood Cancer

Cancer	Incidence Among All Affected Children	
	White Children (%)	Black Children (%)
Leukemia	30.9	24.3
Central nervous system	18.3	21.6
Lymphoma, including Hodgkin	13.8	11.3
Neuroblastoma	6.8	5.4
Soft tissue sarcoma	6.2	8.6
Wilms tumor	5.7	8.1
Bone	4.7	3.6
Eye	2.5	4.1
Germ cell	2.4	4.1
Liver	1.3	—
Other	7.4	8.9

(2) **Point mutations** of proto-oncogenes may occur that alter their product. For example, point mutations of *ras* in acute myelogenous leukemia result in increased *ras* activation and increased cell proliferation.

(3) **Gene amplification** of proto-oncogenes may occur, which enhances the output of their product. For example, amplification of the n-*myc* oncogene in neuroblastoma is associated with a more aggressive tumor and a worse prognosis.

b. **Tumor suppressor genes** regulate the cell cycle or promote apoptosis. They behave in a recessive fashion, because as long as one of two homologous suppressor genes remains, tumor formation is inhibited. Uninhibited cell growth may occur when both suppressor genes are lost. Tumor suppressor genes are lost by **genetic recombination events, point mutations, or deletions** and loss of these genes can occur in either somatic or germ cells. When a gene is lost from germ cells, the condition can be inherited. For example, retinoblastoma is postulated to follow Knudson's **two-hit hypothesis (Figure 16-1)** in which two distinct steps produce genetic abnormalities that result in tumor formation. In hereditary retinoblastoma, the first "hit" is a germline mutation in the Rb gene, passed on from one parent. The second "hit" occurs as a somatic mutation after birth, leading to complete loss of the Rb alleles and resultant dysregulated cell proliferation and tumor formation.

D Predisposing factors Most childhood malignancies are of unknown cause and occur in otherwise healthy children. Certain children, however, are at an increased risk for cancer because of their constitutional makeup or exposure to cancer-causing agents.

1. **Genetic syndromes.** There are several genetic syndromes that carry an elevated risk of developing cancer. For example, **trisomy 21 is associated with a 15-fold increased risk of developing leukemia.** Individuals with overgrowth syndromes (e.g., **Beckwith-Wiedemann) are at increased risk for the development of Wilms tumor.** In addition, children with Fanconi anemia often have short stature, renal and skeletal abnormalities, and a propensity to development of leukemia (see Chapter 15). See **Table 16-2** for a summary of genetic syndromes and associated childhood cancer.

2. **Immunodeficiencies** (see Chapter 9). Children born with congenital immunodeficiencies have a 100-fold increased risk of malignancy, particularly of the lymphoid system. Congenital immunodeficiency disorders that carry an increased risk of cancer include the following:

   a. **Wiskott-Aldrich syndrome** is an X-linked disorder characterized by progressive T-cell dysfunction, eczema, thrombocytopenia, and a propensity to development of lymphomas.

   b. **Common variable immunodeficiency** predisposes affected individuals to stomach cancer and lymphomas, both of which do not usually manifest until adulthood.

   c. **X-linked lymphoproliferative syndrome** in males results in severe infections with the Epstein-Barr virus; if the acute infection does not end fatally, induction of lymphoma occurs.

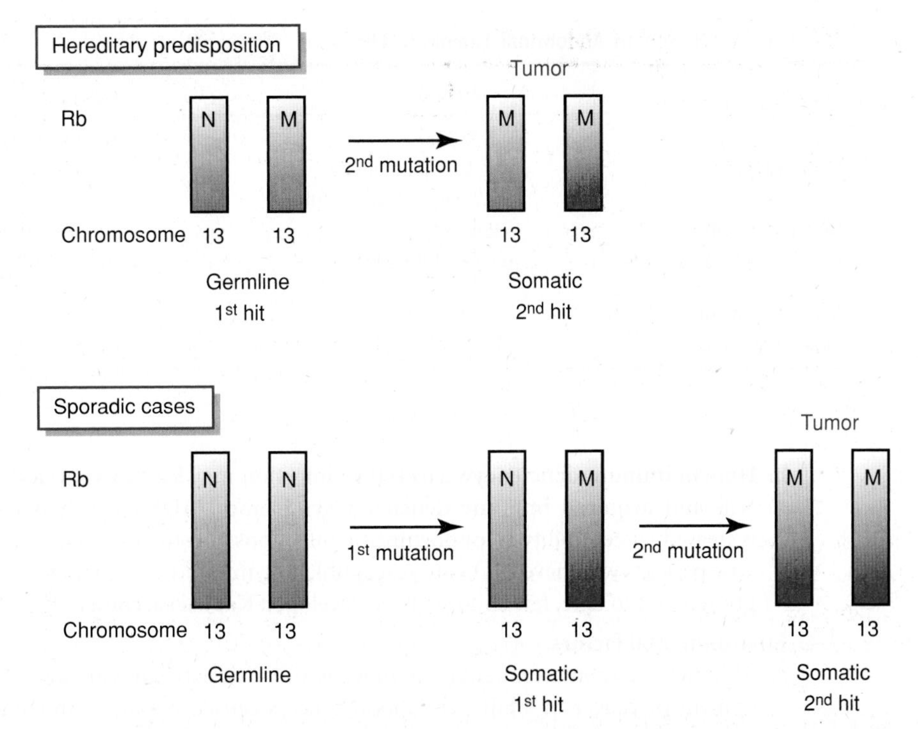

FIGURE 16-1 [Genetic mutations]. The "two-hit" hypothesis was developed by Knudson to explain how inactivation of both copies of a tumor suppressor gene led to the development of retinoblastoma in both hereditary and sporadic cases. In sporadic cases, both copies of the Rb tumor suppressor gene must be independently mutated within the same cell, which is a rare occurrence. In hereditary cases, one of the two genes is already mutated; this mutation makes it much more likely that a tumor will form because only one additional gene must mutate. Rb, retinoblastoma gene; N, normal Rb; M, mutated Rb. (After Knudson AG, Meadows AT, Nichols WW, et al.: Chromosome deletion and retinoblastoma. *N Engl J Med* 295:1120–1123, 1976.)

3. **Infections.** There are primarily two viruses that infect cells of the immune system that have been associated with childhood malignancy.
   a. **Epstein-Barr virus** has been associated with the development of endemic **Burkitt lymphoma.** This malignancy involves a specific chromosomal change involving translocation of a portion of the long arm of chromosome 8—which contains the c-*myc* oncogene—onto the area of another chromosome (14, 2, or 22)—which controls immunoglobulin chain synthesis (a specific B-cell function).

TABLE 16-2 Genetic Syndromes and Associated Childhood Malignancies

Genetic Syndrome	Associated Childhood Malignancies
Trisomy 21	ALL, AML
Ataxia telangiectasia	ALL
Fanconi anemia	ALL, AML
Blooms syndrome	ALL, AML
Beckwith-Wiedemann syndrome	Wilms tumor, hepatoblastoma
WAGR syndrome	Wilms tumor
Familial monosomy 7	AML
Neurofibromatosis type 1	ALL, AML, optic glioma, rhabdomyosarcoma
Tuberous sclerosis	Brain tumors
Li Fraumeni syndrome	Osteosarcoma, rhabdomyosarcoma, retinoblastoma
Nevus basal cell carcinoma syndrome	Medulloblastoma, rhabdomyosarcoma, basal cell carcinoma
Klinefelter syndrome	Dysgerminoma

ALL, acute lymphoblastic leukemia; AML, acute myelodysplastic leukemia; GU, genitourinary; WAGR, Wilms tumor, aniridia, GU abnormalities, mental retardation.

TABLE 16-3 Malignant Abdominal Tumors in Children

Type	Origin	Age
Wilms tumor	Kidney	Infant and young child
Neuroblastoma	Adrenal medulla Sympathetic ganglia	Infant and young child
Hepatoblastoma	Liver	Infant and young child
Non-Hodgkin lymphoma	Lymph node Peyer patch	Older child and adolescent
Germ cell tumor	Ovary	Older child and adolescent
Rhabdomyosarcoma	Primitive mesenchyme	Older child and adolescent

b. **Human immunodeficiency virus** (**HIV**) infection may lead to viral destruction of helper T cells and **acquired immune deficiency syndrome (AIDS),** which is characterized by an increased susceptibility to opportunistic infections and malignancies (see Chapter 9). Pediatric patients who have AIDS are susceptible to lymphoid malignancies such as **Burkitt lymphoma,** but to date, few children have developed **Kaposi sarcoma.**

4. **Environmental factors**
   a. Although many environmental carcinogens and toxic exposures are associated with the development of cancer in adults, childhood cancers caused by environmental factors and toxic exposures are rare.
   b. One known risk factor for childhood cancer is prior treatment of malignancy in a child with chemotherapeutic agents, ionizing radiation, or both.

E Clinical features

1. **Constitutional symptoms.** Fever, night sweats, and unintended weight loss of > 10% may be associated with Hodgkin and other lymphomas, leukemia, and some types of solid tumors, such as Ewing sarcoma or neuroblastoma.
2. **Abdominal masses** (see Table 16-3). The abdomen is the most common site of solid tumor formation. A visible or palpable mass may be detected, though there is often a delay in recognition of an abdominal mass due to the normal protuberant abdomen of young children. Pain may be present, especially if the mass suddenly enlarges because of bleeding within it. The most common malignant neoplasms found in the abdomen include Wilms tumor and neuroblastoma. In addition, **leukemic infiltration** and **metastases** may cause enlargement of the liver, spleen, and intra-abdominal lymph nodes. See Table 16-3 for a list of common and rare tumors found in the abdomen.
3. **Intrathoracic masses**
   a. **Mediastinal masses.** Large masses may cause **wheezing** and hypoxia from severe airway compression, which may lead to a medical emergency. Dysphagia and hoarseness can develop from compression of the esophagus and recurrent laryngeal nerve, respectively.
      (1) **Anterior mediastinal masses** are usually the result of thymic involvement in non-Hodgkin lymphoma or acute lymphoblastic leukemia (*see II B*) but can also result from a thymoma or a germ cell tumor.
      (2) **Middle mediastinal masses** suggest Hodgkin lymphoma or metastatic involvement of leukemia, non-Hodgkin lymphoma, or neuroblastoma.
      (3) **Posterior mediastinal masses** are usually neural tumors, such as neuroblastoma or ganglioneuroma.
   b. **Intrapulmonary lesions** are less common than mediastinal masses and are typically due to **metastatic disease** associated with Wilms tumor, soft tissue or bone sarcomas, germ cell tumors, hepatoblastoma, and Hodgkin lymphoma. Neuroblastoma is the only solid tumor in which pulmonary metastases are rare.
4. **Lymphadenopathy** is usually the response to an infectious or inflammatory stimulus. However, it can also result from the proliferation of neoplastic cells within the lymph node.

a. **Suppuration** strongly suggests an acute bacterial infection. Other findings—such as degree of hardness, matting, or tenderness—cannot reliably distinguish benign from neoplastic adenopathy.

b. **Rapidly enlarging nodes** or nodes in the **supraclavicular region** should increase the suspicion of malignancy.

(1) Leukemias, Hodgkin disease, non-Hodgkin lymphoma, and metastatic solid tumors can all cause nodal enlargement.

(2) Metastases from abdominal tumors often enlarge the left supraclavicular nodes.

(3) Metastases from thoracic tumors often enlarge the right supraclavicular nodes.

5. **Bone pain.** Expansion of the marrow cavity or destruction of cortical bone by leukemic cells, tumor, or metastatic disease can cause considerable pain.

a. If the long bones of the lower extremities are involved, a limp or difficulty in walking may develop.

b. If the skull is involved, proptosis or palpable nodules may develop.

c. Neuroblastoma and the primary bone cancers (i.e., Ewing sarcoma, osteogenic sarcoma) are the most likely solid tumors to produce bone pain, typically worse at night.

6. **Soft tissue masses.** Rhabdomyosarcomas often arise on the trunk or extremities and produce palpable tumors. Bone tumors that break through the cortex and infiltrate the soft tissues can also produce palpable tumors.

7. **Intracranial lesions.** Any space-occupying lesion can produce signs and symptoms of increased intracranial pressure (e.g., papilledema, ocular palsies, headaches, vomiting, lethargy).

a. Primary intracranial malignancies may be infratentorial or supratentorial in location.

b. Discrete intracranial metastatic lesions from solid tumors rarely occur.

c. Leukemic involvement of the central nervous system (CNS) may lead to increased intracranial pressure due to diffuse meningeal infiltration.

8. **Bone marrow failure**

a. **Diffuse replacement** of the normal marrow elements characterizes the acute leukemias and results in anemia, thrombocytopenia, and a paucity of mature and functional leukocytes, especially neutrophils (*see II A 3 a*).

b. **Metastatic infiltration** may result in anemia and leukoerythroblastic changes visible on peripheral smear, consisting of teardrop-shaped, fragmented, and nucleated red blood cells and a shift in the granulocyte series to the left. Tumor cells are often cohesive; clumps of primitive cells in the marrow resulting from solid tumor metastases are termed *syncytia.*

F Staging Current classification systems employ numerical staging; advanced disease is indicated by high numbers and is usually associated with a poor prognosis. Staging systems apply only to solid tumors with a propensity to disseminate and do not apply to the leukemias, which always are disseminated at the time of diagnosis.

1. **Stage I** tumors are **localized** to their organ of origin and, if treated by surgery, must be completely resected with no microscopic or gross disease remaining.

2. **Stages II and III** refer to **more advanced localized** disease than stage I tumors, for which surgical resection does not result in complete tumor removal. Patients with stage II tumors generally have less residual disease after surgery than patients with stage III tumors. For malignancies primary to the lymph nodes, the meaning of stage II and III designations is somewhat different and indicates the degree of spread within the lymphoid system.

3. **Stage IV** is indicative of **disseminated** disease with hematogenous metastases or spread to distant nodes in tumors that are not primary to the lymph nodes.

G Therapeutic strategies Childhood cancers are among the most curable human malignancies. To achieve a cure, therapy often involves multiple disciplines working in concert.

1. **Surgery.** Surgical resection of solid tumors contributes greatly to cure. Very large tumors that cannot initially be resected often can be rendered operable after the size has been decreased by radiotherapy, chemotherapy, or both.

2. **Radiotherapy.** The ionizing radiation beam can be directed at specific tumor locations. Radiotherapy plays an important role in the following situations:

a. **Local control** for selected malignancies including Hodgkin lymphoma, certain brain tumors, sarcomas, and embryonal tumors
b. Reduction in the size of large tumors to render them operable
c. Palliative and curative therapy of discrete metastatic foci
d. Eradication of leukemic cells in sanctuary sites (*see II A 3 d*)

3. **Chemotherapy.** Many different antineoplastic drugs have been developed during the last four decades, and their use is based on the following principles:
a. **Chemotherapy interferes with cell growth and division.**
b. **Chemotherapy produces adverse effects on normal as well as malignant cells.**
c. **Chemotherapy is most likely to effect a cure when the tumor cell burden is small.** However, this modality can also be curative in any of the following situations:
(1) **Primary therapy for disseminated malignancy.** There is no opportunity to control disseminated diseases, such as leukemias, with either surgery or radiotherapy. In addition, metastatic solid tumors also require chemotherapy but are often not as responsive as the leukemias.
(2) **Reduction in bulk disease.** Large solid tumors that cannot initially be removed surgically can sometimes be reduced by chemotherapy to allow an adequate surgical resection.
(3) **Destruction of micrometastases.** Many patients who have nonmetastatic solid tumors are thought to have clinically inapparent spread referred to as **micrometastases,** which, in the absence of systemic therapy, produce gross metastatic disease.

4. **Stem cell transplantation.** Some disseminated malignancies that are not cured by standard doses of chemotherapy and radiotherapy, particularly leukemias, may be cured by high doses if the irreversible toxicity of the therapy can be avoided. Toxicity to bone marrow is the limiting factor in many treatment regimens. If marrow destruction by high therapeutic doses can be circumvented by transplantation of new stem cells, then potentially curative doses of chemotherapy and radiotherapy can be administered.
a. **Types of stem cell transplantation**
(1) In **syngeneic transplantation,** a patient receives stem cells from an identical twin.
(2) In **allogeneic transplantation,** a patient receives stem cells from a related or unrelated donor.
(a) Donors are ideally related to the recipient and typically are siblings, but occasionally they can be other family members. Although the donor and patient are not genetically identical, they must be histocompatible and matched at the major human leukocyte antigen (HLA) loci. If they are not HLA matched, there is an increased risk that the new stem cells will be rejected, referred to as **graft failure,** or that the donated stem cells will mount an immune response against the patient, which manifests as **graft versus host disease (GVHD).** When there is no HLA-matched family member, donors unrelated to the patient can sometimes be found. These unrelated stem cell donors are usually adults. In addition, umbilical cord blood can be cryopreserved and used as a source of stem cells for allogeneic stem cell transplants. Because of the tremendous diversity of HLA antigens, searches for an unrelated donor require access to databases that have information on the HLA types of large numbers of potential donors.
(b) Even with histocompatibility between the donor and recipient of an allogeneic transplantation, there is still a significant risk of GVHD. This can be particularly severe when the donor is not related to the recipient.
(3) In **autologous transplantations,** the patient receives his or her own stem cells.
(a) For these transplantations, the patient's marrow or peripheral blood stem cells must be collected and stored before administering doses of chemotherapy and/or total body radiotherapy, which ablate the marrow.
(b) There is no risk of GVHD with autologous transplantations. Due to concerns for reinfusion of malignant cells, techniques may be employed to **"purge" the marrow in vitro of malignant cells** before it is returned to the patient. Monoclonal antibodies directed against tumor-associated antigens or chemotherapeutic agents are most commonly used.

b. **GVHD**

(1) **Clinical features**

(a) GVHD may produce mild to severe disease involving the skin, gastrointestinal tract, liver, and lungs.

(b) Profound immunodeficiency may develop in patients who have severe forms of GVHD, and they have a high risk of life-threatening infections.

(2) **Prevention**

(a) Risk of GVHD may be reduced with peri- and posttransplantation administration of immunosuppressive agents (e.g., methotrexate, corticosteroids, cyclosporine).

(b) T-cell depletion of stem cells prior to infusion into a recipient may decrease the risk of GVHD. In addition, the use of umbilical cord stem cells is also associated with a lower risk of GVHD.

5. **Long-term complications of therapy.** The increasing numbers of children who survive childhood cancer require surveillance for **late effects** associated with therapy. Some of the complications associated with particular therapeutic modalities are as follows:

a. **Radiotherapy** affects the organs that are in the radiation field.

(1) The **central nervous system** is particularly vulnerable; the following side effects have occurred in patients receiving irradiation to all or part of the brain:

(a) Learning difficulties, especially in young children

(b) Decreased growth due to injury to the hypothalamic/pituitary area

(c) Brain tumors

(2) Patients whose **thyroid glands** are in the radiation field are at risk for:

(a) Hypothyroidism

(b) Thyroid tumors

(3) Patients whose **bones** are in the radiation field are at risk for:

(a) Decreased growth

(b) Development of secondary bone cancers

(4) Radiation to the **gonads** results in sterility.

b. **Chemotherapeutic agents** can injure many organ systems.

(1) The heart can be damaged by anthracyclines (doxorubicin and daunomycin); the effect of these drugs is potentiated if the heart has also been included in a radiation field.

(2) The kidneys can be damaged by carboplatin, cisplatin, and ifosfamide.

(3) Hearing can be decreased by carboplatin and cisplatin.

(4) The bladder can be injured by cyclophosphamide and ifosfamide.

(5) The lungs can be injured by nitrosoureas and bleomycin.

(6) Sterility can be caused by anthracyclines and alkylating agents.

(7) Secondary malignancies, especially leukemia, can develop following exposure to various agents including etoposide, doxorubicin, and cyclophosphamide.

II THE LEUKEMIAS

A General considerations Collectively, these hematologic malignancies account for the greatest percentage of childhood cancer cases (30% of all neoplastic disease in children younger than 15 years of age).

1. **Classification.** Leukemias are classified as **lymphoblastic leukemias,** which are proliferations of cells of lymphoid lineage, and **myeloblastic leukemias,** which are proliferations of cells of granulocyte, monocyte, erythrocyte, or platelet lineage.

a. **Acute leukemias** constitute 97% of all childhood leukemias. If untreated, they are rapidly fatal within weeks to a few months of the diagnosis; however, with treatment, they often are curable.

(1) **Acute lymphoblastic leukemia** (ALL) is the **most common pediatric neoplasm** and accounts for 80% of all childhood acute leukemia cases.

(2) **Acute myeloblastic leukemia** (AML) **is also called acute myelogenous leukemia** and accounts for the remaining 20% of acute leukemia cases in children.

b. **Chronic leukemias** represent 3% of childhood leukemias; even without treatment, patients can survive for many months to years. All chronic leukemias in children are of **nonlymphoid lineage.** The leukemic cells are more mature and functional than the blasts of acute leukemias. Unfortunately, the chronic leukemias evolve into forms of acute leukemia that cannot easily be cured by available chemotherapy.

2. **Epidemiology.** In addition to children who have syndromes associated with chromosomal number or stability abnormalities, or with immunodeficiency states (*see I D 2*), the following individuals are at increased risk for leukemia:
   a. **Identical twins** have a 20% risk of leukemia if it develops in one twin during the first 5 years of life.
   b. In children with solid tumors who have been treated with intense chemotherapy, leukemia may develop as a secondary malignancy.
   c. **Children who have congenital marrow failure states,** such as **Shwachman-Diamond syndrome** (exocrine pancreatic insufficiency and neutropenia) and **Diamond-Blackfan syndrome** (congenital red cell aplasia), have an increased risk of leukemia.

3. **Clinical features**
   a. **Bone marrow failure.** Replacement of the normal hematopoietic elements by the leukemic cell population results in decreased production of red blood cells, normal white blood cells, and platelets. Consequently, most affected patients will have one or more of the following symptoms:
      (1) **Pallor, irritability, or fatigue** secondary to anemia
      (2) **Petechiae, ecchymoses** in the skin**, or epistaxis** secondary to thrombocytopenia. If there is associated disseminated intravascular coagulation (DIC) or extreme leukocytosis (*see II A 5 a* [*4*]), occasionally there may be severe and life-threatening bleeding (e.g., in the CNS).
      (3) **Fever** associated with **infection** due to a paucity of functional white blood cells, especially granulocytes
         (a) Localized signs of infection, such as rales with pneumonia or pus formation in an abscess, may not be apparent in these granulocytopenic patients.
         (b) Infection often quickly disseminates and produces bacteremia and sepsis.
   b. **Reticuloendothelial system infiltration**
      (1) **Lymphadenopathy** is common, especially in ALL, and may be so massive as to resemble that in the lymphomas.
      (2) **Hepatosplenomegaly** may also be present. Both the liver and the spleen can be minimally to massively enlarged.
   c. **Bone pain** (*see I E 5*)
   d. **Involvement of sanctuary sites.** Sanctuary sites are rarely involved at the time of diagnosis but may be involved with the recurrence of disease. These sites are the:
      (1) **CNS,** where involvement manifests as diffuse meningeal infiltration with signs of increased intracranial pressure (*see I E 7 c*)
      (2) **Testes,** one or both of which may be involved, with infiltration producing enlargement that is out of proportion to the child's sexual development

4. **Laboratory findings**
   a. **Peripheral blood.** A normal complete blood count does not preclude a diagnosis of leukemia, but abnormalities frequently are present.
      (1) **Anemia** is present in most patients and is normochromic and normocytic, with a low reticulocyte index indicative of decreased marrow production of red blood cells.
      (2) **Thrombocytopenia** is also very common, though 75% of patients present with platelet counts $> 20{,}000/mm^3$. If the platelet count is $< 20{,}000/mm^3$, there is an increased risk of bleeding.
      (3) **Neutropenia** is often present. Even if the patient has a high total white blood cell count, few of the cells are mature neutrophils. The following distribution of total white blood cells is seen:
         (a) Less than $10{,}000/mm^3$ in 50% of patients
         (b) Between 10,000 and $50{,}000/mm^3$ in 30% of patients

(c) Greater than 50,000/mm^3 in 20% of patients

(4) **Blast cells** are commonly seen on peripheral smear.

b. **Bone marrow** shows extensive replacement of the normal elements by leukemic cells. Even if there are blasts in peripheral blood, a diagnosis of leukemia should always be confirmed by bone marrow examination.

5. **Therapy**

a. **Supportive care.** Treatment of any complications in the child who has newly diagnosed leukemia is essential and lifesaving.

(1) **Transfusion therapy** is often necessary.

(a) Packed red blood cells are used to correct significant anemia.

(b) Platelet concentrates are used for severe thrombocytopenia.

(2) **Treatment of infection** is essential. If a patient becomes febrile, appropriate cultures (blood, urine, sites of local infection) should be obtained promptly, and intravenous administration of broad-spectrum antibiotics should be started immediately thereafter. If there are respiratory symptoms, a chest radiograph should also be obtained to look for infiltrates.

(3) **Metabolic support** is necessary in patients who have large tumor burdens as represented by a high white blood cell count or significant organ infiltration. These patients are at risk for **tumor lysis syndrome** characterized by one or more of the following metabolic abnormalities:

(a) **Hyperuricemia** may develop from the breakdown of purines released by dying leukemic cells. Urate crystal precipitation in the renal tubules may lead to renal insufficiency. This may be prevented by vigorous hydration to promote uric acid excretion. In most cases, allopurinol, a xanthine oxidase inhibitor, is used to block uric acid formation. In cases of severe uric acid elevations, urate oxidase, an enzyme that converts urate into the water-soluble allantoin, has been used to successfully decrease the uric acid to a safe and very low level. Alkalinization of the urine to pH 7 to 7.5 is unnecessary if urate oxidase is used, though using alkalinization to increase uric acid solubility is still considered an optional supportive care measure.

(b) **Hyperkalemia** due to increased cell lysis may also develop and cause serious cardiac arrhythmias if not corrected.

(c) **Hyperphosphatemia** and a reciprocal **hypocalcemia** may result in:

(i) Tetany

(ii) Potentiation of the effect of hyperkalemia on the heart

(iii) Precipitation of calcium phosphate in the renal tubules

(4) **Treatment of hyperviscosity.** White blood cell counts $> 100{,}000/\text{mm}^3$ in patients who have AML can cause significant hyperviscosity, leading to an increased risk of CNS hemorrhagic stroke or pulmonary infarction. The white blood cell count may be lowered by exchange transfusions or leukapheresis.

(5) **Treatment of superior vena cava syndrome.** A mass in the anterior mediastinum may produce compressive symptoms with airway compromise and obstruction of the superior vena cava, which results in a syndrome consisting of facial plethora, venous distention, and increased intracranial pressure. If the mass and compressive symptoms do not decrease with the institution of chemotherapy, radiotherapy to the mass may be effective.

b. **Antileukemic therapy** is administered in distinct phases with distinct objectives (*see II B 5 and II C 3*).

B **Acute lymphoblastic leukemia** is a malignant disease in which abnormal lymphoid blasts accumulate in the bone marrow and replace the normal hematopoietic elements. They are also released into peripheral blood, through which they spread throughout the body and infiltrate all organ systems.

1. **Epidemiology.** ALL is the most common type of childhood leukemia. It is more common in white children than in black children and more common in males than in females (1.2–1.3 times). ALL is associated with a peak incidence in the 3- to 5-year-old age group for white children only.

2. **Etiology.** The malignant lymphoblasts of each patient who has ALL are all thought to be descendants of a single abnormal precursor cell, and as such represent a clone. They demonstrate a

unique pattern of gene rearrangement that is identical in all the cells of the clone, and which distinguishes them from the clones of other ALL patients, and from the innumerable patterns in mature B and T cells.

3. **Classification**
   a. **Morphologic classification** of ALL is based on the following features:
      (1) **Appearance of the leukemic lymphoblasts.** According to the French-American-British (FAB) classification, leukemic lymphoblasts are subdivided into three categories.
         (a) **L1 lymphoblasts** are small, with scant cytoplasm and absent or inconspicuous nucleoli. They are by far the most common type of cells in children who have ALL.
         (b) **L2 lymphoblasts** are larger, with more abundant cytoplasm and one or more prominent nucleoli. They are much less common than L1 cells and are sometimes mistaken for myeloblasts.
         (c) **L3 lymphoblasts** are large, with deeply basophilic and vacuolated cytoplasm and prominent nucleoli. They are rare and usually indicative of a mature B-cell leukemia.
      (2) **Enzymatic evaluation.** Terminal deoxynucleotidyl transferase (TdT) is a unique DNA polymerase that is found in almost all lymphoblasts but only rarely in AML blasts.
      (3) **Histochemical evaluation** shows:
         (a) Absence of surface markers typical of AML blasts
         (b) In many cases, accumulations of glycogen on periodic acid-Schiff stain
   b. **Immunologic classification** regards ALL as a heterogeneous group of malignancies characterized by accumulation of immature lymphoid cells arrested at various stages of development. On the basis of immunophenotype, ALL is divided into the following subtypes (Table 16-4):
      (1) **B-cell precursor ALL** accounts for 84% of all cases. Cells from patients who have this type of ALL are lymphoid precursors that are blocked at very early stages of their development. Early B-cell differentiation antigens are also expressed on the cell surface and these cells cannot synthesize immunoglobulin molecules.
      (2) **Mature B-cell ALL** accounts for 1% of cases and is characterized by cells that lack TdT activity and synthesize complete immunoglobulin molecules, which are expressed on their surface. This is the most mature form of ALL of B-cell lineage and is closely related to Burkitt lymphoma, with which it shares clinical features (e.g., occurrence in older children and teenagers, predilection for males, intra-abdominal mass, and dissemination to the meninges) as well as karyotype features (*see I D 3 a*).
      (3) **T-cell ALL** accounts for the remaining 15% of ALL cases. The malignant cells show evidence of T-cell lineage by expression of various T-cell antigens and rearrangement of the genes for the T-cell antigen receptor. T-cell ALL has a characteristic clinical presentation that includes:
         (a) Occurrence in older children and teenagers
         (b) Predilection for males
         (c) High white blood cell count, often > 100,000/mm^3
         (d) Presence of anterior mediastinal mass
         (e) Early dissemination to meninges and testes

TABLE 16-4 Characteristics of the Different Types of Acute Lymphoblastic Leukemias

Immunophenotype	Age	White Blood Cell Count	Common Karyotype	Other Factors
CD10-negative early pre-B	Infant	High	Translocation	Worst prognosis
CD10-positive early pre-B	Younger child	Low, normal	Hyperdiploidy Cryptic t(12;21)	L1 morphology
Pre-B	Younger child	Low, normal	Translocation	Cytoplasmic immunoglobulin
T-cell	Older child Adolescent	High	Translocation	Mediastinal mass
B-cell	Older child Adolescent	Variable	Translocation	L3 morphology

TABLE 16-5 Prognostic Groups in B-Cell Precursor and T-Cell Acute Lymphoblastic Leukemia as Defined by the Children's Oncology Group

	Standard Risk (All Required)	High Risk (Any Sufficient)
Age	1 through 9 y	Younger than 1 y, 10 y or older
WBC count	< 50,000 mm^3	50,000 mm^3 or higher
t9;22	Absent	Present
t4;11	Absent	Present
Hypodiploidy	Absent	Present

WBC, white blood cell.

4. **Prognosis.** Presenting clinical and laboratory features for each patient who has newly diagnosed ALL determine the probability that the child will remain in remission when treated with current antileukemic therapy. Certain factors (e.g., age, sex, leukemic cell burden as reflected by white blood cell count, and karyotype) are used to determine prognosis. The **Children's Oncology Group** is the major cooperative group treating cancer in infants, children, and adolescents. In the current ALL treatment protocols, this group assigns patients who have acute leukemia into prognostic categories based on their risk of relapse. These categories are standard risk and high risk (Table 16-5); they are based on the following features:
   a. **Standard-risk patients** have an 85% or greater chance of cure.
   b. **High-risk patients** have a < 70% chance of cure.
   c. **Other factors that may determine prognosis**
      (1) Factors believed to carry a worse **prognosis for any type of ALL** include **inadequate therapy, slow response to therapy,** and **male sex.**
      (2) For **B-cell precursor ALL,** certain **karyotypic features** have a strong influence on outcome.
         (a) A **favorable prognosis** is associated with:
            (i) **Presence of the fusion transcript TEL-AML1** in the leukemic cells. It is the most common molecular abnormality in ALL and is produced by the cryptic t(12;21), which usually cannot be detected by cytogenetic analysis but is readily detected by fluorescent in situ hybridization (FISH).
            (ii) **Hyperdiploidy,** especially if there are 53 or more chromosomes within the leukemic cells
         (b) An **unfavorable prognosis** is associated with **pseudodiploidy** due to the presence of certain specific chromosomal translocations within the leukemic cells. They include the Philadelphia chromosome t(9;22); t(4;11), which is seen in most cases of infants with early pre-B-cell ALL; and t(1;19), which is seen in some patients who have pre-B-cell ALL.
         (c) **Hypodiploidy,** due to fewer than 46 chromosomes in the leukemic cells, is also associated with an **unfavorable prognosis.**
      (3) T-cell ALL is generally considered to have a less favorable prognosis and therapy is typically similar to that given to high-risk pre-B-cell leukemia patients.

5. **Therapy**
   a. **Remission induction** is successful in more than 95% of children. This initial phase lasts at least 4 weeks, during which maximal cytoreduction is achieved. If successful, at the conclusion of remission induction, bone marrow should demonstrate normal hematopoiesis and contain < 0.1% blasts; complete blood count values should return to normal; and abnormal physical findings due to leukemia should be gone. At least three drugs—including steroids, vincristine, and asparaginase—are employed. Anthracyclines are added for patients who have a high risk of relapse.
   b. **Consolidation or intensification** consists of continued systemic therapy designed to kill additional leukemic cells to prevent systemic relapse along with CNS-directed therapy to prevent CNS relapse. Intrathecal therapy is the current mainstay of CNS prophylaxis. Radiotherapy

adds to potential CNS toxicity and is reserved primarily for prophylaxis in select high-risk patients and for treatment in patients determined to have CNS leukemic involvement.

c. **Maintenance or continuation therapy** is the longest and last phase of therapy, typically lasting at least 2 to 3 years. The objective in this phase is to continue the remissions achieved in the previous phases and to produce whatever additional cytoreduction is necessary to cure the leukemia.

d. **Delayed intensification** is a 2-month period of aggressive therapy that may be administered once or twice during the first year of therapy; typically patients are given a short period of maintenance therapy followed by this more intense phase. It is designed to eradicate any leukemic cells that escaped destruction during the initial induction and consolidation phases of therapy.

6. **Outcome**
   a. **Continuous complete remission** is the most common outcome for children who have ALL and is especially likely in those with a standard risk of relapse.
   b. **Relapses** still occur in approximately 20% to 25% of patients.
      (1) At least one half of relapses occur while initial chemotherapy is still being administered. Relapse can occur in the:
         (a) Bone marrow, which is the most common site of recurrence
         (b) CNS, which was formerly the most common site of recurrence before CNS prophylaxis
         (c) Testes, which are becoming the most common site of extramedullary relapse
      (2) **Salvage chemotherapy** can sometimes cure children who have:
         (a) Isolated extramedullary relapses in the CNS or testes
         (b) Bone marrow relapses that occur later than 12 months after elective discontinuation of therapy
      (3) **Currently used chemotherapy** regimens frequently produce additional remissions in children who experience bone marrow relapses while receiving chemotherapy or within 12 months of its discontinuation, but these remissions are rarely curative. Most of these patients will ultimately die of their ALL unless they can be treated with bone marrow transplantation. At least one third of children with relapsed ALL who can undergo allogeneic transplantation from an HLA-matched relative are cured of their otherwise fatal disease. Results with other types of bone marrow transplantations (unrelated HLA matched, autologous) are not as good.

C Acute myeloblastic leukemia AML is a malignant disease in which there is accumulation in the marrow of precursors of one or more of the following cell types: Granulocytes, monocytes, erythrocytes, or platelets. These precursor cells also spread to the peripheral blood, through which they spread throughout the body and infiltrate all organ systems.

1. **Epidemiology.** AML accounts for 20% of all childhood leukemia. It is more common in males than in females and more common in black children than in white children. AML has a stable incidence throughout childhood.
2. **Classification.** The FAB classification uses morphologic and histochemical information to subdivide AML into the following subtypes:
   a. **M1 (myeloblastic leukemia without maturation).** The cells are typically very large with abundant cytoplasm and prominent nucleoli.
   b. **M2 (myeloblastic leukemia with differentiation).** The cells have the same histochemical features as M1 cells but also have readily discernible azurophilic granules, which may coalesce into Auer rods.
   c. **M3 (promyelocytic leukemia).** The abundant azurophilic granules in the cells may serve as a source of procoagulant material, which may lead to **DIC.** This form of AML is also associated with a distinct cytogenetic abnormality, t(15;17) (*see I C 2 a [1] [b] [ii]*).
   d. **M4 (myelomonocytic leukemia).** Some of the cells have myeloblastic features by morphology and histochemistry; others may have monocytic features and stain for nonspecific esterase. M4 with eosinophilia (M4Eo) is a distinct subtype associated with an inversion 16 cytogenetic abnormality and typically has a good prognosis.
   e. **M5 (monoblastic leukemia)** is characterized by nonspecific esterase-positive cells, propensity for gum and CNS involvement, and association with DIC.

f. **M6 (erythroleukemia).** The malignant cells are predominantly megaloblastic erythroid precursors, but myeloblasts are also present.

g. **M7 (megakaryoblastic leukemia),** is the most common leukemia seen in children younger than 3 years of age with trisomy 21. This diagnosis is difficult based on morphology alone and often requires flow cytometry.

3. **Therapy**
   a. **Remission induction** requires more intensive chemotherapy than that administered for ALL. Most regimens use at least an anthracycline and cytosine arabinoside. Myelosuppression is severe, and good supportive care is essential. Remission is achieved in 80% of children.
   b. **After remission induction,** the following options are available:
      (1) **Further chemotherapy** consisting of consolidation therapy with intensive systemic therapy and prophylactic therapy to the CNS
      (2) **Allogeneic bone marrow transplantation** if the patient has an HLA-matched related donor
   c. **For acute promyelocytic leukemia (M3),** administration of large doses of *trans*-retinoic acid overcomes the block in differentiation and apoptosis and causes terminal differentiation and death of the leukemic cells. Retinoic acid alone can induce remission, but the remissions are not durable unless cytoreductive chemotherapy is also administered.

4. **Prognosis**
   a. The best chemotherapeutic regimens are curative for slightly less than half of AML patients. M3 AML is associated with an approximately 85% survival with current chemotherapy.
   b. The best allogeneic bone marrow transplantation regimens for those with an HLA-identical related match are curative for up to 60% of these patients.

D Chronic leukemias

1. **Classification.** Two types of chronic leukemias occur during childhood.
   a. **Chronic myeloid leukemia (CML)** is a clonal myeloproliferative disorder arising from a neoplastically transformed stem cell. The neoplastic cells almost invariably contain the **Philadelphia chromosome t(9;22),** resulting in a fusion of the c-*abl* oncogene on chromosome 9 to the breakpoint cluster region (*bcr*) of chromosome 22. The hybrid c-*abl/bcr* region transcribes a novel tyrosine kinase that inhibits apoptosis.
   b. **Juvenile myelomonocytic leukemia (JMML)** is characterized by a proliferation of cells of monocytic and granulocytic origin. It is not a variant CML, and its cells do not contain the Philadelphia chromosome.

2. **Clinical features**
   a. **CML**
      (1) **Symptoms.** CML occurs in older children and teenagers who often present with fatigue, weight loss, bone pain, and increased abdominal girth from massive splenomegaly.
      (2) **Characteristic laboratory findings** include:
         (a) Extreme hyperleukocytosis, which is characterized by a white cell count > 100,000/mm^3, a predominance of more mature granulocytes on peripheral smear, and eosinophilia and basophilia
         (b) Normal to increased platelet count
         (c) Mild anemia
         (d) Extreme myeloid hyperplasia in the bone marrow
         (e) The Philadelphia chromosome
   b. **JMML**
      (1) **Symptoms.** JMML occurs predominantly in children younger than 5 years of age and is more common in male patients presenting with lymphadenopathy, hepatosplenomegaly, desquamative erythematous rash, purpura, and pulmonary infiltrates.
      (2) **Characteristic laboratory findings** include:
         (a) Anemia with characteristics of fetal erythropoiesis
         (b) Thrombocytopenia
         (c) Moderate hyperleukocytosis, which is characterized by a mean white cell count of 60,000/mm^3 and an increase in monocytes and granulocytes in the peripheral blood

(d) An increase in monocytes and granulocytes and a decrease in megakaryocytes in the bone marrow

3. **Prognosis**
   a. **CML** can be subdivided into the following phases:
      (1) During **chronic CML,** the disease manifestations can be well controlled and the majority of both children and adults can sustain long-term remissions.
      (2) During **accelerated CML,** clinical and laboratory findings show marked deterioration, and patient responsiveness to therapy diminishes.
      (3) During **blastic CML,** which is of short duration, the disease acquires the features of a fatal acute leukemia. Blast crisis can be:
         (a) Myeloid, which is more common than lymphoid and usually is unresponsive to further therapy
         (b) **Lymphoid,** which usually is briefly responsive to therapy
   b. **Juvenile CML** is more rapidly fatal, with a median survival of 9 months.

4. **Therapy**
   a. **Chemotherapy** is not curative for CML or JMML. Current therapy for CML includes the use of novel targeted therapy aimed at inhibition of the bcr-abl fusion protein. Since initial use in 1999, the tyrosine receptor inhibitor imatinib mesylate has become the standard up-front therapy for adults with CML and has been successful in inducing long-term remissions for most adult patients. For children, imatinib mesylate has increased in use and is commonly used for patients who do not have an HLA-identically matched donor.
   b. **Bone marrow transplantation** has been curative for both CML and JMML. For children who have CML and an HLA fully matched donor, stem cell transplantation may be considered for curative therapy. Stem cell transplant is much more efficacious if it is done during the chronic phase.

III NON-HODGKIN LYMPHOMAS

Non-Hodgkin lymphomas are a heterogeneous group of diseases characterized by neoplastic proliferations of immature lymphoid cells, which, unlike the malignant lymphoid cells of ALL, accumulate primarily outside the bone marrow.

A Epidemiology

Non-Hodgkin lymphomas represent approximately 6% of all childhood cancers. They occur predominantly in older children and teenagers and have a strong predilection for males.

1. **Childhood non-Hodgkin lymphomas** are most commonly high-grade lesions occurring in extranodal locations.
2. **Burkitt lymphoma** occurs in an endemic form in Africa, with a presentation as a mass in the jaw or abdomen, associated with a prior Epstein-Barr virus infection. Burkitt lymphoma and other closely related forms of B-cell lymphoma also develop in children immunosuppressed by HIV infection (see Chapter 9). The specific chromosomal abnormality consists of translocation of a portion of the long arm of chromosome 8—which contains the c-*myc* oncogene—onto the area of another chromosome (14, 2, or 22)—which controls immunoglobulin chain synthesis (a specific B-cell function).

B Classification

1. **Morphology.** Almost all cases are diffuse lymphomas and are classified as highly aggressive. The following types occur:
   a. In **lymphoblastic non-Hodgkin lymphoma,** the cells resemble those seen in the usual cases of acute lymphoblastic leukemia.
   b. In **nonlymphoblastic non-Hodgkin lymphoma,** the cell morphology can vary from small, such as those seen in small noncleaved lymphoma, to large vacuolated cells, such as those seen in Burkitt lymphoma.
2. **Immunohistology. T-cell origin** is demonstrated in almost half of the cases. The cells generally have a lymphoblastic morphology and contain TdT. **B-cell origin** is demonstrated in most other cases.

C Clinical features Most childhood non-Hodgkin lymphomas are rapidly growing, and thus, symptom duration is short.

1. **Anterior mediastinal masses,** sometimes associated with pleural effusions, are the most common presentation of lymphoblastic lymphomas. They can produce:
   a. Respiratory distress from airway compromise
   b. Superior vena cava syndrome (*see II A 5 a* [5])
2. **Abdominal masses** arise from either abdominal lymph nodes or from intestinal Peyer patches. They can cause:
   a. Abdominal enlargement from a rapidly growing tumor, which sometimes produces pain, ascites, and urinary tract obstruction
   b. Intestinal obstruction, by serving as the lead point for an intussusception
3. **Jaw masses** are a common presentation for endemic Burkitt lymphoma.
4. **Peripheral lymph node enlargement** can be seen with any type of childhood non-Hodgkin lymphoma.
5. **Less common presentations** include:
   a. Obstructing nasopharyngeal tumor
   b. Bone tumor
   c. Skin tumor

D Staging Various systems are employed for classifying different types of childhood non-Hodgkin lymphoma. They all distinguish:

1. **Local disease** of limited bulk, often confined to one side of the diaphragm and carrying a good prognosis
2. **Extensive disease** within the mediastinum or abdomen
3. **Hematogenous dissemination,** especially to the bone marrow (with $<$ 25% involvement) and meninges

E Therapy **Systemic chemotherapy** is needed in all cases to shrink the local tumor and prevent dissemination to distant sites. The intensity and duration of therapy depend on the type of lymphoma and the stage of the disease. In addition to standard nonspecific chemotherapy, the recent addition of the targeted monoclonal anti-CD20 antibody rituximab has drastically improved outcome. **CNS prophylaxis with intrathecal chemotherapy** is usually given. **Radiotherapy** is indicated in treatment sites where there is life-threatening obstruction that does not respond to chemotherapy, or bulk tumor for which chemotherapy alone is judged inadequate.

F Prognosis With appropriate management of the metabolic consequences of rapid cell turnover (*see II A 5 a* [3]) as well as institution of therapy, a favorable outcome is often achieved. Without therapy, rapid and widespread dissemination occurs.

IV HODGKIN LYMPHOMA

Hodgkin lymphoma behaves similarly to the disease that occurs in adults.

A Epidemiology Hodgkin lymphoma accounts for 4% of all childhood cancer. It occurs in older children and teenagers and has a slight female predominance.

B Clinical features

1. **Localized adenopathy,** especially in the cervical region, is the most common presenting symptom.
2. **Systemic "B" symptoms** occur in up to 30% of children and consist of:
   a. Temperature exceeding 100.4°F (38°C)
   b. Drenching night sweats
   c. Weight loss in excess of 10% of body weight in 6 months

C Classification based on histopathology divides Hodgkin disease into:

1. **Lymphocyte predominance,** with many lymphocytes and a few Reed-Sternberg cells

2. **Mixed cellularity,** in which there are more Reed-Sternberg cells admixed with a heterogeneous population of reactive cells
3. **Lymphocyte depletion,** with many Reed-Sternberg cells and a few reactive cells
4. **Nodular sclerosis,** in which dense fibrotic bands separate islands of reactive cells from Reed-Sternberg cell variants (called **lacunar cells**)

D Staging Staging can be assigned by a combination of imaging and laboratory tests. For any given stage, patients are further subdivided into "A" or "B" depending on the absence (A) or presence (B) of systemic symptoms.

1. **Stage I.** Disease is confined to one group of nodes.
2. **Stage II.** Disease is present in more than one group of nodes but is limited to one side of the diaphragm.
3. **Stage III.** Disease involves nodes on both sides of the diaphragm, with the spleen considered a node.
4. **Stage IV.** There is hematogenous spread to the liver, bone marrow, lungs, or other nonnodal sites.

E Therapy and prognosis Prognosis is good and varies from a > 90% cure of stage I disease to an approximately 60% to 70% cure of stage IV disease.

1. **Radiotherapy** can be utilized as primary treatment or in combination with chemotherapy.
2. **Combination chemotherapy** is typically used for all patients with stage II to IV disease, as well as for patients who have localized but bulky disease, such as a large mediastinal mass. Chemotherapy often is given in conjunction with radiotherapy.
3. **Late effects of therapy** are numerous. Most serious are:
   a. Secondary malignancies (e.g., AML, non-Hodgkin lymphoma) in patients treated with combined radiotherapy and nitrogen mustard-derived chemotherapy regimens
   b. Thyroid gland dysfunction (hypothyroidism, benign and malignant tumors) after neck irradiation
   c. Growth disturbances after irradiation
   d. Sterility

V NEUROBLASTOMA

Neuroblastoma is a malignancy of neural crest cells, which, in the course of their normal development, give rise to the paraspinal sympathetic ganglia and the adrenal medulla.

A Epidemiology Its 7% incidence makes neuroblastoma the second most common solid tumor of childhood. Neuroblastoma occurs predominantly in early childhood with two thirds occurring in children younger than 5 years.

B Clinical features are extremely variable and reflect the widespread distribution of neural crest tissue.

1. **Primary sites**
   a. **Abdominal tumors** are the most common presentation, accounting for 70% of the cases; half arise from extra-adrenal tissue and half from the adrenal medulla. Presenting features are:
      (1) Abdominal mass, which often displaces the kidneys anterolaterally and inferiorly
      (2) Abdominal pain
      (3) Systemic hypertension, if there is compression of the renal vasculature
   b. **Thoracic tumors** are the next most common presentation and are located in the posterior mediastinum. Presenting features are:
      (1) Respiratory distress
      (2) Incidental finding on a chest radiograph that was obtained for unrelated symptoms
   c. The presentation of **head and neck tumors** involves palpable tumors that sometimes produce **Horner syndrome.**
   d. **Paraspinal tumors** arise from the paraspinal sympathetic ganglia. They may grow through the neural foramina into the epidural space, where compression of the spinal cord may produce back pain, weakness, or paralysis.

2. **Metastases** are common at diagnosis and often cause the symptoms that lead to the diagnosis of neuroblastoma.
   a. **Nonspecific symptoms** of metastatic disease include:
      (1) Weight loss
      (2) Fever
   b. **Specific symptoms** of metastatic disease include:
      (1) Bone marrow failure (*see I E 8*)
      (2) Cortical bone pain, resulting in a limp if present in the lower extremity
      (3) Proptosis and periorbital ecchymoses from retrobulbar and orbital infiltration
      (4) Liver infiltration, causing hepatomegaly
      (5) Distant lymph node enlargement (*see I E 4*)
      (6) Skin infiltration, causing palpable subcutaneous nodules
3. **Paraneoplastic symptoms** are occasionally seen.
   a. Watery diarrhea may occur in patients who have differentiated tumors that secrete **vasoactive intestinal peptide.**
   b. **Opsoclonus-myoclonus encephalopathy** is a rare manifestation associated with an excellent prognosis.

C **Staging** generally follows the pattern described previously (*see I F*), with the following exceptions:

1. **Stages I** and **II** tumors must not be large enough to cross the midline.
2. **Stage III** tumors cross the midline.
3. **Stage IVS.** This is a special type of metastatic tumor that occurs in infants and carries a much better prognosis than the usual Stage IV tumors. Stage IVS tumors are small primary tumors that occur in young infants who have metastases limited to the skin, liver, and bone marrow but not cortical bone.

D **Tumor markers** are extremely useful in evaluating children who have neuroblastoma.

1. **Urinary markers.** Catecholamines are particularly useful markers and include:
   a. Vanillylmandelic acid (VMA)
   b. Homovanillic acid (HVA)
2. **Serum markers.** Elevation of the following serum markers is often associated with a poor prognosis:
   a. Ferritin
   b. Lactate dehydrogenase
3. **Oncogene marker.** Amplification of the **n-*myc* oncogene** within the tumor cells is also associated with a poor prognosis.

E **Therapy**

1. **Surgery** alone often suffices for stage I and II patients.
2. **Spontaneous regression without any therapy** is common in stage IVS infants.
3. **Aggressive multiagent chemotherapy** regimens can often produce dramatic tumor regression in stage III and IV disease. However, if the patient has poor prognostic features such as n-*myc* amplification or an age of 1 year or older with either stage IV disease or stage III with unfavorable histology, attaining a cure is more difficult.
4. **Autologous stem cell transplantation** has been used for stage III and IV patients who have a poor prognosis and up to 50% of these patients can be cured. Their chances of cure appear to be increased if they are offered posttransplant cis-retinoic acid, an agent that induces terminal differentiation and death of any neuroblastoma cells remaining following transplant.

F **Prognosis** depends on the following factors:

1. **Age.** Infants younger than 1 year of age have the best prognosis.
2. **Stage**
   a. Stage I and II patients and stage IVS infants have a good prognosis.
   b. Most stage III and IV patients have a poor prognosis.

3. **Histopathology** may be an important feature. The degree of differentiation of the tumor cells and the pattern of their growth may, in selected cases, influence prognosis.
4. **Tumor markers** (*see V D*)

VI WILMS TUMOR

Neoplastic embryonal renal cells of the metanephros give rise to this kidney tumor, which is composed of an admixture of cells (blastemic, epithelial, and stromal) in varying proportions. The epithelial cells form tubules.

A Epidemiology Wilms tumor accounts for 6% of all childhood cancers. It is predominantly a tumor that occurs during the first 5 years of life, with an approximately equal incidence throughout each of those 5 years. Occurrence is equal in males and females.

B Clinical features Most children with newly diagnosed Wilms tumor have localized disease and appear well.

1. **Asymptomatic abdominal mass** is by far the most common presentation, usually detected on routine physical examination or by a caretaker bathing the patient.
2. **Hypertension** occurs in approximately one fourth of all patients and may be related to elaboration of renin by tumor cells or, less frequently, to compression of the renal vasculature by the tumor.
3. **Microscopic hematuria** may be seen on routine urinalysis.
4. **Abdominal pain,** especially with hemorrhage into the tumor, is less commonly present. There may be associated fever and anemia.
5. **Genetic factors** (*see I D 1*) and associated abnormalities include:
   a. **Aniridia**
      (1) Children who have sporadic (as opposed to hereditary) aniridia are at increased risk for development of Wilms tumor. In many of these children, a deletion in the 11p13 region can be demonstrated.
      (2) Children who have both sporadic aniridia and the chromosome deletion have an almost 50% chance for development of Wilms tumor.
      (3) Children who have the Wilms tumor, aniridia, genitourinary anomalies, and mental retardation (**WAGR**) syndrome have deletions at 11p13 that involve genes for iris development (PAX6) and genitourinary tract development (WT1).
   b. Hemihypertrophy
      (1) Children with **Beckwith-Wiedemann syndrome** are at an increased risk of developing hepatoblastoma, adrenal cortical carcinoma, and Wilms tumor. These children have abnormalities at 11p15.

C Staging is similar to that for other solid tumors (*see I F*). An additional stage, stage V, designates those 5% of patients who have tumor in both kidneys. Most patients have relatively localized disease; only 10% to 15% of patients have distant metastases at diagnosis.

D Diagnosis

1. **Appropriate imaging studies,** including ultrasound, computed tomography (CT) scan, or magnetic resonance imaging (MRI), are used to define the site of origin within the kidneys and evaluate the contralateral kidney for tumor.
2. **Search for distant metastases** is undertaken. Sites may include:
   a. Lungs
   b. Liver
   c. Bone (in patients whose tumors have an unfavorable histology)

E Therapy Dramatic advances in survival have occurred with the use of combined modality therapy.

1. **Surgery** involves removal of the primary tumor (by nephrectomy except in the case of bilateral tumors where at least part of one kidney must be preserved), local lymph nodes, and selected metastases.

2. **Radiotherapy** involves treatment of residual local disease and selected metastatic foci.
3. **Chemotherapy** varies in duration and intensity, depending on the patient's stage and histology.

F Prognosis Patients with localized disease and a favorable histology have a > 90% chance of survival. Poor prognosis patients have a < 70% chance of survival.

1. **Stage**
   a. Patients who have distant metastases (stage IV) have the worst prognosis.
   b. Stage V patients often do well with individualized management of their bilateral tumors.
2. **Histopathology**
   a. Ninety percent of patients have a favorable histology, and most, in absence of distant metastases, do very well.
   b. Ten percent have unfavorable histologies and often do poorly, even if their disease is localized. They usually have:
      (1) Anaplastic Wilms tumor
      (2) Clear cell sarcoma and rhabdoid tumor

VII RHABDOMYOSARCOMA

Rhabdomyosarcoma arises from the embryonal mesenchyme from which skeletal muscle originates.

A Epidemiology Rhabdomyosarcoma is the most common soft tissue sarcoma and accounts for 3.5% of cancer in children younger than 15 years old.

B Pathology Rhabdomyosarcoma can have a more favorable **embryonal** histologic subtype or a more unfavorable **alveolar** subtype.

C Clinical features Rhabdomyosarcoma is heterogeneous in presentation. The following are common sites of occurrence:

1. **Head and neck** (38%)
   a. **Orbit tumors** have a rapid onset of symptoms due to their confinement by the bony orbit. Their presentation involves:
      (1) Exophthalmos
      (2) Ptosis
      (3) Eyelid swelling
   b. **Nasopharyngeal** and **middle ear tumors** are associated with:
      (1) Discharge
      (2) Polypoid mass
      (3) Airway obstruction
      (4) Chronic otitis media
      (5) Spread to the adjacent meninges, causing increased intracranial pressure and cranial nerve palsies
   c. **Neck tumors** cause:
      (1) Mass
      (2) Pain
      (3) Cervical and brachial plexus palsy
2. **Genitourinary tract** (21%)
   a. **Bladder** and **prostate tumors** cause:
      (1) Urinary obstruction
      (2) Hematuria
   b. **Vaginal** and **uterine tumors** cause:
      (1) Vaginal bleeding
      (2) Polypoid tumor with glistening membrane (**sarcoma botryoides**, or "cluster of grapes") extruding from the vaginal orifice
3. The presentation of **extremity tumors** (18%) involves solid masses on the upper or lower extremities.

4. **Miscellaneous presentations.** Twenty-one percent occur with a mass or obstructing lesion in the following locations:
   a. Trunk
   b. Retroperitoneum
   c. Paratesticular region
   d. Perianal region
   e. Gastrointestinal and biliary tracts

D Therapy

1. **Surgery.** Complete excision is optimal when possible for locations where disfigurement will not result.
2. **Radiotherapy** is used for local tumors and metastases. It is also indicated for patients who have parameningeal head and neck tumors. This prevents meningeal spread and greatly decreases the risk of recurrence in the CNS.
3. **Chemotherapy** is used as an adjuvant to other therapy in patients who have localized disease to prevent development of metastatic disease. It can also be used to decrease the size of a tumor to improve the ability to attain a complete surgical resection.

E **Prognosis** has dramatically improved over the years by judicious use of all therapeutic modalities.

1. Children with primary tumors of the orbit have an **excellent** (90%) survival rate without need for disfiguring surgery.
2. Children who have primary tumors of the genitourinary tract have long-term survival as high as 75%.
3. **Poor** prognosis is still seen with:
   a. Extremity tumors
   b. Retroperitoneal tumors
   c. Metastatic disease

VIII BONE TUMORS

Primary malignant bone tumors account for 5% of childhood cancer. Two highly malignant tumors predominate: Osteogenic sarcoma and Ewing sarcoma.

A **Osteogenic sarcoma** is a malignant tumor of the bone-producing mesenchyme.

1. **Epidemiology.** Osteogenic sarcoma is the most common primary malignant bone tumor seen in pediatric patients. It occurs mainly in adolescents and is twice as common in males as in females.
2. **Clinical features**
   a. Pain and swelling are common.
   b. Systemic manifestations are rare.
   c. The most common tumor sites in decreasing order of frequency include the **distal femur, proximal tibia, and proximal humerus.**
   d. **Metastases** occur in the lungs and bone.
   e. **Radiographic findings** include destructive lesions with periosteal reaction, with a characteristic radial **"sunburst"** as the tumor breaks through the cortex and new bone spicules are produced.
3. **Therapy**
   a. **Chemotherapy** is of great importance and clearly improves disease-free survival. Chemotherapy is typically given prior to surgery (**neoadjuvant chemotherapy**), followed by continuation of chemotherapy after surgery (**adjuvant chemotherapy**).
   b. **Surgery** plays a key role and, if cure is to be attained, must involve a complete resection. **Limb salvage** procedures are favored and involve the use of cadaveric or synthetic bone grafts. **Amputation** is performed when limb salvage is not possible.
4. **Prognosis.** Patients with nonmetastatic disease at diagnosis, treated with both surgery and chemotherapy, have an overall survival of approximately 65%. However, patients with metastatic disease at diagnosis do not fare as well with $< 20\%$ disease-free survival.

B **Ewing sarcoma** is an undifferentiated sarcoma of uncertain histogenesis, which arises primarily in bone. A possible neurogenic origin has been suggested for the Ewing sarcoma's cells and a more primitive form of Ewing sarcoma has historically been referred to as a primitive neuroectodermal tumor (PNET). A t11:22 translocation is associated with this tumor and leads to the fusion of the transcription factor gene FLI1 on chromosome 11 to the EWS gene on chromosome 22. A new fusion protein is produced, which leads to tumor formation. In 25% of patients, the Ewing sarcoma arises in the soft tissues of the extremities and paravertebral region rather than in bone, and is referred to as **extraosseous Ewing sarcoma.**

1. **Epidemiology.** Ewing sarcoma is seen primarily in adolescents and is 1.5 times more common in males than females. It is rarely seen in blacks.
2. **Clinical features.** Pain and localized swelling are the most common presenting complaints and **constitutional symptoms** including fatigue, fever, and weight loss are more frequently associated with this tumor than any other sarcoma. Any bone can be affected, though the most likely sites are the **femur, humerus, and pelvic bones.** Other long bones, ribs, and the scapula may also be involved.
3. **Diagnosis**
   a. Radiographs characteristically show "onion skinning," a destructive lesion associated with periosteal elevation or a soft tissue mass.
   b. Evaluation for metastatic disease should include studies of the lungs, other bones, and bone marrow.
4. **Therapy**
   a. **Chemotherapy** plays an important role in reduction of primary tumor bulk, prevention of metastatic disease, and treatment of patients with metastases at diagnosis.
   b. **Surgery** plays a crucial role in local tumor therapy. Patients will undergo surgery when they have tumors that can be completely surgically resected without major morbidity.
   c. **Radiotherapy** is employed when tumors cannot be completely surgically resected.
5. **Prognosis**
   a. The overall survival for patients with nonmetastatic tumors treated with chemotherapy and either radiotherapy or surgery is 65%.
   b. The prognosis is worse for patients who have:
      (1) Metastatic disease at diagnosis
      (2) Tumors of the pelvic bones

IX BRAIN TUMORS

Collectively, brain tumors **are the second most common form of childhood cancer,** accounting for 20% of the total. They are of diverse types, each with unique characteristics, locations, and growth rates.

A Special problems in management

1. The blood–brain barrier limits the delivery of chemotherapy by the systemic route.
2. The developing brain of infants and young children is vulnerable to the toxicity of therapeutic modalities.
3. The proximity of some tumors to important areas of brain function precludes their extensive surgical resection.
4. There is a tendency for the tumors to spread within rather than outside the neuraxis.

B Classification

1. **Location.** Two thirds of brain tumors arise below and one third arise above the tentorium.
2. **Histology.** Most brain tumors fall into two distinct groups:
   a. **Tumors of glial origin**
      (1) **High-grade astrocytomas** arise primarily above the tentorium; their presentation involves:
         (a) Focal neurologic deficits

(b) Signs of increased intracranial pressure (*see I E 7*)
(c) Focal seizures
(2) **Low-grade astrocytomas** arise primarily below the tentorium in the cerebellum; their presentation involves:
(a) Signs of increased intracranial pressure
(b) Signs of cerebellar dysfunction (e.g., ataxia, nystagmus)
(3) The presentation of **brainstem gliomas** involves:
(a) Multiple cranial nerve palsies
(b) Ataxia
(c) Long tract signs
(4) **Ependymomas** develop more commonly below the tentorium and involve symptoms of increased intracranial pressure when they obstruct the fourth ventricle.

b. **Tumors of neuroepithelial origin**
(1) **Medulloblastoma** is the most common malignant brain tumor in children; its characteristic presentation is that of a cerebellar tumor causing:
(a) Signs of increased intracranial pressure secondary to obstruction of the fourth ventricle, preventing cerebrospinal fluid (CSF) flow through it and causing hydrocephalus. Patients have the following symptoms:
(i) Headache
(ii) Vomiting
(iii) Lethargy
(b) Ataxia due to cerebellar dysfunction
(c) Propensity for rapid spread throughout the neuraxis by the CSF pathways, which is more common in young children and carries a poor prognosis
(2) **Primitive neuroectodermal tumors** of the CNS are much less common than medulloblastomas and are highly malignant. Their presentation is that of cerebral masses with symptoms similar to those of cerebral astrocytomas.

C Therapy

1. Surgery plays an important role in the management of tumors whose location permits resection.
   a. Resectable tumors include many cerebellar and cerebral tumors.
   b. Brainstem gliomas usually are not resectable, and their location often makes even biopsy hazardous.
2. **Radiotherapy** plays a major role in the management of tumors in all locations and is indicated for most tumors except completely resected low-grade astrocytomas. Unfortunately, the doses delivered are often associated with significant toxicity, which is especially severe in young children (*see I G 5 a [1]*).
3. **Chemotherapy** is a relatively recent addition to the armamentarium and has shown promise in:
   a. Prolonging survival of patients who have high-grade astrocytomas
   b. Increasing the cure rate of patients who have medulloblastoma
   c. Controlling tumor growth in infants and young children so that radiotherapy can be postponed to a somewhat later age, when it may be less toxic to the developing nervous system

D Prognosis

1. The prognosis is **excellent** for patients with completely resected low-grade astrocytomas.
2. The prognosis is **good** for many medulloblastomas, particularly if they:
   a. Occur in children older than 4 years of age
   b. Are relatively small in size
   c. Have not spread
3. The prognosis is **poor** for:
   a. Brainstem gliomas
   b. Medulloblastomas that occur in young children, are large in size, and spread into the CSF and to distant sites in the neuraxis

BIBLIOGRAPHY

American Cancer Society, Inc.: Cancer Facts and Figures 2005. Atlanta, American Cancer Society, Inc., 2005.

Pui CH, Relling MV, Downing JR: Acute lymphoblastic leukemia. *N Engl J Med* 350(15):1535–1548, 2004.

Quesnel S, Malkin D: Genetic predisposition to cancer and familial cancer syndromes. *Pediatr Clin North Am* 44:791–808, 1997.

Ries LA, Kosary CL, Hankey BF, et al., eds.: SEER Cancer Statistics Review, 1973–1996. Bethesda, MD, National Cancer Institute, 1999. Also available online. Last accessed December 18, 2006.

Rubnitz JE, Crist WM: Molecular genetics of childhood cancer: implications for pathogenesis, diagnosis and treatment. *Pediatrics* 100:101–108, 1997.

Xie Y, Davies SM, Xiang Y, et al.: Trends in leukemia incidence and survival in the United States (1973–1998). *Cancer* 97(9):2229–2235, 2003.

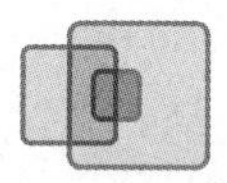

Study Questions

Directions: *Each of the numbered items or incomplete statements in this section is followed by answers or completions of the statement. Select the ONE lettered answer or completion that is BEST in each case.*

1. A 17-year-old male who has hemophilia A and is seropositive for HIV presents with a large left supraclavicular mass that has grown over a 3-week period. He has received many transfusions in the past but does not have a factor VIII inhibitor. The mass does not regress with factor VIII therapy. Which of the following is the most likely diagnosis?

A Non-Hodgkin lymphoma
B Metastatic neuroblastoma
C Kaposi sarcoma
D Acute myelogenous leukemia
E Hemorrhage into tissues in the supraclavicular region

2. A 2-year-old boy is initially seen with a large left-sided abdominal mass, which, on intravenous pyelogram, appears to arise within the left kidney and distort and displace the collecting system. On chest radiography, multiple pulmonary nodules are present. Which of the following is the most likely diagnosis?

A Neuroblastoma
B Wilms tumor
C Non-Hodgkin lymphoma
D Rhabdomyosarcoma
E Hepatoblastoma

QUESTIONS 3–5

An 8-year-old girl presents with fever, numerous bruises over the entire body, and pain in both legs. Physical examination reveals pallor; ecchymoses and petechiae on the face, trunk, and extremities; a soft midsystolic murmur; and the spleen palpable at 2 cm below the left costal margin. Findings on complete blood count (CBC) include a hemoglobin of 6.3 g/dL; white blood cell count (WBC) of 2800/mm^3 (10% neutrophils, 1% bands, 2% monocytes, 87% lymphocytes); and platelet count of 29,000/mm^3.

3. Which of the following is the most appropriate initial diagnostic test?

A Heterophile antibody
B Bone marrow aspiration
C Erythrocyte sedimentation rate
D Skeletal survey
E Liver and spleen scan

4. The patient described above has a bone marrow aspiration revealing replacement by precursor B-cell lymphoblasts with L1 morphology, typical of acute lymphoblastic leukemia. Based on the bone marrow results and initial presentation described above, which of the following risk group categories should this patient be placed into?

A High risk
B Standard risk
C Undetermined risk
D No risk

5. The patient develops cough and fever to 103°F (39.5°C). Which of the following is the most appropriate initial therapy for this patient?

- A Administer aspirin for the fever
- B Start narrow-spectrum intravenous antibiotics
- C Start oral antibiotics
- D Administer codeine to suppress the cough
- E Start broad-spectrum intravenous antibiotics

QUESTIONS 6–8

A 2-year-old boy initially presents with bilateral proptosis and periorbital ecchymoses, a large right flank mass, and pain in the lower back and right arm. Evaluation reveals moderate anemia, a large right-sided mass that is distinct from the right kidney, clumps of primitive cells in the bone marrow, and bone scan that demonstrates increased activity in the right humerus, left and right orbits, and L1 to L3 vertebrae.

6. Which of the following is the most likely diagnosis?

- A Langerhans cell histiocytosis
- B Rhabdomyosarcoma
- C Neuroblastoma
- D Wilms tumor
- E Lymphoblastic lymphoma

7. Which of the following laboratory findings is most commonly seen in patients with this boy's diagnosis?

- A c-*myc*-immunoglobulin translocation (8;14) in the involved cells
- B Amplification of n-*myc* oncogene in the involved cells
- C Elevation of α-fetoprotein (AFP) or human chorionic gonadotropin (hCG)
- D bcr-abl translocation (9;22) in the involved cells
- E Abnormalities of the 11p13 or 11p15 locus

8. The patient experiences increased back pain and is unable to walk. Neurologic examination reveals decreased strength in the lower extremities. Which of the following is the most appropriate initial management?

- A Analgesic therapy for bone metastases with a nonsteroidal anti-inflammatory agent
- B Lumbar puncture
- C Imaging studies to evaluate the dorsolumbar epidural space
- D Careful, serial neurologic examinations
- E Physical therapy to decrease lumbar muscle spasm and increase strength of lower extremity muscles

9. A 15-year-old adolescent boy complains of worsening deep right thigh pain that has woken him from sleep every night for the past week. A radiograph reveals a destructive mass in the distal femur with a "sunburst" pattern visible on the radiograph. A biopsy of this lesion confirms the diagnosis of osteogenic sarcoma and staging evaluation confirms nonmetastatic disease. Which of the following is the most appropriate therapy for this patient?

- A Surgical resection alone
- B Chemotherapy alone
- C Radiation therapy alone
- D A combination of surgery and chemotherapy
- E A combination of surgery and radiation therapy

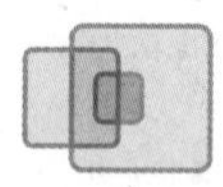

Answers and Explanations

1. The answer is A (*I D 3 b; III A-C*). The most likely diagnosis is non-Hodgkin lymphoma. The boy described in this case has infection with HIV and may, as a consequence, develop AIDS-associated, aggressive B-cell lymphoma. Kaposi sarcoma occurs less commonly than lymphoma in pediatric patients who have AIDS. Metastatic neuroblastoma can have this type of presentation, but the boy's age, HIV infection, and hemophilia make this disease unlikely. Acute myelogenous leukemia usually does not produce this degree of adenopathy, and would be unusual in a hemophiliac patient with HIV infection. Hemorrhage always is a possible diagnosis in a patient who has hemophilia, but failure of the mass to respond to appropriate treatment and absence of an inhibitor interfering with response to treatment makes this very unlikely.

2. The answer is B (*VI B, D*). The most likely diagnosis is Wilms tumor. The classic radiographic appearance of Wilms tumor is an abdominal mass that occurs within the kidney, distorting and displacing the renal collecting system; metastases to the lungs are noted on chest radiography. Neuroblastoma arises above the kidney and displaces it anterolaterally and inferiorly and rarely metastasizes to the lungs. B-cell non-Hodgkin lymphomas often arise in the abdomen but usually not from the kidney, and they do not produce nodular pulmonary metastases. Rhabdomyosarcomas may arise in the retroperitoneum, but they are much rarer than Wilms tumor and are extrarenal. They do spread to the lungs. Hepatoblastomas most commonly arise in the right rather than left lobe of the liver and produce right-sided masses. They would not distort the intrarenal architecture. They do, however, metastasize to the lungs.

3–5. The answers are 3-B (*I E 8 a; II A 3 a-c, 4 b*), **4-B** (*II B 4 a; Table 16-4, 16-5*), and **5-E** (*II A 3 a [2], [3], 5 a [2]*). This child's presentation is typical of acute lymphoblastic leukemia. She has signs and symptoms of anemia and thrombocytopenia as well as bone pain and splenomegaly, and her CBC values indicate pancytopenia. In this situation, bone marrow aspiration is the most appropriate test to see whether the bone marrow can produce adequate numbers of blood cells and, if not, whether the marrow is aplastic or replaced by malignant cells. Heterophile antibody testing would be useful only if infectious mononucleosis was a strong possibility. Splenomegaly, immune thrombocytopenia, and hemolytic anemia can be seen with mononucleosis, but leukopenia and bone pain would not be expected to occur with a typical Epstein-Barr virus infection. The erythrocyte sedimentation rate is not a specific enough test to be useful in this patient and would not provide a diagnosis. Skeletal survey may show leukemic lines, but their presence or absence cannot substitute for bone marrow examination, which is much more definitive and provides material for diagnosis of the specific type of leukemia. Liver and spleen scan would show splenic enlargement but would not provide a specific diagnosis.

A low WBC count, age of 8 years, and L1 morphology of lymphoblasts are typical of standard-risk ALL. There are no high-risk features in this patient, such as a high WBC or age younger than 1 year or equal to or older than 10 years. Even with standard-risk ALL, relapse occurs in 10% of patients and, therefore, risk is certainly greater than zero.

Aspirin should not be used as an antipyretic in a thrombocytopenic patient because salicylates interfere with platelet function and would worsen the bleeding tendency. Prompt institution of intravenous broad-spectrum antibiotics, however, is mandatory in the febrile, neutropenic patient. The use of narrow-spectrum antibiotics would not be appropriate in this situation since patients are at risk of both Gram-positive and Gram-negative microorganisms. Oral antibiotics would not be appropriate for empiric treatment for presumed bacteremia in a neutropenic patient. Administration of codeine would not be an appropriate first step in this patient with fever and neutropenia. In addition, use of medication to suppress a cough would generally not be recommended due to concern for decreased clearance of pulmonary secretion. Blood and urine cultures should be obtained before initiating antibiotic therapy. A chest radiograph should also be performed to detect any infiltrates.

6–8. The answers are 6-C (*V B 1 a, 2 b*), **7-B** (*II D 1 a; V D 3*), and **8-C** (*V B 1 d*). This is a typical presentation of stage IV neuroblastoma, with the primary tumor arising from one of the paravertebral sympathetic ganglia and metastasizing to bone marrow, cortical bone, and the retro-orbital tissues. Langerhans cell histiocytosis may have a somewhat similar presentation and involve multiple bones, but it usually involves one rather than both orbits; also, the right flank mass and tumor clumps in the marrow of this patient are not characteristic of Langerhans cell histiocytosis. Rhabdomyosarcoma may arise in the orbit but is usually unilateral; the tumor also rarely is associated with systemic metastases at initial diagnosis. Wilms tumor would produce a right renal mass and would metastasize to the lungs rather than to bone and bone marrow. Lymphoblastic lymphoma usually arises in the anterior mediastinum or peripheral nodes. Even if it were to involve widespread dissemination, abdominal rather than thoracic mass would be unusual, and lymphoblasts rather than tumor clumps would be seen in the bone marrow.

The Philadelphia chromosome contains translocation (9;22) and is seen in chronic myelogenous leukemia, not neuroblastoma. c-*myc*–immunoglobulin translocation (8;14) is the most common cytogenetic abnormality seen in Burkitt lymphoma. AFP and hCG are tumor markers that may be elevated in patients diagnosed with germ cell tumors. Abnormalities of the 11p13 or 11p15 locus are seen in patients with Wilms tumor. Increased urinary excretion of catecholamine metabolites (e.g., vanillylmandelic acid) is common in neuroblastoma. In many cases of neuroblastoma, the cells demonstrate amplification of the n-*myc* oncogene, and elevated levels of ferritin are detected in serum. The presence of either or both of these findings often portends a worse prognosis. Patients with marrow metastases from neuroblastoma often have leukoerythroblastic changes that are demonstrable on peripheral blood smear.

The development of back pain, inability to walk, and decreased lower extremity strength indicates a medically emergent situation in which the tumor has grown posteriorly through the intervertebral foramina into the epidural space. In this location, the tumor can compress the spinal cord and produce irreversible damage from ischemia to the cord. Prompt evaluation with an MRI or CT scan is needed to detect the tumor in the epidural space. Lumbar puncture would not be useful unless it were combined with myelography to detect the encroachment on the cord. Institution of analgesic therapy or physical therapy would be inappropriate in this situation, as would serial neurologic examinations. Speed in establishing a diagnosis and preventing permanent cord damage is critical.

9. The answer is D (*VIII A 3*). Osteogenic sarcoma is the most common malignant bone tumor in children and most commonly affects adolescent males. The best option for patients with nonmetastatic disease is treatment with a combination of chemotherapy and surgery and is associated with an overall survival of approximately 65%. Surgery alone for nonmetastatic disease is associated with $< 15\%$ overall survival and is not considered to be an appropriate option for adolescents or young adults with this diagnosis. Chemotherapy is not considered to be a curative therapy when used alone and radiation is not an effective therapy for osteogenic sarcoma.

chapter **17**

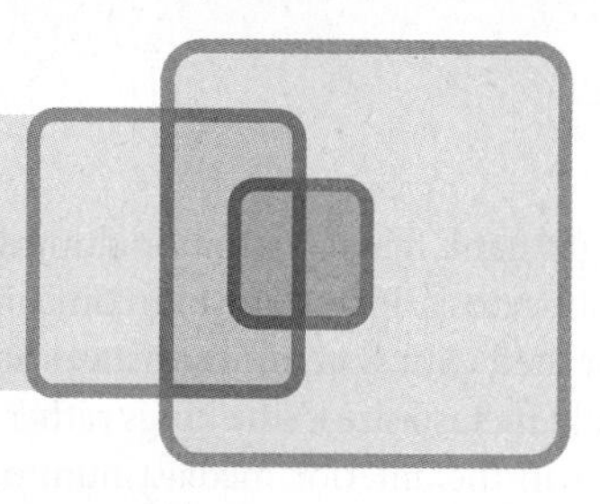

Endocrine and Metabolic Disorders

ELIZABETH D. ESTRADA

I GROWTH DISORDERS

A Normal growth

1. The regulation of growth in children and adolescents is a complex process influenced by multiple factors, including the individual genetic makeup, nutritional status, endocrine milieu, presence of underlying illnesses, and environmental conditions.
2. Growth velocity varies during childhood and adolescence, being the fastest during the first year of life, approximately 25 cm. The rate of growth then decreases, averaging 5 cm/year after age 6 until puberty (see Chapter 4).
3. After the age of 2 years and before the onset of puberty, most children grow in parallel to a percentile channel on growth charts and any deviation should prompt further assessment of growth abnormalities (see Chapters 1, 4, and 5).

B Endocrine regulation of growth

1. **Growth hormone (GH)** is an anabolic polypeptide hormone that stimulates growth of all tissues. Its most striking effect is on the growth of long bones.
   a. GH release from the anterior lobe is stimulated by the hypothalamic peptide, **growth hormone–releasing hormone (GHRH)** and **ghrelin,** and is inhibited by somatostatin.
   b. Other substances and factors play a role in GH release, and many form the basis of testing for abnormalities of GH secretion, including sleep, exercise, hypoglycemia, amino acids (e.g., arginine), β-adrenergic blockers, sex hormones, and other drugs (e.g., L-dopa, clonidine).
2. Fifty percent of GH circulates bound to **growth hormone–binding protein (GHBP).** This protein is cleaved from the extracellular portion of the **GH receptor (GHR).**
3. GH action on long bone growth is mediated through another polypeptide hormone, **insulin-like growth factor 1 (IGF-1),** which is mostly generated in the liver. Besides the systemic effect of the liver-secreted IGF-1, there are growth promoting autocrine and paracrine effects of IGF-1 secreted by bone and muscle. Low IGF-1 levels stimulate the secretion of growth hormone from the pituitary gland.
4. **IGF-binding proteins (IGFBPs)** are a family of six proteins that bind IGF-1. They are produced in the liver under the influence of GH. Almost all circulating IGF-1 is bound to IGFBP, particularly **IGFBP-3.**

C Short stature

The main causes of growth failure may be divided into endocrine abnormalities, variants of normal growth, and primary growth abnormalities.

1. **Endocrine causes of short stature**
   a. **Abnormalities of the GH–IGF-1 axis leading to IGF-1 deficiency.** With the recent discoveries of IGF-1 production defects and the availability of IGF-1 for pharmacologic treatment, a new terminology based on the etiology of IGF-1 deficiency has been adopted as follows.
      (1) **Hypothalamic-pituitary defects causing GH deficiency (GHD)**
         (a) Abnormal GH secretion could occur as an isolated deficiency or in combination with other pituitary hormone deficiencies (**panhypopituitarism**). Congenital anatomic

abnormalities such as septo-optic dysplasia, holoprosencephaly, or midline defects that disrupt the formation of the hypothalamus or pituitary gland may be found. Malignant tumors as well as benign intracranial lesions that damage the hypothalamic-pituitary axis are a common cause of GHD. These include craniopharyngioma, germinomas, meningiomas, and Rathke cleft cysts. Growth hormone deficiency can also be acquired as result of trauma, radiotherapy, and infections or infiltrative processes such as histiocytosis.

(b) Because GH does not appear to be necessary for fetal growth, affected newborns are of normal size. Growth velocity slows after 6 to 12 months of age, so that by 2 years of age, height is below the fifth percentile. Symptomatic hypoglycemia and prolonged jaundice may occur in the newborn period.

(2) **IGF-1 deficiency due to GH receptor/postreceptor abnormalities.** In these conditions, although GH secretion is normal, patients are not able to produce normal amounts of IGF-1. A typical example of growth hormone resistance is the condition known as Laron syndrome. These patients have an inherited GHBP deficiency, which leads to GH unresponsiveness. Abnormally high GH, low IGF-1, and low GHBP levels are found in the serum. To date, many other defects of the GHR, GH signaling cascade, or IGF-1 synthesis have been identified as a cause of IGF-1 deficiency.

b. **Primary hypothyroidism** (*see III B 2*) causes marked growth failure and marked retardation of skeletal maturation. Because primary hypothyroidism is easily treatable, all children with short stature should have thyroid function tests measured—even in the absence of obvious symptoms—to rule out any degree of hypothyroidism.

c. **Cushing disease** (*see IV A 2*) is a very rare cause of short stature in children. However, **hypercortisolism** (from either exogenous treatment with pharmacologic doses of steroids or endogenous oversecretion) may have a profound growth-suppressing effect. Usually other features of Cushing syndrome are evident. Increasing use of potent inhaled steroids for treatment of moderate to severe asthma is being increasingly recognized as a cause of growth failure.

2. **Variants of normal growth**

a. **Constitutional delay of growth and puberty** is one of the most frequently found diagnoses among children visiting an endocrinologist with the complaint of short stature. It is more commonly found among boys than among girls, perhaps because of greater social value placed on height for boys than girls. These patients are typically known as "late bloomers." It probably represents a variant of normal growth. Usual findings are as follows:

(1) Growth velocity is normal, which results in a curve that is parallel to the fifth percentile.

(2) Puberty is delayed and is usually reflected by significantly delayed skeletal maturation. Because these children fail to enter puberty at the usual age, their short stature and sexual immaturity are accentuated at this time compared to those of normally developing peers.

(3) There is often a family history of delayed puberty in other family members.

b. **Familial short stature.** Also called **genetic short stature,** this probably represents a heterogenous group of conditions. Short stature is usually found in at least one parent or immediate relative. It should be remembered that short stature in a parent may reflect a multitude of factors that may have affected the parent's height and should not be assumed to be "normal." These children establish growth curves at or below the fifth percentile by 2 to 3 years of age. They are otherwise completely healthy. Bone age, IGF-1, and GH levels in these children are normal. Therefore, puberty occurs at the usual age and thus limits potential for growth late into adolescence.

c. **Idiopathic short stature (ISS).** This controversial term denotes a child growing below the third percentile of the normal growth charts who is otherwise healthy and has normal bone maturation, normal GH production, and normal genetic potential. Recent evidence indicates that some of these children may in fact have abnormalities of IGF-1 production or the short stature homeobox (SHOX) gene, among others. The evolving knowledge will hopefully provide tools for better understanding and classification of ISS, which, in turn, will lead to better treatment of this population.

3. **Primary (syndromic) growth failure** has been used to describe a large, diverse group of children who have normal endocrine function but inherent limitations on skeletal growth. The cause of

short stature in these children is usually easily identified on the basis of abnormal body proportions (skeletal dysplasias), dysmorphic features (chromosome abnormalities), and other characteristics of the history or physical examination. Special attention should be given to the evaluation of **girls who have short stature.** Although a short girl who has all of the physical stigmata of **Turner syndrome** may be easily identified, the features may sometimes be quite subtle (see Chapter 8). Therefore, girls with short stature should have a karyotype done.

4. **Chronic systemic disease**
   a. The impact of chronic systemic disease on growth is well known. The mechanism is probably related to a combination of nutritional deficits, increased metabolic demands, and production of inflammatory factors associated with the disease process.
   b. Some chronic diseases may show minimal symptoms and yet have a significant effect on growth. The most recognized chronic diseases that may manifest as short stature are inflammatory bowel disease (Crohn disease) and celiac disease (see Chapter 11). Also, renal disease associated with renal tubular acidosis or uremia, cyanotic congenital heart disease, poorly controlled diabetes mellitus, and severe rheumatoid arthritis have deleterious effects on growth.

D **Evaluation** Short stature can generally be ascribed to several broad categories of medical problems. On the basis of previous growth and medical records; the current medical, nutritional, family, and social history; and the physical examination, the laboratory evaluation focuses on a relatively small number of tests of both diagnostic and prognostic significance. Assessment includes:

1. **Plotting of growth.** Assessment of growth in childhood begins with accurate and serial measurements that are plotted on the appropriate growth chart (see Chapter 4).
2. **History.** Information that may have a bearing on the child's growth should be gathered.
   a. Birth history and birth weight are important considerations since intrauterine growth retardation may be a clue to the diagnosis.
   b. Review of symptoms referable to each organ system must be obtained.
   c. Growth records should be carefully reviewed.
   d. Information about genetic potential for height may be gathered by recording the heights of parents, siblings, and other relatives. A family history of other medical problems is also relevant.
   e. The child should be questioned sensitively about the impact of short stature on his or her relationships with peers, participation in sports, and other social activities. Parents' perceptions should also be noted in these matters.
3. **Physical examination.** The following aspects should receive special attention during a physical examination:
   a. **Height and weight.** Accurate **recumbent length** for children birth to 24 months of age and **standing height** for children 2 to 18 years of age should be obtained. In addition to height, **arm span** and **upper-to-lower body segment ratio** may be measured.
   b. Dysmorphic features in a pattern suggestive of a specific syndrome and obesity should be noted. Children with abnormalities of the GH–IGF-1 axis leading to IGF-1 deficiency usually present with truncal adiposity, frontal bossing, a flat nasal bridge, and a high-pitched voice.
   c. **Skin** is examined for abnormal pigmentation or cyanosis, and the skin and hair texture are noted for possible clues to hypothyroidism.
   d. **Head, ears,** and **eyes** are examined for midline defects (e.g., clefts) and ocular or dental anomalies. Visual field examination is performed. Funduscopy is performed to look for optic nerve abnormalities, which might indicate increased intracranial pressure or an underlying central nervous system (CNS) abnormality associated with growth hormone deficiency.
   e. The **thyroid** is palpated to determine its size and consistency and the presence of nodules.
   f. **Chest** and **heart** are examined for evidence of chronic cardiopulmonary disease or heart murmur.
   g. **Abdomen.** Tenderness or bloating may indicate chronic gastrointestinal disease, such as celiac disease or inflammatory bowel disease.
   h. **Genitalia.** Anomalies of the genitalia, such as undescended testes and micropenis in boys, should be noted. For example, male infants with pituitary abnormalities and GH deficiency may have microphallus secondary to intrauterine gonadotropin deficiency. Tanner staging should be documented.
   i. **Neurologic examination** is performed to rule out underlying CNS disease, especially any tumor that might cause GH deficiency.

4. **Laboratory evaluation and imaging studies**
   a. Laboratory evaluation should be guided by the clinical findings. Accordingly, screening tests to assess kidney and liver function, hematologic conditions, inflammatory bowel disease, celiac disease, and thyroid functions should be ordered. In girls with short stature, a karyotype should be ordered to exclude Turner syndrome, even in the absence of dysmorphic features. The diagnosis of GH deficiency is not clear-cut and is currently a subject of debate and research. Because GH is secreted episodically, with the major surge coming after sleep onset, GH levels are low throughout most of the day and it is not possible to differentiate the normal low basal GH level from disease states associated with absent or diminished GH secretion. GH **provocative tests** have been developed in which GH levels are measured after exercise, insulin-induced hypoglycemia, and arginine infusion, as well as following L-dopa, glucagon, and clonidine administration. The validity of these tests is currently under evaluation since several problems are associated with the interpretation of the results, including the definition of abnormal response levels, individual variability in response, and the effect of sex steroids, among others. Measurement of IGF-1 and IGFBP-3 levels is preferred for evaluation of GH/IGF-1 deficiencies. They are low in cases of GH receptor/postreceptor abnormalities. Although they show no diurnal variations, the levels are affected by nutritional status, age, and Tanner stage; therefore, appropriate normative ranges should be used.
   b. **Bone age,** as assessed by a plain film of the left hand and wrist, is usually delayed in cases of hormonal abnormalities, constitutional delay, and chronic illnesses. Bone age may be used to "predict" the adult final height in children with familial or idiopathic short stature.
   c. **Magnetic resonance imaging (MRI)** of the pituitary gland may identify abnormalities of the hypothalamic-pituitary areas causing GH deficiency.
5. **Therapy**
   a. For children deemed **GH deficient, recombinant human GH** is given by subcutaneous injection every day. Accelerated growth velocity on GH treatment results in catch-up growth in most children.
   b. Subcutaneous **recombinant human IGF-1** has been used for treatment of severe IGF-1 deficiency (Laron syndrome) since the 1990s. It was recently approved by the U.S. Food and Drug Administration (FDA) for less severe forms of IGF-1 deficiency. There are studies under way to assess the long-term effectiveness of IGF-1 treatment in the less severe forms.
   c. Treatment of underlying illnesses is needed to restore normal growth, as well as hormone replacement in cases of **hypothyroidism** and **hypocortisolism.**
   d. GH treatment has resulted in greater adult stature in some cases of pathologic short stature (Turner syndrome) and in improved body composition (Prader-Willi syndrome).
   e. Although in 2003 the FDA approved GH treatment for patients with **ISS,** the use of GH in this population is still in debate. More research is needed to identify the patients who would benefit from this intervention.

E Tall stature Occasionally, children appear to be growing too rapidly. Children who are growing above the 95th percentile should be examined carefully for signs of precocious puberty or adrenal androgen excess (*see IV A 3*).

1. Most children have **familial tall stature.** Occasionally, girls in early adolescence who have familial tall stature may request treatment to reduce final adult stature. High-dose estrogen may induce premature epiphyseal fusion and reduce final height.
2. Other causes of tall stature are GH excess (causing **acromegaly** and **gigantism**), hyperthyroidism, Marfan syndrome, and homocystinuria.

II DISORDERS OF PUBERTY

A Precocious puberty Development of secondary sexual characteristics before the expected age of onset for gender and race (see Chapter 5) is considered precocious.

1. **Premature thelarche** refers to the frequent finding of **isolated breast development** in very young girls. The usual age of onset is 12 to 24 months. It has been postulated that premature thelarche is caused by transient bursts of estrogen from the prepubertal ovary or increased sensitivity to low levels of estrogen. Gonadotropins and serum estrogen levels are found in the prepubertal range.

Linear growth acceleration and advanced skeletal maturation are not present. Breast development does not progress, and no other signs of puberty develop.

2. **Idiopathic premature adrenarche** describes the **early appearance of sexual hair.** This is a benign condition believed to be caused by early maturation of adrenal androgen secretion (adrenarche). Levels of adrenal androgens are found to be normal for pubertal stage. Bone age is not usually significantly advanced. Children who have premature adrenarche with clinical evidence of significant androgen effect (e.g., advanced bone age, growth acceleration, hirsutism, acne) must be evaluated for other causes of increased androgen production, such as congenital adrenal hyperplasia or adrenal tumor.
3. **Precocious isosexual puberty,** in which usual pubertal changes appear at an earlier age than normal, may be divided into two types: Central or gonadotropin dependent and peripheral or gonadotropin independent.
   a. **Central or gonadotropin-dependent precocious puberty** (**GDPP**) is **true puberty** beginning at an abnormally early age. It appears to be more common in girls than in boys. In girls, there rarely is underlying CNS disease, and it is therefore considered idiopathic. In contrast, there is a significant incidence of CNS pathology, especially tumors, in boys who have central precocious puberty. A variety of diseases of the CNS have been associated with GDPP, including tumors (e.g., glioma, pinealoma, hamartoma), hydrocephalus, head injury, congenital malformation, and infection.
      (1) **Clinical features** are progressive development of secondary sex characteristics, accompanied by a growth spurt. If the GDPP is secondary to a CNS problem, abnormal neurologic findings on history or physical examination may be present. Because sex steroids stimulate growth while promoting epiphyseal fusion, precocious puberty causes tall stature in childhood, premature closure of the epiphyses, and adult short stature.
      (2) **Diagnosis** is based on evidence of growth acceleration, significantly advanced bone age, and pubertal levels of gonadotropins and estrogen or testosterone.
      (3) **Therapy.** Goals are to diminish secondary sexual characteristics, inhibit menses in girls, and slow down growth velocity and skeletal maturation to a normal prepubertal rate. Long-acting analogues of gonadotropin-releasing hormone (GnRH) that inhibit gonadotropin release have provided effective treatment of GDPP.

   b. **Peripheral or gonadotropin-independent precocious puberty** (**GIPP**) is a rare cause of precocious sexual development. The sex hormones are secreted from peripheral sources. Examples of GIPP are McCune-Albright syndrome, familial male precocious puberty (testitoxicosis), Leydig cell tumors, and ectopic human chorionic gonadotropin (hCG) production by germ cell tumors. Levels of gonadotropins are low, and there is no increase in gonadotropins after GnRH infusion. GIPP does not respond to treatment with analogues of GnRH. The treatment is geared to the underlying cause.

B **Delayed puberty** The absence of secondary sex characteristics by 13 years of age in girls and by 14 years in boys is considered delayed. Normal secondary sex characteristics but absence of menarche by 15 years of age is also considered delayed **(primary amenorrhea).** Delayed puberty may be secondary to a variety of underlying endocrine and systemic diseases, such as hypothyroidism, sickle cell anemia, rheumatoid arthritis, inflammatory bowel disease, chronic renal failure, and others. Primary causes of delayed puberty include:

1. **Constitutional delay of puberty** is a designation reserved for otherwise healthy children in whom late but otherwise normal puberty occurs. It is less commonly diagnosed in girls than in boys. These children are frequently short but growing at normal prepubertal growth velocities. Bone age is often significantly delayed; however, there is no evidence of other endocrine or systemic disease. There is frequently a strong history of delayed puberty or menarche in adult family members.
2. **Gonadal failure.** In these conditions, gonadotropin levels are found elevated by the usual age of puberty because of the lack of estrogen/testosterone feedback on the hypothalamic-pituitary axis.
   a. **Primary ovarian failure. Turner syndrome** (see Chapter 8) is the most common cause of primary ovarian failure. **Prepubertal surgical removal** or **irradiation** of the ovaries for treatment of cancer may also cause primary ovarian failure. **Autoimmune ovarian failure** may

occur in association with other autoimmune diseases, adrenal insufficiency, thyroiditis, hypoparathyroidism, and type 1 diabetes.

b. **Primary testicular failure.** In **Klinefelter syndrome** (see Chapter 8), a common cause of testicular failure, puberty may begin at the usual age and secondary sex characteristics acquired. However, these boys have small, firm testes and often have gynecomastia. Congenital bilateral anorchia or **"vanishing testes"** syndrome presents in boys with normal male sexual differentiation and apparent cryptorchidism. However, no testes are found on surgical exploration. Because they have normal male karyotype and external genitalia and there are no müllerian remnants internally, it is presumed that testes must have been present in early fetal life and subsequently "vanished." Other causes of testicular failure include **chemotherapy, irradiation, surgical excision, trauma,** and **infection.**

3. **Hypogonadotropic hypogonadism** may be difficult to distinguish from constitutional delay of puberty because, in each situation, gonadotropin levels are low and the response to GnRH stimulation is also minimal. This disorder is often part of other recognizable syndromes.
   a. **Kallmann syndrome** involves anosmia with hypogonadotropic hypogonadism.
   b. **Hypopituitarism** may include gonadotropin deficiency as one of several deficient pituitary hormones.
   c. **Hypothalamic** and **pituitary tumors** include adenoma, microadenoma (especially one secreting prolactin), craniopharyngioma, and pinealoma.
   d. **Anorexia nervosa** may cause delayed puberty or, in older adolescents, secondary amenorrhea due to gonadotropin deficiency.
   e. **Prader-Willi syndrome** (see Chapter 8) is characterized by short stature, obesity, mental retardation, and hypogonadotropic hypogonadism.

4. **Diagnosis**
   a. A careful **history** and **physical examination** should be taken, including height and weight. Tanner staging of pubertal development should be performed. Assessment for the presence of dysmorphic features, anosmia, or signs of other endocrine or systemic disease is important.
   b. **Laboratory studies** include an evaluation of skeletal maturation (bone age) as well as follicle-stimulating hormone (FSH), leuteinizing hormone (LH), prolactin, thyroid function tests, and testosterone or estrogen levels. Studies to exclude systemic diseases should also be obtained. A karyotype is essential in the diagnosis of Turner, Klinefelter, and other syndromes. Depending on the clinical situation, computed tomography (CT) or MRI scan of the head and testing of other pituitary hormones may be indicated.

5. **Therapy.** Treatment with appropriate sex steroid replacement for adolescents who have a permanent cause of delayed puberty should be instituted at the usual age of puberty. For adolescents who have constitutional delay of puberty, smaller doses of the appropriate sex steroid may be used for a short course of treatment. This will initiate some development of secondary sex characteristics and be psychologically beneficial.

C Polycystic ovary syndrome (PCOS or ovarian hyperandrogenemia) PCOS is the most common cause of androgen excess in female adolescents with hyperandrogenemia. It occurs in 5% to 10% of women with a trend of increasing incidence.

1. **Presentation.** These patients usually present with menstrual irregularities, signs of hyperandrogenism (hirsutism, acne), chronic anovulation that leads to infertility, obesity, and acanthosis nigricans. The risk of cardiovascular disease, diabetes, and metabolic syndrome is significantly increased in women with PCOS.

2. **Etiology**
   a. PCOS is a multifactorial disorder characterized by high androgen levels of ovarian and adrenal origin and **insulin resistance,** which leads to hyperinsulinemia. Insulin enhances LH-stimulated androgen production from the ovaries. It also decreases the hepatic production of sex hormone–binding globulin (SHBG), therefore increasing the fraction of circulating unbound testosterone or **free testosterone,** the bioactive metabolite.
   b. **Obesity** is frequently associated with PCOS. When present, obesity worsens the clinical presentation of PCOS by increasing insulin resistance. The increased insulin resistance associated with puberty may explain why there is an increased expression of PCOS during adolescence.

3. **Diagnosis.** The diagnosis of PCOS is mainly based on the clinical features. Measurements of testosterone, free testosterone, SHBG, and adrenal androgens are indicated to confirm the biochemical abnormalities. Screening for lipid disorders and glucose tolerance abnormalities is also indicated.

4. **Treatment.** In adolescent patients with PCOS, lowered levels of insulin induced by treatment result in decrease androgen levels. Lifestyle changes aiming for weight loss in obese patients are an important part of the treatment. Pharmacologic treatment with insulin sensitizers, oral contraceptives, and antiandrogenic agents should be used according to the presenting features.

III DISORDERS OF THE THYROID GLAND

A Assessment of thyroid function The assessment of a patient with possible thyroid disorder involves measurement of thyroid hormones, markers of thyroid autoimmunity, and imaging of the thyroid gland. The most commonly used tests are the following:

1. **Hormones**
   a. **Total thyroxine (T_4)** reflects the total amount of all circulating forms of the hormone, including free and protein-bound T_4. Consequently, total T_4 may be affected by processes that change thyroxine-binding globulin (TBG) levels independently of thyroid function. For example, increased estrogen as found in patients taking oral contraceptives stimulates production of TBG, thereby increasing the total T_4 level by raising the T_4 bound to TBG. The free T_4 in this case would be normal and no clinical abnormality should be found.
   b. **Free T_4** measurement is largely replacing measurement of total T_4 because it is not affected by alterations of protein binding.
   c. **Triiodothyronine (T_3)** is particularly useful in diagnosing hyperthyroidism. Some forms of hyperthyroidism are primarily due to T_3 excess, particularly in the case of autonomous thyroid nodules.
   d. **Thyroid-stimulating hormone (TSH)** measurement is most valuable in the diagnosis of primary hypothyroidism (elevated TSH). In newer, ultrasensitive assays, very low levels of circulating TSH can be distinguished from normal levels and may be supportive of a diagnosis of hyperthyroidism.

2. **TBG** is produced in the liver and may be measured directly by radioimmunoassay. Several genetic forms of TBG excess or deficiency exist. They are all associated with abnormal total thyroid hormone concentration but with a clinically euthyroid state.

3. **Thyrotropin receptor stimulating antibodies (TRAbs)** are a heterogeneous group of immunoglobulins that stimulate thyroid hormone production by binding to the TSH receptor on thyroid cells. The most commonly measured antibodies are **TSH binding inhibitory immunoglobulin (TBII)** and **TSH receptor stimulating immunoglobulin (TSI)**. The presence of TBII and TSI correlates with disease activity in Graves disease and their measurement may be useful in predicting the likelihood of clinical remission.

4. **Thyroid gland imaging**
   a. **Sodium pertechnetate (^{99m}Tc) scanning** of the thyroid is the most commonly used functional thyroid imaging technique used in children. It is most useful for identification and localization of thyroid tissue in cases of congenital hypothyroidism.
   b. **Ultrasonography** of the thyroid gland is useful for characterization of cystic and solid lesions.

B **Hypothyroidism** may occur at birth (**congenital hypothyroidism**) or be acquired at any time during childhood or adolescence. Because of the importance of thyroid hormone for normal brain growth and development in the first 2 years of life, the clinical considerations are different for infants than for older children and adolescents.

1. **Congenital hypothyroidism (CH)** is one of the most common preventable causes of mental retardation. When the diagnosis is delayed, a high proportion of children suffer **permanent neurologic impairment.** CH is primarily caused by a developmental thyroid defect (thyroid agenesis or dysgenesis). Defective biosynthesis of thyroid hormone may also cause the disorder. Transient congenital hypothyroidism may occur as a result of transplacental passage of maternally

ingested goitrogens (e.g., iodide expectorants, antithyroid drugs, or maternal antithyroid antibodies).

a. Clinical features are not usually apparent at birth because of the protection from transplacental passage of maternal thyroid hormone. Often the first symptom is prolonged neonatal **jaundice.** Physical findings develop over time in the untreated infant, including coarse facies with large, open fontanelles; large, protruding tongue; hoarse cry; umbilical hernia; cool, dry, mottled skin; hypotonia; and delayed development.

b. **Diagnosis** is made by documenting decreased free T_4 and elevated TSH. A thyroid scan may be helpful in ascertaining the cause of CH.

c. **Screening.** Because congenital hypothyroidism is a relatively common problem (occurring in 1 in 4000 births) and because of the recognition of the critical role of thyroid hormones in neurologic development, techniques for newborn screening for hypothyroidism were developed in the 1970s. Newborn screening for hypothyroidism has become widely applied. Neurologic function and intelligence are preserved in children treated from birth.

d. **Therapy.** Thyroid hormone replacement should be instituted after confirming blood tests are drawn.

2. **Acquired hypothyroidism.** When symptoms appear after the first year of life, hypothyroidism is presumed to be acquired. It is more common in girls than in boys, as are most thyroid diseases.

a. **Etiology.** The most common cause is **autoimmune destruction** of the thyroid secondary to chronic lymphocytic thyroiditis (Hashimoto thyroiditis). Children with certain chromosomal disorders (Down, Turner, or Klinefelter syndromes) or other autoimmune disorders (type 1 diabetes mellitus) have an increased incidence of autoimmune thyroid diseases. Other causes include pituitary/hypothalamic disorders causing **central hypothyroidism.** Goitrogen or drug ingestion, such as iodide cough syrup, antithyroid drugs, lithium, and anticonvulsants, can also cause hypothyroidism.

b. **Clinical features. Slow linear growth** is the hallmark of hypothyroidism in childhood. Puberty is usually delayed. Other symptoms include cold intolerance, decreased appetite, inactivity, and constipation. Affected children may have coarse, puffy facies; immature body proportions; stocky habitus; paucity of speech and spontaneous movement; dull, dry, thin hair; and rough, dry skin with a pale, waxy hue. Deep tendon reflexes show delayed relaxation time ("hung" reflexes).

c. **Diagnosis** is made on the basis of documentation of decreased serum concentrations of free T_4. TSH levels are elevated in the case of primary hypothyroidism. In case of secondary or tertiary hypothyroidism (pituitary or hypothalamic dysfunction, respectively), TSH levels are found low or normal. The presence of circulating thyroid autoantibodies implies an autoimmune basis for the disease.

d. **Therapy.** Thyroid hormone replacement therapy is indicated. Serum free T_4 and TSH should normalize with treatment.

C Hyperthyroidism

1. **Graves disease** is the most common cause of hyperthyroidism. It is an **autoimmune disorder** in which enlargement and hyperfunction of the thyroid gland is stimulated by circulating thyroid-stimulating immunoglobulins that binds to TSH receptors on thyroid cells. Thus, thyroid hyperfunction is not TSH dependent.

a. **Clinical features.** The onset of symptoms is **insidious.** Weight loss, palpitations, frequent loose stools, fatigue, heat intolerance, interrupted sleep, hyperactivity, and deterioration in school performance are the most common symptoms. On physical examination, tachycardia and fidgety appearance are usually present. The thyroid gland is usually diffusely enlarged, smooth, firm but not hard, and nontender. The skin is velvety smooth, warm, flushed, and moist. A fine tremor of outstretched fingers may be seen. Proximal muscle weakness may be present. **Graves ophthalmopathy** is present in about 60% of patients. It is caused by lymphocytic infiltration of the extraocular eye muscles and retrobulbar soft tissue and may cause exophthalmos. Its course may proceed independent of treatment of the hyperthyroidism.

b. **Diagnosis.** Increased serum concentrations of free T_4 and total T_3 and low levels of TSH confirm the diagnosis of hyperthyroidism. The presence of TSI and TBII confirms the diagnosis of Graves disease. Thyroid scanning is only helpful if a hyperfunctioning nodule is suspected.

c. **Therapy**

(1) Initial treatment consists of antithyroid medication, either **propylthiouracil** or **methimazole.** Approximately 5% of patients experience side effects (e.g., skin rash, arthralgias, drug-induced hepatitis) while on antithyroid medication. In 40% to 50% of children with Graves disease, the disease goes into remission; antithyroid medication may then be discontinued after 12 to 24 months of treatment. Relapse rates are 30% to 40%.

(2) **Permanent treatment is achieved with either radioactive iodine (RAI)** or **subtotal thyroidectomy.** RAI is considered a safe and effective treatment modality for Graves disease in children older than 10 years. **Surgery** may be selected for recurrent hyperthyroidism after a course of medical treatment or if the patient is noncompliant with medical therapy. The choice of surgery versus RAI depends on the availability of an experienced thyroid surgeon and the desire of the family after a thorough discussion of risks and benefits of each modality. Most children eventually become hypothyroid after either treatment, requiring thyroid hormone replacement.

2. **Neonatal Graves disease**

a. Some infants born to women who have Graves disease exhibit neonatal hyperthyroidism, which is caused by transplacental passage of TRAbs. Symptoms are jitteriness, stare, hyperactivity, increased appetite, and poor weight gain. Tachycardia is present, and thyromegaly may be detectable. Thyroid hormone levels are elevated and TSH levels are suppressed.

b. Therapy with antithyroid medications is recommended. Initially, infants should be monitored closely for signs of congestive heart failure. Neonatal Graves disease usually resolves during the first several months of life.

3. **Other causes** for hyperthyroidism in children are rare but include an autonomous hyperfunctioning "hot" thyroid nodule and subacute thyroiditis.

IV DISORDERS OF THE ADRENAL GLAND

A Disorders of the adrenal cortex

1. **Hypoadrenocorticism.** Adrenal insufficiency can be the result of an abnormality of the adrenal glands (primary hypoadrenocorticism) or deficiency of adrenocorticotropic hormone (ACTH; secondary hypoadrenocorticism), or due to hormone resistance to ACTH or cortisol. **Primary adrenal insufficiency** may be congenital or acquired. The most common causes are described in Table 17-1.

TABLE 17-1 Causes of Adrenal Insufficiency

Primary Adrenal Insufficiency
Autoimmune
Addison disease
Autoimmune polyglandular syndromes
Infections
Tuberculosis, fungal infections
Sepsis
AIDS
Congenital adrenal hyperplasia
Adrenal hemorrhage or infarction
Unresponsiveness to ACTH
Secondary Adrenal Insufficiency
Withdrawal from glucocorticoid therapy
Hypopituitarism
Tumors, irradiation of central nervous system

ACTH, adrenocorticotropic hormone; AIDS, acquire immune deficiency syndrome.

a. **Symptoms** of chronic adrenal insufficiency include weakness, fatigue, nausea, vomiting, weight loss, growth failure, and salt craving.

b. **Physical findings** include postural hypotension and increased pigmentation, especially over joints, scar tissue, lips, nipples, and the buccal mucosa. The congenital forms can present with hypoglycemia in the neonatal period.

c. **Acute adrenal insufficiency** is characterized by vomiting, dehydration, hypotension, and shock that may be triggered by intercurrent illness, surgery, or trauma.

d. **Diagnosis.** The characteristic electrolyte abnormalities are hyponatremia, hyperkalemia, metabolic acidosis, and hypoglycemia. The serum cortisol level is low ($< 5\ \mu g/dL$) and fails to rise after an injection of ACTH.

e. **Therapy**

(1) **Treatment of adrenal crisis.** Diagnostic studies should not delay treatment of this life-threatening illness. Rehydration and correction of electrolyte abnormalities are needed immediately, along with acute administration of intravenous glucocorticoid in stress doses.

(2) **Long-term treatment** of adrenal insufficiency consists of maintenance doses of oral glucocorticoid and mineralocorticoid. The glucocorticoid dosage must be increased to stress doses during significant intercurrent illness, trauma, or surgery to prevent acute adrenal insufficiency.

2. **Hypercortisolism or Cushing syndrome** is a group of signs and symptoms that develop as a result of excessive cortisol, due to either endogenous overproduction of cortisol or exogenous treatment with glucocorticoids or ACTH.

a. **Etiology**

(1) **Bilateral adrenal hyperplasia** is the most common cause in children older than 7 years of age. This condition is usually caused by chronic oversecretion of ACTH by a **pituitary tumor.**

(2) **Adrenal tumors** may also cause Cushing syndrome. Most adrenal tumors are benign adenomas, although in younger children the possibility of malignancy is greater.

b. **Clinical features.** The classic manifestations of Cushing syndrome in childhood are slow growth, truncal obesity, rounded "moon" facies, buffalo hump, purple striae, and acne. Hypertension and muscle weakness are common. These features are not often found in children, most commonly presenting with obesity and short stature.

c. **Diagnosis.** A **24-hour urine collection** for measurement of free cortisol is the most discriminating test. Elevated serum cortisol levels and absence of the normal diurnal variation may be present but are difficult to interpret in the obese, stressed, or hospitalized child. An MRI of the pituitary and adrenal areas is also warranted.

d. **Therapy.** Surgical excision of the pituitary adenoma or adrenal tumors is the treatment of choice. Some children have been treated with pituitary irradiation. Chemotherapy for malignant metastatic disease may be indicated.

3. **Congenital adrenal hyperplasia (CAH)** results from an enzymatic defect in the **adrenal steroidogenesis** pathway. The clinical characteristics of CAH depend on which enzyme in the pathway of cortisol synthesis is deficient (Figure 17-1). ACTH secretion is increased due to the lack of negative feedback from cortisol. In certain forms of CAH, like 21-hydroxylase deficiency, oversecretion of ACTH stimulates excessive production of precursors that are shunted to androgens. The following are the most common forms of CAH:

a. **21-Hydroxylase deficiency** is the most common form of CAH. The clinical presentation varies and includes the classic salt-wasting form, the simple virilizing form, and the nonclassic presentation, also called late onset. The **clinical symptoms** result from the excess of precursors and subsequent increased androgen production, as well as glucocorticoid and mineralocorticoid deficiencies.

(1) **Virilization** of the genitalia is found at birth in female infants with classic or simple virilizing forms. It is induced by exposure to high androgen levels during early pregnancy. The nonclassic form manifests in adolescents or adult females with signs and symptoms of androgen excess (i.e., menstrual irregularities, hirsutism, acne).

(2) **Salt wasting** is secondary to mineralocorticoid deficiency; therefore, it is present only in the classic form of CAH. Hyponatremia, hyperkalemia, metabolic acidosis, and often hypoglycemia develop in the first 2 to 4 weeks of life in the untreated child.

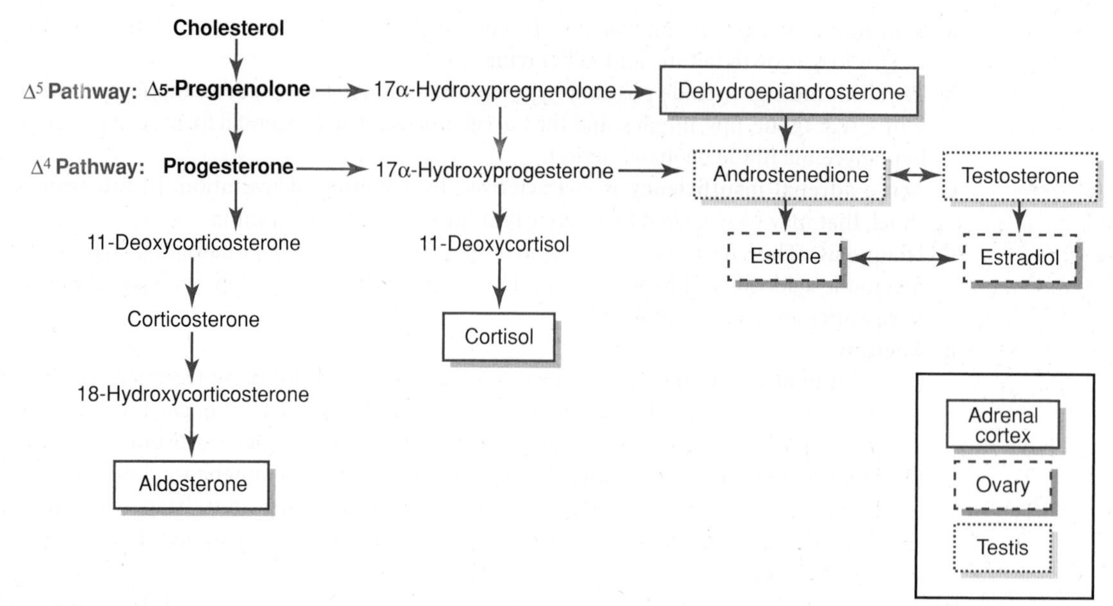

FIGURE 17-1 Summary of steroidogenesis in the adrenal cortex, ovary, and testis (Reprinted from Bullock J, Boyle J, Wang M: *NMS Physiology,* 3rd ed. Baltimore, Williams & Wilkins, p 491.)

(3) **Diagnosis** rests on measurement of markedly elevated levels of 17-hydroxyprogesterone (17 OH-P) and androgens in the serum. In the nonclassic form, basal levels of 17 OH-P may be only modestly elevated. However, the excessive rise of 17 OH-P after ACTH stimulation is diagnostic.

(4) **Genetics.** This form of CAH is inherited as an autosomal recessive trait. The gene is located in the human leukocyte antigen (HLA) major histocompatibility complex on the short arm of chromosome 6. **Newborn screening** for CAH due to 21-hydroxylase deficiency has been adopted by many states and countries.

(5) **Therapy** consists of the replacement of cortisol to correct cortisol deficiency and to suppress ACTH and androgens overproduction. In the salt-wasting forms, mineralocorticoid replacement is indicated.

b. **11-Hydroxylase deficiency** is the second most common form of CAH, accounting for approximately 5% to 8% of cases. In this disorder, precursors are shunted toward overproduction of androgens and mineralocorticoids, resulting in virilization, hypertension, and hypokalemia. The **diagnosis** is based on the measurement of increased levels of androstenedione, testosterone, 11-deoxycortisol, and deoxycorticosterone in serum. Renin and aldosterone are suppressed.

B Disorders of the adrenal medulla

1. **Catecholamines** exert widespread metabolic effects on glycogenolysis, lipolysis, and gluconeogenesis, as well as effects on the cardiovascular system. The physiologic effects on vasodilation and cardiac muscle contractility are mediated through α- and β-adrenergic receptors on target cell surfaces. The major clinical problems arising from the adrenal medulla are **tumors.**

2. **Pheochromocytoma** is a rare tumor of chromaffin tissue. The most common site of occurrence is the adrenal medulla, but the tumor may also occur in extra-adrenal sites in the chest and abdomen. Most tumors in childhood are benign. Morbidity and mortality result from the effects of overproduction of catecholamines.

   a. **Clinical features.** Hypertension, headache, vomiting, pallor, and sweating are prominent.

   b. **Diagnosis** is based on finding of elevated levels of catecholamines and their metabolites (e.g., metanephrine, normetanephrine) and vanillylmandelic acid (VMA) in a 24-hour urine sample. **Imaging studies** including ultrasonography, CT, or MRI scanning may be obtained. ^{123}I-metaiodobenzylguanidine scintigraphy is helpful in imaging the adrenal medulla as well as extra-adrenal chromaffin tissue.

   c. **Therapy** for pheochromocytoma is surgical excision.

V DISORDERS OF SEX DEVELOPMENT

The term *disorders of sex development* (DSD) refers to congenital conditions in which development of chromosomal, gonadal, or anatomic sex is atypical. Table 17-2 summarizes proposed revised nomenclature.

A **Abnormal sexual differentiation** results in a newborn who appears sexually ambiguous.

1. **46,XY DSD** refers to infants who are 46,XY males (with testes) but who appear to have signs of **incomplete masculinization,** including hypospadias, a small phallus, and a poorly developed scrotum with or without descended testes. This can be caused by a variety of endocrine disorders involving testosterone synthesis, metabolism, or action at the cellular level and gonadal dysgenesis.
   a. **Androgen insensitivity syndromes (testicular feminization syndrome)**
      (1) **Complete androgen insensitivity** presents as an XY male infant with testes who appears unambiguously female because of complete resistance to androgen action at the cellular level. The first clue to this disorder may be the discovery of testes in inguinal hernia sacs in early childhood. Some children may initially be seen as female adolescents with primary amenorrhea. Internal female organs do not develop because the testes produce antimüllerian factor (AMF) in utero. If the testes are not removed before the time of puberty, female breasts develop from the increased conversion of testosterone to estrogen.
      (2) In **partial androgen insensitivity,** the affected XY individual has ambiguous genitalia. Because it is inherited as an X-linked recessive trait, a family history of infertile or cryptorchid relatives may exist.
   b. **Defects in androgen synthesis**
      (1) **5α-Reductase deficiency i**mpairs conversion of testosterone to dihydrotestosterone (DHT). Boys are born with ambiguous genitalia because DHT is necessary for masculinization of the male external genitalia. The diagnosis may be made in childhood by finding an increased ratio of testosterone to DHT.
      (2) **Defects in testosterone synthesis** are very rare and may be caused by one of five enzyme deficiencies inherited as autosomal recessive traits. Some of them result in defects in cortisol synthesis as well, and therefore are classified as forms of **congenital adrenal hyperplasia.**
2. **46,XX DSD** refers to infants who are 46,XX females (with ovaries) but who appear masculinized at birth. Exposure of the female infant to increased androgen during the critical period of 8 to 12 weeks' gestation causes a variable degree of labioscrotal fusion, formation of a urogenital sinus, and clitoral enlargement. Exposure after the 12th week cannot cause labioscrotal fusion, but it can induce clitoral enlargement. Some infants appear to be cryptorchid males at birth.
   a. **Congenital adrenal hyperplasia.** Defects that cause masculinization of the female genitalia are 21-hydroxylase deficiency, 11-hydroxylase deficiency, and 3β-hydroxysteroid dehydrogenase deficiency. This is the more common cause of ambiguous genitalia (*see IV A 3*).

TABLE 17-2 Proposed Revised Nomenclature for Disorders of Sex Development (DSD)

Previous Intersex	Proposed DSD
Male pseudohermaphrodite Undervirilization of an XY male Undermasculinization of an XY male	46,XY DSD
Female pseudohermaphrodite Overvirilization of an XX female Masculinization of an XX female	46,XX DSD
True hermaphrodite	Ovotesticular DSD
XX male or XX sex reversal	46,XX testicular DSD
XY sex reversal	46,XY complete gonadal dysgenesis

Based on Hughes IA, Houk C, Ahmed SF, et al., LWPES1/ESPE2 Consensus Group: Consensus statement on management of intersex disorders. *Arch Dis Child* 91:554–562, 2006.

b. **Maternal androgen** or **progestin exposure.** Exogenous ingestion of androgenic substances is a rare cause of virilization of female newborns. Occasionally, a virilizing tumor or disease during pregnancy in the mother may cause this syndrome.

3. **Abnormal gonadal differentiation or sex chromosome DSD**
   a. **Ovotesticular DSD** occurs when there is both ovarian and testicular tissue present in the gonads. In approximately 80% of patients, the karyotype is 46,XX, and in the remainder is 46,XX/46,XY mosaicism. The exact cause is unknown. Ovotesticular DSD may be suspected in an infant who has ambiguous genitalia, an XX karyotype, and normal serum 17-hydroxyprogresterone levels, thus ruling out CAH. The final diagnosis rests with surgical exploration and demonstration of gonads containing both ovarian and testicular tissue.
   b. **Mixed gonadal dysgenesis** involves a karyotype of 45,X/46,XY. There is a spectrum of appearance of the external genitalia from completely male to completely female. The gonads may appear as streak ovaries to dysgenetic testes and are often asymmetric. Because of the 45,X cell line, some somatic features of Turner syndrome may be present. Diagnosis is made by karyotyping.
   c. **Other defects in external genital development** include hypospadias, cloacal exstrophy, and microphallus. **Microphallus** describes males who have an abnormally small but well-differentiated penis. Standards are available for assessing stretched penile length from infancy through adulthood. Male genital growth depends on fetal pituitary gonadotropin stimulation of the fetal testis.

B Management of the child with ambiguous genitalia

1. **Complete diagnostic evaluation** should be undertaken as soon as possible after birth by a multidisciplinary team of specialists in endocrinology, surgery or urology, genetics, psychiatry, neonatology, and medical ethics. It is important to arrive at the most specific diagnosis possible for a variety of therapeutic and management considerations. Parents should be encouraged to delay naming and announcing the child's sex until diagnostic workup is complete. A careful family and pregnancy history and physical examination are the basis for further testing. Infants must be monitored closely for evidence of salt wasting and glucocorticoid deficiency while awaiting diagnostic test results.
   a. **Physical examination.** The size of the phallus, position of the urethra, palpable gonads (usually testes), and other dysmorphic or asymmetric features should be noted.
   b. **Laboratory studies** initially include chromosome analysis and evaluation of 17-hydroxyprogesterone, testosterone, gonadotropins, serum electrolytes, and AMF levels. Radiographic contrast study of the urogenital sinus is often helpful to delineate the presence of a vagina and cervix, and occasionally fallopian tubes may be seen. **Pelvic imaging** may demonstrate the presence of ovaries and a uterus.
2. **Gender assignment.** Initial gender uncertainty is unsettling and stressful for families. Expediting a thorough assessment and decision is required. Factors that influence gender assignment include:
   a. Diagnosis
   b. Genital appearance
   c. Surgical options
   d. Need for life-long replacement therapy
   e. Potential for fertility
   f. Views of the family and cultural practices
3. **Surgical management.** Only surgeons with expertise in the management of children with DSD should be involved. Emphasis is on **functional outcome** rather than a strictly cosmetic appearance.
4. **Psychosocial management.** Psychosocial care provided by mental health staff with expertise in DSD should be an integral part of management in order to promote positive adaptation and psychosexual maturation. This expertise can facilitate team decisions about gender assignment/reassignment, timing of surgery, and sex hormone replacement.
5. **Sex steroid replacement.** Appropriate hormonal replacement at the usual age of puberty should be provided. Hormonal induction of puberty should attempt to replicate normal pubertal maturation to induce secondary sexual characteristics, a pubertal growth spurt, and optimal bone mineral accumulation.

VI HYPOGLYCEMIA

A Neonatal hypoglycemia The newborn is at special risk for hypoglycemia because counterregulatory mechanisms to maintain euglycemia are immature at birth, especially in low-birth-weight and premature infants. Blood glucose levels below 50 to 60 mg/dL during the neonatal period deserve to be evaluated and treated (see Chapter 6).

B Childhood hypoglycemia Hypoglycemia beyond the neonatal period is quite rare. The symptoms are produced by two major underlying mechanisms: An adrenergic response to hypoglycemia causes sweating, hunger, tremors, pallor, and palpitations; and a lack of glucose available to the brain causes weakness, drowsiness, bizarre behavior, and loss of consciousness and seizures.

1. **Etiology**
   a. **Ketotic hypoglycemia is** the most common cause of hypoglycemia in children 1 to 4 years of age. The child typically presents with one or more episodes of early morning hypoglycemia with large amounts of ketones in the urine. The child is otherwise well. Episodes are associated with a decreased intake of food due to intercurrent illness. The **etiology** of ketotic hypoglycemia appears to be a diminished tolerance for fasting, perhaps related to smaller muscle mass, which limits substrate availability. Growth hormone and cortisol levels are appropriately high, and insulin levels are appropriately low. Gluconeogenic mechanisms are preserved. Treatment consists of avoidance of fasting by eating frequent, small meals, particularly during illness. Symptoms usually disappear after the age of 6 to 8 years.
   b. **Growth hormone deficiency** and **hypocortisolism** may manifest as symptomatic hypoglycemia.
   c. Certain **hepatic enzyme deficiencies,** which result in impaired glycogenolysis or gluconeogenesis, may occur during infancy. These deficiencies include glycogen storage disease types I, III, and IV; hereditary fructose intolerance; fructose 1,6-diphosphatase deficiency; and galactosemia. The presence of marked hepatomegaly with failure to thrive and hypotonia should suggest one of these defects; the actual diagnosis may require liver biopsy for assay of the specific enzyme.
   d. **Hyperinsulinism** in the older child may be the manifestation of an insulin-secreting tumor. The child usually becomes hypoglycemic after fasting for 6 to 12 hours. Ketones are not present in the urine. Insulin levels are inappropriately high and sometimes markedly elevated during hypoglycemia.
2. The **differential diagnosis of hypoglycemia** is best made by obtaining a detailed history and physical exam. A "critical" blood sample, obtained during a documented episode of hypoglycemia, should be analyzed to identify the cause of hypoglycemia. In the absence of this blood sample, a fasting test is performed by monitoring blood glucose throughout a **24-hour fast.** If the blood glucose level falls below 45 mg/dL, blood for measurement of insulin, glucose, cortisol, GH, and other metabolites is obtained, as well as urine for ketones (Figure 17-2).

VII DIABETES MELLITUS AND INSULIN RESISTANCE SYNDROME

Diabetes mellitus is a heterogeneous group of metabolic disorders characterized by hyperglycemia and abnormal energy metabolism, caused by abnormalities of insulin secretion, insulin resistance, or both. The chronic hyperglycemia of diabetes is associated with long-term damage, especially the eyes, kidneys, nerves, heart, and blood vessels.

A Classification The American Diabetes Association (ADA) has recommended a classification of diabetes based on the etiology of the disease, abandoning past classifications that were based on the treatment required (insulin, non–insulin dependent) or the age at onset of the disease (juvenile, adult onset).

1. **Type 1 diabetes mellitus (T1DM)** includes cases that are primarily insulin deficient due to β-cell destruction, either secondary to an autoimmune process or of unknown etiology. These are now called **type 1A** and **type 1B,** respectively. T1DM does not include those forms of β-cell destruction for which non–autoimmune-specific causes can be assigned (e.g., cystic fibrosis). T1DM is the most common endocrine-metabolic disease in childhood, occurring in 1 in 500 children and adolescents. It is also the most common form of diabetes in children.

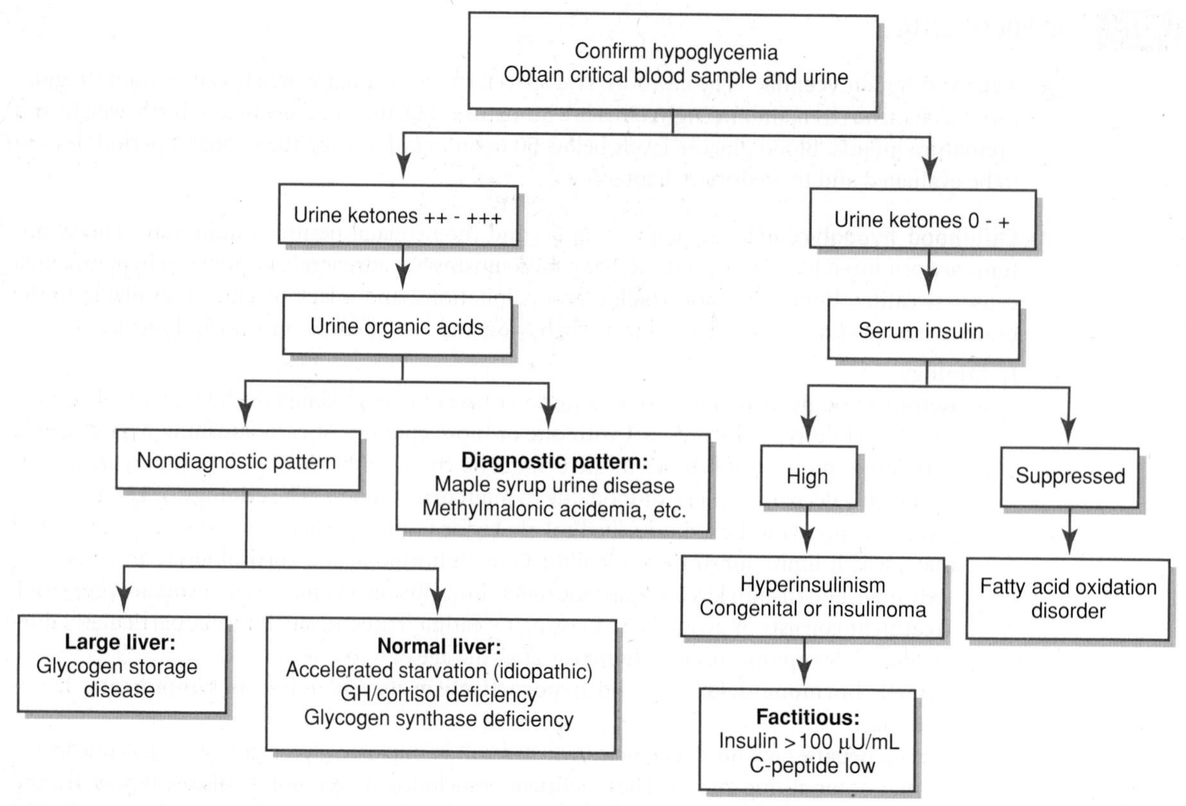

FIGURE 17-2 Algorithm for diagnosis of hypoglycemia. GH, growth hormone. (From Wolfsdorf J, Weinstein D: Hypoglycemia in children. In: *Pediatric Endocrinology,* 5th ed. Edited by Lifshitz F. New York, Informa Healthcare USA, 2007, pp 291–327.)

2. **Type 2 diabetes (T2DM)** results from insulin resistance and an insulin secretory defect. It is the most prevalent form of diabetes in adults. T2DM was a rare entity in pediatrics until the 1990s, but it currently accounts for 10% to 50% of newly diagnosed children with diabetes.

B **Diagnosis** Although in most cases the diagnosis of T1DM and T2DM in children may be based on the clinical presentation, the differentiation between the two may be challenging and only the course of the disease over time clarifies the diagnosis.

1. Typically, children with **T1DM** present in an **acute** manner with a short history of polyuria, polydipsia, or weight loss, or in diabetes ketoacidosis. Islet cell autoimmunity is present and insulin production is very low. Family history of T1DM is found in 5% to 10% of cases.
2. Children with **T2DM** present with an **insidious** course or without symptoms, often being diagnosed during a routine screening. The majority of these children are obese, have a family history of diabetes, and belong to a high-risk ethnic group (e.g., Hispanic, Black, Native American). Increased insulin levels and signs of insulin resistance, such as acanthosis nigricans, are present. There is no evidence of autoimmunity. Certain factors make the distinction between T1DM and T2DM difficult. For example, children with T1DM may be obese at presentation. Insulin levels at diagnosis may be low in a child with T2DM because of glucotoxicity affecting β-cell function. Islet cell autoimmunity has been reported in increasing numbers of cases of T2DM.

C **Definition of diabetes and prediabetes** The diagnostic criteria for diabetes based on the results of an oral glucose tolerance test or random blood glucose findings were recently revised by the ADA. The term **prediabetes** has been chosen to include the states of impaired glucose tolerance and impaired fasting glucose. This decision was partly based after the recognition that these conditions are risk factors for cardiovascular disease and stroke. The criteria are described in Table 17-3.

TABLE 17-3 Criteria for the Diagnosis of Diabetes and Prediabetes

	Diabetes	Prediabetes: Impaired Fasting Glucose	Prediabetes: Impaired Glucose Tolerance
Fasting glucose	≥ 126 mg/dL	110–126 mg/dL	
2-Hour glucose during OGTT[a]	≥ 200 mg/dL		140–200 mg/dL
Random	≥ 200 mg/dL plus symptoms of diabetes[b]		

OGTT, oral glucose tolerance test.
[a]OGTT using a glucose load containing 1.75 g/kg of glucose, up to a maximum of 75 g.
[b]Symptoms of diabetes include polyuria, polydipsia, and unexplained weight loss.

D Type 1 diabetes mellitus

1. **Etiology**
   a. Although the precise cause of T1DM is unknown, the pathologic process that ultimately results in the loss of insulin secretion by the β-cells is related to an **autoimmune destruction** of these cells.
   b. There is an increased frequency of certain **HLAs** that confer greater risk for the development of T1DM (HLA genotypes DR3, DR4, DQB0302, DQB0201). Diabetes risk is increased in relatives of T1DM patients compared to the general population. Among first-degree relatives, the risk is approximately 5% before age 20 years and 10% by age 60 years. Concordance for identical twins is 30% to 50%.
   c. The variability in the incidence of T1DM, even in the genetically predisposed subject, as well as its rising incidence, suggests the participation of **environmental factors** as triggers in the development of disease. Multiple factors have been suggested to increase the risk of T1DM including viruses, cow's milk antigens, lack of exposure to infection during infancy, and vaccinations. There are many studies under way to better define the role of these and other agents in the etiology of T1DM.
2. **Pathophysiology**
   a. When 90% of the functioning β-cells have been destroyed, **loss of insulin secretion** becomes clinically significant and hyperglycemia ensues. In the state of insulin deficiency, levels of counterregulatory hormones (i.e., glucagon, epinephrine, growth hormone, and cortisol) are elevated. These hormones stimulate lipolysis, fatty acid release, and ketoacid production.
   b. When the blood glucose concentration is persistently above the renal threshold for glucose reabsorption (i.e., 180 mg/dL), **glucosuria** develops, which causes an osmotic diuresis with increased urine output (polyuria) and increased fluid intake (polydipsia).
   c. **Ketones** are produced in abundant amounts when insulin deficiency is severe. If insulin treatment is not initiated, **diabetic ketoacidosis** develops. This deranged metabolic state is characterized by hyperglycemia, metabolic acidosis (ketoacidosis), dehydration, and lethargy, which may progress to coma and death.
3. **Clinical features.** Typically symptoms are **polyuria, polydipsia, nocturia** or **enuresis,** and **weight loss,** and, with increasing insulin deficiency, ketone bodies accumulation occurs. Nausea, abdominal pain, and vomiting are symptoms of **diabetic ketoacidosis** that contribute to severe dehydration.
4. **Diagnosis** in the symptomatic child rests on documentation of fasting or random hyperglycemia. Glucosuria and ketonuria are usually found.
5. **Therapy.** The immediate goal of treatment is to **restore fluid and electrolyte losses,** either orally or intravenously, and to **reverse the catabolic state** by replacing insulin. The long-term goal is to achieve the best possible metabolic control to prevent the development of complications. The rapidly developing technology resulting in "designer" insulins, different insulin delivery devices, and continuous glucose monitoring systems has made the management of childhood diabetes more successful, although it remains challenging for the children and their families.

TABLE 17-4 Insulin Types

Insulin Type	Onset	Peak	Duration
Rapid Analogues: Lispro, Aspart, glulisine	15–30 min	30–90 min	3–5 h
Short Regular human insulin	30–60 min	2–3 h	4–6 h
Intermediate NPH human insulin	1–4 h	5–14 h	10–16 h
Long Analogues: Glargine, detemir	1–2 h	None	20–24 h

a. **Insulin replacement** is the foundation of T1DM treatment. In recent years, human insulins produced by recombinant DNA technique and synthetic insulin analogues have become available, improving our ability to tailor the insulin regimen to the individual needs of the patients. Insulin analogs result from minor changes to the human insulin molecule that affect the speed of absorption into the circulation. The types of insulin currently available can be classified according to their pharmacokinetic profile, which determines the onset, peak, and duration of action (Table 17-4). Insulin regimens can be divided in two main categories:

(1) **Basal/bolus.** This regimen aims to mimic the physiologic insulin secretion pattern. Basal insulin is given to maintain a small amount of insulin in the circulation. Additionally, **boluses** of insulin are given at meal times in proportion to the amount of carbohydrates to be consumed and the premeal blood glucose. This regimen can be delivered by injections using a combination of long-acting/peakless insulin as basal, and rapid-acting insulin for the boluses before meals. Therefore, the patient receives several injections a day. The continuous subcutaneous insulin infusion pump is another method that can be used. The pump is preprogrammed to deliver basal amounts of rapid-acting insulin continuously at varying basal rates. Meal-time boluses are delivered through the pump as well. Although the carbohydrate ratios and corrections are programmed into the pump memory, the patient needs to activate the mechanism at each meal. These regimens offer flexibility of meal timing and content, but require a more motivated family to cope with multiple injections and pump operation. Another advantage of pump therapy is the ability to modify the amount of basal insulin delivered according to levels of physical activity to avoid hypoglycemia.

(2) **Split/mixed regimens.** Also called "conventional therapy," this consists of two injections of a combination of intermediate-acting insulin and rapid- or short-acting insulin. The patient then is required to follow a meal plan consisting of three meals and three snacks to try to match the peak of insulin action with food intake. During and after periods of heavy exercise, increased food intake may be required to avoid hypoglycemia. The disadvantages of these regimens compared to basal/bolus is that the timing and carbohydrate content of the meals are fixed, they are associated with a higher frequency of hypoglycemia, and most patients are not able to achieve near-normal glycemia.

(3) Besides the regimens described above, multiple combinations of long-, intermediate-, and short-acting insulins are currently used according to the children's and families' needs, lifestyle, expectations, and ability to cope with the demands of different regimens.

b. **Blood glucose monitoring** is key to achieve optimal diabetes control. Blood glucose levels are used to decide insulin dose at meal times, as well as to adjust insulin doses overall. **Continuous glucose monitoring devices** that are inserted subcutaneously are currently available, although data on their use and accuracy in children are still limited.

c. **Diet.** Children on basal/bolus regimens should follow a balanced meal plan that promotes normal growth and weight gain. For children on the split/mixed regimens, food intake must match the time course of insulin absorption. Meals and snacks must be roughly equivalent in carbohydrate content from day to day and should be eaten on time. A specialized diabetes nutritionist should help guide the child and family with meal planning.

d. **Exercise.** Children who have T1DM should be encouraged and not restricted to exercise regularly. Because strenuous exercise may result in hypoglycemia, extra food may be eaten before exercise or pump rates adjusted accordingly.

e. **Patient education.** Children who have T1DM and their families should be educated on diabetes management by an experienced multidisciplinary team composed of educators, nutritionists, physicians, and psychosocial support personnel. Education is an ongoing process, and periodic reinforcement is important as the child grows older and more independent of the family. The diagnosis of diabetes arouses strong emotional responses in both the child and family members, including grief, anger, guilt, resentment, and fear; therefore, psychological support and counseling are important.

f. **Medical follow-up.** Regular follow-up visits every 3 to 4 months are indicated. **Hemoglobin A_{1c}** measurement as an objective index of blood glucose control over the preceding 3 months should be part of routine monitoring. Because of the increased risk of autoimmune disease in children who have T1DM, periodic assessment of thyroid function and for celiac disease should be performed.

6. **Complications** of T1DM can be divided into **immediate complications,** which include hypoglycemia and diabetic ketoacidosis, and **late complications,** which are those generally associated with a long duration of T1DM.

a. **Hypoglycemia** is the most common complication and a limiting factor in bringing glucose to near-normal levels. It occurs from a relative excess of insulin to carbohydrate availability (low carbohydrate intake or increased consumption due to exercise). Typical symptoms of hypoglycemia may be related to sympathetic discharge (e.g., sweating, tremulousness, hunger) and should be readily recognizable by the child or family. More severe symptoms (e.g., lethargy, bizarre behavior, slurred speech, unconsciousness, seizures) are caused by glucose deprivation to the CNS. These may occur in combination with sympathetic symptoms or alone.

b. **Diabetic ketoacidosis** is caused by relative or absolute insulin deficiency, most commonly due to **omission of insulin doses.** The condition may also be triggered by intercurrent illness, which may be associated with some degree of insulin resistance. Patients present with severe acidosis secondary to ketone bodies accumulation and dehydration. Potassium urinary loses increase because of acidosis, leading to total body potassium depletion. However, the measured serum potassium at presentation may be high because in the presence of acidosis, potassium is pulled from the intracellular compartment.

c. **Late complications of T1DM** are related to chronic hyperglycemia; improved glycemic control results in a decreased rate of development of complications. Efforts to maintain near-normal blood glucose levels must be balanced with the increased risk of hypoglycemia, especially in children and adolescents. Complications associated with a long duration of diabetes include **microvascular disease** of the eye **(retinopathy),** the kidney **(nephropathy),** and the nerves **(neuropathy).** These problems may be seen in the older adolescent patient. The other major category of late complications is **large vessel atherosclerotic disease,** which leads to premature myocardial infarction and stroke. Children and adolescents who have had diabetes for more than 5 years should have yearly surveillance for complications.

E Type 2 diabetes There is evidence that the incidence of T2DM has increased dramatically in the pediatric population over the past 10 to 15 years. The rise in the incidence of T2DM has paralleled the increased prevalence of childhood obesity. Clearly, Black, Hispanic, and Native American children are at most risk. Considering that T2DM in adults can remain undiagnosed for years due to the lack of overt symptoms or that it could be misclassified as type 1, it is likely that the magnitude of T2DM in the pediatric population is underestimated for the same reasons.

1. **Etiology**

a. T2DM results from the confluence of **insulin resistance** and the **failure of the β-cell** to produce sufficient insulin to compensate for the decreased insulin sensitivity. Initially there is compensatory hyperinsulinemia, but as the disease progresses, a relative β-cell "failure" develops with consequent overt hyperglycemia and diabetes. Insulin resistance is in part **genetically determined.** It is well known that insulin sensitivity varies among ethnic groups, which may in part explain the higher prevalence of T2DM in these groups. As well, the fact that puberty enhances insulin resistance may be the underlying explanation to the more dramatic increase of T2DM in adolescents. Pathophysiologic events such as obesity, hyperlipidemia, and hyperglycemia also contribute to decreased responsiveness to insulin.

b. **Genetics.** T2DM is a **polygenic** disease. Multiple loci have been associated with T2DM in adults but the frequency of a particular susceptibility locus varies between different populations. Among these loci, some are associated with abnormalities of insulin action on target cells and others are associated with abnormalities of insulin secretion from the β-cell.

c. **The fetal environment** may also play a role in the later development of obesity and T2DM. Intrauterine growth retardation has been associated with an increased risk of insulin resistance in children and T2DM in adults. Fetal undernutrition appears to lead to a permanent reduction in glucose transport into the cells in response to insulin that is responsible for the postnatal development of decreased insulin sensitivity.

2. **Clinical presentation**

a. The presentation of T2DM in children is usually **insidious,** and most children with T2DM are actually identified incidentally after detection of glycosuria or hyperglycemia during routine evaluations. A minority of patients present more acutely with the typical symptoms of diabetes. Some black adolescents can present in frank ketoacidosis. Additionally, a small portion of children with T2DM may present with hyperosmolar coma. There is a preponderance of females over males (ratio of 1.7:1). The hallmark of T2DM in children is obesity, which is reported in almost 100% of cases.

b. **Acanthosis nigricans,** a cutaneous marker of insulin resistance, is also very common (85%–90% of cases) (Figure 17-3). This condition is characterized by hyperpigmented, thickened skin, with a velvety texture. Acanthosis is usually found around the neck and axillae.

c. All comorbidities associated with childhood obesity may be present in the patient with T2DM. These include hypertension, dyslipidemias, polycystic ovary syndrome, nonalcoholic fatty liver disease, obstructive apnea, orthopedic complications, and others.

3. **Screening.** Screening for T2DM in children is recommended only for the at-risk population, according to the criteria outlined in Table 17-5. The screening should probably be repeated before the recommended 2 years if the child goes through puberty or gains weight significantly.

4. **Treatment.** Intensive glucose control decreases the risk for the development of diabetes complications. Therefore, the overall goal of the treatment in the child with diabetes should be the achievement of near-normal glycemia. The treatment of T2DM in children is stepwise, similar to the treatment of adults with T2DM. Multicenter trials addressing the treatment of T2DM in the pediatric population are under way.

a. **Lifestyle modification** is the cornerstone of the treatment to promote weight loss. Changing eating habits and patterns of physical activity in adolescents can be difficult to implement and even more difficult to maintain. A **multidisciplinary team approach** is necessary for the management of these patients. Nutritionists, behavioral modification specialists, and exercise trainers are desirable members of the team. A supportive family that helps with the availability

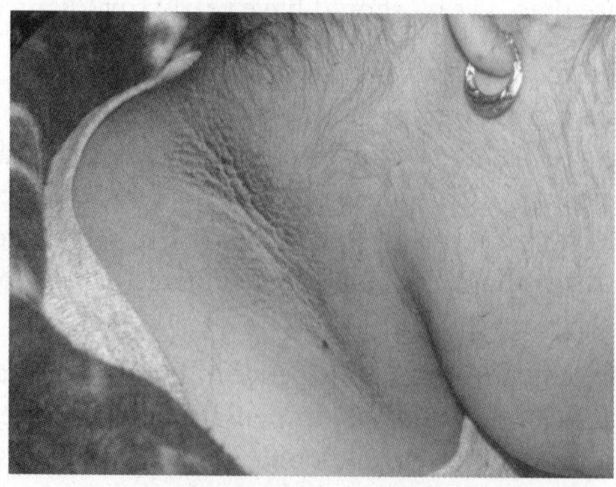

FIGURE 17-3 Acanthosis nigricans. (From Goodheart HP. *Goodheart's Photoguide of Common Skin Disorders,* 2nd ed. Philadelphia, Lippincott Williams & Wilkins, 2003.)

TABLE 17-5 American Diabetes Association Guidelines for Screening Children for Type 2 Diabetes Mellitus

- Overweight children (defined as BMI > 85th percentile for age and sex, weight for height > 85th percentile, or weight > 120% of ideal [50th percentile] for height)

Plus any two of the risk factors listed below:

  - Have a family history of type 2 diabetes in first- and second-degree relatives
  - Belong to a certain race/ethnic group (American Indians, Blacks, Hispanic Americans, Asians/South Pacific Islanders)
  - Have signs of insulin resistance or conditions associated with insulin resistance (acanthosis nigricans, hypertension, dyslipidemia, PCOS)
- Age of test initiation: Starting at age 10 y or at onset of puberty if it occurs at a younger age
- Frequency of testing: Every 2 y
- Preferred test: Fasting plasma glucose and 2-h plasma glucose are both suitable. The fasting plasma glucose is preferred because of its lower cost and greater convenience. Fasting is defined as no consumption of food or beverage other than water for at least 8 h before testing
- Testing may be considered in other high-risk patients according to clinical judgment

BMI, body mass index; PCOS, polycystic ovary syndrome.
Based on American Diabetes Association: Type 2 diabetes in children and adolescents. *Diabetes Care* 23(3):381–389, 2000.

of healthy food choices and activities that promote more exercise is key to success. Cultural and economic factors should be taken into account during counseling.

b. **Pharmacologic treatment.** Children who are not responsive to diet and exercise or present with severe hyperglycemia require pharmacotherapy. Oral hypoglycemic drugs that were previously reserved for adults are now being used in the pediatric patient with T2DM. **Metformin** is the only oral antidiabetic drug approved by the FDA for use in children and is the medication recommended by the ADA for the treatment of pediatric T2DM.

c. **Insulin therapy** is needed when the natural progression of the disease has reached insufficient insulin secretion by the pancreatic β-cells. It is usually added to the therapy when diet, exercise, and oral medications cannot achieve optimal glycemic control.

5. **Complications** associated with T2DM include increased risk of cardiovascular disease, retinopathy, end-stage renal disease, and vascular insufficiency of the lower extremities. Some of these complications may be already present at diagnosis and the incidence increases with duration of illness. The long-term effect of early-onset T2DM in children on morbidity and mortality is not yet known.

F Insulin resistance syndrome Insulin resistance syndrome (IRS), also called **metabolic syndrome** or **syndrome X,** consists of the cluster of hyperinsulinemia, glucose intolerance, hypertension, increased very-low-density lipoproteins (VLDLs), increased triglycerides, decreased high-density-lipoproteins (HDLs), and obesity. IRS may affect 50% of the adult population in the United States, with even higher prevalence among the high-risk ethnic groups (Blacks, Hispanics, and Native Americans). IRS is also rising in children in parallel to the rising incidence of obesity. This syndrome confers a very high risk for T2DM and cardiovascular disease in the affected patients. Early manifestations of syndrome X have been demonstrated in children. Clinical features at presentation include high insulin levels; obesity, particularly of central distribution with increased waist-to-hip ratio; acanthosis nigricans; acne; hirsutism; hypertension; dyslipidemia (particularly increased LDLs and triglycerides, decreased HDLs); PCOS; hepatic steatosis; and premature adrenarche. Most of these children have family history of obesity, T2DM, hypertension, and early cardiovascular disease. **Treatment** is geared to weight loss with lifestyle modification. Pharmacotherapy should be used to target the individual aspects of IRS.

VIII CALCIUM AND BONE DISORDERS

Normal mineral metabolism and skeletal development depends mainly on the interactions of three organs—the intestines, kidneys, and bones—and three hormones—parathyroid hormone (PTH), vitamin D, and calcitonin.

A Disorders of parathyroid hormones

1. **Hyperparathyroidism** is rare in childhood. The disorder may be **primary or secondary. Primary** hyperparathyroidism could be due to an adenoma or hyperplasia of the parathyroid gland, which may be isolated or occur as part of **multiple endocrine neoplastic syndromes. Secondary** hyperplasia of the parathyroid gland also occurs from exposure to chronic hypocalcemia, as in cases of chronic renal disease, liver disease, and lack of vitamin D.
   a. **Clinical features.** Symptoms are related to hypercalcemia and include nausea, vomiting, constipation, lethargy, confusion, and weakness. Hypertension and renal colic secondary to kidney stones are common.
   b. **Diagnosis**
      (1) Elevated serum levels of calcium, low serum levels of phosphorus, and increased phosphorus elimination in the urine are found. PTH levels are elevated.
      (2) **Radiographs** of bone show subperiosteal bone resorption that is especially evident in the clavicles.
   c. **Therapy** involves excision of the tumor if an adenoma is found, or subtotal parathyroidectomy for gland hyperplasia. Treatment of underlying conditions is needed in secondary hyperparathyroidism.
2. **Hypoparathyroidism**
   a. **Idiopathic hypoparathyroidism** may occur in the neonatal period or at any time during childhood. The cause may be autoimmune.
      (1) **Clinical features.** Symptoms are caused by low serum levels of calcium and include seizures, tetany, numbness of the face and extremities, and carpopedal spasm.
      (2) **Diagnosis.** Serum calcium levels are low and phosphorus levels are high; the PTH levels are inappropriately low, indicating lack of PTH response to hypocalcemia.
   b. **Pseudohypoparathyroidism** also manifests as symptomatic hypocalcemia, but PTH levels are very high, indicating **PTH unresponsiveness** due to a receptor or postreceptor defect. Patients with pseudohypoparathyroidism may have distinctive skeletal and facial characteristics, including short stature; round face; a short, thick neck; and short metacarpals. Cognitive impairment to a variable degree is common.
   c. **Therapy**
      (1) **Vitamin D** (calcitriol) is the treatment for idiopathic hypoparathyroidism and pseudohypoparathyroidism. Calcitriol stimulates increased calcium absorption in the intestine.
      (2) **Oral calcium supplementation** may speed the restoration of normal calcium levels. These children should have serum calcium and phosphorus levels monitored frequently to avoid hypercalcemia and potential nephrocalcinosis and renal damage.

B Rickets

Rickets is characterized by bone lesions that are caused by **failure of osteoid,** the growing cellular matrix of bone, **to become mineralized.** The undermineralized bone is less rigid and the growing, remodeling bone bends and twists abnormally.

1. **Clinical features.** Characteristic physical findings are bowing of the legs, thickening of the costochondral junction (rachitic rosary), knobby prominence of the wrists and knees, and growth failure. In infants, craniotabes (thinning of the skull bones) and fractures are common. The radiographic manifestations are readily visible in views of the wrists and knees, with widening of the space between the metaphysis and epiphysis. The epiphyses are cupped, widened, and irregular or frayed.
2. **Classification.** Rickets may be caused by **vitamin D deficiency** (decreased intake, absorption, or metabolism of vitamin D) or **lack of adequate calcium and phosphorus** for normal bone mineralization (deficient mineral intake or increased losses by the kidneys).
   a. **Nutritional rickets.** Lack of vitamin D in the diet results in decreased calcium absorption in the intestine. Hypocalcemia stimulates PTH secretion, which then causes increased reabsorption of calcium from bone and decreased renal reabsorption of phosphorus.
      (1) **Etiology.** Nutritional rickets occurs in children who have low vitamin D intake, for example, unsupplemented breast-fed infants older than 6 months of age. Often other factors are present in these infants, such as decreased exposure to sunlight due to dark skin pigmentation, urban living conditions, and the winter season.

(2) **Diagnosis.** Serum calcium and phosphorus levels are low, and the alkaline phosphatase level is high due to active bone resorption from secondary hyperparathyroidism.

(3) **Therapy.** High-dose vitamin D therapy is indicated until the biochemical and radiologic findings improve.

b. Rickets associated with abnormal metabolism of vitamin D

(1) **Vitamin D–dependent rickets,** an autosomal recessive disease, is caused by absence of the renal enzyme 1 α-hydroxylase, which converts 25-hydroxyvitamin D_3 to the active metabolite 1,25-dihydroxyvitamin D_3. Therefore, 25-hydroxyvitamin D_3 levels are normal, whereas 1,25-dihydroxyvitamin D_3 levels are low. **Therapy** with physiologic doses of 1,25-dihydroxyvitamin D_3 is curative.

(2) **Vitamin D–resistant rickets** is associated with a hereditary defect of the vitamin D receptor causing unresponsiveness to the vitamin. These patients typically present with hypocalcemia, rickets, and alopecia, and vitamin D levels are elevated in the serum. Some of these patients respond to very large doses of vitamin D therapy.

(3) **Chronic illnesses,** such as **chronic renal or liver disease,** may result in rickets because of impaired hydroxylation of vitamin D into its active metabolite or decreased vitamin D absorption from the intestine.

(4) **Chronic anticonvulsant therapy.** Phenobarbital and phenytoin cause increased metabolism of calcidiol and may be associated with rickets.

c. Rickets due to mineral deficiency

(1) **Hypophosphatemic rickets** results from several hereditary conditions that lead to rickets in children and osteomalacia in adults. These include X-linked hypophosphatemic rickets (XLH), autosomal dominant hypophosphatemic rickets (ADHR), and hereditary hypophosphatemic rickets with hypercalciuria (HHRH). These diseases are characterized by phosphate wasting in the urine due to a defect in phosphate reabsorption. Mutations in different genes have been identified in each condition. Biochemical abnormalities and radiographic signs of rickets are evident in the first few months of life. Subsequently, these children have severe rickets and short stature. **Therapy** consists of high oral doses of phosphate to replace renal losses.

(2) **Rickets of prematurity (metabolic bone disease of the premature infant).** Infants born prematurely have decreased bone mineralization compared to full-term infants because they do not benefit from the major skeletal accretion of calcium and phosphorus occurring in utero during the last trimester. Human milk and standard infant formulas that provide adequate calcium and phosphorus for the full-term infant are not adequate for the needs of the premature infant. Severe osteopenia and rickets that results in fractures may present in premature infants not supplied with the right balance of minerals. In these infants, serum calcium levels are normal, and phosphorus levels are low. 1,25-Dihydroxyvitamin D_3 levels are elevated, probably because of the hypophosphatemic stimulus. Fortifying human milk or formulas with additional calcium and phosphorus results in improvement in bone mineralization and healing of fractures and rickets. Adequate intake of vitamin D should be monitored.

IX ANTIDIURETIC HORMONE AND ITS ABNORMALITIES

A **Diabetes insipidus (DI)** is a condition marked by the inability to concentrate urine appropriately despite a normal kidney function. With loss of antidiuretic hormone (ADH) secretion, 24-hour urine output may reach 5 to 10 L/day. Urine osmolality remains low (approximately 100 mOsm/L, specific gravity 1.000).

1. **Etiology.** DI usually occurs accompanied by anterior pituitary hormone deficiency (as in septo-optical dysplasia). It may also occur after head trauma, after surgical interruption of the pituitary stalk (e.g., for craniopharyngioma), and with tumors and infections of the CNS. A rare familial form of idiopathic DI exists. The differential diagnosis of DI also includes **"psychogenic water drinking,"** which is found in children with a history of other neurotic behaviors.
2. **Clinical features.** Patients with DI present with polyuria and polydipsia. Polyuria persists even when they are water deprived. Caloric intake diminishes, and growth and weight gain may fall off. Neurologic and visual complaints may be present if DI is secondary to a tumor.

3. **Diagnosis.** Children with DI present with high serum sodium levels and a dilute fasting urine as result of excessive water loss. A **water deprivation test** must be done to confirm the diagnosis. During the water deprivation test, the child is not allowed to eat or drink while weight, urine output, urine specific gravity and osmolality, and serum sodium and osmolality are monitored. The test is terminated when 5% of body weight is lost, or the serum osmolality rises to 300 mOsm/L or more, and urine osmolality remains dilute (< 250 mOsm/L). Documentation of responsiveness to ADH by giving an ADH analogue at the end of the test is important in differentiating ADH-deficient diabetes insipidus from nephrogenic diabetes insipidus. Children with compulsive (psychogenic) water drinking will show ability to concentrate urine during the water deprivation test.
4. **Therapy** with an ADH analogue (DDAVP) intranasally every 12 to 24 hours provides relief of symptoms of polyuria and polydipsia.

B **Syndrome of inappropriate antidiuretic hormone (SIADH)** SIADH causes expansion of the vascular volume and hyponatremia, which may lead to lethargy, confusion, and seizures. In children, SIADH is occasionally associated with pulmonary and CNS disease (e.g., pneumonia, bacterial meningitis). It is also associated with some chemotherapeutic agents (e.g., vincristine, cyclophosphamide). **Therapy** involves fluid restriction. Symptomatic hyponatremia is treated with infusion of 3% sodium chloride solution.

BIBLIOGRAPHY

American Diabetes Association: Diagnosis and classification of diabetes mellitus. *Diabetes Care* 30(Suppl 1): S42–S47, 2007.

American Diabetes Association. Type 2 diabetes in children and adolescents. *Diabetes Care* 23(3):381–389, 2000.

Fisher D: Thyroid disorders in childhood and adolescence. In: *Pediatric Endocrinology,* 2nd ed. Edited by Sperling M. Philadelphia, 2002, pp 187–209.

Glaser N, McFeely M, Jones K: Non-insulin dependent diabetes mellitus in childhood. *J Invest Med* 43:134A, 1995.

Grimberg A, Lifshitz F: Worrisome growth. In: *Pediatric Endocrinology,* 5th ed. Edited by Lifshitz F. New York, Informa Healthcare USA, 2007, pp 1–50.

Hughes IA, Houk C, Ahmed SF, et al., LWPES1/ESPE2 Consensus Group: Consensus statement on management of intersex disorders. *Arch Dis Child* 91:554–562, 2006.

LaFranchi S, Hanna C: The thyroid gland and its disorders. In: *Principles and Practice of Pediatric Endocrinology.* Edited by Kappy M, Allen D, Geffner M. Springfield, IL, C Thomas, 2005, pp 279–356.

New M, Ghizzoni L, Lin-Su K. An update in congenital adrenal hyperplasia. In *Pediatric Endocrinology,* 5th ed. Edited by Lifshitz F. New York, Informa Healthcare USA, 2007, pp 227–245.

Report of the Expert Committee on the Diagnosis and Classification of Diabetes Mellitus: [Report]. *Diabetes Care.* 26(Suppl 1):S4–S20, 2003.

Rosembloom AL: Obesity, insulin resistance, beta cell autoimmunity, and the changing clinical epidemiology of childhood diabetes. *Diabetes Care* 26:2954–2956, 2003.

Wolfsdorf J, Weinstein D: Hypoglycemia in children. In *Pediatric Endocrinology,* 5th ed. Edited by Lifshitz F. New York, Informa Healthcare USA, 2007, pp 291–327.

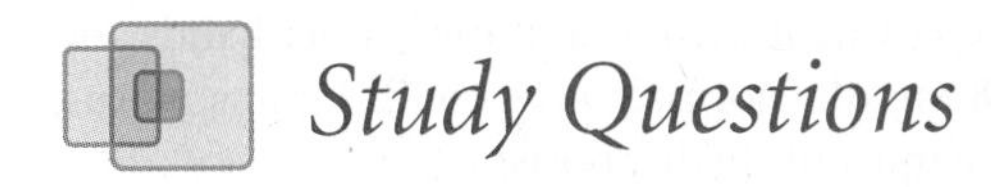

Study Questions

Directions: *Each of the numbered items or incomplete statements in this section is followed by answers or completions of the statement. Select the ONE lettered answer or completion that is BEST in each case.*

1. A 5-year-old boy is discovered to have pubic hair during his prekindergarten physical examination. Additional findings include accelerated height velocity and acne. A bone age study showed advanced skeletal maturation. Which of the following is the most likely diagnosis?

A Idiopathic premature adrenarche
B Hyperprolactinemia
C Growth hormone excess
D Hypothalamic hamartoma
E Kallmann syndrome

2. A 10-year-old girl diagnosed with type 1 diabetes at age 5 years was maintained in relatively good control until a year ago when she began to experience frequent episodes of ketoacidosis. Her parents are extremely concerned and are determined to uncover the source for the deterioration in their daughter's diabetes management. Fortunately, before instituting any major alterations in the child's routine, the parents schedule a meeting with the pediatrician. They admit feeling totally confused as to whether the child's recent problems have anything to do with eating, exercise, undiagnosed associated conditions, or recent onset of pubertal changes. They request help before deciding whether changes in medication or lifestyle management are indicated to improve overall diabetes control and prevent the occurrence of further episodes of DKA. The pediatrician obtains further history, which further raises his suspicion about the etiology of the recurrent episodes of DKA. Which of the following is the most common factor underlying the development of diabetic ketoacidosis in a child known to have type 1 diabetes?

A Overeating
B Excessive exercise
C Omission of insulin doses
D Hypothyroidism
E Puberty

3. A full-term male infant is noted to have circumoral cyanosis and twitching of his left hand at 12 hours of age. On physical examination, he is found to have absent pupillary response to light and a small penis. Which of the following is the most likely diagnosis?

A Hypocalcemia
B Hypoglycemia
C Congenital hypothyroidism
D Congenital heart disease
E Idiopathic epilepsy

4. A 12-year-old boy is referred to his pediatrician by his teacher for poor attention span, deteriorating school performance, and frequent trips to the bathroom. According to the pediatrician's records, the boy has lost 5 lbs (2.25 kg) since his previous visit 6 months earlier. On physical examination, the boy's resting pulse is 110 beats per minute and blood pressure is 130/50 mm Hg. His thyroid gland is approximately twice the normal size. Which of the following is the most likely diagnosis?

A Hashimoto thyroiditis
B Medullary carcinoma of the thyroid
C Type 1 diabetes
D Juvenile hypothyroidism
E Thyrotoxicosis

5. A 14-month-old infant is brought to the emergency department with "cramping" of her hands and feet. Initial laboratory studies show the following: Ca, 7.8 mg/dL (normal, 9–11 mg/dL); phosphorus, 2.8 mg/dL (normal, 4.5–6.0). Which of the following is the most likely diagnosis?

- A Hypoparathyroidism
- B Pseudohypoparathyroidism
- C Vitamin D deficiency (rickets)
- D Cow's milk tetany
- E Chronic renal insufficiency

Directions: *Each set of matching questions in this section consists of a list of 4 to 6 lettered options followed by several numbered items. For each numbered item, select the ONE lettered option that is most closely associated with it. Each lettered option may be selected once, more than once, or not at all.*

QUESTIONS 6–10

For each of the following patients, select the diagnosis that most likely accounts for his or her puberty-related finding(s).

- A Delayed puberty
- B Central precocious puberty
- C Normal development
- D Premature adrenarche
- E Premature thelarche

6. A 7-year-old boy has pubic hair

7. An 8½-year-old girl has breast budding

8. An 8-year-old boy has enlarged testicles and pubic hair

9. A 16-year-old girl has recent onset of menarche

10. A 5-year-old girl has breast enlargement and no pubic hair

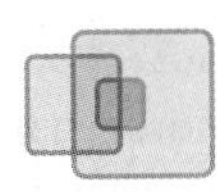

Answers and Explanations

1. The answer is D (*II A 3 a*). This 5-year-old boy demonstrates signs of precocious sexual development. The cause of his disorder could be gonadotropin-dependent precocious puberty secondary to a hypothalamic tumor. Children with idiopathic premature adrenarche present with early appearance of pubic hair, but they have normal growth velocity and bone age. The boy described in this case also has other signs of virilization, like acne, which are not found in idiopathic premature adrenarche. Growth velocity and tall stature are features of growth hormone excess, but early signs of puberty are not consistent with this diagnosis. Hyperprolactinemia causes galactorrhea, not virilization. Kallmann syndrome is associated with anosmia and delayed puberty due to hypogonadotropic hypogonadism.

2. The answer is C (*VII D 6 b*). Central to the development of diabetic ketoacidosis is absolute or relative lack of insulin, most commonly due to omitted insulin doses. Inappropriate actions, such as withholding insulin during intercurrent illness—especially when vomiting—may play a role in an uninformed patient. The key to explaining the problem seen in this patient is the change in diabetes management that occurred over the previous 12 months. Determined to foster increasing autonomy, the parents had gradually relaxed the rules and increasingly allowed the girl to administer her insulin on her own, without direct supervision by an adult in the household. When the parents confronted her, she reluctantly confessed to having "skipped" injections "now and then." In the end, the explanation for deterioration in her control was consistent with the key factor, lack of insulin, which underlies most episodes of DKA. Overeating may cause excessive hyperglycemia, but as long as the patient continues his or her usual insulin dose, there should be enough insulin present to suppress ketogenesis and subsequent ketoacidosis. Exercise may cause hypoglycemia but does not lead to hyperglycemia or accumulation of ketones. Hypothyroidism does not affect insulin utilization or requirements. Although insulin sensitivity decreases during puberty, ketoacidosis should not develop unless the patient's insulin is extremely low.

3. The answer is B (*I D 3 d and h, VI A and B 1 b*). The cyanosis and focal seizures in this infant are caused by hypoglycemia related to congenital hypopituitarism. The physical findings of microphallus and lack of light response suggest the syndrome of septo-optic dysplasia, which frequently is associated with deficiency of GH, ACTH, TSH, and arginine vasopressin (ADH). Hypoglycemia should be anticipated in infants with these findings. Low cortisol and GH levels during hypoglycemia confirm the diagnosis of congenital hypopituitarism. Hypoglycemia resolves with appropriate hormone replacement. Hypocalcemia is a cause of neonatal seizures but would not explain the other findings. Seizures are not characteristic of congenital hypothyroidism. Congenital heart disease may result in cyanosis but would not explain the other findings. Idiopathic epilepsy is an unlikely etiology for neonatal seizures and would similarly not account for the other findings.

4. The answer is E (*III C 1 a*). The 12-year-old boy described in the question has symptoms of thyrotoxicosis (Graves disease), particularly weight loss, deterioration of behavior and school performance, and tachycardia. Medullary thyroid carcinoma presents as an asymptomatic nodule or mass in the neck. In children with juvenile hypothyroidism, school performance is not impaired, and clinical symptoms include lethargy and constipation. Hashimoto thyroiditis usually presents as an asymptomatic goiter. Transient symptoms of thyrotoxicosis very rarely are present in Hashimoto thyroiditis. Insulin-dependent diabetes mellitus would not account for thyromegaly, widened pulse pressure, and tachycardia.

5. The answer is C (*VIII B 2 a*). This infant has carpopedal spasm associated with hypocalcemia—a low serum calcium level with a low serum phosphorus level due to lack of vitamin D—until proven otherwise. A careful dietary history for an infant at this age may reveal lack of vitamin D (solely breast-fed or milk avoidance with juice substitution). Other inherited forms of rickets are also possible diagnoses. Lack of parathyroid hormone action (hypoparathyroidism or pseudohypoparathyroidism) may manifest as carpopedal spasm. However, biochemical measures in these conditions show a low calcium level and an elevated phosphorus level. Cow's milk tetany occurs in very young infants (2–4 weeks of age) who are fed high phosphorous-containing formulas or cow's milk. Chronic renal insufficiency may be associated with renal osteodystrophy. However, the phosphorous level is usually elevated due to renal failure.

6–10. The answers are 6-D (*II A 2*), 7-C (*II A1*), 8-B (*II A 3 a*), 9-A (*II B*), and 10-E (*II A 1*) and 6-D—10-E (Figure 5-5, Figure 5-6). Appearance of pubic hair due to adrenarche (rise of adrenal androgens) is considered normal after age 7 years in girls and 9 years in boys. Based on recent data breast development is considered normal by many experts after age 7½ years in White girls and 6½ years in Black and Hispanic American girls. Testicular enlargement is the first sign of puberty in boys. It occurs once the hypothalamic-pituitary-gonadal axis is activated, therefore the denomination of "central" puberty. If this happens before the age of 9 years, it is considered precocious. Absence of menses by the age of 15 is considered delayed (primary amenorrhea), which may be due to hormonal or systemic abnormalities and should be investigated. Premature thelarche is a nonprogressive benign condition that refers to the frequent finding of isolated breast development in girls under age of 2 years. Gonadotropins and serum estrogen levels are in the prepubertal range. Unlike the cases of true precocious puberty, these girls have normal growth rate and bone age.

chapter **18**

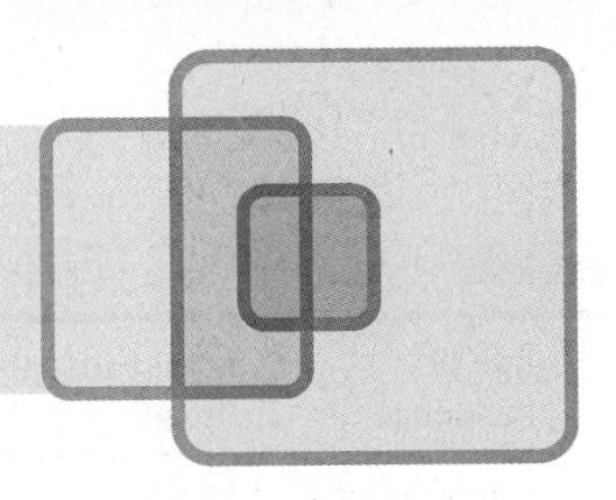

Neurologic Diseases

CAROL R. LEICHER

I GENERAL PRINCIPLES OF PEDIATRIC NEUROLOGIC DIAGNOSIS

The common neurologic conditions seen in the ambulatory setting include (a) headaches; (b) abnormal development (motor, cognitive, language); (c) seizures; and (d) movement disorders (tics). The general principles of pediatric neurologic diagnosis apply to the evaluation of any patient who has a neurologic disorder.

A History

1. A well-performed history should emphasize whether the neurologic problem being analyzed is:
   a. Focal or diffuse
   b. Acute or insidious
   c. Static or progressive
2. An attempt should be made to obtain eyewitness accounts of "spells" or suspect behaviors. Special attention should be given to the developmental history and school function.

B Physical examination

Special aspects of the pediatric neurologic examination include evaluation of the developmental reflexes (Table 18-1), measurement of head circumference, assessment of developmental milestones, and search for birthmarks, which can signal a neurologic defect.

C Diagnostic studies

Useful procedures, depending on the clinical problem, can include:

1. **Lumbar puncture** and cerebrospinal fluid (CSF) examination (e.g., for infectious, metabolic, and degenerative diseases)
2. **Electroencephalography (EEG)** (for epilepsy)
3. **Electromyography (EMG)** and nerve conduction studies (for motor unit diseases)
4. **Measurement of cortical evoked potentials** (for assessment of central nervous system [CNS] function)
5. **Neuroimaging studies**
   a. **Skull radiography** (e.g., for depressed skull fracture)
   b. **Computed tomography (CT) scan** (useful in emergencies and detection of calcification and blood or bony abnormalities)
   c. **Magnetic resonance imaging (MRI) scan** (for evaluating anatomic abnormalities, especially in the midline structures; optimal for assessing gliosis or other abnormalities of gray and white matter; new techniques [magnetic resonance angiography] also permit assessment of the cerebral vasculature)
   d. **Arteriography** (for vascular disease)
   e. **Positron emission tomography (PET) scan** (research tool for assessment of brain metabolism)
6. **Biopsies** of muscle, peripheral nerve, skin, liver, bone marrow, rectal mucosa, and, rarely, brain (for evaluation of a degenerative disease)

TABLE 18-1 Evaluation of Developmental Reflexes

Reflex	Test Position	Stimulus	Age at Response	Age at Disappearance Onset		Significance
Moro	Support head and shoulders 30 degrees above horizontal	Allow head to drop to horizontal	Extension of upper extremities at shoulders and elbows	28 wk gestational age	6 mo	**Absence** suggests severe myopathy or severe CNS abnormality **Persistence** suggests CNS abnormality
Asymmetric tonic neck	Supine with head in midline	Passive or active neck rotation to left or right	Extension of arm and leg on face side, with flexion of arm and leg on occipital side	37 wk gestational age	6 mo—never obligatory[a]	If **obligatory** or **persistent**, suggests CNS pathology
Parachute	Support infant in vertical position	Sudden tip of upper body downward	Arms extend to break fall	8–9 mo	Persists	Should be symmetric; if **not developed** at appropriate time suggests CNS abnormality
Sucking	Any	Finger or pacifier placed in mouth	Sucking	37 wk gestational age	Not applicable	**Absence** suggest either CNS or muscle dysfunction
Rooting	Any	Touching side of mouth with cheek	Head turns	37 wk gestational age	3 mo	**Absence** suggests CNS depression
Grasping (palmar)		Finger in palm	Grasps finger	20 weeks' gestational age	4–5 mo	**Absence** suggests CNS dysfunction
Placing	Held upright	Touching dorsum of foot	Places foot onto surface	37 wk gestational age	Covered by voluntary action	**Absence** suggests CNS dysfunction

CNS, central nervous system.
[a]An obligatory reflex is defined as a tonic neck posture that is maintained beyond 30 seconds after the head is turned.

II ALTERED STATES OF CONSCIOUSNESS

When assessing a child's altered state of behavior or decreased responsiveness, the developmental age and typical responses to various stimuli must be considered (determined by history).

A Definitions

1. **Delirium** is an altered state of behavior in which the patient appears alert, but is confused, is irritable, and has inappropriate reactions to stimuli.
2. **Coma** is a state of unarousable unresponsiveness. This is a consequence of bilateral cerebral dysfunction or involvement of the periventricular gray matter in the brainstem. Assessment of a patient in coma should include a description of the stimulus used and the response observed. Inexact terms (e.g., "stupor," "lethargy," "semi-coma") are best avoided. The **Glasgow Coma Scale** is a reliable tool in this evaluation (Table 18-2).

B Etiology

There are many possible causes of delirium and coma (Table 18-3).

TABLE 18-2 Glasgow Coma Scale: Determination of Scores[a]

Best Verbal Response		Eyes Open	
Oriented	5	Spontaneously	4
Confused	4	To speech	3
Inappropriate words	3	To pain	2
Incomprehensible sounds	2	None	1
None	1		
Motor response			
Obeys commands	5		
Able to localize pain	4		
Flexion to pain	3		
Extension to pain	2		
None	1		

[a]Scoring is as follows: 3–7, severe head injury; 8–11, moderate head injury; 12–14, mild head injury.

C Diagnosis

1. **History.** The patient history must be obtained rapidly, usually while the child is being stabilized. Particular attention should be paid to the events leading to altered consciousness, past medical conditions, and availability of toxins.
2. **Physical examination.** In addition to establishing the patient's standing on the Glasgow Coma Scale, special attention should be given to the following areas:
   a. **Eyes.** Pupil size and reaction to light may suggest the presence of a toxic substance or a brainstem injury. Abnormal extraocular movements, as elicited by the "doll's eye" maneuver or caloric testing, will suggest brainstem damage. Papilledema suggests elevated intracranial pressure.
   b. **Motor status.** Spontaneous movements should be observed and carefully recorded. The presence of decorticate or decerebrate posturing or seizures should be specifically noted.
   c. **Respiratory pattern.** The rate of respiration as well as breathing abnormalities (e.g., Cheyne-Stokes respiration, central neurogenic hyperventilation, Biot breathing) should be noted.

TABLE 18-3 Etiology and Clues to Delirium and Coma

Causes	Diagnostic Clues
Infection—meningitis, encephalitis	Fever, nuchal rigidity, history of preceding illness, exanthem
Cerebrovascular disease—arteriovenous malformation, stroke	Focal neurologic signs, nuchal rigidity
Trauma	Scalp or facial bruises, hemotympanum (blood behind the eardrum), papilledema
Metabolic disorders—abnormalities of electrolytes, glucose, oxygen content; cyanosis	Signs of dehydration, acetone on breath; laboratory evaluation is necessary to establish the etiology
Toxic (poisoning)—one of the most common causes of altered consciousness in toddlers and adolescents	Breath may smell of the ingested agent, such as cleaning fluids, alcohol; parents should be questioned on medications available in the home
Postictal state—depressed level of consciousness secondary to an unwitnessed seizure	History of seizures; abnormal electroencephalogram may be helpful

3. **Laboratory studies.** Tests to be ordered are determined by the history and physical examination.
   a. **Blood** should be analyzed for metabolic abnormalities (e.g., hypoglycemia).
   b. **Urine** should be analyzed for the presence of toxic substances, heavy metals, sugar, and acetone.
   c. **CT scan** screens for most emergency conditions (i.e., hemorrhage, mass lesions, blunt trauma); MRI scan provides more detailed information about other intracranial lesions.
   d. **EEG** can help diagnose seizures as the cause of the coma (*see IV C*).
   e. **Lumbar puncture** should be performed if an infection is suspected.

D Therapy

1. **Supportive treatment** includes establishing an airway, maintaining hydration, and decreasing intracranial pressure. Hyperventilating the patients is the quickest way to lower intracranial pressure. Medications (e.g., mannitol, steroids) are also helpful.
2. **Specific treatment** depends on the cause of the delirium or coma.

III DISORDERS OF MOTOR FUNCTION

A Motor function in children may be the result of static injury or progressive disorders at all levels of the neural axis. Motor difficulties may result from cerebral dysfunction or may be the result of spinal cord injury, neuropathy, or muscle disease. The nature of the motor symptoms is determined by the part of the nervous system that is affected.

B Cerebral palsy

1. **Definition.** "Cerebral palsy" is a descriptive term that refers to abnormal control of motor movements due to a nonprogressive (static) lesion of the immature brain. The lesion or lesions may occur prenatally, perinatally, or postnatally.
2. **Etiology and risk factors.** The cause of cerebral palsy is unknown in approximately 70% of patients. Approximately 20% of cases can be correlated with risk factors, including prematurity, cerebral anoxia, and trauma. Specific causes include embryologic malformations and infection.
3. **Clinical features**
   a. **Typical clinical patterns.** The classification system for cerebral palsy considers the number of limbs involved and the type of motor abnormality (Table 18-4).
   b. **Injuries to the brain** that result in motor problems may have other, more widespread effects. Problems associated with cerebral palsy include epilepsy in approximately 30% of patients, mental retardation or learning disabilities in approximately 40% to 50%, behavior problems in at least 20%, and strabismus in approximately 40% of patients.

TABLE 18-4 Anatomic and Physiologic Classifications of Cerebral Palsy

Anatomic Classification
Diplegia: The lower limbs are more affected than the upper limbs
Hemiplegia: One side of the body is involved more than the other, and the arm is usually affected more than the leg
Quadriplegia: All four limbs are similarly affected
Double hemiplegia: Both sides of the body are affected, the arms more than the legs
Paraplegia: Both legs are affected; the arms are spared
Physiologic Classification
Spasticity: An increase in muscle tone
Dyskinesia: A collective term for several movement disorders:
Chorea: Abrupt, jerky movements
Athetosis: Slow, writhing, continuous movements in the extremities
Dystonia: Writhing movements leading to sustained, bizarre postures of the trunk and extremities
Ataxia: An incoordination of movement; commonly associated with hypotonia, at least during the first few years of life

4. **Diagnosis**
   a. **History.** The patient is initially seen with a history of a motor delay, but he or she is not losing skills that have been attained.
   b. **Physical examination.** Findings on physical examination place the lesion in the CNS and commonly include any or all of the following:
      (1) Hyperactive reflexes
      (2) Abnormal movements of chorea, athetosis, or dystonia
      (3) Abnormal absence or persistence of infantile reflexes (see Table 18-1)
   c. **Differential diagnosis.** Distinguishing cerebral palsy from a progressive neurologic disorder may be difficult early on because the infant is in the initial stages of developing skills, and a loss of minimal skills may be impossible to determine. If a progressive disease is of concern, screening tests are available for a number of the inherited metabolic disorders.

5. **Therapy.** Early on, physical therapy programs are usually indicated. When the patient reaches the toddler or school-age stage, orthopedic intervention (e.g., special shoes, braces, surgery) is often necessary. The treatment of associated problems (e.g., learning disabilities, seizures) is no different for cerebral palsy patients than for children who are impaired in other ways.

C Disorders of the motor unit (neuromuscular disorders) Common to all patients who have motor unit diseases are weak muscles. Most of the diseases in this category are progressive, and many are genetic.

1. **Anterior horn cell disorders** affect the primary motor neurons in the spinal cord resulting in weakness and areflexia. These are genetic disorders, usually recessive, but also occasionally of autosomal dominant or X-linked inheritance.
   a. **Spinal muscular atrophies** are autosomal recessive diseases primarily, although rare autosomal dominant and X-linked types have been described. **Amyotrophic lateral sclerosis** (involves the corticospinal tract as well) typically affects adults, although juvenile and familial forms have been described. The clinical presentation is variable, from profound weakness noted at birth to presentation as onset of weakness in later childhood or even adolescence. The characteristic clinical features are weakness, areflexia, and muscle fasciculations. There is generally progression of weakness over time, although this may be very slow. Diagnosis is established through genetic testing, electrophysiologic studies, and/or muscle biopsy. Treatment at this time is supportive, with orthopedic management, respiratory support, and nutritional support.
   b. **Arthrogryposis multiplex congenita** is a nonprogressive disease characterized by muscle weakness and contractures of at least two joints. Although the clinical findings are present at birth, the condition seldom is familial. A viral or toxic cause primarily affecting the anterior horn cells is suspected in most cases. In others, a uterine problem (e.g., amniotic bands) is suspected. Diagnosis is established by physical examination. The extent of the contractures determines how disabled the patient will be and how amenable the problem will be to surgical correction.
   c. **Poliomyelitis** is rarely seen but must be considered in the differential diagnosis of muscle weakness secondary to anterior horn cell disease.

2. **Peripheral neuropathies.** Trauma, infections, postinfectious states, toxins (e.g., lead), and genetic factors all may affect the axon, the myelin (via the Schwann cell), or both. Neuropathies generally present with symptoms of weakness affecting the distal extremities initially. Sensation may also be affected. In chronically progressive neuropathies, there may also be orthopedic abnormalities such as foot deformities or joint contractures.
   a. **Hereditary sensory** and **motor neuropathy (HSMN)** is the most common progressive neuropathy of childhood. This is a group of genetic disorders that may affect myelin or axons, and often presents with foot deformities or hand muscle weakness. There are autosomal dominant, autosomal recessive, and X-linked forms of the disorder. The diagnosis is generally established with electrophysiologic and genetic testing. Treatment consists of orthopedic intervention and physical therapy.
   b. **Guillain-Barré syndrome** and other postinfectious, presumably autoimmune neuropathies are discussed in *X E*. Other peripheral neuropathies are less common and include brachial

and lumbar plexus neuropathies, hereditary sensory/autonomic neuropathies, giant cell neuropathy, Leber optic atrophy, and neuroaxonal dystrophy.

3. **Diseases of the neuromuscular junction. Myasthenia gravis** is usually a sporadic disease, although familial cases have been described. It is an autoimmune disease in which antibodies develop against the acetylcholine receptor protein at the motor end-plate. This may occur in neonates who are born to mothers with myasthenia gravis as the result of transplacental antibodies. The patients may have fluctuating weakness in the extremities and ptosis is also common. Patients who have myasthenia gravis show normal muscle strength after receiving 2 to 10 mg of edrophonium chloride; the involved muscles weaken 1 to 5 minutes later. Occasionally, a repetitive nerve stimulation test, which causes rapid muscle fatigue, helps to establish the diagnosis. Pyridostigmine, an anticholinesterase agent, is helpful in more than 50% of patients. Immunosuppressant therapy with corticosteroids may be necessary. Plasmapheresis and thymectomy may benefit some patients.

4. **Diseases of muscle** may be the result of inflammatory disorders (Chapter 9) or may be the result of abnormalities in muscle proteins that result in abnormal contractile function or decreased integrity of the muscle membrane with cell death.
   a. **Muscular dystrophies** are disorders characterized by progressive weakness, usually affecting the proximal muscles with gradual involvement of all muscles.
      (1) **Duchenne (pseudohypertrophic) muscular dystrophy,** the most common, is an X-linked disease caused by abnormalities in the gene that produces dystrophin, a structural protein of muscle. Symptoms typically begin at 2 to 4 years of age. Independent walking may be delayed; affected children never run normally and never walk up stairs using alternating feet. A positive Gower sign (Figure 18-1) indicates weakness of the lower back and pelvic girdle muscles. The patients are typically wheelchair bound by 12 years of age and die, usually from congestive heart failure or pneumonia, before 25 years of age. The diagnosis is generally made with genetic testing or muscle biopsy, and the serum creatine phosphokinase (CPK) is 10 to 20 times normal. There are no specific treatments available for this disorder, but steroids (prednisone) can delay the course of the disease. Aggressive management of the orthopedic, respiratory, and cardiac difficulties has resulted in longer survival of these patients.
      (2) **Limb-girdle dystrophies** are clinically similar to Duchenne muscular dystrophy, but may have more indolent courses and are the result of defects in other structural proteins of muscle.
   b. **Congenital myopathies** are disorders of muscle that result from defects in the contractile proteins. These present with weakness in the neonatal period, often involving the face, muscles of glutition, and eye muscles. They may be static or slowly progressive. Muscle biopsy is necessary to establish the diagnosis and genetic diagnosis is possible in some forms. Specific disorders, usually named for the histologic finding, include **central core disease, nemaline myopathy,** and **myotubular myopathy.**
   c. **Myotonic muscle disorders.** Myotonia is the failure of voluntary muscles to relax after a contracture. The examiner can demonstrate myotonia by percussing the patient's tongue or thenar eminence. These disorders may present in the neonatal period or later in childhood and are characterized by progressive weakness and cramping.
   d. **Metabolic myopathies.** Several genetic abnormalities in carbohydrate or lipid metabolism cause identifiable myopathic syndromes; the underlying enzyme deficiencies have been elucidated in many of these disorders.

IV SEIZURES AND EPILEPSY

A Definitions

1. **Seizures** represent abnormal neural discharges in the cerebral cortex that result in abnormal function. The nature of the clinical manifestation depends on the region(s) of the brain affected by the discharge. Seizures may be the result of a known cerebral insult or may arise without detectable cerebral disturbance.

2. **Epilepsy** is a condition in which the patient is subject to recurrent, unprovoked seizures.

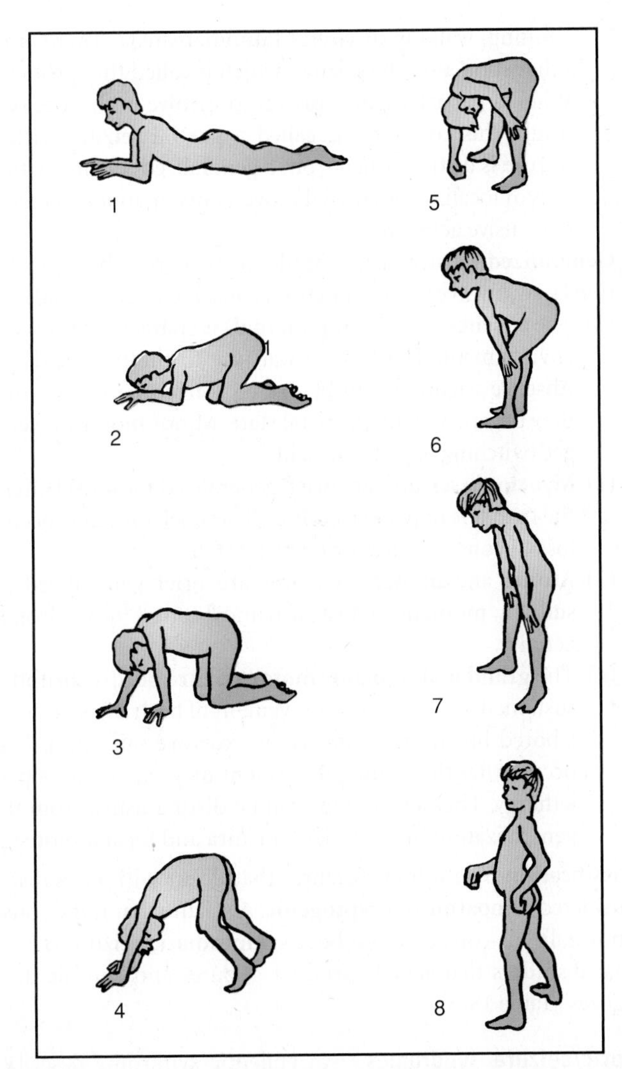

FIGURE 18-1 Gowers sign. A patient who has mild hip weakness uses this maneuver to arise from the floor. Rather than assuming a squatting position, the patient first pushes off the floor (*1, 2, 3*), forming an arch with buttocks at the apex (*4*), then pushes against the knee with the nonfloor hand (*5*), and "walks" the hands up the legs (*6, 7*) to assume the standing position (*8*).

3. **Status epilepticus** is a prolonged seizure lasting more than 30 minutes or a series of seizures without return to consciousness for more than 30 minutes.
4. An **epileptic** or **seizure syndrome** describes a seizure type(s) that occurs in association with characteristic EEG findings, demographic characteristics, and prognosis. There are several epileptic or seizure syndromes in childhood.

B **Classification** There are several ways to classify seizures. By classifying seizures by type or cause, it is possible to recognize certain clinical patterns and determine appropriate diagnostic testing and treatment.

1. **Classification by seizure type**
   a. **Partial** seizures arise from a localized portion of the cerebral cortex. Because of the limited cortical involvement, consciousness may not be affected by the seizure activity.
      (1) A **simple partial seizure** may have motor manifestations or sensory manifestations, depending on the location of the seizure discharge, without loss of consciousness.
      (2) In **complex partial seizures,** there is a greater degree of cortical involvement. In addition to the motor and sensory phenomena, consciousness is clouded or lost. The motor manifestations of this seizure type are often complex and semipurposeful (i.e., picking at

clothing, walking in circles [automatisms]). There is usually a period of confusion or exhaustion after the seizure, which is called the "postictal" state.

(3) When a partial seizure spreads to involve both sides of the brain, a full convulsion may result; this condition is called a **partial seizure with secondary generalization.** This seizure is distinguished from a generalized seizure by the aura, or focal onset, which consists of localized abnormal movements or abnormal sensations preceding the generalized convulsive activity.

b. Generalized seizures arise simultaneously from both cerebral hemispheres. The manifestations may involve motor function, consciousness, or both.

(1) The **absence** seizure (or **petit mal**) is characterized by staring and loss of awareness of the environment. There is no warning to the patient that the seizure is about to happen. Absence seizures are brief—rarely longer than 30 seconds—and terminate as abruptly as they began, with no postictal state. Minor motor movements, such as eye blinking or finger twitching, may be present.

(2) **Myoclonic** seizures are brief, generalized motor seizures consisting of symmetric jerks of the trunk or upper extremities. These seizures may occur in flurries. There is no apparent loss of consciousness or postictal state.

(3) **Atonic** and **akinetic** seizures are brief generalized seizures characterized by either sudden, momentary loss of truncal tone ("head-drop seizures") or sudden freezing of activity.

(4) The **grand mal** or **major motor seizure** begins abruptly with no warning. There may be sustained tonic or clonic movement of both sides of the body. The patient may experience labored breathing, cyanosis, or excessive salivation. Urinary or fecal incontinence may occur. After the seizure, the patient may experience a period of confusion, headache, and lethargy. This seizure type can be distinguished from the partial seizure with secondary generalization by the lack of an aura and focal motor signs.

2. **Classification by etiology.** Seizures that occur without a discernible cerebral abnormality are considered **idiopathic** or **cryptogenic.** A seizure that is the consequence of a discernible cerebral abnormality is considered to be a **symptomatic** seizure. This category is further divided into those disorders that acutely produce seizures and chronic disorders associated with recurrent seizures (Table 18-5).

C Epileptic/seizure syndromes An epileptic syndrome describes a particular type or types of seizure associated with typical EEG findings and patient characteristics. The concept of the epileptic syndrome is useful diagnostically and in treatment because it allows for accurate prognostic statements to be made and also helps in choosing appropriate anticonvulsant therapy.

1. **Absence seizures (petit mal) of childhood.** This idiopathic syndrome is thought to be inherited as an autosomal recessive trait in children who are otherwise normal. The onset is between 4 and 10 years of age.

TABLE 18-5 Etiology of Seizures

Acute Symptomatic Seizures	Chronic Symptomatic Seizures
Metabolic disturbances (hypoglycemia, hypoxia, electrolyte disturbances)	Cerebral malformations
Intoxications (cocaine, tricyclic antidepressants, antipsychotics)	Acquired cerebral injuries
Tumors	Neurocutaneous syndromes
Fever	Inborn errors of metabolism
Head injury	
CNS infections (meningitis, encephalitis)	
Vascular accidents (CVA, AVM)	

AVM, arteriovenous malformation; CNS, central nervous system; CVA, cerebrovascular accident.

a. **Seizure type.** The seizures are generalized, 10 to 20 seconds in duration, and characterized by staring, with minimal clonic activity (*see V B 1 b [1]*).

b. **EEG findings.** The characteristic findings are bursts of 3-cycle-per-second spike waves. These bursts of abnormal brain activity may be precipitated by using hyperventilation or a strobe light. During the episodes, the patient will often not hear or be able to answer a question.

c. **Prognosis.** Sixty percent of children with this syndrome will have remission of seizures by late adolescence. Children with concurrent grand mal seizures are more likely to have lifelong epilepsy.

d. **Treatment.** Ethosuximide or valproate is the drug of choice for this type of epilepsy. Clonazepam may be useful as a second-line medication. Phenobarbital, phenytoin, and carbamazepine are not effective.

2. **Benign focal epilepsy of childhood.** This is one of the most common idiopathic epileptic syndromes of childhood. The age of onset is 4 to 10 years. This syndrome is not associated with underlying cerebral disorders.

a. **Seizure type.** If the patient is awake, the typical seizure is a focal seizure, involving the face, pharynx, and possibly the arm. The patient is conscious but is unable to speak and may drool. Nocturnal seizures may be generalized convulsive seizures, but they may also have focal motor involvement or involvement of the pharyngeal muscles. Gagging is a common symptom of the nocturnal seizures in this syndrome.

b. **EEG findings.** The interictal EEG shows discharges in either one or both central and midtemporal electrodes, corresponding to the prerolandic gyrus. These discharges may be limited to the sleep portion of the recording.

c. **Prognosis.** This syndrome has a high remission rate, with 99% resolution by 16 years of age.

d. **Treatment.** Carbamazepine and phenytoin are the most commonly used anticonvulsants for this disorder.

3. **Infantile spasms.** This syndrome may be symptomatic (e.g., tuberous sclerosis) or idiopathic. The onset is typically from 4 to 18 months of age.

a. **Seizure type.** Infantile spasms are massive myoclonic seizures, with either forceful flexion or extension of the trunk. The spasms occur in clusters at short intervals for periods of 30 minutes or more. The child may cry or be extremely irritable during these periods.

b. **EEG findings.** The EEG pattern, called "hypsarrhythmia," shows extreme disorganization of the background activity, with very-high-voltage and frequent, multifocal spike-wave discharges.

c. **Prognosis.** If not treated, the outcome of this syndrome is poor, with lifelong epilepsy and severe neurodevelopmental disability. Idiopathic infantile spasms are more likely to respond to aggressive treatment, and 40% of patients may have excellent outcome. Treatment outcome for the symptomatic forms of infantile spasms is less successful and may reflect the severity of the underlying disorder. The spasms may progress to akinetic or atonic seizures later in life.

d. **Treatment.** Intramuscular adrenocorticotropic hormone (ACTH) is the most effective treatment for infantile spasms. This is administered for a 4- to 8-week period. Valproate and clonazepam may also be useful as secondary agents.

4. **Juvenile myoclonic epilepsy** is an idiopathic form of seizure disorder that typically begins in adolescence.

a. **Seizure type.** There are three types of possible seizures: Grand mal or major motor, absence, and myoclonic.

b. **EEG findings.** The interictal abnormality is generalized spike and wave (4.5–5 Hz).

c. **Prognosis.** Although the seizures are usually readily controlled with medication, the rate of relapse is high. Treatment is usually lifelong.

d. **Treatment.** Valproate is the drug of choice. Phenytoin or carbamazepine can also be used in combination with clonazepam.

D **Febrile seizures** are worthy of special consideration because they are so common. They are not typically considered to be epileptic because they are provoked events, not spontaneous. This seizure type is typically seen in infants from 6 months to 3 years of age, but may occur until 6 years. This is a frequent syndrome, affecting between 3 and 8 per 1000 children. The seizures occur in the context of a febrile illness, often an upper respiratory tract infection or otitis media.

1. **Seizure type.** The classic seizure type is a brief generalized seizure lasting < 5 minutes.

2. **EEG findings.** The interictal EEG is usually normal. If an EEG is done shortly after the seizure, background slowing may be present.
3. **Prognosis.** The risk of recurrent febrile seizures is 30%. In a small number of children, afebrile seizures and, ultimately, epilepsy will subsequently develop. Abnormal neurologic examination results and the presence of atypical seizure features (focal involvement, prolonged seizure, or multiple seizures in 24 hours) are risk factors for the development of epilepsy.
4. **Treatment.** Because most of the seizures are brief and nonrecurrent, **fever control** is the only warranted therapy. If a child has multiple or prolonged febrile convulsions, rectal Valium may be used to terminate the seizures when they occur. Rarely, chronic anticonvulsant therapy is used. Phenobarbital and valproate have been shown to be effective for this purpose. Phenytoin and carbamazepine are not effective for prophylaxis of febrile seizures.

E Diagnosis The diagnosis of seizures or epilepsy is usually made on the basis of the description of the event. This is usually obtained from an observer, but in the case of the partial seizure, the patient may be able to relate some of his or her own symptoms. The physical and neurologic examination may provide clues to the diagnosis in patients who have symptomatic epilepsy, but the results of these examinations are usually negative in patients who have idiopathic epilepsy. Provocative maneuvers, such as hyperventilation, may allow the physician to observe an event. This is particularly useful in diagnosing absence seizures. **Ancillary tests** include the following:

1. An **EEG** is the most commonly ordered test in the evaluation of epilepsy. An EEG is the recording of the electrical activity at the surface of the cortex. The resting patterns of the brain change according to location of the electrodes on the scalp and the brain state. During a seizure, the brain generates high-voltage, chaotic activity that peaks rapidly, which gives the appearance of a "spike" or "sharp wave." The cells giving rise to the clinical seizure may produce a sustained abnormal discharge—the "ictal" pattern—which accompanies the clinical seizure. Between clinical seizures, shorter discharges may be recorded; this is called the interictal pattern. Since most seizures occur infrequently, it is much more common to record interictal abnormalities than ictal abnormalities. The chances of recording an abnormality can be increased by recording during sleep or using provocation modalities such as hyperventilation or stimulation with a strobe light.
2. In the event that a routine EEG captures no abnormality or fails to define the nature of the clinical event, **video-telemetry** may be helpful. This modality consists of simultaneously recording EEG while videotaping patient behavior for a prolonged period of time. This combination technique increases the likelihood of capturing an event and defining the nature of the abnormality.
3. Neuroimaging procedures such as **CT** or **MRI** are useful in the evaluation of symptomatic seizures. An imaging study should be performed in the case of a partial seizure or when the neurologic examination findings are positive. When the clinical history and EEG findings are consistent with an idiopathic epileptic syndrome, such as absence seizures of childhood, an imaging study is not required. CT is often more readily available in emergencies and is adequate for evaluating the presence of most mass lesions, hemorrhage, or gross cerebral abnormalities. MRI is superior in the evaluation of subtle cerebral abnormalities and white matter changes.

F Treatment Once the presence of seizures and epilepsy has been established, treatment usually consists of the use of anticonvulsant medication. Not every child who has a seizure will be started on anticonvulsants. The decision will be based on the circumstances of the seizure and the prognosis for further seizures.

1. **Counseling.** The child who has epilepsy should lead as normal a life as possible. Physical and social activities should be encouraged. Family and teachers may need counseling to provide the needed psychological support.
2. **Anticonvulsant medication.** The choice of drug is based on the seizure type and EEG findings. Blood levels are guidelines only: Some patients need lower drug doses, whereas others need and can tolerate higher doses. Medication must be increased slowly to avoid side effects (e.g., lethargy) and withdrawn slowly to avoid precipitating seizures.
3. **Diet.** A ketogenic diet is used for grand mal or absence seizures that are difficult to control with medication; this diet is most effective in children 2 to 5 years of age.

4. **Surgery.** When drug treatment is unsuccessful, surgical excision of the epileptic focus can be considered. However, most patients who undergo surgery still require anticonvulsant medication.

G **Prognosis** Anticonvulsant medication can control seizures in 35% to 50% of patients. Adequate control is less likely when seizures begin early in life, occur frequently, are mixed in type, and are associated with mental retardation or abnormal results on neurologic examination. If a patient is seizure free for at least 2 years, discontinuing medication should be considered.

V NONEPILEPTIFORM PAROXYSMAL DISORDERS

A **Headaches** are one of the most common neurologic symptoms of childhood. Pain in the head results from inflammation or compression of blood vessels, muscles, periosteum/sinuses, or nerve roots. Although there are different headache syndromes described in children, there is frequently significant crossover of symptoms. It is important to exclude headaches caused by systemic illness or increased intracranial pressure.

1. **Migraine** is characterized by recurrent attacks of headache that are pulsatile in character and sometimes unilateral; these headaches are often accompanied by neurologic disturbances as well as nausea, vomiting, and photophobia. Migraine attacks may be precipitated by stress or ingestion of certain foods or substances, such as chocolate, peanuts, tyramine (found in aged cheese, chicken liver, and beer), nitrites, and quinine.
   a. **Clinical features** and **diagnosis**
      (1) In **classic migraine,** the patient has an **aura** preceding the attack (visual scotoma, flashing lights). The headache is unilateral, pulsatile, and associated with gastrointestinal upset and photophobia. The patient will frequently report relief with sleep. The physical examination findings are typically negative. In approximately 75% of patients, a positive family history exists.
      (2) In **common migraine,** the headache tends to be diffuse rather than unilateral, and no aura is present. Nausea and vomiting are variably present.
      (3) There are several forms of **complicated migraine,** such as hemiplegic migraine or basilar artery migraine. In these disorders, there are a variety of neurologic symptoms such as weakness, visual deficits, or cranial nerve palsies that accompany the headache.
      (4) **Cyclic vomiting**—recurrent attacks of pernicious vomiting without systemic illness—is thought to be a childhood variant of migraine. This condition can occur in infants and toddlers and can result in hospitalization for dehydration. Metabolic evaluation of these patients is unrewarding, and as they grow older, more typical migraine attacks with prominent headache may occur.
   b. **Diagnosis** of migraine headaches is made on the basis of the history, which reveals the typical characteristics, and by the presence of a normal neurologic examination, with no signs of increased intracranial pressure or focal neurologic abnormality. An imaging procedure (CT or MRI) is warranted only when the examination results are abnormal or the history reveals atypical features.
   c. **Therapy.** Many drugs have been tried in the management of migraine, including vasoconstrictors (ergotamine); serotonin antagonists (cyproheptadine); serotonin agonists (sumatriptan); drugs that prevent reuptake of norepinephrine (amitriptyline); prostaglandin inhibitors (aspirin, ibuprofen); membrane stabilizers (phenytoin); calcium channel blockers; and other agents (e.g., propranolol).
   d. **Prognosis** is extremely variable, and no helpful predictive factors have been found. The patient can go into remission for years, only to have the migraine return decades later.
2. **Tension headaches** are caused by prolonged contraction of scalp and cervical muscles.
   a. The **clinical characteristics** of tension headaches are generalized or "band-like" pain described as constant, squeezing, or aching. There is no associated nausea or photophobia. The headaches are precipitated by stress, fatigue, or exertion. These headaches may be episodic or chronic.
   b. As with migraine headache, the major **diagnostic tools** are the history and physical examination. Neuroimaging studies should be reserved for atypical cases or children who have abnormal

examination findings. In a child who has chronic, disabling headaches, depression or school phobia should be considered in the differential diagnosis.

c. **Treatment** consists of analgesic medications, rest, and removal of stressful circumstances, if possible. Amitriptyline (10–40 mg) is an effective medication for the management of chronic headaches. Biofeedback or relaxation exercises may also be helpful.

3. **Headaches** may be a symptom of **increased intracranial pressure.** These headaches are caused by traction on the intracranial arteries. Hydrocephalus, CNS tumors, and CNS infections can all cause increased intracranial pressure. **Pseudotumor cerebri** is a syndrome that is associated with papilledema and increased intracranial pressure without a structural lesion or infection. It may be caused by obesity, vitamin intoxication, or certain drugs.
   a. The **location** of such headaches may be occipital or frontal. Papilledema is a common sign of increased intracranial pressure. Sixth-nerve palsy, limitation of upward gaze, or increased head size may also be seen. Vomiting is commonly associated with these headaches.
   b. The **diagnosis** is established by a neuroimaging procedure (CT or MRI). If the results of these studies are normal, a lumbar puncture is indicated to exclude infection or CNS neoplasm.
   c. **Treatment** requires management of the underlying disorder. Multiple lumbar punctures or use of acetazolamide may be necessary in the management of pseudotumor cerebri.

B Sleep disorders

1. **Sleepwalking (somnambulism), sleeptalking,** and **night terrors** are common in children younger than 5 years of age. These disorders occur in stage 4 (deep) sleep. There is no recollection of the event the following day. An EEG sometimes is necessary to rule out a seizure disorder. Diazepam may be helpful if the sleepwalking is a danger to the patient.
2. **Narcolepsy** is characterized by paroxysmal attacks of irrepressible sleep. Hypnagogic hallucinations, cataplexy (sudden loss of body tone precipitated by strong emotion), and sleep paralysis are also seen in these patients. This disorder most commonly occurs in the second decade, although it has been reported in younger children. The characteristic abnormality on EEG consists of a shortened latency from full alertness to onset of rapid eye movement sleep. Narcolepsy is treated by regulating nighttime sleep schedules and allowing for brief daytime naps, if possible. When the symptoms are severe, stimulants may be helpful.

C Other paroxysmal disorders

1. **Syncope** (fainting, with loss of consciousness) occurs because of decreased blood flow in the posterior circulation of the brain secondary to vagal stimulation. It is essentially a benign disorder and is treated by reassurance. However, cardiac arrhythmias must be considered as a possible cause.
2. **Breath-holding spells** occur between 3 months and 6 years of age. The child initially cries and then holds his or her breath, turns cyanotic, and becomes limp. Occasionally, the patient has a short-lived tonic seizure. This is a benign disorder; reassurance is the treatment.

VI MOVEMENT DISORDERS

A

There are several disorders involving involuntary movements that occur in childhood (see Table 18-4). These are usually associated with abnormalities of the basal ganglia. **Chorea** is a quick involuntary movement affecting any part of the body. These movements are variable, as opposed to **tics,** which are also usually brief muscle movements, but have a stereotyped quality. **Dystonia** is a more prolonged abnormal movement, which results from simultaneous contracture of agonist and antagonist muscles. **Myoclonus** is characterized by rapid muscle jerks. Movement disorders may be transient and symptomatic, or chronic and progressive.

B Symptomatic movement disorders

1. **Drug-induced movements.** Medications can produce multiple types of abnormal movements (Table 18-6).
2. **Systemic disorders**
   a. **Sydenham chorea (rheumatic chorea).** Chorea is one of the cardinal symptoms of rheumatic fever (see Chapter 9). The child has choreic movements of the extremities and face. Hypotonia

TABLE 18-6 Abnormal Movements Related to Medications

Movement	Medication Type
Chorea	Anticonvulsants Stimulants Phenothiazines
Tics	Stimulants
Dystonia	Phenothiazines Haloperidol Metoclopramide

and emotional lability may also be seen. Recovery is gradual and usually complete. The patient must be treated for rheumatic fever, and the chorea may respond to diazepam, haloperidol, or phenobarbital.

b. Lupus erythematosus may occasionally occur with chorea. The symptoms are indistinguishable from Sydenham chorea, and the diagnosis is established by serologic testing. Treatment with corticosteroids is indicated (see Chapter 9).

C Idiopathic or genetic movement disorders

1. **Tic disorders** are a common symptom of childhood. Tics are brief, repetitive, nonpurposeful movements such as head nodding, eye blinking, facial grimaces, or involuntary noises. Tics typically present from 5 to 10 years of age but have been described in toddlers. Tics may be associated with the use of medications such as stimulants and are exacerbated by anxiety or excitement.
   a. The most common presentation of tics is **simple tic disorder.** This is a single tic type that may be present for a variable amount of time and then disappears. Often, a child with a simple tic may have recurrences of that tic at certain times, such as at the beginning of the school year.
   b. **Gilles de la Tourette syndrome** is a chronic tic disorder characterized by multiple and vocal **tics** that have been persistent for at least 12 months. The tics typically fluctuate over time and may worsen as a result of medications or stress. In addition to tics, patients with chronic tic disorders have a high frequency of coexistent conditions such as attention deficit hyperactivity disorder (50%–70%), learning disability (40%–50%), and obsessive-compulsive disorder (40%–50%). Dopamine antagonists such as haloperidol and pimozide are the most effective medications for tic suppression, but these agents produce significant side effects. Clonidine and clonazepam have also been used for tic control, but they are less effective. Approximately 30% of children will have lifelong symptoms. Another 30% experience complete remission of symptoms, and the rest have milder symptoms as they enter adulthood. Prognosis depends on the severity of tics and associated disorders.

VII CEREBROVASCULAR DISORDERS

Stroke is an uncommon cause of acute neurologic dysfunction in children.

A Vascular occlusion

1. **Thrombosis.** Arterial thrombosis can occur as a result of cerebral arteritis, trauma, or a congenital vascular abnormality (e.g., carotid artery stenosis). **Hypercoagulable states** (see Chapter 15) are increasingly recognized as producing arterial and venous occlusion, resulting in neurologic deficits. Differential diagnoses include systemic vascular disorders such as periarteritis nodosa, sickle cell anemia, and systemic lupus erythematosus. Vascular occlusion must also be differentiated from Todd paralysis (which occurs up to 24 hours after a focal seizure) and hemiplegic migraine. Todd paralysis and hemiplegic migraine are distinguished by the patient's recovery without sequelae.
2. **Embolism.** Cerebral embolism is seen in patients who have congenital heart disease (see Chapter 12). These patients may experience embolism through right-to-left shunting or as a result of cardiac catheterization or open heart surgery.

B Hemorrhage Intraventricular hemorrhage in the neonate is discussed in Chapter 6.

1. **Angiomas** and other malformations of blood vessels are uncommon as causes of intracranial hemorrhage in children.
2. **Arteriovenous malformation** (AVM) is the most common of the brain angiomas. AVM rarely is hereditary.
   a. **Clinical features**
      (1) **Seizure** is the most common presentation. Rupture of an AVM causes sudden symptoms, which may include coma, nuchal rigidity, and paresis.
      (2) **Malformation** of the Galen vein usually does not manifest as a CNS hemorrhage. Rather, the presenting problems may be congestive heart failure in the newborn period, hydrocephalus at 6 months of age, and seizures at 18 months of age.
   b. **Diagnosis** of AVM is established by a contrast CT or MRI scan. Arteriography is necessary to determine the extent of the malformation.
   c. **Therapy.** Surgery is considered if the AVM is accessible. Embolization techniques are used for surgically inaccessible lesions. Even without operative intervention, 85% of these patients are alive 5 years later.

VIII DISEASES AFFECTING BOTH THE SKIN AND CENTRAL NERVOUS SYSTEM

Neurocutaneous disorders (**phakomatoses**) are disorders that commonly have lesions of the skin, brain, and eyes. Most of these disorders are inherited.

A Neurofibromatosis is an autosomal dominant disease with variable expression. There are two distinct forms of neurofibromatosis, although other variant forms also exist. It is estimated that 1 in 3000 people have at least a very mild variety of this disease.

1. **Clinical features and diagnosis**
   a. **Neurofibromatosis-1 (NF-1; von Recklinghausen disease).** The diagnosis of NF-1 is established by the presence of two or more of the following:
      (1) Six or more café au lait spots larger than 5 mm in greatest diameter in prepubertal individuals and larger than 15 mm in postpubertal individuals
      (2) Two or more neurofibromas of any type, or one plexiform neurofibroma
      (3) Freckling in the axillary or inguinal region
      (4) Optic glioma
      (5) Two or more Lisch nodules (pigmented hamartomas of the iris)
      (6) A distinctive osseous lesion (e.g., sphenoid dysplasia or thinning of the long bone cortex with or without pseudoarthrosis)
      (7) A first-degree relative who has NF-1 according to the preceding criteria
   b. **Neurofibromatosis-2 (NF-2).** Diagnosis of NF-2 is established by the presence of:
      (1) Bilateral eighth-nerve masses seen with appropriate imaging techniques, or
      (2) A first-degree relative who has NF-2 and either unilateral eighth-nerve mass or two of the following: Neurofibroma, meningioma, glioma, schwannoma, or juvenile posterior subcapsular lenticular opacity
   c. **Important considerations.** Screening for visual change, hearing loss, and learning disabilities should be routine. Screening MRI scans are also used to monitor optic nerve glioma. Patients with NF-1 may have seizures and cognitive deficits.

B Tuberous sclerosis (Bourneville disease) is an autosomal dominant disease of variable expression, which affects approximately 1 person in 30,000.

1. **Clinical features.** Tuberous sclerosis is characterized by the triad of skin lesions, seizures, and mental retardation.
   a. **Skin lesions** are seen by 3 years of age in 40% of patients. The lesions include flat, hypopigmented "ash-leaf" spots (visible under a Wood lamp), shagreen patches (unevenly thickened skin areas), and café au lait spots. During the second decade, angiokeratomas appear on the face. Retinal hamartomas are noted in 50% of patients.
   b. **Epilepsy** may begin early in life and may be difficult to control.

c. **Periventricular tumors** may occur, leading to hydrocephalus and, if large enough, causing the patient's death. Autistic features are noted in approximately 10% to 15% of patients.

d. **Cysts** and **malignant tumors** may develop in the heart, kidneys, pancreas, and peritoneal cavity.

2. **Therapy and prognosis.** The various clinical problems are treated as they are in patients who do not have tuberous sclerosis. Prognosis is related to the severity of the seizure disorder and the cognitive dysfunction.

C **Sturge-Weber syndrome** is most likely a sporadic disease, although familial cases have been described.

1. **Clinical features.** A port-wine stain (capillary hemangioma) occurs unilaterally in a trigeminal distribution (over the forehead and, often, the maxillary area); occasionally this hemangioma is bilateral. Glaucoma develops later in 50% of patients. A seizure disorder is likely.
2. **Therapy and prognosis.** Anticonvulsant therapy is often unsuccessful, and surgical removal of the damaged cortex is necessary. Prognosis is related to the ease of seizure control.

D **von Hippel-Lindau disease** is an autosomal dominant disorder characterized by vascular tumors in the cerebellum and spinal cord. Associated retinal hemangiomas are seen in 50% of patients, and renal carcinoma is seen in 45%. The skin is not involved in this syndrome.

E **Ataxia-telangiectasia (Louis-Bar syndrome)** is an autosomal recessive disease affecting the cerebellum, skin, and immune system.

1. **Clinical features.** The ataxia typically develops during the first 5 years of life. It is distinguished from cerebral palsy because the ataxia is progressive; it is distinguished from Friedreich ataxia because of the absence of peripheral neurologic abnormalities such as decreased reflexes and sensory loss. The telangiectasias, most apparent on the conjunctiva and ears, become prominent during the second 5 years of life. Lung infections secondary to immunoglobulin A deficiency develop by approximately 10 years of age, and malignant lymphomas begin to develop at approximately 15 to 20 years of age.
2. **Therapy and prognosis.** Treatment is symptomatic. The disease is progressive, and death usually results from infection or malignancy.

IX DEGENERATIVE CENTRAL NERVOUS SYSTEM DISEASES

A General approach to the patient who has a degenerative CNS disease

1. **Clinical features.** Degenerative CNS diseases are characterized clinically by a deterioration of function over an extended period of time. Most of the diseases are genetic, and many have a metabolic basis (Table 18-7). The clinical condition may start with seizures or losses in motor, cognitive, or language skills. These losses may be subtle and difficult to recognize in the very young child. The clinical symptoms are determined by those areas or systems of the brain that are involved.

TABLE 18-7 Degenerative Disease of the Nervous System

Degenerative Diseases of Basal Ganglia	Degenerative Diseases of Cerebellum, Brainstem, and Spinal Cord	Degenerative Diseases of White Matter	Degenerative Diseases of Gray Matter
Wilson Disease	Friedreich ataxia	Metachromatic leukodystrophy	Tay-Sachs disease
Hallervorden-Spatz syndrome	Hereditary cerebellar ataxia	Adrenoleukodystrophy	Gaucher disease
Huntington chorea (juvenile)	Familial spastic paraplegia	Pelizaeus-Merzbacher disease	Niemann-Pick disease
Lesch-Nyhan syndrome	Abetalipoproteinemia	Canavan disease	Neuronal ceroid lipofuscinosis
Fahr disease		Alexander disease	Fabry disease
		Krabbe disease	Menke disease
			Rett syndrome

a. **Degenerative diseases of the basal ganglia.** The major abnormalities noted in these diseases are movement disorders (e.g., tremor, chorea, athetosis, dystonia).

b. **Degenerative diseases of white matter.** These diseases commonly start with loss of motor function accompanied by **spasticity** and **visual impairment.** Dementia and, occasionally, seizures appear as late manifestations.

c. **Degenerative diseases primarily affecting gray matter.** Many of these diseases are **neuronal storage diseases,** in which a lipid (usually a ganglioside or other sphingolipid) accumulates in cerebral neurons. Patients with gray matter diseases typically have **seizures** and **dementia.**

2. **Diagnosis**

a. **History.** In evaluating the patient who has a suspected neurodegenerative disease, a careful and probing history is necessary. An infant may show a lack of normal motor and social development and may have recurrent episodes of altered consciousness or unexplained vomiting. A toddler may show a loss of motor, cognitive, or social milestones. An older child may have problems with schoolwork.

b. **Laboratory studies** may aid in the diagnosis of degenerative CNS diseases.

(1) **Urine screening** should include:

(a) Quantitative determination of amino acids (for phenylketonuria, maple syrup urine disease, and other aminoacidopathies)

(b) Quantitative determination of organic acids for disorders of fatty acid metabolism

(c) Quantitative determination of bile acids for disorders of peroxisomal function, such as Refsum disease or neonatal adrenoleukodystrophy

(2) **Blood screening** should include tests for fasting blood sugar, ammonium, lactate, and pyruvate levels; pH and carbon dioxide partial pressure; and lysosomal enzymes.

(3) **Radiography** of the skull and vertebral bodies may be helpful.

(4) **Fibroblast evaluation.** Fibroblasts in skin and other tissues should be evaluated for microscopic abnormalities and missing enzymes.

X POSTINFECTIOUS, PRESUMED AUTOIMMUNE NEUROLOGIC DISORDERS

(See Chapter 10 for a discussion of acute CNS infections.) The neurologic disorders discussed in this section are presumed to have an immunologic basis. Many are clearly preceded by an infectious (usually viral) disease, and the infectious agent is presumed to initiate a cell-mediated autoimmune reaction. In some diseases, the immune response occurs shortly after the original infection, and in other diseases it does not occur until years later. In some of the disorders discussed here, no preceding infection has been identified, but clinicopathologic evidence strongly suggests an autoimmune, postinfectious cause.

A **Slow virus infections** are characterized by a lapse of months to years between the initial viral infection of the host and the appearance of a progressive CNS disease that primarily involves dementia, seizures, and motor deficits. The most common slow viral infection in children is **subacute sclerosing panencephalitis (SSPE),** which is caused by the measles virus or a measles-like virus that has been isolated from the brain. A similar syndrome can be seen in patients with congenital infection. This can occur with natural infection or rarely after vaccination. With widespread vaccination for childhood illnesses, the incidence of these disorders has declined significantly.

B **Acute disseminated (parainfectious) encephalomyelitis** occurs several days after certain viral infections (e.g., measles, chickenpox, influenza [rarely], rubella, or mumps) or after vaccination for smallpox, rabies, or influenza. A cell-mediated autoimmune reaction to myelin basic protein is the presumed cause.

1. **Clinical features and diagnosis.** The patient becomes irritable and lethargic, even comatose. The CSF commonly shows a slight increase in lymphocytes and an increase in protein.

2. **Prognosis.** Many patients recover completely, but mental retardation, seizures, or even death can ensue.

3. **Postpertussis vaccination encephalopathy** is controversial and deserves special comment. Within hours to a few days after whole-cell pertussis vaccination, approximately 1 in 300,000 patients may develop encephalopathy that, if not fatal, leaves the patient with mental retardation

and a severe seizure disorder. Nevertheless, the argument for pertussis vaccination of infants is quite strong, because the complications of pertussis itself are more common in this age group than are the reactions to the vaccine (see also Chapter 1). Furthermore, recent research has suggested that the incidence of postvaccine encephalopathy may be much lower than previously thought. The routine use of acellular pertussis vaccine instead of whole-cell pertussis vaccine has further diminished concerns for the development of encephalopathy.

C Presumed autoimmune diseases affecting the cerebellum

1. **Acute cerebellar ataxia** occurs in young children 1 to 2 weeks after a nonspecific respiratory tract infection. A brain tumor, intoxications, and an occult neuroblastoma must be excluded as causes. The disease is self-limited, with recovery occurring in two thirds of patients within 6 months.
2. **Myoclonic encephalopathy (Kinsbourne syndrome)** usually starts by 6 months of age and causes irregular, rapid eye movements (opsoclonus) as well as polymyoclonus and ataxia. In some cases, the cause is a neuroblastoma or a tumor of the brainstem or cerebellum. Treatment with ACTH, which is usually needed for several years, has been helpful in suppressing the symptoms. Approximately half of the children who are afflicted are mildly retarded.

D Other presumed autoimmune postinfectious CNS diseases

1. **Reye syndrome** is characterized by encephalopathy and acute liver dysfunction with fatty infiltration of the liver and kidney in individuals who are usually between 2 and 16 years of age. The incidence has dropped dramatically in the past decade, corresponding to the association of the disease with aspirin ingestion and subsequent warnings.
2. **Multiple sclerosis** currently is thought to be the result of an autoimmune reaction to an infectious agent that occurs in genetically susceptible people. It is primarily a disease of young adults, but has been diagnosed as early as 2 years of age. A demyelinating disease noted for its exacerbations and remissions, multiple sclerosis in children often manifests as ataxia, spasticity, and visual disturbances; however, seizures and cognitive deficits may also be seen. MRI scan will demonstrate areas of demyelination, and abnormal levels of immunoglobulins can be detected in CSF.
3. **Transverse myelitis (transverse myelopathy)** is a presumed autoimmune disease that affects the spinal cord, causing sudden back pain followed by rapidly progressing weakness and loss of sensation below the level of the lesion. The disease may occur at any age but the mean age of onset is 9 years. The sensory level determined on neurologic examination as well as loss of bladder and bowel function distinguishes this disorder from Guillain-Barré syndrome. A space-occupying lesion should be ruled out by CT or MRI scan.

E Presumed autoimmune, postinfectious diseases of peripheral nerves

1. **Guillain-Barré syndrome,** the most common of these disorders in children, is a postinfectious demyelinating polyneuropathy. Lymphocytes sensitized to the basic protein of myelin have been identified in this disease, which supports the presumed autoimmune pathogenesis.
   a. **Clinical features**
      (1) Typically, 2 weeks after a viral infection or an immunization, weakness insidiously begins to develop in the distal muscles of the lower extremities, occasionally with accompanying paresthesias.
      (2) The weakness progresses upward and centrally over a period of 2 to 4 weeks, so that the diaphragm and cranial nerve musculature may eventually become involved. A plateau lasting approximately 4 weeks then develops, followed by gradual recovery, which may take up to 1 year.
      (3) At the height of the clinical manifestations, the CSF shows an elevated protein level without an elevation in the white blood cell count.
   b. **Therapy** is supportive until the patient loses ambulation, at which time plasmapheresis is indicated. Respiratory difficulties may require assisted respiration. Steroid therapy, plasmapheresis, or intravenous γ-globulin is recommended for patients whose condition is chronically progressive (worsening 4–6 weeks after onset) or relapsing.

c. **Prognosis.** Approximately 10% to 15% of patients have residual deficits, such as weakness of the distal foot muscles that necessitates orthoses (e.g., special shoes, braces). Another 10% have a relapse, usually within the first year after recovery. Fatalities are rare, but they can occur.

2. **Other presumably autoimmune, postinfectious neuropathies** include **Bell palsy** (facial nerve palsy) and **sixth-nerve palsy. Gradenigo syndrome** (sixth-nerve palsy associated with pain in the distribution of the fifth cranial nerve) is secondary to osteomyelitis of the petrous ridge of the sphenoid bone. **Brachial plexus neuropathies** have been associated with influenza vaccination.

BIBLIOGRAPHY

Fenichel GM: *Clinical Pediatric Neurology: A Signs and Symptoms Approach,* 4th ed. Philadelphia, Elsevier/WB Saunders, 2005.

Goebel HH (ed): Pediatric neuromuscular disorders. *Semin Pediatr Neurol* 3(2):53–161, 1996.

Kuban KCK, Leviton A: Cerebral palsy. *N Engl J Med* 330:188–195, 1994.

Swaiman K: *Pediatric Neurology Principles and Practice.* Philadelphia, Mosby Elsevier, 2006.

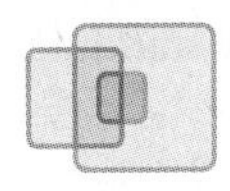

Study Questions

Directions: *Each of the numbered items or incomplete statements in this section is followed by answers or completions of the statement. Select the ONE lettered answer or completion that is BEST in each case.*

1. A 13-year-old female presents with 6 months of severe headaches. The headaches are unilateral and throbbing. She reports that at the onset of the headache, she frequently sees "spots" in her field of vision. During the headache itself she experiences nausea and sensitivity to light. Findings on general physical examination including neurologic and funduscopic exams are entirely normal. Which of the following is the most likely diagnosis?

A Migraine headache
B Tension headache
C Cerebral aneurysm
D Cerebral tumor
E School avoidance

2. A 5-year-old female is noted to have episodic staring. The spells can occur at any time and occasionally interrupt activity. Several adults have witnessed the child during a spell and describe that "she stares, her eyelids flutter, and she stops speaking." The episodes last for approximately 10 to 15 seconds. Afterwards the child resumes speaking about whatever she had been saying before the spell began. Her development has been entirely normal and she is currently doing well in kindergarten with no behavioral concerns. Her neurologic examination is normal. Which of the following is the most likely diagnosis?

A Breath-holding spells
B Partial complex seizures
C Daydreaming
D Migraine headaches
E Absence seizures

3. A 2-year-old male is brought in for evaluation of spells. If he falls down or bumps his head while playing he will begin to cry and seem unable to catch his breath. He turns red in the face and then his eyes roll up and he loses consciousness. Sometimes he will arch and then go limp. He recovers consciousness within 30 seconds and afterwards seems tired. He has a normal neurologic examination. Which of the following is the most likely diagnosis?

A Tonic-clonic seizures
B Temper tantrums
C Myoclonic seizures
D Breath-holding spells
E Narcolepsy

4. A 6-year-old boy is seen for toe-walking and frequent falls. He has had progressive gait difficulty over the past year. On examination he has enlarged calf muscles and tight Achilles tendons. He walks on the balls of his feet and has lumbar lordosis. When getting up from the ground, he needs to push off on his thighs to stand. Reflexes are diminished. Which of the following is the most likely diagnosis?

A Cerebral palsy
B Guillain-Barré syndrome
C Multiple sclerosis
D Duchenne muscular dystrophy
E Arthrogryposis multiplex congenita

5. While recovering from varicella, a 4-year-old boy manifests gait ataxia. When examined, he is alert and afebrile, with no meningismus or complaint of headache. The boy has no diplopia or facial weakness, but does have difficulty reaching for objects because of an intention tremor. Deep tendon reflexes are normal, and plantar responses are flexor. He walks with a wide-based gait and sways while standing still. Which of the following is the most likely diagnosis?

- A Guillain-Barré syndrome
- B Varicella encephalitis
- C Acute cerebellar ataxia
- D Ataxia-telangiectasia
- E Reye syndrome

6. An 18-month-male child has a 30-second episode of loss of consciousness associated with tonic stiffening of his body and twitching of his arms and legs. His eyes are partially open and deviated upwards. Afterwards he is limp and sleepy. On arrival in the emergency room he is found to have a rectal temperature of 104°F. He is sleepy but able to respond with symmetric motor function and reflexes and normal cranial nerve function. He has otitis media. His development thus far has been normal and his father had similar episodes at this age. Which of the following is the most likely diagnosis?

- A Febrile seizure
- B Epilepsy
- C Syncope
- D Night terrors
- E Meningitis

7. A 7-year-old child is seen in the clinic for evaluation of motor delay. The examination reveals limited voluntary movements as well as slow, writhing, continuous movements of the arms and legs whenever the patient initiates a motor movement. At rest, these movements are not seen. Which of the following physiologic classifications best describes this child's motor deficit?

- A Spasticity
- B Athetosis
- C Dystonia
- D Ataxia
- E Hypotonia

8. An 11-year-old male presents with difficulty walking. He had been fine until 7 days ago when he noticed some tingling in his feet. Over the next few days he began tripping more and he had difficulty climbing the stairs at school. This morning he had difficulty getting out of a chair. His past history is unremarkable except for a recent viral illness. On examination, he is alert, with normal mental status. He has normal strength in his arms but he is weak in his lower extremities. Reflexes are absent. He has normal sensation in his extremities but has hand and feet paresthesias. He has difficulty walking. Which of the following is the most likely diagnosis?

- A Muscular dystrophy
- B Cerebral palsy
- C Guillain-Barré syndrome
- D Myasthenia gravis
- E Intoxication

9. A 4-month-old male infant is observed to have marked floppiness. His parents believed that he was normal until 2 months of age, when they were concerned by his failure to support his head. On examination, the infant is alert and tracks readily. He has a social smile. Facial grimace is normal, but there are fasciculations of the tongue. His motor examination shows truncal weakness with slip-through on vertical suspension and decreased movement in the lower extremities. No deep tendon reflexes are appreciated. Which of the following is the anatomic site most affected in this child?

- A Upper motor neuron
- B Anterior horn cell
- C Peripheral nerve
- D Neuromuscular junction
- E Muscle

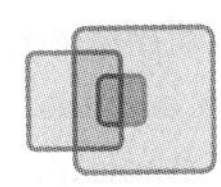

Answers and Explanations

1. The answer is A (*V A 1 a*). Migraine headaches are characterized by throbbing pain that is often but not always unilateral. Photophobia and nausea are common and there may be associated visual phenomena such as scotomas. A positive family history is common. Neuroimaging studies are normal. Tension headache is typically bilateral, squeezing in character, without nausea or visual symptoms. Cerebral aneurysms present with sudden onset of severe headache with photophobia and meningismus. There may also be abnormalities on neurologic examination. Cerebral tumor may present with headache if there is increased intracranial pressure. Papilledema and abnormal findings on neurologic examination are usually present. School avoidance often presents as daily headaches, worse in the morning when it is time to go to school. These headaches are often refractory to medical intervention.

2. The answer is E (*IV B 1 b [1], C 1*). Absence seizures are characteristically brief in duration (5–15 seconds), with staring and minimal motor symptoms and with no postictal confusion. Most children with absence seizures are developmentally and neurologically normal. Breath-holding spells are usually provoked by fear or pain and are associated with loss of tone and consciousness. Partial complex seizures can be associated with staring, but usually there are other manifestations, often motor automatisms. These spells typically last 30 seconds to several minutes and there is postictal confusion. Migraine headaches may be associated with confusion but headache is usually present. Daydreaming is staring that can easily be interrupted by stimulation.

3. The answer is D (*V C 2*). Breath-holding spells are a form of infantile syncope, provoked by fear, pain, or frustration. There is usually color change (pallor or cyanosis) followed by loss of consciousness, loss of tone, and occasionally tonic stiffening. Temper tantrums are not characterized by loss of consciousness and involve directed aggressive behavior and/or prolonged crying. Myoclonic seizures are brief, bilateral twitching or stiffening, usually without observable loss of consciousness. A tonic-clonic seizure is spontaneous, marked by loss of consciousness, stiffening, and then repetitive twitching movements, followed by postictal depression. Narcolepsy may produce attacks of sudden loss of tone, caused by surprise or sudden emotion, but with no loss of consciousness.

4. The answer is D (*III C 4 a [1]*). Duchenne muscular dystrophy is a progressive myopathy caused by defects in the gene that produces dystrophin, a structural protein of myocytes, found on the X chromosome. Boys typically become symptomatic in the first decade with proximal weakness, muscular hypertrophy, and progressive gait difficulties. Ultimately wheelchair dependence, cardiomyopathy, and respiratory failure occur, resulting in death. Cerebral palsy is the result of injury to the developing brain, which results in motor dysfunction. Muscle tone may be increased or decreased; reflexes are usually increased. Guillain-Barré syndrome is a rapidly progressive form of weakness caused by postinfectious demyelination of peripheral nerves. There is usually ascending weakness from the legs to the arms, trunk, and even cranial nerves. Areflexia is common. Multiple sclerosis is an intermittent or progressive central nervous system disorder caused by an autoimmune process. Motor signs in this disorder usually have the features of an upper motor neuron disorder with weakness, abnormal tone, and increased reflexes. Arthrogryposis multiplex congentia is a non-progressive disorder characterized by muscle weakness and contractures of at least two joints with findings present at birth. A viral or toxic cause primarily affecting anterior cells is suspected in most cases.

5. The answer is C (*X C 1*). Acute cerebellar ataxia is a postinfectious encephalomyelitis that often manifests primarily as cerebellar dysfunction. Other symptoms, such as cranial neuropathies, confusion, or pyramidal tract weakness, can also be seen. Guillain-Barré syndrome is a demyelinating neuropathy; clinically, areflexia and ascending limb weakness are noted. Varicella encephalitis is usually seen during the acute phase of the illness and is associated with fever and, often, seizures. Reye syndrome may occur with varicella but occurs with signs of acute increased intracranial pressure and confusion. Ataxia-telangiectasia is a slowly progressive disorder and does not present with acute deterioration.

6. The answer is A (*IV D*). Febrile seizures occur from 6 months to 6 years of age. They are precipitated by a fever and typically are brief and generalized. The prognosis for this seizure type is good. A diagnosis of epilepsy requires more than one seizure, without a clear provocative event, such as fever. Syncope may be associated with brief twitching and loss of consciousness. Pallor is usually seen and high fever is unusual. Night terrors, or parasomnias, occur during sleep and are characterized by screaming and flailing, as though the child was frightened. The child, once wakened, is generally not confused and usually returns to sleep. Meningitis can cause a fever and a brief seizure, but should be associated with meningismus and irritability or altered mental status.

7. The answer is B (*III B 4 b, Table 18-4*). Athetosis refers to slow, writhing, continuous movements in the extremities, which are seen in many diseases, but most commonly in patients who have cerebral palsy. Chorea, athetosis, spasticity, dystonia, ataxia, and hypotonia are physiologic classifications for the abnormal muscle tone or movement disorders commonly seen in children who have cerebral palsy. When classifying a patient's disorder, both the anatomic location of the abnormality and the physiologic characteristic of the abnormality are considered.

8. The answer is C (*X E 1*). Guillain-Barré syndrome or postinfectious polyneuropathy is rapidly progressive demyelinating polyneuropathy that typically follows a viral illness. There is ascending paralysis with areflexia. Since large myelinated sensory fibers may be affected, there may be paresthesias and decreased proprioception. Respiratory failure and autonomic instability may occur. Muscular dystrophy is a gradually progressive myopathy with increasing weakness over the course of years. There are no sensory abnormalities. Cerebral palsy is a chronic disorder that is not associated with progressive weakness. Myasthenia gravis is a neuromuscular disorder with fluctuating weakness. Ptosis and ophthalmoplegia are common presenting signs. Intoxication generally presents with mental status changes. Rarely, heavy metal poisoning, such as mercury and lead, can produce peripheral neurologic symptoms, but this occurs more gradually with other systemic symptoms.

9. The answer is B (*III C 1 a*). This child has spinal muscular atrophy, with characteristic weakness, areflexia, and fasciculations of the tongue. The anterior horn cell is the site of the abnormality. This disorder is slowly progressive, leading ultimately to respiratory compromise.

Index

Page numbers followed by "f" indicate figures; those followed by "t" denote tables.